Manual of Cardiovascular Diagnosis and Therapy

Fifth Edition

D1343727

Manual of Cardiovascular Diagnosis and Therapy
Fifth Edition

Joseph S. Alpert, M.D.

Head, Department of Medicine
Robert S. and Irene P. Flinn Professor of Medicine
Department of Medicine
University of Arizona Health Sciences Center
Tucson, Arizona

Gordon A. Ewy, M.D.

Head, Section of Cardiology
Director, Sarver Heart Center
Professor of Medicine
Department of Medicine
University of Arizona Health Sciences Center
Tucson, Arizona

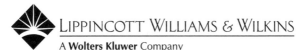

LIPPINCOTT WILLIAMS & WILKINS
A **Wolters Kluwer** Company
Philadelphia · Baltimore · New York · London
Buenos Aires · Hong Kong · Sydney · Tokyo

Acquisitions Editor: Ruth W. Weinberg
Developmental Editor: Denise Martin
Production Editor: Jeff Somers
Manufacturing Manager: Benjamin Rivera
Cover Designer: Patricia Gast
Compositor: Circle Graphics
Printer: RR Donnelley

© 2002 by LIPPINCOTT WILLIAMS & WILKINS
530 Walnut Street
Philadelphia, PA 19106 USA
LWW.com

Printed in the USA

Library of Congress Cataloging-in-Publication Data

Alpert, Joseph S.
    Manual of cardiovascular diagnosis and therapy / Joseph S. Alpert, Gordon A. Ewy.—
5th ed.
        p. ; cm.
    Includes bibliographical references and index.
    ISBN 0-7817-2803-7 (alk. paper)
        1. Cardiovascular system—Diseases—Handbooks, manuals, etc. I. Ewy, Gordon A.,
1933- II. Title.
        [DNLM: 1. Cardiovascular Diseases—diagnosis—Handbooks. 2. Cardiovascular
Diseases—therapy—Handbooks. WG 39 A456ma 2002]
    RC667 .A39 2002
    616.1—dc21
                                                                            2002069380

10 9 8 7 6 5 4 3 2 1

CONTENTS

PREFACE

Six years have passed since we published the last edition of this concise guide to the diagnosis and therapy of patients with cardiovascular disease. During this time, many important clinical trials and scientific observations have been reported in the medical literature. This new edition of the *Manual of Cardiovascular Diagnosis and Therapy* contains much information based on the results of these advances. The Manual will again be of considerable use to practicing physicians, house officers, and medical students in this challenging era of managed medical care.

Dr. Gordon Ewy and I acknowledge the inspiration and assistance of our cardiology colleagues at the University of Arizona and throughout the world. We appreciate the considerable support afforded us by Mrs. Barbara Raney, Mrs. Jane Barth, and Mrs. Debra Young. Of course, none of this would be possible without the understanding, succor, and assistance of our spouses, Helle and Priscilla. We also acknowledge the dependable support of Mrs. Ruth Weinberg and Lippincott Williams & Wilkins.

We hope that this new edition will be as helpful to our colleagues and trainees as previous editions have been.

Joseph S. Alpert, MD
Gordon A. Ewy, MD
Tucson, Arizona

I. INTRODUCTION TO THE CARDIOVASCULAR SYSTEM

1. PHYSICAL EXAMINATION OF THE CARDIOVASCULAR SYSTEM

I. Introduction. "The secret of patient care is caring for the patient." This quote from Peabody is one that every physician needs to take to heart. Once patients find a physician who cares, they are more likely to receive the best medicine. Many physicians, however, are caring but are not trained observers. Skill in obtaining the medical history and in performing the cardiovascular examination are other essential steps to good patient care. A careful physical examination of the cardiovascular system provides important information. Together with a thorough history, the cardiovascular physical examination provides the initial database that the physician uses to suggest further diagnostic tests and therapeutic interventions.

This chapter focuses on diagnostic aspects of physical examination of the cardiovascular system and provides general guidelines for evaluating physical findings. Descriptions of the actual techniques of physical examination and theories concerning the origins of heart sounds are beyond the scope of this manual. Detailed descriptions of physical examination findings for various cardiac diseases are found in the chapter for each entity.

II. Observations, palpation, and percussion
  A. General observation. A trained observer can gain much from simple observation of the patient. General observation is often the first clue to a variety of cardiovascular diseases or conditions. Hyperthyroidism (atrial fibrillation), hypothyroidism (pericardial effusion), trisomy 13 syndrome (mitral regurgitation secondary to atrioventricular canal defect), straight back or pectus excavatum (mitral valve prolapse), neurofibromatosis (pheochromocytoma), and Marfan's syndrome (aortic root disease) are some clues, but there are many others. One look can suggest whether the patient is stable or severely ill. Often a house officer will present a patient, giving me a mental image of that patient. Then, after walking into the patient's room, the first look will change my differential diagnosis completely.
  B. Jugular venous pulse (JVP). The JVP is also evaluated by observation. Two types of information are obtained from the JVP: the venous wave form and the central venous pressure (CVP).
    1. Technique of examination. The JVP is best observed in the right side of the neck. The internal jugular vein is located just below the sternocleidomastoid muscle (Fig. 1.1). This muscle divides in its origin from the clavicle. This division into its two heads and the clavicle form the internal jugular bulb, a landmark that is essential for all hospital physicians to know, as this bulb affords easy assess via venipuncture to the central venous system. To accurately interpret the jugular venous pressure and waveform, the patient's head must be positioned so that the sternocleidomastoid muscle is relaxed. If a pillow is present, the head can be tilted too far forward. In most patients, the physician has to remove the patient's pillow, and position the patient's chin somewhat to the left, to observe the venous pulsations of the internal jugular vein. (Be sure to fluff the pillow before returning it under the patient's head.) A common misconception is that the external jugular vein cannot be used to evaluate the patient's JVP as it has venous valves, however, so do the internal jugular veins. Therefore, if the pulsations are obvious in the external jugular veins, they can be used as well as the internal jugular veins. With normal CVP, the JVP is assessed with the patient's trunk flat or slightly raised. With elevated CVP, the patient's trunk must be raised higher, sometimes to as much as 90 degrees (or the patient can be sitting upright). The JVP is accentuated by turning the patient's head away from the examiner and shining a flashlight obliquely across the skin overlying the vein.

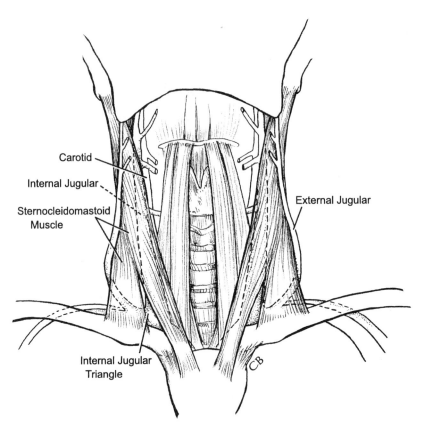

FIG. 1-1. Superficial anatomy of the neck. Variations in the jugular venous pressure produce pulsations of the skin over the sternocleidomastoid muscle and over the internal jugular triangle, the area at the base of the neck bounded inferiorly by the clavicle and laterally by the two heads of sternocleidomastoid muscles as they arise from the clavicle. Accordingly, to see these low-pressure pulsations, the neck muscles must be relaxed.

In the mid and lower neck, the internal jugular veins lie lateral to the carotid artery. Pulsations of the smaller external jugular vein may be easier to observe, especially in patients who have had chronically elevated venous pressure, because the external jugular veins are superficial.

2. Wave form of the JVP. The traditional teaching is that two waves per heartbeat are generally visible in the JVP: the A wave and the V wave (Fig. 1.2). The A wave represents an increased venous pressure that results from atrial contraction and occurs in timing with the first heart sound (S1). The V wave follows the A wave and represents continued venous return to the right atrium while the tricuspid valve is closed. The V wave occurs in timing with the second heart sound (S2). The drop in pressure following the A wave is called the X descent, and the fall in pressure after the V wave is denoted as the Y descent (Fig. 1.2). Rarely, another small wave, the C wave, transmitted from the carotid, follows S1. The JVP waves may also be timed with simultaneous palpation of the carotid artery. The A wave immediately precedes the carotid pulse;

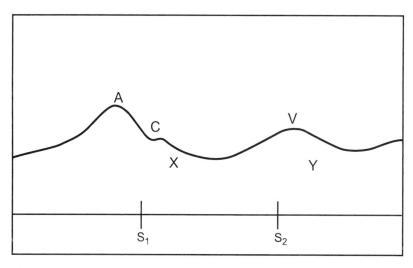

FIG. 1-2. The normal jugular venous pulsations as classically illustrated. The venous pulsations are said to consist of two main waves, the A and V waves. The A wave due to atrial contraction, begins before systole and peaks near the first heart sound (S1). The A wave is followed by the X descent, due to atrial relaxation. The V wave is caused by continuous venous return to the right atrium. It peaks just after the second heart sound (S2) and is terminated by the fall of the right atrial pressure after the opening of the tricuspid valve. Occasionally the X descent is interrupted by a C wave, which is caused by transmitted carotid artery pulsations. This wave, although recordable with some techniques, is seldom visible unless the carotid pulsations are prominent.

the V wave follows the pulse. Rarely, difficulty may be experienced in differentiating venous and arterial pulsations in the neck. Several observations and findings may be helpful: (i) the arterial pulse is more localized and palpable, whereas palpation will obliterate a venous pulse; (ii) compression with the edge of one's hand at the base of the neck over the internal jugular bulb will not alter arterial pulses but will obliterate the venous pulsations; and (iii) arterial pulses do not change with respiration or with alternations in the patient position, whereas venous pulses will often disappear when the patient assumes an upright posture (either sitting upright or standing).

In normal individuals, however, distinct A and V waves are not visible! This little known fact has convinced many physicians that they cannot interpret the jugular venous waveform; try as they might, they cannot see what has been classically described in older textbooks as distinct A and V waves. The reason is because with a normal or slow heart rate, there is another wave, the H wave. At slower heart rates, diastole is longer. Following the V wave, venous blood continues to return to the right heart, and the venous pressure gradually increases, forming the H wave (Fig. 1.3). The atrial contraction that produces the A wave is normally not strong, so the A wave is but a small increase on the slowly rising H wave. The dominant motion of the normal JVP is the X descent. The normal V wave is also very small and is followed by the slowly rising H wave. Therefore, in normal individuals there are no distinct A or V waves! When the A wave is obvious, it is abnormal. When the V wave is obvious, it also is abnormal. In normal individuals, the major venous motion is a collapsing motion in systole (Fig. 1.3). This is

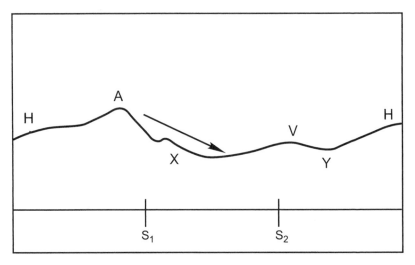

FIG. 1-3. Illustration of the normal jugular venous pulsations. The normal jugular pulsations are not as classically illustrated. This is because in normal individuals with a slow heart rate, there is another wave, the H wave that begins after the Y descent and continues until atrial contraction. The H wave is caused by continued filling of the right atrium during diastole that is interrupted by the A wave because of atrial contraction. In normal patients, the A and V waves are not very prominent. Therefore, the dominant venous motion is the systolic X descent (arrow), occurring between the first and second heart sound. If you observe this gentle collapse of the venous pulsation during systole, the jugular venous pulsations are normal. In fact, if one can appreciate a distinct A wave and a distinct V wave, they are abnormal.

best timed by looking at the right side of the neck while palpating the left carotid artery.

There are only a few abnormalities of the venous waveform. The A wave is increased when there is increased resistance to right atrial contraction, such as right ventricular hypertrophy, infiltration, or scaring. The A wave is absent in atrial fibrillation. The V wave is increased in tricuspid regurgitation—a very common abnormality in patients with cardiovascular disease. The venous wave of tricuspid regurgitation starts early in systole and is sometimes referred to as a CV wave, or because it is a prominent wave occurring in systole, it is sometimes referred to as an S wave (Fig. 1.4). Because the regurgitant jet of tricuspid insufficiency in the absence of pulmonary hypertension is not forceful, a murmur is not generated. Therefore, in the majority of patients, the only way to diagnose tricuspid regurgitation at the bedside is by observing a large venous pulsation that occurs in systole, that is, between S1 and S2 (Fig. 1.4).

It is important not to miss the prominent X and Y descents in the elevated venous pulsations of patients with restrictive heart disease or constrictive pericardial disease. Although very rare, many a patient has been misdiagnosed for years because the physician did not appreciate the classic venous pulsations of these conditions.

3. Determination of CVP. In the absence of obstruction, the JVP is a reflection of both right atrial venous pressure or CVP and right atrial hemodynamics. The CVP can be estimated by observing the vertical distance from the mean height of the venous pulsations to the angle of Lewis, the sternal angle. When estimating the venous pressure, one is

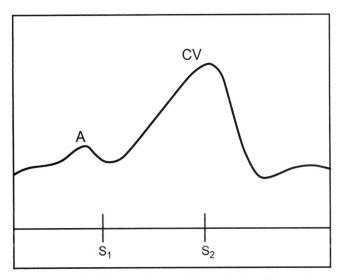

FIG. 1-4. Illustration of a CV wave of tricuspid regurgitation. The most common abnormality of the jugular venous pulsation is the absence of the A wave due to atrial fibrillation. The second most common abnormality of the jugular venous pulsation is the presence of a CV wave due to tricuspid regurgitation. This pulsation is called a CV wave as it begins early in systole, at the timing of the normal C wave, and continues and peaks in timing of the V wave. Its height is determined by the amount of regurgitation and the size of the right atrium.

measuring hydrostatic pressure. Hydrostatic pressure is measured vertically, regardless of the configuration of the container. This concept is applicable in the clinical estimation of the venous pressure because venous pressure is measured as the vertical distance between the venous pulsation at the top of the column of venous blood and the reference point. The reference point for the estimation of the height of the venous pressure is the sternal angle. This angle can be felt as a transverse ridge formed by the articulation of the manubrium and the body of the sternum. Sir Thomas Lewis demonstrated that this angle bears a constant relation to the mean right atrium when the patient is in a supine, upright, or any intermediate position (Fig. 1.5). In the individual with normal CVP, the mean of the venous pulsations is about 2 cm above the sternal angle. This would make the CVP or mean right atrial pressure 7 cm of blood. A common mistake is to always estimate the venous pressure with the patient's thorax elevated at 30 or 45 degrees. It is true that if the venous pulsations are not visible with the patient in this position, the venous pressure is not significantly elevated. However, the patient needs to have the thorax raised or lowered to the position at which the venous pulsations are best seen; then the venous waveform and the venous pressure are estimated. In some pathologic conditions (e.g., cardiac tamponade, constrictive pericarditis), CVP may be so high that the venous pressure is above the angle of the jaw, even with the patient sitting bolt upright. It is important to not use the mean height of the JVPs when estimating the height of the venous pressure in patients with large central venous waves. In such patients, the reference point is the base of the central venous wave, as this point corresponds to the right ventricular end-diastolic pressure. If the tricuspid valve were surgically removed, the

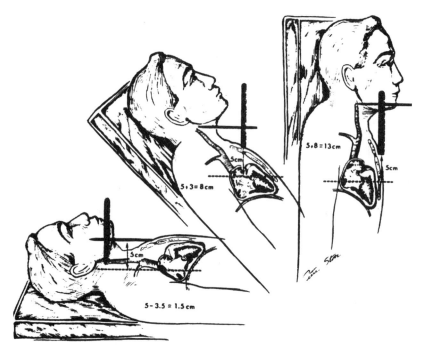

FIG. 1-5. Illustration of three different individuals (although they look the same) with different jugular venous pressures. Note that there is no pillow. To estimate the jugular venous pressure, one places the individual in the position in which the top of the venous pulsations are best seen. The reference point for estimating venous pressure is the sternal angle. This is because the sternal angle is approximately 5 cm above the mid right atrium with the patient supine, sitting upright, or any position in between. The mid right atrium is the phlebostatic axis for the human circulation.

Normal individuals have to be placed in the near supine position to see the venous pulsations, as the normal mean venous pressure averages about 5 cm. In this illustration, the venous pressure is low in the supine individual, 3.5 cm below the sternal angle, giving an estimated central venous pressure of 1.5 cm.

In most patients with elevated jugular venous pressure, the patient has to be examined with the head of the bed or examining table elevated to see the top of the venous pulsations. In this illustration the individual is place at a 45-degree angle. The venous pressure is 3 cm above the angle of Lewis, so the estimated venous pressure is 8 cm. In actual practice, when the venous pulsations are visible above the clavicle with the patient's upper body raised to 45 degrees, the venous pressure is elevated. In patients with markedly elevated jugular venous pressure, the patient has to be sitting bolt upright to appreciate the top of the venous pulsations. In this illustration, the top of the venous pulsations are seen at 8 cm above the sternal angle, so the estimated venous pressure is 13 cm.

RV contraction would be reflected into the right atrium. To give such a patient diuretics to decrease the venous pressure to normal would put the patient into shock. Therefore, with severe tricuspid regurgitation and a large central venous wave, the venous pressure is estimated from the onset of the central venous wave and from not the mean height of the venous waves, as it is in normal individuals. The technique for estimation of central venous or jugular venous pressure is illustrated in Fig. 1.5.

During inspiration, the height of the JVP typically declines (although amplitude of the X and Y descents will increase). In certain pathologic conditions—such as chronic constrictive pericarditis, congestive heart failure, right ventricular dysfunction, or infarction—the JVP actually increases with inspiration. This important clinical finding is known as **Kussmaul's sign.**

C. Abdominojugular (hepatojugular or abdominal jugular) test. During the past century, the hepatojugular or abdominojugular reflux generally has been an accepted method for diagnosing occult right ventricular failure, and thus, it is not surprising that the abdominojugular test is positive in patients with acute right ventricular infarction. Recent studies have shown that in patients with chronic congestive heart failure, a positive abdominojugular test is a reflection of increased pressure in both the left and right atria. In the absence of another explanation, such as an acute right ventricular infarction, when the abdominojugular test is positive, the pulmonary arterial wedge pressure is greater than 15 mm Hg. The reason for this observation is not completely understood, but it is thought to relate to a marked increase in venous pressure throughout the body, so that pressure on the veins of the abdomen increases the pressure throughout the venous system. Another explanation is that this phenomenon results from pericardial restraint. Abdominal pressure results in increased venous return to the right atrium. Acute or subacute ventricular dilation causes pericardial restraint, so that the patients have the hemodynamics of acute or subacute constrictive pericarditis. In such patients, abdominal pressure increases not only the right atrial (and jugular venous pressure) but also the pulmonary arterial wedge pressure.

Thus, the abdominojugular test is invaluable in diagnosing and monitoring patients with heart failure. In patients with acute left ventricular decompensation, the pulmonary venous system is engorged and the patient has both pulmonary congestion on the chest radiograph and pulmonary rales on auscultation. With chronic congestion, however, the pulmonary lymphatics clear this congestion, and the patient can have a markedly elevated pulmonary arterial wedge pressure and clear lung fields on chest radiograph and no rales on auscultation. If a patient with chronic heart failure has rales and pulmonary congestion on chest radiograph, one can be sure that the pulmonary arterial wedge pressure is markedly elevated. Therefore, the abdominojugular test is an invaluable method of diagnosing and monitoring patients with actual or suspected heart failure. Because heart failure is the most common hospital discharge diagnosis of patients over the age of 65 years, familiarity with this test is essential.

A positive abdominojugular test is defined as an increase in the jugular venous pressure with midabdominal pressure, followed by an abrupt drop in the pressure of 4 cm after the release of 10 seconds of firm midabdominal pressure. To convey the amount of pressure applied, an adult blood pressure cuff is used. The bladder of an unrolled adult blood pressure cuff is placed flat on the patient's mid abdomen. The bladder is inflated with air by six full-bulb compressions. Enough pressure is the applied to generate 20 mm Hg (the examiner's hand should be flat with the fingers slightly spread). With experience, even this simple method of pressure quantification is not necessary. It is important that the patient breathes normally throughout the test. Straining can raise the intrathoracic pressure and give a false-positive test. Figure 1.6 is a schematic representation of positive and negative responses. Figure 1.7 shows the increase in right atrial pressure in a patient with a pos-

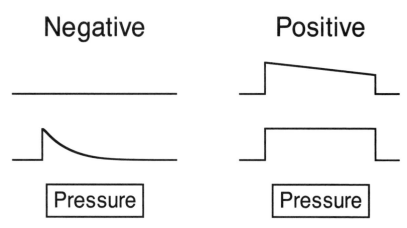

FIG. 1-6. Schematic representations of negative (left) and positive (right) response of jugular venous pressure to ten seconds of abdominal pressure. The application of firm abdominal pressure on the patient's abdomen with the examiner's hand while the patient is relaxed and breathing normally, will not result in an increase in the jugular venous pressure in normal individuals (upper left). On occasion, the patient will strain when abdominal pressure is applied but will relax with sustained pressure, and the jugular venous pressure will return to normal (lower left). As is illustrated on the right, a positive test is a 4 cm or greater fall in the jugular venous pressure with abrupt cessation of firm midabdominal pressure.

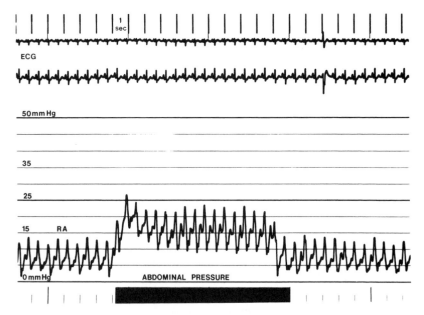

FIG. 1-7. Simultaneous recording of 1-second timelines (top), ECG, and right atrial pressures before, during, and after 10 seconds of midabdominal pressure. Note the abrupt and sustained increase in right atrial pressure during midabdominal pressure and the abrupt drop in right atrial pressure with release of midabdominal pressure. This is a positive abdominojugular test.

itive abdominojugular test. Figure 1.8 shows the increase in both the right atrial and pulmonary arterial wedge pressures in a patient with a positive abdominojugular test.

D. Arterial pressure pulse. The central arterial pressure pulse is characterized by a rapid rise to a rounded shoulder peak with a less rapid decline. Information about the adequacy of ventricular contraction and possible obstruction of the left ventricular outflow tract may be assessed by palpation of the carotid artery.

By the time the pulse wave is transmitted to peripheral arteries, much of this initial information is lost; however, pulsus alternans and pulsus paradoxus are best evaluated in peripheral arteries. In patients with unexplained hypertension, simultaneous palpation of radial and femoral arterial pulses helps to rule out coarctation of the aorta.

A variety of pathologic conditions alters the characteristics of the carotid pulse. These conditions, and the corresponding modifications of the carotid pulse, are listed in Table 1-1.

Auscultation over both carotid pulses is essential in every patient in the cardiovascular disease age group. Finding a carotid bruit, followed by appropriate Doppler duplex scan, can find asymptomatic carotid artery stenosis. Appropriate therapy can prevent a stroke.

E. Precordial palpation. Information concerning the location and quality of the left ventricular impulse is available through precordial palpation. In addition, intensity of murmurs may be gauged by palpating associated thrills.

Palpation is best accomplished using the fingertips, with the patient in either a supine or left lateral decubitus position. Simultaneous auscultation

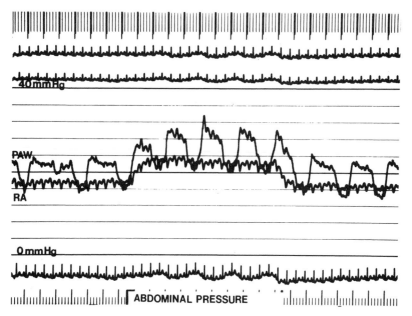

FIG. 1-8. Simultaneous recording of one second time lines (top), ECG (two leads), pulmonary arterial wedge (PAW), and right atrial (RA) pressures before, during, and after 10 seconds of midabdominal pressure. Note the increase not only in right atrial pressure during midabdominal pressure but also the increase in pulmonary arterial wedge pressure with abdominal pressure, and the abrupt decrease in right atrial pressure with release of midabdominal pressure. This is a positive abdominojugular test.

TABLE 1-1. CLINICAL INFORMATION DERIVED FROM ABNORMAL JUGULAR VENOUS PULSATIONS

Finding	Comment/significance
Markedly raised central venous pressure, accentuated X and Y descents	? Cardiac tamponade ? Constrictive pericarditis ? Endocardial fibroelastosis ? Severe right-heart failure
Large A waves	? Pulmonary valvular stenosis ? Hypertension ? Various arrhythmias in which atria contract against closed AV valve (e.g., junctional rhythm, AV dissociation)
Absent A wave	Atrial fibrillation
Large V wave	Tricuspid regurgitation

can aid in the timing of events. A list of abnormalities detected by precordial palpation, and their significance, is found in Table 1-2. When palpating for thrills, the area of the palm of the hand just at the junction of the fingers is the most sensitive area. This can be proven by stroking the inside of the opposite hand from the tips of the finger to the base of the palm with the fingernail of the other hand.

   III. Auscultation

      A. S1. S1 occurs at the time of closure of the mitral and tricuspid valves. S1 is frequently split (with mitral closure preceding tricuspid), but this event is of

TABLE 1-2. CLINICAL INFORMATION DERIVED FROM ABNORMALITIES IN CAROTID PULSE

Finding	Comment/significance
Pulsus bisferiens (two systolic peaks)	Found in aortic regurgitation and hypertrophic obstructive cardiomyopathy
Pulsus parvus (small, weak pulse)	Any condition causing diminished left ventricular stroke volume or narrow pulse pressure (hypovolemia, mitral/aortic valve stenosis, restrictive pericarditis, recent myocardial infarction); may also be caused by atherosclerosis of the carotid artery or diseases of the aortic arch
Pulsus tardus (delayed systolic peak of pulse)	Aortic outflow obstruction
Pulsus paradoxus (larger than normal decrease in systolic arterial pressure during inspiration)	Pericardial tamponade, airway obstruction, superior vena caval obstruction; may be seen in asthma or chronic obstructive pulmonary disease
Pulsus alternans (consistent alternation in pulse pressure amplitude despite regular rhythm)	Severe left ventricular decompensation for any reason; after paroxysmal tachycardia; for several beats after a premature beat

little clinical relevance other than it may mimic other causes of extra sounds around the timing of the S1. More important is variation in the intensity of the first sound. S1 varies with the P–R interval of the ECG. The shorter the P–R interval, the louder the S1. The best example of S1 variation with P–R interval occurs in complete heart block, in which atrial and ventricular contractions are dissociated.

S1 may be loud and "snapping" in quality in mitral stenosis, indicating both that the valve is pliable and that it remains wide open at the beginning of isovolumic contraction. Conversely, a diminished or absent S1 in mitral stenosis suggests a rigidly calcified valve that cannot "snap" shut. Other situations in which S1 may be diminished include long P–R intervals, poor sound conduction through the chest wall, and poor ventricular function, resulting in a slow rise of left ventricular pressure.

B. S2. In contrast to S1, in which splitting is less important than changes in intensity, S2 reveals variations in both splitting and intensity that provide important clinical information.

S2 occurs at the time of closure of the aortic and pulmonic valves. In normal circumstances, aortic closure precedes pulmonic closure (A2 followed by P2). In normal circumstances, the split in S2 is maximal at the end of **inspiration** and minimal or single at the end of **expiration.** This phenomenon reflects an underlying movement of P2 with respect to a relatively constant A2. During inspiration, right ventricular filling increases and P2 is delayed, causing the widely split S2. During expiration, less right ventricular filling occurs and P2 "closes" toward A2 or occurs simultaneously, causing a diminished split in S2. This "normal splitting" of S2 is invariably present in individuals under 30 years of age, provided heart rates are not markedly accelerated. It is best appreciated over the "pulmonic area" and can be heard best with the diaphragm of the stethoscope.

1. Fixed splitting of S2. Fixed splitting of S2 occurs when the pulmonic component (P2) of S2 is delayed in both inspiration and expiration. Fixed splitting of S2 is classically found in patients with an atrial septal defect, but it is also present in clinical settings in which the right ventricle is acutely or chronically overloaded and right ventricular ejection is delayed. This is caused by acute right heart pressure overload (e.g., pulmonary embolism) and chronic biventricular failure when left ventricular systolic ejection time is shortened and right ventricular contraction is delayed because of elevated right ventricular pressures.

    Wide splitting of S2 (e.g., P2 is delayed but still moves somewhat closer to S1 with expiration) occurs in patients with right bundle branch block and pulmonary artery stenosis. Wide splitting can also occur in early phases of heart failure.

2. Paradoxical splitting of S2. Paradoxical splitting of S2 is said to be present when S2 splits on expiration and closes on inspiration. Although fixed splitting denotes delay in normal closure of the pulmonic valve, paradoxical splitting denotes delayed closure of the aortic valve. Delay in the closure of the aortic valve can be caused by either an electrical delay (left bundle branch block) or a mechanical delay (atrial septal defect). This important clinical sign never occurs in the absence of cardiac disease. The most common states in which paradoxical splitting is encountered are significant aortic stenosis and left bundle branch block. Paradoxical splitting may occur in patients with coronary artery disease, hypertension, or both. Alterations in the intensity of S2 can also yield important clinical information. A2 is frequently decreased in aortic stenosis. The presence of a normal A2 when aortic stenosis is clinically suspected raises the question of outflow obstruction at a site other than the valve. A2 is increased in systemic hypertension and can become tambour- or drumlike in quality when the aortic root is dilated. P2 may be augmented in pulmonary hypertension and diminished in pulmonic stenosis. Finally, P2 may appear unusually loud in thin-chested individuals without cardiac disease.

A summary of clinical information derived from alterations in S2 is found in Table 1-3.

C. **S3.** The third heart sound (S3, or ventricular gallop) is low-pitched and best heard at the apex with the stethoscope bell. To hear an S3, the patient should be placed in the left lateral position. The apex is located by palpation. The bell of the stethoscope is then placed over the apex with just enough force to make an air seal. Firm pressure on the bell of the stethoscope will stretch the skin, making a diaphragm and filtering out low-frequency sounds. The cadence of the S3 has been likened to the *y* in *Kentucky.* An S3 is the result of a mismatch between rapidity of ventricular filling and ventricular compliance. An S3 is normal variant, particularly in children and young adults, in whom filling is rapid and ventricular compliance is normal. The S3 is lost as one gets older, only to return in patients with heart failure, when the filling may be normal or slow, but there is a decrease in ventricular compliance.

A loud, early diastolic sound is often heard in constrictive pericarditis. This sound is earlier, louder, and of higher frequency than that of an S3, but the physiology is the same abrupt deceleration of blood filling the left ventricle.

D. **S4.** The fourth heart sound (S4, or atrial gallop) is a low-frequency presystolic sound. The S4 is the result of a forceful atrial contraction into a stiff or noncompliant ventricle. It is absent in atrial fibrillation and in patients with enlarged poorly contracting atria. Its cadence has been likened to the soft *a* of *appendix.* It is a low-pitched sound that is also best heard with the stethoscope bell. It is loudest at the apex and may also be accentuated by placing the patient in the left lateral decubitus position. The presence of an S4 implies effective atrial contraction; it is never heard in atrial fibrillation. An S4 may be heard in any condition that causes reduced ventricular compliance: aortic stenosis, systemic hypertension, coronary artery disease, hypertrophic

TABLE 1-3. CLINICAL SIGNIFICANCE OF ABNORMALITIES IN PRECORDIAL PALPATION

Finding	Comment/significance
Left ventricular thrust	Left ventricular hypertrophy
Displacement of left ventricular pulse downward and to the left	Left ventricular dilatation; left ventricular failure; volume overload (aortic regurgitation or decompensated mitral regurgitation)
Presystolic impulse	Pressure overloaded states (hypertension, aortic stenosis)
Double systolic impulse	Hypertrophic obstructive cardiomyopathy
Systolic bulge (dyskinetic impulse)	Coronary artery disease; recent myocardial infarction (most commonly felt above and medial to the point of maximal impulse)
Parasternal lift	Mitral regurgitation (occurs after the left ventricular apical impulse); right ventricular dilatation (mitral stenosis, pulmonary embolism)
Thrills	Aortic stenosis; pulmonic stenosis; ventricular septal defect; severe mitral regurgitation

cardiomyopathy, acute mitral regurgitation, and myocardial infarction. Right-sided S4 can be present in patients with primary pulmonary hypertension and pulmonic stenosis.

An S4 is always pathological and a very useful clinical tool. If a patient is seen with hypertension and has an S4, it is not necessary to confirm three separate occasions that the blood pressure is elevated. However, every duplication of sounds around S1 is not an S4. A split S1 is high frequency and best heard over the tricuspid area. An ejection click is a high-frequency sound best heard at the apex and at the base, over the aortic area, the pulmonary area, or both. Very early midsystolic clicks have the same characteristics as ejection sounds (ESs), except clicks change their systolic timing when one is listening to the patient in both the standing and squatting positions.

E. Snaps, clicks, and other adventitious sounds

1. Opening snap (OS). An OS of the mitral valve is heard in patients with mitral stenosis and a pliable mitral valve. The OS arises from the snapping of the mitral valve toward the left ventricle in early diastole. The OS is best heard in the fourth intercostal space halfway between the apex and the left sternal border. The interval between S2 and the OS is related to the severity of mitral stenosis. The more severe the stenosis, the shorter the S2–OS interval.

2. ESs. ESs are high-pitched sounds occurring in early systole. Previously called ejection clicks, they are now referred to as ESs, so as not to confused them with midsystolic clicks (see below). ESs can be either valvular or vascular in origin. A common cause of a valvular ES is from a bicuspid aortic valve. A stenosed pulmonary valve also produces an ES. The interesting phenomenon of the pulmonary ES is that it is the only right-sided event that gets louder with expiration. Another cause of ESs is dilatation of the aorta or pulmonary artery. With ejection into a widened artery, the forward velocity decreases and the lateral force produces a sound.

3. Midsystolic clicks. Midsystolic clicks occur in patients with prolapse of the mitral or tricuspid valve. The clicks may result from sudden tensing of the chordae tendineae or snapping of the prolapsing leaflet. The clicks may be single or multiple and may occur at any time during systole. When they are very early, they can be confused with ESs. To tell the difference, the patient should be listened to in both the standing and squatting positions. ESs do not move with changes in ventricular volume caused by these maneuvers, whereas systolic clicks do.

F. Systolic murmurs. Systolic murmurs are classified according to their time of occurrence, sound quality, and duration. The most fundamental distinction is between systolic ejection murmurs (SEMs) and regurgitant murmurs. SEMs occur during the time blood is ejected from the ventricle and thus occur in early and midsystole. SEMs begin after S1 and are usually crescendo-decrescendo ("diamond-shaped"), ending before S2.

In contrast, regurgitant murmurs, classically pansystolic, begin with S1, extend to S2, and are characteristically uniform in intensity. As explained below, however, not all regurgitant murmurs are pansystolic.

1. SEMs. SEMs begin after the semilunar (aortic and pulmonic) valves open at the end of isovolumic systole (Fig. 1.9). Their intensity parallels the velocity of blood being ejected through the stenosis, peaking in midsystole with mild stenosis and late in systole with severe stenosis. SEMs are caused by sclerosis or stenosis of the aortic or pulmonic valve; by increased velocity of ejection within the ventricle, as in hypertrophic cardiomyopathy; or by increased cardiac output owing to, for example, pregnancy, anemia, thyrotoxicosis, and arterial venous shunts. SEMs are generally louder at the base of the heart and radiate to the neck. One exception is the murmur of severe aortic stenosis, in which the high-frequency "cooing," or seagull, component is best heard at the apex. Another exception is the murmur caused by increased intraventricular velocities owing to enhanced contractility of a hypertrophic ventricle.

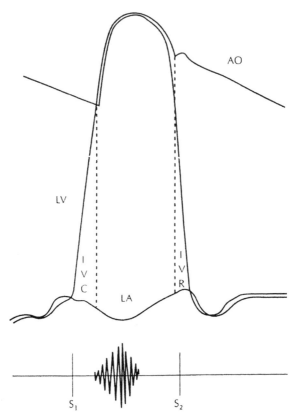

FIG. 1-9. Illustration of simultaneous aortic (Ao), left ventricular (LV), and left atrial pressure (LA) pressure curves during one cardiac systole, with simultaneous phonocardiographic recording of a systolic ejection murmur (SEM). Systolic ejection murmurs have a distinct period of silence between the first heart sound and the onset of the murmur. During the isovolumetric contraction (IVC) period, for example, the time between the closure of the atrioventricular (AV) valves and the opening of the semilunar valves, all valves are closed. If the valves do not leak or obstruct, these is no murmur right after the first heart sound or right before the second heart sound.

2. Regurgitant murmurs. Regurgitant murmurs occur when blood flows through a ventricular septal defect, or retrograde through the mitral or tricuspid valve. These murmurs are classically pansystolic. The even intensity and long duration of these murmurs reflect the large pressure difference across the orifice where the sound originates. The murmur continues as long as pressure in the chamber of origin exceeds that in the recipient chamber. When one hears a pansystolic murmur, the patient has mitral regurgitation, tricuspid regurgitation, or a ventricular septal defect.

   The characteristics of the murmur of mitral regurgitation are that it begins with the S1 (as soon as the pressure in the left ventricle increases above the pressure in the left atrium) and does not end until after S2. Even at the time of S2, the pressure in the left ventricle is higher than that of the left atrium (Fig. 1.10). Unfortunately, not all regurgitant

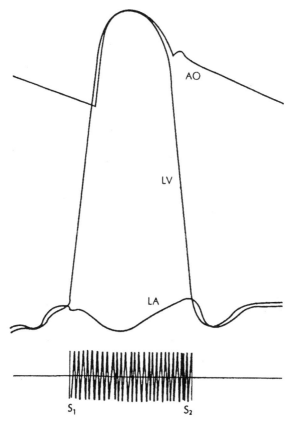

FIG. 1-10. Illustration of simultaneous aortic (Ao), left ventricular (LV), and left atrial pressure (LA) pressure curves during one cardiac systole, with simultaneous phonocardiographic recording of a pansystolic or holosystolic regurgitant murmur. A pansystolic or holosystolic murmur is one that begins with the first heart sound and continues through the second heart sound. A holosystolic or pansystolic murmur is always regurgitant, because the murmur involves both the isovolumetric periods, a time when all valves are closed.

murmurs are pansystolic. However, any murmur that begins with S1 (Fig. 1.11)—and thus, during the isovolumic contraction period when, all valves are closed—is regurgitant. Likewise, any murmur that extends through S2—and thus, during the isovolumic relaxation period— is regurgitant (Fig. 1.12). Thus any murmur that touches S1, S2, or both is regurgitant.

3. Late systolic murmurs. Late systolic murmurs begin in midsystole and extend to or through S2. They may be heard in mitral valve prolapse (frequently accompanied by midsystolic clicks)

4. Summary. Systolic murmurs arising from the right side of the heart generally increase with inspiration, whereas those originating on the left side decrease or do not change. Systolic murmurs in adults most often suggest cardiac disease. Even the so-called "innocent murmur of the elderly" has been shown to be associated with an adverse prognosis. Many systolic murmurs are totally innocent (as in pregnant women,

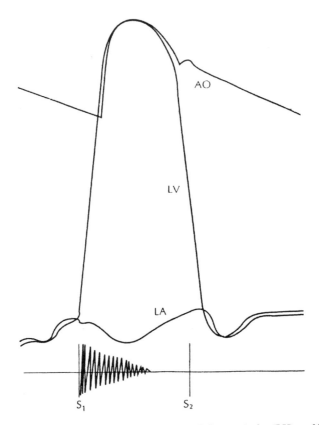

FIG. 1-11. Illustration of simultaneous aortic (Ao), left ventricular (LV), and left atrial pressure (LA) pressure curves during one cardiac systole, with simultaneous phono-cardiographic recording of an early systolic regurgitant murmur. A murmur that begins with the first heart sound is always regurgitant, because the murmur involves the isovolumetric contraction period, a time when all valves are closed.

growing children, and individuals with abnormal chest configuration). Others suggest the presence of noncardiac disease (high-output states such as anemia or thyrotoxicosis). In general, systolic murmurs do not require endocarditis prophylaxis.

G. Diastolic murmurs. Diastolic murmurs are either high frequency or low frequency. They occur in either early or late systole.

1. Early diastolic murmurs. High-frequency early diastolic murmurs begin immediately after S2. The most common cause is aortic regurgitation. The murmur is usually high pitched and blowing in quality, with a decrescendo configuration. The intensity of the murmur reflects the size of the valvular leak, the acoustic properties of the chest, and the pressure difference across the valve. The murmur of pulmonary insufficiency is high frequency only if pulmonary hypertension is present. The murmur of congenital pulmonary insufficiency is a low-frequency diastolic murmur best heard along the left sternal border.

2. Mid and late diastolic murmurs. Mid and late diastolic murmurs are produced by forward flow of blood through the atrioventricular (mitral

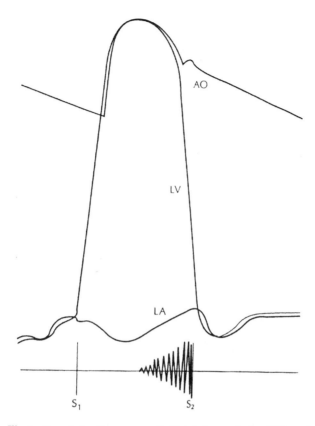

FIG. 1-12. Illustration of simultaneous aortic (Ao), left ventricular (LV), and left atrial pressure (LA) pressure curves during one cardiac systole, with simultaneous phono-cardiographic recording of a late systolic regurgitant murmur. A murmur that continues to or through the second heart sound is always regurgitant, because the murmur involves the isovolumetric relaxation period, a time when all valves are closed.

and tricuspid) valves. They arise from either augmented blood flow or a stenosed valve. As a rule, the murmur is low pitched and rumbling in quality. It does not begin until the valve from which it originates opens (sometimes with an audible snap), and ventricular pressure has fallen below atrial pressure in early diastole. Conditions in which mid or late diastolic murmurs may arise include (i) mitral or tricuspid stenosis, (ii) atrial myxomas, (iii) mitral regurgitation (increased flow in diastole, as all the blood that was regurgitated into the left atrium during systole along with the normal forward flow must cross the mitral valve in diastole), and (iv) large left-to-right shunts (increased flow across the tricuspid valve in patients with atrial septal defect and across the mitral valve in patients with ventricular septal defect).

H. Continuous murmurs. Murmurs are considered continuous when they envelop S2. Most continuous murmurs are audible throughout systole and diastole. They arise when a continuous pressure differential allows blood to flow constantly from a high-pressure to a low-pressure area, as may occur in a variety of congenital defects, such as patent ductus arteriosus or coronary arteriovenous fistula. An analogous phenomenon is the *venous hum*. This continuous, medium-pitched murmur results from increased velocity of venous blood flow. It is usually heard in the lower anterior portion of the neck. Venous hum is accentuated by deep inspiration in most patients and may be obliterated by the Valsalva maneuver or by pressure on the internal jugular vein. Venous hums are common in children and in patients with high-flow states such as thyrotoxicosis.

IV. Physiologic and pharmacologic manipulation of heart sounds and murmurs. Various physiologic and pharmacologic maneuvers are available to accentuate heart sounds and murmurs. A partial listing of these maneuvers, together with their physiologic consequences, is found in Table 1-4. Maneuvers that are useful in the analysis of specific murmurs and heart sounds are listed in Table 1-5.

Finally, physiologic and pharmacologic manipulations may help untangle difficult problems in differential diagnosis when normal auscultatory findings are ambiguous. A listing of some diagnostic problems and appropriate maneuvers is found in Table 1-6.

TABLE 1-4. MANIPULATION OF HEART SOUNDS AND MURMURS

Maneuver	Physiologic consequence	Comment
Physiologic maneuvers Respiration	Inspiration: right-heart filling increased, left-heart filling decreased	Right-heart murmurs increased; left-heart murmurs decreased or unchanged
Rapid changes in position (e.g., elevation of legs, standing, squatting)	Mechanical changes; changes in RV filling (RV filling increased by lying, leg elevation, or squatting; venous return decreased by standing)	Gallop sounds, murmurs of pulmonic and aortic stenosis, all increased by lying, leg elevation, or squatting; IHSS murmur increased by standing
Valsalva maneuver	Initially causes sharp rise in blood pressure (phase I), then impairs venous return and blood pressure drops (phase II)	During phase II, murmurs of pulmonic and aortic stenosis and mitral regurgitation diminish, whereas murmurs of IHSS increase
Pharmacologic maneuvers Phenylephrine	Raised systemic arterial pressure	Murmur of aortic regurgitation and mitral regurgitation increased
Isoproterenol	Increased myocardial contraction	Murmur of IHSS increased
Amyl nitrite	Potent vasodilator; decreased systolic pressure; reflex increase in heart rate	Murmurs of aortic and mitral regurgitation decreased; all ejection murmurs increased; VSD murmur decreased

RV, right ventricular; IHSS, idiopathic hypertrophic subaortic stenosis; VSD, ventricular septal defect.

TABLE 1-5. MANEUVERS FOR ANALYSIS OF HEART SOUNDS AND MURMURS

Condition	Maneuver
Aortic stenosis	Valvular: midsystolic murmur louder with sudden squatting, leg raising, or amyl nitrite; fades during Valsalva maneuver Hypertrophic subvalvular: systolic murmur louder with sitting or squatting, during Valsalva maneuver, or with amyl nitrite; softens with sudden squatting or leg elevation
Aortic regurgitation	Blowing diastolic murmur increases with sudden squatting; fades with amyl nitrite Austin Flint murmur fades with amyl nitrite
Mitral stenosis	Diastolic murmur made louder with tachycardia, exercise, left lateral position, coughing, or amyl nitrite
Mitral regurgitation	Rheumatic: systolic murmur louder with sudden squatting; softer with amyl nitrite Midsystolic to late systolic mitral valve prolapse: late systolic murmur becomes mid- or holosystolic with upright position, with amyl nitrite, and during Valsalva maneuver; midsystolic click occurs earlier with these maneuvers; murmur fades with lying flat
Pulmonic stenosis	Midsystolic murmur increases with amyl nitrite, except with marked right ventricular hypertrophy; also may increase with first few beats after Valsalva release
Pulmonic regurgitation	Congenital: early or middiastolic murmur (harsh, low-pitched) increases on inspiration and with amyl nitrite Pulmonary hypertensive: high-frequency early diastolic blowing murmur not influenced by respiration; inconstant response to amyl nitrite
Tricuspid stenosis	Middiastolic and presystolic murmurs increase during inspiration and with amyl nitrite
Tricuspid regurgitation	Systolic murmur increases during inspiration and with amyl nitrite
Ventricular septal defect	Small defect without pulmonary hypertension: murmur fades with amyl nitrite Large defect with hyperkinetic pulmonary hypertension: murmur louder with amyl nitrite Large defect with severe pulmonary vascular disease: little change with above agents
Gallop rhythm	Ventricular filling sounds: ventricular gallop and atrial gallop are accentuated by lying flat with passive leg raising; decreased by sitting or standing; right-sided gallop sounds usually increased during inspiration, left-sided during expiration Summation gallop may separate into ventricular gallop (S3) and atrial gallop (S4) sounds when heart rate slowed by carotid sinus massage
Ejection sounds	Ejection sound in pulmonic stenosis fades and occurs closer to the first heart sound (S1) during inspiration

Source: Adapted from Dohan MC, Criscitiello MG. Physiological and pharmacological manipulations of heart sounds and murmurs. *Mod Concepts Cardiovasc Dis* 1970;39:121.

TABLE 1-6. MANEUVERS TO DIFFERENTIATE AUSCULTATORY FINDINGS

Auscultatory problem	Maneuver
Systolic murmur of valvular aortic stenosis vs. hypertrophic subaortic stenosis	Sudden squatting, Valsalva maneuver
Systolic murmur of valvular aortic stenosis vs. midsystolic to late systolic mitral valve prolapse	Sudden standing, amyl nitrite
Systolic murmur of valvular aortic stenosis vs. mitral regurgitation	Amyl nitrite, isometric hand grip, variation in cycle length
Diastolic rumble of mitral stenosis vs. Austin Flint murmur	Amyl nitrite
Diastolic murmur of mitral stenosis vs. tricuspid stenosis	Respiration
Systolic murmur of mitral regurgitation vs. tricuspid regurgitation	Respiration
Ejection sound in pulmonic stenosis vs. aortic stenosis	Respiration
Small ventricular septal defect vs. pulmonic stenosis	Amyl nitrite
S4 plus S1 vs. separation of two components of S1	Respiration, sudden standing, lying with passive leg raising
S2 plus opening snap vs. wide separation of S2 components	Respiration

S1, first heart sound; S2, second heart sound; S3, third heart sound; S4, fourth heart sound.
Source: Adapted from Dohan MC, Criscitiello MG. Physiological and pharmacological manipulations of heart sounds and murmurs. *Mod Concepts Cardiovasc Dis* 1970;39:12.

SELECTED READINGS

Butman SM, Ewy GA, Standen JR, et al. Bedside cardiovascular examination in patients with severe chronic heart failure: importance of rest and inducible jugular venous distension. *J Am Coll Cardiol* 1993;22:968–974.

Ewy GA. Bedside evaluation of precordial pulsations *Cardiology in Practice* 1984; July/August:127.

Ewy GA. The abdominojugular test: technique and hemodynamic correlates. *Ann Intern Med* 1988;109:456–460.

Ewy GA, Marcus FI. Bedside estimation of the venous pressure. *Heart Bull* 1968;17:41.

Ewy GA, Rios JC, Marcus, FI. The dicrotic arterial pulse. *Circulation* 1969;39:655–661.

Harvey, W. *Proctor cardiac pearls.* Cedar Grove, NJ: Laennec Publishing, 1993

Marcus FI, Ewy GA, O'Rourke RA, et al. The effect of pregnancy on the murmurs of mitral and aortic regurgitation. *Circulation* 1970;41:795–805.

American Heart Association. Examination of the Heart: *Part one, "The Clinical History"* by ME Silverman; part two, "Inspection and palpation of venous and arterial pulses" by NO Fowler; part three, "Precordial pulsations" by JW Hurst and RC Schlant; and part four, "Auscultation" by JJ Leonard, FW Kroetz, DF Leon, et al. Palles, Texas: American Heart Association.

2. NONINVASIVE EXAMINATION OF THE HEART

I. **Introduction.** The use of noninvasive techniques in the diagnosis of cardiac disease has expanded during recent decades. New techniques have been developed and old ones improved, providing added sensitivity and specificity. Positive aspects of noninvasive techniques include (i) expanded diagnostic information at decreased risk to the patient, (ii) ability to screen larger populations for cardiac disease, and (iii) capability of monitoring clinical progression with serial studies. Negative aspects include (i) confusion about which tests to use in a given clinical setting (with subsequent overuse of worthless or redundant procedures) and (ii) increased cost.

This chapter briefly reviews major noninvasive techniques and discusses their clinical applicability and limitation. Further information on the diagnostic use of each technique is found in chapters on specific cardiac diseases. Because roentgenographic techniques and ECG are covered in detail in other chapters and are familiar to most physicians, they will not be treated separately here.

II. Noninvasive techniques

  A. Echocardiography

    1. **Technique.** The human ear is unable to discern sounds with frequencies higher than 20,000 Hz. Sound with a frequency greater than 20,000 Hz is called ultrasound. Ultrasound used in cardiac diagnosis is very high frequency (1.6 to 2.25 million Hz). The sound waves are both emitted and received by the same transducer. Sound waves are reflected at interfaces between media of different acoustic impedances. Echocardiograms are generated by ultrasonic beams that traverse cardiac structures with definable anatomic shapes (chamber walls, interventricular septum) or characteristic motions (cardiac valves). The echocardiograms are then recorded on videotape or laser disc. These images can be played back and forth, over and over again, for analysis of ventricular wall motion and size, valvular function, and the presence or absence of pericardial effusion. Other observations that can be made during an echo study include visualization of the proximal portion of the coronary arteries, the presence of cardiac tumors or thrombus, and the size and integrity of the great cardiac vessels. Using specialized probes, the interior aspect of the coronary arteries and the aorta can be examined by means of intravascular ultrasound. With this latter technique, atherosclerotic plaques and arterial dissection can be detected.

      a. **Doppler echocardiography.** This technique is usually combined with most standard echocardiographic studies. The technique uses the Doppler principle that when the ultrasonic wave is reflected by a moving object, the frequency of the reflected beam is altered. Doppler echocardiography discloses patterns of blood flow within the heart and great cardiac vessels, as well as gradients and regurgitant jets involving the cardiac valves. Therefore, the severity of valvular stenosis and regurgitation can be determined.

      b. **Transesophageal echocardiography.** With this technique, a cross-sectional echo transducer is placed at the end of the flexible endoscope, and high-quality cross-sectional images are obtained through the esophagus. Doppler information may also be obtained with this technique. Transesophageal echocardiography has proved useful in specific patients in whom the standard echocardiogram cannot be obtained from the usual position, for example, patients with chest wall deformities or severe chronic obstructive pulmonary disease. This technique is also particularly helpful in assessing possible aortic dissection, vegetations of endocarditis, and prosthetic valve function. Esophageal echocardiography has also proved useful in monitoring left ventricular function during surgical procedures and during the postoperative period.

   c. Contrast echocardiography. Intravascular bubbles can be picked up with a high degree of sensitivity by ultrasound. Almost any liquid injected intravascularly will result in microbubbles. Tracing these bubbles by ultrasound then allows visualization of intracardiac shunts and heightened clarity of endocardial borders and even myocardial perfusion. Liquids that have been used for this purpose include normal saline, 5% dextrose in water, and indocyanine green dye. Specially designed echocardiographic contrast fluids produce exceptionally clear images and are increasingly used during echocardiographic studies. This technique confirms the presence of abnormal flow patterns within the heart and increases the accuracy of various intracardiac chamber measurements. It is likely that in the near future, contrast echocardiographic techniques will enable us to measure myocardial perfusion with considerable accuracy.

   d. Dobutamine echocardiographic stress test. This is a test to assist in the diagnosis of atherosclerotic coronary artery disease (CAD) and in determining the viability of injured and/or ischemic myocardium in patients with severe CAD. Left ventricular function is monitored during graded increases in heart rate that develop during infusion of increasing doses of dobutamine. The test is said to be positive for myocardial ischemia when new left ventricular hypokinesis or akinesis is observed during dobutamine infusion. The test is said to be positive for the presence of stunned or hibernating myocardium, namely, transiently injured but viable myocardium, when wall motion improves during the dobutamine infusion.

2. Clinical uses of echocardiography. The clinical conditions in which echocardiography provides useful information are as follows:

Evaluation of cardiac performance (left and right ventricles and atria)
Mitral stenosis
Mitral regurgitation, mitral valve prolapse, and flail mitral valve leaflet
Left ventricular outflow obstruction
Hypertrophic obstructive cardiomyopathy
Aortic stenosis and regurgitation
Diseases of the aorta and aortic root
Aortic dissection
Dilatation of the aortic root
Endocarditis
Pericardial effusion and cardiac tamponade
Pulmonary valvular disease and pulmonary hypertension
Congenital heart disease (all forms)
Prosthetic heart valves
Cardiac tumors
Viability of myocardium in patients with severe CAD
Tricuspid valve disease
Intracardiac thrombus
Intracardiac shunts
Myocardial abscess
Ventricular aneurysm and pseudoaneurysm
Cardiac involvement in patients with systemic diseases, for example, systemic lupus erythematosus or amyloidosis
Monitoring of cardiac function during chemotherapy for various malignancies

   a. Evaluation of cardiac performance. Considerable information concerning cardiac performance is available from the echocardiogram. Left and right ventricular and atrial sizes can be assessed by means of an echocardiographic study. Noninvasive ejection fraction and indexes of contractility may be measured, and segmental wall motion abnormalities may be detected. Wall thickness and changes of thickness during systole can also be determined.

b. Mitral stenosis. Initial observations in the late 1950s showed that echocardiography demonstrated characteristic anterior mitral valve leaflet motion abnormalities. Echocardiographic examination allows for direct visualization of the mitral valve orifice and computation of its area. Cross-sectional echocardiography may even provide a more accurate method than does angiography for evaluating mitral valve orifice size in patients with combined mitral stenosis and regurgitation. Doppler studies are useful for measuring the mitral valve gradient, estimating the valve area, and detecting the presence of concomitant mitral regurgitation.

c. Left ventricular outflow obstruction. Subvalvular, valvular, and supravalvular aortic stenoses produce identifiable echocardiographic patterns. Echocardiography may provide useful information in a variety of other diseases of the aorta and aortic root, such as dilatation of the aortic root or aortic dissection. Doppler helps to identify and quantitate aortic regurgitation.

d. Mitral regurgitation. Doppler echocardiography discloses useful information in patients with mitral regurgitation. The volume of regurgitant blood can be quantitated. Cross-sectional echocardiography assesses left ventricular size and function. The pulmonary arterial systolic pressure can be measured. The echocardiographic image of the mitral valve helps distinguish a rheumatic origin, subacute bacterial endocarditis, and mitral valve prolapse.

e. Mitral valve prolapse. Echocardiograms in patients with auscultatory findings of mitral valve prolapse usually show posterior displacement of the valve leaflets at end systole. Echocardiography is the procedure of choice for screening populations and for identifying asymptomatic or minimally symptomatic individuals with mitral valve prolapse.

f. Flail mitral valve leaflet. A flail mitral valve leaflet may be difficult to distinguish by echocardiography from a vegetation caused by infectious endocarditis (IE). In both, coarse fluttering of the valve leaflet may be observed. Often the valve will be seen to prolapse into the left atrium during systole. Flail leaflets tend to exhibit both systolic and diastolic fluttering. Cross-sectional echocardiography reveals that the flail leaflet may be distinguished from mitral valve prolapse; in the former, the tip of the leaflet prolapses into the left atrium during systole, and in the latter, the body of the valve prolapses.

g. IE. The minimum size of vegetation that can be visualized by echocardiography is approximately 2 mm in diameter. Although failure to demonstrate a vegetation does not rule out IE, the echocardiographic demonstration of vegetation has diagnostic and prognostic significance. Positive echocardiographic evidence of vegetation correlates well with the ultimate need for surgical replacement of the valve. Echocardiography demonstrates which valve(s) is involved in patients with IE. Transesophageal echocardiography identifies a valvular vegetation in nearly all patients with proven IE.

h. Pericardial effusion. Echocardiography is a very sensitive diagnostic modality for the detection of pericardial effusion. Pericardial effusions as small as 50 ml may be identified by echo.

i. Pulmonary valvular disease. Echocardiographic analysis of pulmonic valve structure and function provides useful information in patients with pulmonary hypertension or pulmonic stenosis. Echocardiography allows the clinician to estimate pulmonary arterial systolic pressure.

j. Congenital heart disease. Echocardiography is the noninvasive diagnostic method of choice to identify most congenital cardiac conditions.

Specific echocardiographic findings for various congenital anomalies are discussed in the later chapters of this book and in entire textbooks.

  k. Echocardiography in systemic conditions with cardiovascular involvement. Echocardiography can provide important diagnostic information in a variety of systemic diseases in which cardiac involvement is suspected, for example, systemic lupus erythematosus or amyloidosis.

Echocardiography is also used for serial monitoring of cardiac function in therapies with cardiovascular side effects. Some of the potential uses of echocardiography are given in Table 2-1.

B. Vectorcardiography (VCG)
  1. Technique. VCG displays ventricular electrical activity as a "loop" derived from two simultaneously recorded scalar ECGs. The scalar ECGs are obtained at right angles to each other on the thorax. They generate a composite electrical signal that is focused on an oscilloscope and moved along two perpendicular axes by two pairs of perpendicularly oriented charged plates. The VCG loop represents the composite electrical activity in a given two-dimensional plane of the heart.
  2. Clinical uses. The chief use of VCG is to clarify confusing scalar ECG findings.

In some situations, VCG adds important information; however, it should be used selectively. VCG can contribute important additional information in approximately 5% of all ECG tracings. Conditions in which VCG may prove helpful include the following:
  a. Ischemic heart disease. VCG can confirm or deny the presence of myocardial infarction (MI). ECG findings such as nondiagnostic Q waves, concomitant inferior MI, left anterior hemiblock, or an R wave in V1 may pose diagnostic problems. VCG can be helpful in each of these settings.
  b. Ventricular enlargement. VCG may prove helpful when ECG shows equivocal evidence of ventricular enlargement. VCG is particularly useful when ECG suggests either right or left ventricular enlargement and biventricular enlargement is suspected clinically. VCG is not superior to ECG in assessing hypertrophy secondary to pressure overload.

TABLE 2-1. USE OF ECHOCARDIOGRAPHY FOR DEFINING CARDIAC COMPLICATIONS OF SYSTEMIC DISEASES OR TREATMENT

Disease or treatment	Use of echocardiography
Chronic renal disease	To assess left ventricular function, myocardial wall thickness, and presence or absence of pericardial effusion
Malignancy	Cardiac involvement with metastatic disease; malignant pericardial effusion
Chronic anemia, hemochromatosis	Abnormalities in left ventricular wall motion
Embolic stroke	Mitral stenosis; possible atrial myxoma
Rheumatologic disorders	Detection of pericardial involvement in conditions causing polyserositis
Connective tissue disease	Detection of aortic root dilatation or mitral valve prolapse in Marfan's syndrome or rheumatoid spondylitis
Doxorubicin (Adriamycin) administration	Serial assessment of left ventricular function

c. Intraventricular blocks. VCG adds little to ECG in uncomplicated cases of complete right or left bundle branch block. VCG may be helpful, however, in the following situations: (i) right bundle branch block and left anterior hemiblock, (ii) prolonged QRS after MI, and (iii) suspected Wolff-Parkinson-White syndrome.

C. Nuclear medicine techniques

1. Cold spot scanning

   a. Technique. Cold spot scanning takes advantage of the fact that normal myocardial cells take up certain radioactively labeled potassium analogs and exchange them for intracellular potassium. Damaged or dead myocytes will not do this. Thus, abnormal zones of myocardium will show up as areas of relatively decreased tracer uptake or "cold spots."

   The two tests most commonly performed are the thallium 201 and radiolabeled sestamibi examinations.

   b. Clinical uses. Cold spot scanning is used to detect areas of cell necrosis (MI) or ischemia. Studies are performed either at rest, after exercise, or after intravenous dipyridamole, adenosine, or dobutamine. Specific clinical uses for cold spot scanning include the following:

   (1) Equivocal evidence of ischemia on ECG exercise tolerance testing (ETT) or in patients with a markedly abnormal baseline ECG.

   (2) Patients unable to exercise in whom a diagnosis of CAD is being entertained.

   (3) Evidence of graft closure in patients who have undergone coronary bypass surgery.

   (4) Suspected MI with equivocal clinical and laboratory findings.

   (5) Risk stratification following MI

   When thallium or sestamibi scanning is used to clarify a clinical diagnosis of CAD ETT results, the patient must exercise vigorously at the time the isotope is injected and for 30 to 45 seconds afterward. Several studies have shown that the use of exercise thallium scanning in conjunction with the traditional ETT protocol is significantly more sensitive than either technique alone. A form of thallium or sestamibi scanning in use in some institutions combines scanning with intravenous dipyridamole, a potent coronary vasodilator. After it is administered, areas distal to fixed coronary arterial obstructions will show relative hypoperfusion and decreased tracer uptake. Dipyridamole radionuclide scans are particularly useful in patients who, for one reason or another, cannot exercise. These scans have been found to be highly accurate and useful in patients with peripheral vascular disease and claudication. Intravenous infusions of adenosine or dobutamine can also be used for this type of scan.

   c. Limitations. The use of cold spot scanning is limited in a variety of clinical settings. A cold spot may represent three different situations: a viable, but ischemic, myocardial zone; an acute infarction; or a chronic infarction. It may be difficult to distinguish among these three alternatives. Furthermore, cold spot imaging relies on the physician's interpretation of relative differences in radionuclide uptake. Global ischemia from three-vessel disease may be overlooked because of a uniform decrease in tracer uptake. False-positive images have also been reported in 10% of patients with normal coronary arteries. Finally, the uptake of radioactive tracer into myocardial cells may be altered by medication. Both digitalis and beta-blockade have been shown to diminish thallium 201 uptake in experimental settings.

2. "Hot spot" scanning

   a. Technique. In contrast to cold spot imaging, which relies on the ability of normal cells to accumulate radioactive tracer, hot spot scanning takes advantage of the fact that damaged myocardial cells accumulate certain radioactively labeled agents. The most commonly used tracer for hot spot imaging is technetium 99m stannous pyrophosphate (99m Tc–PYP). This agent accumulates in irreversibly damaged myocardium.

b. Clinical uses. The chief use of hot spot scanning is in the detection of irreversible myocardial damage secondary to MI. Hot spot scanning can also provide important clinical information in other clinical settings:

   (1) Myocardial contusion (secondary to blunt trauma)
   (2) Myocardial infarction after cardiac surgery
   (3) Right ventricular infarction

   Hot spot scanning is sometimes used in the detection of MI. Experimental studies in dogs have shown that 99m Tc–PYP scintiscans can detect infarctions as small as 3 g. In humans, infarcts must be 5% of the ventricle or larger to be reliably detected. 99m Tc–PYP scintiscans are more sensitive than is ECG in the diagnosis of acute MI in the presence of left bundle branch block. 99m Tc–PYP localizes in necrotic myocardium regardless of etiology. Thus, false-positive hot spot scans may occur in such conditions as myocarditis, myocardial abscess, cardiac trauma, and old MI. These conditions cannot be distinguished from each other by 99m Tc–PYP scanning.

   Timing is important in hot spot scanning. 99m Tc–PYP scans are generally negative during the first few hours after infarction and should not be obtained until at least 12 hours after the onset of infarction. If infarction is suspected, and the initial technetium scan is negative, repetition of the scan at 48 to 72 hours increases the likelihood of positive findings. Technetium scanning is very sensitive for transmural infarction. More than 95% of transmural infarcts are demonstrated by hot spot scans. 99m Tc–PYP scanning is less sensitive in nontransmural infarction. Labeled antimyosin antibodies can also be used to detect myocardial necrosis with a high degree of accuracy.

c. Limitations. The chief limitation in hot spot scanning is lack of specificity. In addition, interobserver differences in interpretation may occur.

3. Gated blood pool scanning

a. Technique. Gated blood pool scanning labels the blood passing through the cardiac chambers. Human serum albumin or red blood cells labeled with technetium 99m are usually used. Images are made by a scintillation camera, which is gated in response to a preselected event in the ECG (multigated acquisition scans). The image in multigated acquisition scanning can be displayed either as a series of still pictures or in movie format.

b. Clinical uses. The main use of gated blood pool scanning is assessment of left ventricular function. Gated blood pool scanning may be helpful in other clinical situations as well:

   (1) Assessing prognosis in patients with acute MI
   (2) Evaluating treatment in patients with CAD
   (3) Distinguishing between diffuse left ventricular hypokinesis and left ventricular aneurysm in patients with congestive heart failure after MI
   (4) Detecting right ventricular failure
   (5) Detecting intracardiac shunts in patients with congenital heart disease or septal rupture after MI. Exercise gated blood pool scanning may provide useful information in patients with aortic regurgitation or CAD. In patients with CAD, exercise gated blood pool scanning can show functional capacity and ischemically induced wall motion abnormalities

4. Positron emission tomography (PET)
   a. Technique. Over the past 20 years, PET has evolved as an imaging technique with a variety of clinically useful applications. PET scanning depends on biologically active positron-emitting radiopharmaceuticals and their ability to image biologic phenomena. The PET imaging protocols vary according to the type of radiopharmaceutical being used and the type of detector.
   b. Clinical uses. The chief use of PET scanning is assessment of myocardial ischemia and/or viability. Specific indications for PET scanning include:
      (1) Diagnosis of CAD
      (2) Assessment of myocardial blood flow
      (3) Assessment of myocardial metabolism
      (4) Assessment of myocardial viability in patients with CAD

D. Computed tomography (CT) of the heart. Increasingly sophisticated CT equipment has led to its increased utility in the diagnosis of cardiovascular disease. Equipment is now available with rapid scanning capability (1 to 4 seconds), and when this is gated with an ECG scan, times of 0.1 second can be achieved. Contrast enhancement typically is used to allow differentiation between the myocardium and intracavitary blood. CT scanning has been successfully used to identify constrictive pericarditis, pericardial effusion, and coronary artery calcification.

CT is particularly useful in diagnosing anomalies of the aortic arch and great vessels. CT scanning is very accurate in identifying cardiac tumors and intracavitary thrombus. The role of CT scanning in sizing MI remains uncertain, although it is under active investigation. Contrast-enhanced CT scanning may be useful in diagnosing and monitoring small aortic dissections. CT scanning has also been used to assess patency of coronary artery bypass grafts.

Electron beam CT scanning identifies coronary arterial calcification with great accuracy. Because coronary arterial atherosclerosis is associated with coronary arterial calcification, a number of cardiologists use this test to identify patients with early evidence of CAD. There is considerable controversy concerning the role that electron beam CT should play in the evaluation of patients with suspected CAD. Large-scale clinical trials currently underway should help define the utility of this technique in the near future.

Spiral CT scanning with intravenous contrast agent administration is commonly used to identify pulmonary embolism. The technique appears to be as accurate as ventilation/perfusion (V/Q) lung scanning for the diagnosis of pulmonary embolism. Large-scale clinical trials currently underway will help to define the eventual role of this diagnostic modality in the diagnosis of acute pulmonary embolism.

E. Magnetic resonance imaging (MRI). MRI scanning can disclose both tomographic and metabolic information about the heart and other structures without the use of radiation. MRI can be useful in evaluating myocardial ischemia, myocardial mass, ventricular volumes, anatomic relationships, and the presence of pericardial constriction and regurgitant valvular lesions. At the present time, other modalities such as echocardiography can disclose the same information more simply and with less expense. It is likely, however, that MRI will become increasingly useful in the future as new, more efficient, and more rapid MRI devices are produced. One possible use for MRI in the future would be a totally noninvasive coronary arteriogram. Such images are currently beyond the capability of current MRI machines but may be available in the near future.

F. Digital subtraction angiography. This technique, which involves digital processing of a fluoroscopic image after an intravenous injection of contrast material, is a relatively noninvasive technique for evaluating vascular anatomy. It is already a standard technique for evaluating peripheral vascular disease. Its application to coronary anatomy has awaited the development of gating techniques to eliminate the problem of cardiac motion. The exact role of digital subtraction angiography in evaluating CAD remains to be determined.

G. Exercise tests and Holter monitors. Exercise testing is discussed in Chapter 15 and earlier in this chapter under nuclear medicine tests. Holter or ambulatory electrocardiographic monitoring is discussed in Chapter 3.

SELECTED READINGS

Aurigemma G, Orsinelli D, Sweeney A. Echocardiography in the ICU. In: Rippe JM, Irwin RS, Fink MP, et al., eds. *Intensive care medicine.* Boston: Little, Brown and Company, 1995.
A comprehensive chapter on the use of echocardiography in the intensive care unit setting.

Beller GA, Zaret BL. Contributions of nuclear cardiology to diagnosis and prognosis of patients with coronary artery disease. *Circulation* 2000;101:1465–1478.
A review of the various nuclear techniques for identifying patients with CAD and for defining their prognosis.

Camici PG, Rosen SD. Does positron emission tomography contribute to the management of clinical cardiac problems? *Eur Heart J* 1996;17:174–181.
A review of the results of studies involving PET in patients with CAD.

Cheitlin MD, Alpert JS, Armstrong WF, et al. ACC/AHA guidelines for the clinical application of echocardiography. *Circulation* 1997;95:1686–1744.
An extensive review of indications and applications of echocardiography.

The clinical role of magnetic resonance in cardiovascular disease: task force of the European Society of Cardiology, in collaboration with the Association of European Paediatric Cardiologists. *Eur Heart J* 1998;19:19–39.
A thorough review of all aspects of cardiovascular MRI.

Daniel WG, Mugge A. Transesophageal echocardiography. *N Engl J Med* 1995;332:1268–1279.
A thorough review of the indications and results obtained from transesophageal echo studies.

Geleijnse ML, Elhendy A, Fioretti PM, Roelandt JRTC. Dobutamine stress myocardial perfusion imaging. *J Am Coll Cardiol* 2000;36:2017–2027.
Dobutamine stress echo is a safe and accurate means of assessing severity and prognosis in patients with CAD.

Mandalapu B, Amato M, Stratmann HG. Technetium Tc 99m sestamibi myocardial perfusion imaging: current role for evaluation of prognosis. *Chest* 1999;115:1684–1694.
A summary of the value of sestamibi scanning in patients with CAD.

Nagel E, Underwood R, Pennell D, et al. New developments in non-invasive cardiac imaging: critical assessment of the clinical role of cardiac magnetic resonance imaging. *Eur Heart J* 1998;19:1286–1292.
A review of the indications and results obtained with cardiac MRI.

Nissen SE, Yock P. Intravascular ultrasound. Novel pathophysiological insights and current clinical applications. *Circulation* 2001 103:604–616.
A thoughtful review of the indications and results obtained with intravascular ultrasound in patients with CAD.

Usher BW, O'Brien TX. Recent advances in dobutamine stress echocardiography. *Clin Cardiol* 2000;23:560–570.
A review of the technique and results obtained with dobutamine stress echo.

Vanzetto G, Ormezzano O, Fagret D, et al. Long-term additive prognostic value of thallium-201 myocardial perfusion imaging over clinical and exercise stress test in low to intermediate risk patients: study in 1137 patients with 6 year follow-up. *Circulation* 1999;100:1521–1527.
The incremental predictive value of thallium 201 stress testing over standard ECG stress testing is maintained over a 6-year follow-up period.

3. ARRHYTHMIAS

I. Introduction. Cardiac arrhythmias can arise in a wide variety of settings and can pose difficult diagnostic and management problems. Their clinical importance ranges from life-threatening problems that demand immediate attention to incidental findings that do not require treatment. Over recent decades, data from electrophysiologic studies (EPS) have fostered a new understanding about the etiology of various arrhythmias and have provided an important new diagnostic tool. Significant advances have also been made in pharmacologic management of arrhythmias, and a wide variety of new antiarrhythmic medications have become available. A detailed description of the ECG recognition of arrhythmias is beyond the scope of this manual and is covered in a number of standard ECG and general cardiology texts. The present chapter focuses on four topics: (i) general approach to the patient with an arrhythmia, (ii) recognition of specific arrhythmias, (iii) pharmacologic treatment of rhythm disorders, and (iv) electrical treatment of rhythm disorders.

II. Approach to the patient with cardiac arrhythmia
    A. Etiology. Cardiac arrhythmias may occur in either the presence or the absence of underlying structural heart disease. Certain arrhythmias, however, are more likely to occur in patients with heart disease and serve as clues to the etiology of the cardiac condition. When arrhythmias occur in the setting of organic heart disease, the rhythm disturbance should not be treated in isolation. Often, arrhythmias cannot be controlled unless the underlying cardiac problem is discovered and treated. Structural cardiac disease may actually provoke the arrhythmia.

    Conduction disturbances (second- and third-degree atrioventricular [AV] block) may be caused by fibrosis, calcification, or both in the vicinity of the AV node. Atrial arrhythmias (atrial fibrillation [AF], atrial flutter) may be caused by mechanical obstruction to atrial emptying or left ventricular dysfunction with subsequent left atrial dilatation. Ventricular tachycardia and ventricular fibrillation (VF) may accompany a variety of organic heart diseases.

    Arrhythmias do not always imply underlying structural disease of the heart. Rhythm disturbances that can occur without demonstrable underlying structural heart disease include first-degree AV block, bundle branch block, atrial and ventricular premature contractions, sinus arrhythmia, sinus bradycardia, and sinus tachycardia. Systemic diseases that cause circulatory disturbances may provoke arrhythmias. Diseases in this category include endocrine disease (particularly thyrotoxicosis or pheochromocytoma), systemic infection, rapid development of hypercapnia or hypoxemia, and metastatic neoplasm to the heart. Drug toxicity often provokes arrhythmia. Drugs usually implicated are digitalis, antiarrhythmic agents, catecholamines, some psychotropic agents, and methylxanthines (e.g., aminophylline).

    Inherited diseases such as the prolonged Q–T syndrome may be the cause of arrhythmias.

    Electrolyte disturbances are also a common cause of rhythm disturbance and should be strongly considered in any hospitalized patient. Hyperkalemia, hypokalemia, hypomagnesemia, hypercalcemia, and hypocalcemia can all provoke arrhythmias.

    B. Pathophysiology. Modern concepts of arrhythmogenesis are based on an understanding of the anatomy of the cardiac conduction system and the electrical basis of the cardiac action potential.
        1. Anatomic considerations. In normal circumstances, the pacemaker function of the cardiac electrical system is performed by the sinus node. This structure lies less than 1 mm from the epicardial surface at the junction of the right atrium and the superior vena cava. The sinus node consists

of a variety of densely packed cells, including nodal cells, transitional cells, and atrial myocardial cells. Its blood supply is drawn from the sinus node artery, which originates from the right coronary artery in approximately 55% to 60% of individuals and from the left circumflex coronary artery in 40% to 45%. Pacemaker activity within the sinus node cells results from spontaneous depolarization of these specialized cells. An electrical wave of depolarization then spreads through both atria, possibly aided by specialized atrial conducting pathways. The wave of electrical depolarization then arrives at a complex structure called the atrioventricular junctional area. This area consists of nodal approaches, the AV node itself, and the bundle of His (penetrating portion of the AV bundle). This structure derives blood supply from both the posterior descending artery and the left anterior descending artery and is thus less vulnerable to ischemic insult than is the sinus node. The electrical impulse is propagated next to the left and right bundle branches (branching portions of the AV bundle). Considerable anatomic variability exists in this structure. In some individuals, the left bundle consists of two discrete branches, and in others, a branching network exists. The right bundle is generally anatomically discrete and remains unbranched as it travels down the right side of the interventricular septum. The left bundle branch consists of two final arborizations, the left anterior hemibundle and the left posterior hemibundle. Compared with the left posterior branch, the left anterior branch of the left bundle is almost invariably thinner and more susceptible to injury. Therefore, left anterior hemiblock is much more common than left posterior hemiblock. The final specialized electrical conducting tissue is the network of terminal Purkinje fibers. These fibers are connected to the ends of the AV branch bundles and form a rich network of interwoven connections that allow for the transmission of the electrical impulse simultaneously to both the entire left and right ventricular endocardial surfaces.

2. Electrophysiologic principles. The phospholipid bilayer of the cellular membrane is responsible for maintaining a transmembrane electrical potential. During electrical quiescence (in diastole) the intracellular potential is 50 to 95 mV. In a spontaneously depolarizing cell, for example, a pacemaker cell in the sinus or AV node, this potential drifts toward 0 mV until it reaches a threshold level, at which point the cell depolarizes in an all-or-none fashion. In contrast to nerve tissue in which the depolarization-repolarization process may occur in several milliseconds, the process takes several hundred milliseconds in cardiac tissue. The action potential in cardiac tissue is divided into five phases: phase 0, rapid depolarization; phase 1, early rapid repolarization; phase 2, plateau; phase 3, late rapid repolarization; and phase 4, resting potential and diastolic depolarization.

   The swings in electrical current are largely caused by rapid influx of Na^+ and outflux of K^+ ions, actions that are controlled by the Na^+/K^+ ion pump.

3. Mechanisms of arrhythmogenesis. Most arrhythmias are now believed to be caused by abnormalities in (i) impulse formation (disordered automaticity); (ii) impulse conduction in which a wave of depolarization reenters repolarized cardiac tissue, thereby setting up an abnormal recurrent circular route of cardiac depolarization; or (iii) both mechanisms. Disordered automaticity has been demonstrated in human ventricular cells from patients undergoing aneurysmectomy for recurrent ventricular tachycardia (VT). Disordered conduction appears to underlie the reentry mechanism now thought to cause most supraventricular tachycardias and VTs, fibrillation, and flutter.

   a. Impulse formation/automaticity. Cells in the cardiac conduction system are able to maintain an electrical potential across their cell membranes. The cells depolarize in an all-or-none fashion when an impulse of sufficient magnitude to exceed their threshold potential arrives. Some electrically active cells in the myocardium have the additional property of automaticity. They will depolarize spontaneously without external stimulation. The cells with the most rapid spontaneous depolarization control depolarization of the entire conduction system. Under normal conditions, these cells are located in the sinus node. Their rate of discharge may be influenced by any condition that (i) alters the magnitude of the threshold potential, (ii) changes the slope of spontaneous depolarization (phase 4), or (iii) alters the maximum potential at the end of repolarization. Parasympathomimetic autonomic agents or stimuli causing vagal discharge slow phase 4 depolarization, thereby slowing heart rate. Sympathomimetic agents or sympathetic nerve discharge increases heart rate by shortening spontaneous depolarization. Temperature reduction slows phase 4 depolarization, as do stretch (e.g., in atrial dilatation), hypercapnia, and hypoxia. Increased extracellular calcium increases the transmembrane potential and slows depolarization of automatic cells. Decreased extracellular calcium has the opposite effect.

Once depolarization occurs in automatic pacemaker cells, it travels through the conduction system and depolarizes other electrically active cells. As noted, arrhythmias arise from disturbances in cardiac automaticity or conduction. Disturbances in automaticity may reflect either depression of the normal pacemaker cells in the sinus node or increased automaticity in an accessory focus. Disturbances in automaticity are caused by hypocalcemia, hypercalcemia, hypokalemia, hyperkalemia, hypercapnia, acidosis, alkalosis, myocardial fiber stretch, norepinephrine, epinephrine, and various drugs, for example, digitalis and antiarrhythmic agents.

b. Conduction. Any condition that decreases the amplitude of the action potential (hypercalcemia, calcification of the conducting fibers, ischemia) can cause disturbance in cardiac conduction. Either heart block or a reentry rhythm may occur in this setting.

c. Clinical responses associated with arrhythmias. Efficient pumping action of the heart results from normal contraction induced by normal electrical activity. Alterations in this sequence can hinder cardiac function by a variety of mechanisms, including (i) loss of appropriately timed atrial contraction, (ii) increase in myocardial oxygen consumption (particularly in tachycardias), and (iii) inefficient ventricular contraction (loss of proper sequence). The circulatory response to these disturbances may pose particular problems in patients with underlying cardiac disease and diminished cardiac reserve.

d. Diagnostic approach to arrhythmias. Three general techniques are available to the physician to aid in the diagnosis of an arrhythmia: history, physical examination, and ECG techniques.

  (1) History. Patients often describe sensations accompanying an abnormal cardiac rhythm, such as "pounding," "racing," or "skipping beats." The patient may be able to tap out the rhythm with his or her hand. History of any cardiac disease should be sought. Any medications the patient is taking should be considered. Any previous experience that the individual has had with rhythm disturbances should be thoroughly explored, together with the treatment attempted and its efficacy. Family history of rhythm disturbance should be ascertained.

  (2) Physical examination. A complete physical examination should be undertaken with emphasis on the heart and peripheral vasculature.

    Pulse should be palpated for at least a full minute, and both rate and regularity should be noted. The intensity of the first heart sound (S1) may provide information about the relation of atrial to ventricular contraction. The longer the P–R interval, the softer is S1. Observation of the jugular venous pulse may prove helpful. In situations in which the atria and ventricles contract independently (AV dissociation), giant A waves (cannon waves) may be observed when the right atrium contracts against a closed tricuspid valve.

Several provocative maneuvers may bring out arrhythmias not discernible during the initial examination of the patient. Carotid sinus massage elicits a vagal discharge, which primarily affects the atrial and AV nodal conduction system. Ventricular tachycardia is not influenced by this maneuver. Atrial flutter or atrial tachycardia sometimes slows temporarily. Paroxysmal atrial tachycardia can be broken by carotid sinus massage. Mild exercise may provoke arrhythmias that are absent at rest. Psychological stress (asking the patient to perform difficult mathematical problems rapidly) has also been used to unmask arrhythmias.

(3) ECG. A complete description of the ECG recognition of arrhythmias is beyond the scope of this manual. Several excellent texts have been written on this topic (see Selected Readings). Patients in whom arrhythmias are suspected should have a 12-lead ECG with a rhythm strip lasting at least 2 to 3 minutes. Infrequent arrhythmias can be recognized with the aid of a 24-hour ambulatory ECG recording or more sophisticated long-term ECG monitoring systems, such as portable event recorders or even subcutaneous implantable ECG recording devices.

(4) Exercise testing. Exercise testing can be of use in the diagnostic workup of arrhythmias. More than 50% of patients with coronary artery disease (CAD) will develop ventricular premature contractions (VPCs) with exercise; however, more than 30% of normal individuals will also develop VPCs with exercise. Ventricular ectopy, particularly multiform VPCs, and VT are more likely to occur with exercise in patients with CAD. Patients whose clinical history suggests exercise-induced arrhythmia should undergo exercise testing. Because considerable variability occurs in the frequency of VPCs between exercise tests, a decrease in exercise-induced VPCs after therapy is of uncertain significance. Failure to reproduce sustained VT after therapy may be of greater prognostic significance. Ambulatory 24-hour ECG monitoring is more sensitive in ascertaining ventricular ectopy than is exercise testing, although each technique misses some serious arrhythmias, and event recording devices may be required to identify very infrequent rhythm disturbances. Both ambulatory ECG recording and exercise testing may be required to identify infrequent arrhythmias in selected patients with ischemic heart disease.

(5) Long-term ECG monitoring. Ambulatory 24-hour ECG monitoring (Holter monitoring) may be helpful in quantitating arrhythmias and relating rhythm disturbances to symptoms. More than 50% of patients with ischemic heart disease will display VPCs when monitored for 24 hours. The following rhythm disturbances have been reported to carry a poor prognosis in patients with CAD: (i) frequent VPCs (greater than 10 per minute), (ii) frequent multiform VPCs, (iii) frequent ventricular couplets, (iv) R-on-T phenomenon, and (v) sustained or nonsustained VT. The exact significance of each of these phenomena is still debated, and in the absence of symptoms, most clinicians do not treat ventricular ectopy, except for VT. Because spontaneous variability of up to 90% in number of VPCs may occur between

two 24-hour ambulatory studies in the same patient, a decrease in VPC count after therapy is of uncertain significance.

Supraventricular tachycardias, bradyarrhythmias, and intermittent heart block may also be detected with this test. Various long-term ECG monitoring systems are now available, including transtelephonic, portable event recording devices, and subcutaneous implantable ECG recorders.

(6) Signal-averaged ECG. This technique summates and amplifies ECG information from the terminal phase of the QRS complex.

Persistent electrical activity following the end of the QRS complex reflects ongoing depolarizations in the myocardium during early diastole, so-called after-depolarizations. Patients with this persistent electrical activity in the myocardium during early diastole are at increased risk for developing malignant ventricular arrhythmias or sudden death. Individuals with a positive signal-averaged ECG reading and a low left ventricular ejection fraction (less than 40%) are at higher risk for developing malignant ventricular arrhythmias and should be considered for EPS.

(7) His bundle electrogram. This technique involves the use of a transvenous electrode catheter positioned in the right ventricle near the tricuspid valve. Characteristic atrial (A), His bundle (H), and ventricular (V) depolarizations are recorded and intervals timed. The technique is useful in determining the type and severity of AV block and in identifying ectopic foci within the His-Purkinje system.

(8) EPS. This invasive procedure is usually performed in the electrophysiology laboratory. Multipolar electrode catheters are introduced into either the venous or arterial circulation and advanced to various intracardiac positions to monitor electrical activity within the heart or to provoke arrhythmias. The procedure also has been used to identify patients who are high risk for sudden cardiac death.

Arrhythmias can also be terminated, at least temporarily, by various pacing modes employed during an EPS. In selected patients, specialized radiofrequency catheters can be used to destroy (ablate) small zones of myocardium that are involved in the genesis of specific arrhythmias.

Failure to elicit an arrhythmia during an EPS is not proof that the patient will not develop a rhythm disturbance at another time. In addition, false-positive EPSs do occur. EPS may be particularly helpful in the following settings: sinus node dysfunction, AV block (to determine the site and the severity of the block), intraventricular conduction disturbances, preexcitation syndromes (particularly Wolff-Parkinson-White syndrome to identify and eventual ablate bypass tracts), supraventricular tachycardia, VT, unexplained syncope or palpitations, and survivors of sudden cardiac death.

(9) Direct cardiac mapping. Mapping electrical activity directly from the surface of the heart is occasionally performed to map bypass tracts in the Wolff-Parkinson-White syndrome or reentrant circuits in patients with sustained VT. A prior EPS is essential, because anesthesia may alter cardiac electrical properties.

III. Approach to specific arrhythmias
   A. Rhythm disturbances arising in the sinus node and atrium
      1. Sinus tachycardia. Sinus tachycardia is defined as a normal sinus mechanism with a heart rate of more than 100 beats per minute. Sinus tachycardia must be distinguished from ectopic atrial rhythms (paroxysmal atrial tachycardia, atrial flutter). Sinus tachycardia typically does not

exceed 170 beats per minute. Sinus tachycardia is usually the result of noncardiac conditions such as infection, hypovolemia, anxiety, pain, gastrointestinal (GI) discomfort, or fecal impaction (Fig. 3.1). Such remediable causes should be actively sought. In the seriously ill patient, volume status may be accurately assessed by measuring left-heart filling pressures with a pulmonary arterial catheter (see Chapter 6). Correction of hypovolemia usually alleviates sinus tachycardia. Carotid sinus massage is likely to be helpful in distinguishing sinus tachycardia from ectopic atrial rhythms. If volume status is believed to be normal, serial doses of an intravenous (IV) beta-blocker—e.g., metoprolol, atenolol, propranolol, or esmolol—may be administered to slow the heart rate. Slowing the heart rate in this manner is important when rapid heart rate is deleterious (e.g., after myocardial infarction [MI]). The standard treatment of sinus tachycardia, however, is correction of the underlying abnormality (e.g., fever, hypovolemia) causing this rhythm disturbance.

2. Sinus bradycardia. Sinus bradycardia is defined as a normal sinus mechanism with a ventricular response of less than 60 beats per minute. Sinus bradycardia is often a normal finding in highly trained athletes. In elderly patients, it may represent sinus node disease. Sinus bradycardia may occur with myxedema or elevated intracranial pressure (Fig. 3.2).

The decision concerning therapy of sinus bradycardia is based on the presence or absence of symptoms or hemodynamic embarrassment. If signs of hypoperfusion are present (chest pain, heart failure, low blood pressure), the treatment of choice is IV atropine (0.6- to 1.0-mg boluses, up to a 2-mg total dose) until bradycardia is relieved. Low-dose IV dobutamine or aminophylline can also speed the sinus rate when indicated.

3. Sinus arrhythmia. Sinus arrhythmia involves cyclical acceleration and deceleration of the heart rate during inspiration and expiration. Sinus arrhythmia is present in many healthy young adults and is of no pathologic significance. No treatment is necessary.

4. Sinoatrial block. Sinoatrial block involves regular, normal depolarization of the sinus node with failure of the electrical impulse to reach the atria or ventricles. Causes of sinoatrial block include ischemia, electrolyte disturbances, antiarrhythmic drugs, digitalis, and fibrosis of the sinoatrial node. Treatment entails discontinuing potentially offending drugs and correcting any electrolyte disturbance.

5. AF. In AF, normal contraction of the atria is lost, and a rapid and irregular series of stimuli bombard the AV node. Many impulses stop at the AV node; those passing through it elicit a ventricular response that is generally rapid and irregularly irregular (random). AF may be either chronic or paroxysmal (Fig. 3.3).

Chronic AF almost always implies underlying cardiac disease. Common etiologies include congestive heart failure, mitral stenosis, ischemic heart disease, constrictive pericarditis, and chronic hypertension. Paroxysmal AF may arise in healthy individuals (so-called lone fibrillators), in pa-

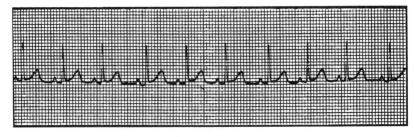

FIG. 3-1. Sinus tachycardia with a heart rate of 125 beats per minute.

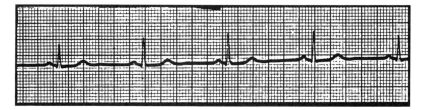

FIG. 3-2. Sinus bradycardia with a heart rate of 55 beats per minute.

tients with preexcitation syndromes, and in the setting of an acute illness such as infection or acute MI.

Treatment of AF depends on the rate of the ventricular response and the hemodynamic consequences of the arrhythmia. For ventricular responses of more than 140 beats per minute with hemodynamic compromise, cardioversion is the treatment of choice (for details, see Section **V.A.**).

Digitalis glycosides should be withheld if cardioversion is contemplated. For ventricular rates between 90 and 140, IV diltiazem, a beta-blocker, or digoxin may be given until the ventricular response is slowed to 70 to 80 beats per minute.

The clinician faces two potential therapeutic strategies when faced with a patient who has AF. The first strategy emphasizes drug therapy to keep the patient in sinus rhythm. This is accomplished by means of anti-arrhythmic drug therapy. Agents commonly used include beta-blockers, sotalol, amiodarone, propafenone, disopyramide, and flecainide. This strategy is called "maintenance of sinus rhythm." Patients usually receive concomitant anticoagulant therapy with warfarin to prevent the formation of clots that might embolize from the fibrillating left atrium. Patients who cannot tolerate warfarin are given daily aspirin, which is only half as effective as warfarin in preventing arterial embolism in patients with AF. If the patient remains in stable sinus rhythm for 6 months, some clinicians discontinue anticoagulant therapy.

The second therapeutic strategy for these patients is to allow AF to persist and to control the heart rate with combinations of agents such as beta-blockers, verapamil, diltiazem, and digoxin. This strategy is known as "rate control" and should be accompanied by life-long anticoagulation with warfarin to prevent arterial embolism. Once a patient has been in AF for a long period of time (e.g., more than 6 to 12 months), it is unlikely

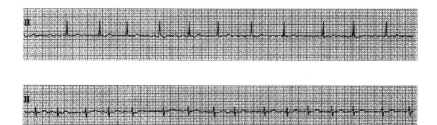

FIG. 3-3. Two examples of atrial fibrillation. Note the irregular random nature of the heart rate.

that sinus rhythm can be restored, even with aggressive antiarrhythmic therapy.

At the present time, it appears that both strategies are of equal benefit. The strategy selected depends on a variety of factors, including the patient's clinical status and the presence of comorbid conditions. Here are two examples of patients with AF who required different therapeutic strategies: The first patient is 85 years old and has had multiple admissions for colonic bleeding with no identified source. The patient is very sedentary and quite weak, having suffered two MIs in the past. He has severe chronic obstructive pulmonary disease. He is on many medicines and has many drug intolerances. This patient is not a good candidate for antiarrhythmic or anticoagulant therapy because of his general medical condition, his drug intolerances, his sedentary lifestyle, and his recurrent episodes of GI bleeding. He should have rate control therapy with digoxin combined with a small dose of beta-blocker or diltiazem. He should also receive daily aspirin if tolerated. If aspirin precipitates GI bleeding, then no anticoagulant therapy is indicated.

The second patient is 64 years old and has recently retired. He is very active and plays golf and tennis almost everyday in the retirement community where he lives. He manages a large stock portfolio with his computer on a daily basis. He has mild angina, but this has been well controlled with medication and an angioplasty 2 years earlier. Maintenance of sinus rhythm should be attempted for this patient by using one of the pharmacological agents described above. Probably, one should try beta-blockers first, and if these fail, then one might consider sotalol, propafenone, and amiodarone, in that order. The patient should be anticoagulated with warfarin. Please note that amiodarone can result in marked increases in warfarin effect when the two drugs are administered simultaneously. Careful monitoring of the International Normalized Ratio (INR) is essential when these two drugs are combined.

6. Atrial flutter. Atrial flutter results from rapid atrial contractions at a rate of 280 to 350 beats per minute (usually 300 per minute), with variable AV block (2:1, 3:1, or 4:1) causing a ventricular response of 75 to 150 beats per minute. The diagnosis is made by observing the regular sawtooth pattern of atrial contractions on the ECG (usually leads II and V1) (Fig. 3.4).

Exercise may increase the ventricular response suddenly and stepwise. Carotid sinus massage often diminishes the ventricular rate temporarily and in step fashion. Atrial flutter rarely occurs in the absence of organic heart disease. Underlying etiologies include heart failure, ischemic heart disease, mitral stenosis, and atrial septal defect. Atrial flutter can complicate thyrotoxicosis or chronic obstructive pulmonary disease. Treatment of atrial flutter is either pharmacologic or electrical; electrical cardioversion is the preferred therapy. Digitalis is rarely effective with a protocol similar to that already indicated for AF (0.25-mg IV doses repeated q3–4h). Diltiazem and beta-blockers are more often used to slow the ventricular response. Digoxin generally converts atrial flutter to fibrillation, which, in turn, frequently spontaneously reverts to

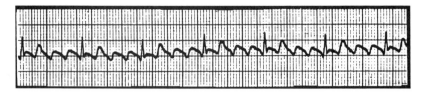

FIG. 3-4. Atrial flutter with a flutter rate of 300 beats per minute and a ventricular rate of 75 beats per minute (4:1 atrioventricular block).

sinus rhythm. If spontaneous reversion to sinus rhythm does not occur, antiarrhythmic drug therapy may be administered, for example, oral propafenone, sotalol, or other agent. Acute episodes of atrial flutter may convert to sinus rhythm after therapy with IV or oral beta-blockers or IV procainamide (1 gm IV over 40 to 60 minutes, followed by 2 to 4 mg per minute IV infusion). Electrical cardioversion is usually successful in converting atrial flutter to sinus rhythm. Low levels of electrical energy are needed (generally 25 to 50 J). Rapid atrial pacing may also convert atrial flutter to sinus rhythm. Verapamil, administered as an initial IV bolus of 5 to 10 mg followed by a constant infusion of 5 g/kg per minute may effectively slow the ventricular response and may result in reversion to sinus rhythm if the atrial flutter is of recent onset. Intravenous diltiazem can have the same beneficial effect.

An occasional patient remains in atrial flutter, with the heart rate controlled by the same agents used to control rate in AF. Chronic atrial flutter patients should be anticoagulated with warfarin to prevent arterial embolism. The risk for arterial embolism, however, is less with atrial flutter than with AF.

7. Paroxysmal supraventricular tachycardia (PSVT). Evidence from His bundle studies has shown that PSVT arises from sustained reentry mechanisms involving the sinus node, atrium, and/or AV node (Fig. 3.5).

The vast majority of patients with PSVT will have a reentrant circuit that involves the AV node. The term *reciprocating tachycardia* has been suggested as an alternative to PSVT. PSVTs usually develop suddenly. Patients frequently experience the symptom of rapid, regular, forceful heartbeat and become anxious. Supraventricular tachycardias with aberrant conduction may be difficult to distinguish from VT. Heart rate greater than 170, AV dissociation, and QRS longer than 0.14 second all favor VT. Patients often develop their own methods for terminating these arrhythmias, including carotid sinus pressure, gagging, placing their face in cold water, or performing the Valsalva maneuver. The physician should institute one or more of these modalities, particularly if such maneuvers have previously succeeded in terminating the arrhythmia. A typical treatment sequence for PSVT begins with reassurance. The patient should lie down. Carotid sinus massage or another vagal maneuver, for example, performing a Valsalva maneuver, is tried next. Placing the patient's face in cold water also may terminate this arrhythmia by activating the so-called diving reflex. Verapamil, administered as a IV bolus of 5 to 10 mg (or IV diltiazem), will successfully terminate more than 90% of PSVTs that involve AV nodal reentry within 2 minutes. Intravenous adenosine induces transient AV block and is also highly effective in interrupting PSVT. Adenosine is administered as a 6-mg IV bolus and is repeated if initially unsuccessful. If all of the above-mentioned maneuvers fail and the patient appears hemodynamically compromised, direct current cardioversion should be performed. Electrical energies between 10 and 50 J are generally success-

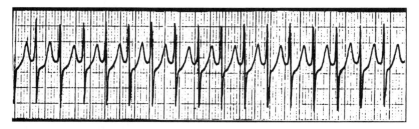

FIG. 3-5. Supraventricular tachycardia at a heart rate of 240 beats per minute.

ful, although higher energy levels occasionally may be required. An alternative pharmacologic approach involves the use of IV beta-blockers such as metoprolol, atenolol, or propranolol. Rapid atrial pacing has also been successfully used to treat this rhythm and is particularly useful if digitalis toxicity is suspected.

8. Atrial tachycardia with block. Atrial tachycardia with block has elements that make it resemble both PSVT and atrial flutter. The atrial rate is generally between 130 and 250 beats per minute; 2:1 AV block is common. The exact mechanism of this arrhythmia is not known. By far, the most common etiology is digitalis intoxication. Carotid sinus massage may aid in making the diagnosis (same response as with PSVT) and, in some instances, may terminate the arrhythmia. Digitalis-induced atrial tachycardia generally responds to potassium administration. Digitalis administration should be discontinued. Phenytoin, 250 mg IV over 5 minutes, may also be effective. If the patient is hemodynamically compromised and digitalis intoxication is suspected because of a high serum digoxin level, Fab fragments that specifically bind to digoxin (Digibind) should be administered.

9. Multifocal atrial tachycardia. Multifocal atrial tachycardia is an irregular atrial tachycardia (heart rate greater than 100 beats per minute) distinguished by ECG evidence of at least three morphologically different P waves with three different P–R intervals. Atrial premature beats and AV block may also be present. The rhythm generally reflects advanced cardiac or pulmonary disease. Treatment should be directed to the underlying disease and correction of any associated hypoxia or electrolyte disturbance.

10. Sick sinus syndrome (brady-tachy syndrome). The sick sinus syndrome is characterized by episodes of both bradycardia and supraventricular tachycardia. It reflects sinoatrial node dysfunction. Underlying etiologies include rheumatic heart disease, atherosclerosis, and degeneration/fibrosis of the sinus node in elderly patients. Patients may experience syncope (during bradycardiac episodes) or angina (during tachycardia). The treatment of choice is permanent pacing to control the bradycardia and beta-blockade or other antiarrhythmic agent, for example, propafenone, sotalol, or amiodarone to control the tachycardia.

11. Ectopic atrial contractions. Arising from an abnormal focus in the atrium, ectopic atrial beats usually occur prematurely. They may be conducted aberrantly and may be difficult to distinguish from VPCs. Definitive diagnosis requires demonstration of P waves on the ECG. Premature ectopic beats with the same QRS morphology as the associated sinus mechanism, however, are likely the result of an atrial premature beat. His bundle recordings may be helpful in difficult diagnostic situations. Common underlying etiologies for ectopic atrial contractions include congestive heart failure; electrolyte disturbances; drugs such as aminophylline, albuterol, and caffeine; and hypoxia. Ectopic atrial contractions have little clinical significance in their own right but often presage more sustained atrial arrhythmias.

B. Rhythm disturbances arising at the AV node or ventricle

1. AV junctional rhythm. The AV junctional rhythm is an escape rhythm. It arises in the bundle of His if impulses from the sinus node fail to arrive in time to prevent the AV junctional pacemaker from firing. The ventricular rate is 40 to 60 beats per minute and regular. QRS complexes on ECG are indistinguishable from those with the normal sinus mechanism (Fig. 3.6).

In some instances, this rhythm is a manifestation of digitalis toxicity. The rhythm is usually regarded as a protective safety device and does not require treatment unless the rate is too slow to provide effective circulation (usually below 50 beats per minute). For slow ventricular rates, atropine or a temporary pacemaker may be considered.

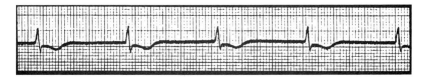

FIG. 3-6. Junctional rhythm at a heart rate of 52 beats per minute.

2. AV junctional tachycardia. Junctional tachycardia usually involves a ventricular response of 100 to 140 beats per minute (Fig. 3.7). With this rhythm disturbance, the inherent automaticity of the AV junction exceeds that of the sinus node. Underlying etiologies include digitalis toxicity, acute rheumatic fever, and MI.

   Treatment includes administration of potassium and withholding of digitalis preparations. Carotid sinus massage may also be effective. Antiarrhythmic therapy with lidocaine, beta-blockers or phenytoin may be required if the initial maneuvers are not successful or if the clinical situation is precarious. If it is certain that the underlying etiology is not digitalis toxicity, cardioversion with low-watt energy may be attempted.

3. Junctional ectopic beats. His bundle studies have shown that not all cells in the AV junction are capable of automatic electrical activity. Ectopic beats may arise in the low atrium, His bundle, or several areas of the AV node. The ECG morphology of the junctional ectopic beats depends on where the ectopic focus lies (Fig. 3.8). Underlying causes include digitalis toxicity, congestive heart failure, hypokalemia, and hypoxia. Treatment involves correction of these abnormalities.

4. VPCs. VPCs may arise from one or more ectopic foci located in the ventricle, and they can occur in healthy individuals (Fig. 3.9). Their frequency increases with age. They may arise as an escape phenomenon in bradycardias or from an accelerated focus in the ventricle.

   Underlying conditions that may provoke VPCs include ischemia, hypoxia, MI, congestive heart failure, abnormal ventricular repolarization (prolonged Q–T syndrome), mitral valve prolapse, cerebrovascular accident, antiarrhythmic drugs, digitalis toxicity, and hypokalemia. VPCs sometimes occur in a regular coupling sequence with normal beats (bigeminy, trigeminy). Treatment of VPCs should focus on treatment of underlying disorders and suppression of patterns of ectopic activity that are likely to degenerate into more dangerous rhythms such as VT. Generally accepted criteria for treatment of VPCs in the setting of acute ischemia are as follows:

   Runs of VPCs (nonsustained VT)

   Frequent VPCs with the R wave of the VPC falling on the T wave of the preceding beat (R-on-T phenomenon)

   Frequent multifocal VPCs

   The rationale for treating these patterns involves prevention of VF. It is important to understand, however, that in acute ischemia, VF occurs

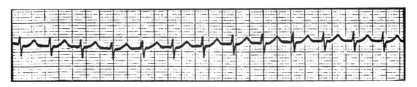

FIG. 3-7. Junctional tachycardia at a heart rate of 140 beats per minute.

PJC

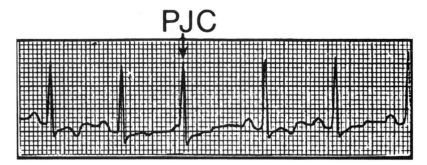

FIG. 3-8. A premature junctional contraction—labeled PJC. Note the absence of a P wave in front of the QRS complex.

in the absence of warning arrhythmias in more than 50% of cases. Moreover, lidocaine therapy in this setting has not been shown to reduce infarct-associated mortality. Intravenous lidocaine can precipitate grand mal seizures.

Various treatments are available. In normal individuals, withholding cigarettes or coffee may suppress ectopic activity. Sedation may play a role in anxious individuals. Pharmacologic agents include beta-blockers, disopyramide, lidocaine, amiodarone, sotalol, propafenone, procainamide, phenytoin, mexiletine, tocainide, and moricizine. Clinical information for each of these medications is presented in Section **IV.B**.

5. VT. VT is defined as three or more sequential extrasystoles at a rate ranging from 120 to 250 beats per minute. It is a dangerous arrhythmia

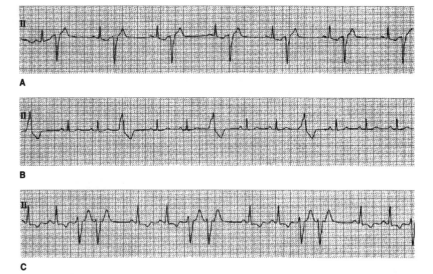

FIG. 3-9. Three examples of premature ventricular contractions (PVC). The top strip demonstrates a bigeminal rhythm, with every other beat a PVC. The middle strip demonstrates a trigeminal rhythm, with every third beat a PVC. The bottom strip demonstrates PVC couplets.

because of its propensity to degenerate into VF (see Chapter 8). A variety of forms of VT may occur. The QRS complexes may be uniform or random (multiform, pleomorphic) or may vary in alternate complexes (bidirectional VT) or in a repetitive manner (torsades de pointes). When VT lasts longer than 30 seconds or causes hemodynamic collapse requiring its termination, it is termed sustained. Nonsustained VT (NSVT) lasts less than 30 seconds and stops spontaneously. Common underlying causes include ischemia, acute MI (the rhythm occurs in 16% to 40% of patients after MI), congestive heart failure, antiarrhythmic drugs, and digoxin. VT occasionally occurs in presumably healthy individuals without evidence of underlying cardiac disease. VT is often difficult to distinguish from supraventricular tachycardias with aberrant conduction. The presence of dissociated P waves is strong evidence for VT; however, the presence of a P wave associated with each ventricular complex does not provide definitive evidence of supraventricular tachycardia with aberrant conduction, because each of these P waves may represent retrograde conduction from the previous ventricular depolarization during VT. Occasionally, His bundle recordings will be needed for definitive diagnosis. If the His bundle depolarization is dissociated from ventricular depolarization, the arrhythmia is VT. More often, however, the His bundle tracing is obscured in the QRS deflection. Bidirectional VT is a rare but very dangerous form of this arrhythmia characterized by alternating electrocardiographic complexes with left and right axis deviation (Figs. 3.10 and 3.11). Treatment of VT depends on the gravity of the clinical setting. VT occurring after MI should be terminated immediately with electrical countershock, followed by administration of antiarrhythmic therapy (generally IV lidocaine). If the patient is awake and appears to be tolerating the arrhythmia, a brief trial of IV lidocaine may be used as a first approach (100 mg lidocaine IV followed by an additional 50 mg in 2 minutes). If the arrhythmia persists, countershock is required. Once VT has been abolished, a loading dose of 100 mg IV lidocaine should be given (if not already administered before cardioversion) and an IV drip (2 to 3 mg per minute) started. This infusion should be continued for 24 hours. If not contraindicated or already administered, IV beta-blockade should be initiated. In the nonacute setting, the major decision involves which patients with VT require treatment. Patients with sustained VT should be treated whether or not structural heart disease is present. Even nonsustained VT should be treated if ischemic heart disease is present. Patients with nonsustained VT and no ischemic heart disease may be treated with close observation.

   a. Internal cardioverter/defibrillators (ICDs). The approach to the long-term management of VT has been altered by data from randomized controlled trials of patients with CAD, cardiac arrest, and sustained and nonsustained VT. At this time, there have been four major trials

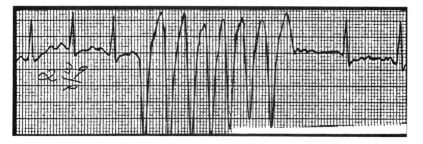

FIG. 3-10. A seven-beat run of nonsustained ventricular tachycardia.

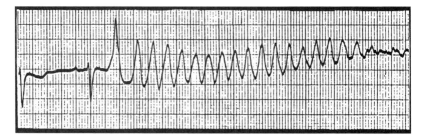

FIG. 3-11. A premature ventricular contraction occurs during the middle of the T wave (so-called R-on-T phenomenon) precipitating an episode of sustained, rapid ventricular tachycardia that degenerates into ventricular fibrillation.

using implantable ICDs. These trials are CIDS (Canadian Implantable Defibrillator Study), the AVID (Antiarrhythmics Versus Implantable Defibrillators) trial, MADIT (Multicenter Automatic Defibrillator Implantation Trial), and the CASH (Cardiac Arrest Study Hamburg) trial. The multicenter CIDS used over 600 patients with documented or likely cardiac arrest or VT. These patients were randomized to either ICD or amiodarone therapy. CIDS demonstrated a small nonsignificant mortality advantage for the ICD patients, but the cost benefit analysis revealed a very high cost per year of life saved by the ICDs. The authors concluded that ICD implantation was *not* a cost-effective therapy in these patients. In the MADIT and AVID trials, however, the opposite conclusion was made: ICD implantation resulted in statistically significant reductions in mortality during follow-up, and ICD therapy was cost-effective.

A number of points should be made about these studies. First, the patient populations in the various trials have all been different. For example, the CIDS patients had resuscitated VF or VT or unmonitored syncope, whereas the CASH patients had all been resuscitated from cardiac arrest secondary to sustained malignant ventricular arrhythmias. Patients in the MADIT trial were post-MI with a left ventricular ejection fraction of less than 35% and a positive cardiac EPS. Each subgroup of arrhythmia patients has a different long-term prognosis; therefore, the results of each trial relates to the relative risk for sudden death of the particular patients studied in that trial. One should clearly be cautious in drawing universal conclusions from the results of any one trial. Indeed, a cost analysis of the MADIT trial concluded that ICD implantation was cost-effective—approximately $28,000 per life-year gained compared with approximately $150,000 per life-year gained in the CIDS trial, which concluded that ICD implantation was not cost effective. Second, 17% of the amiodarone patients in the CIDS trial crossed over and received an ICD during the more than 6-year follow-up period. This crossover could have confounded that study to some degree. Finally, the quality of life analysis from the CIDS trial demonstrated that patients assigned to the ICD group had better functioning on five of the seven domains of life quality that were monitored during the trial.

In conclusion, at the present time, the clinician should carefully consider the long-term prognosis of any patient identified with sustained or nonsustained VT. One should examine the state of left ventricular function and comorbid conditions before considering ICD implantation. There are clearly many patients with VT in whom ICD implantation is potentially life saving and cost-effective.

  b. EPS. Many cardiac electrophysiologists feel that patients with VT should undergo an EPS to risk stratify these patients. Although some trials have demonstrated the usefulness of EPS in identifying patients who are high risk for sudden death, other trials have demonstrated the opposite, namely, EPS is not predictive of sudden death/cardiac arrest. In this confusing arena, it is important for the clinician to treat each patient individually with a careful clinical risk assessment before therapy is selected. Such an assessment should include an examination of such factors as age, comorbid conditions, left ventricular function, the presence of clinical heart failure, the underlying cardiac disease, and the patient's psychological status.

  c. Drug therapy. If antiarrhythmic drug therapy is selected for a patient with VT, the most effective drug would appear to be amiodarone. At times, amiodarone is combined with other drugs, for example, beta-blockers. Combination therapy with several drugs may succeed if a single agent is unsuccessful. Occasionally, surgical intervention involving ventriculotomy, aneurysmectomy, and coronary artery bypass is combined with implantation of an ICD. After such procedures, patients are frequently still maintained on antiarrhythmic agents.

6. Accelerated idioventricular rhythm (AIVR). AIVR is characterized by three or more bizarre, widened QRS complexes that occur at a rate similar to the sinus rate. The rate is almost always less than 100 beats per minute. AIVR may be caused by digitalis toxicity. It is common after MI (13% to 30% of patients with MI have this rhythm at some point), particularly inferior MI. (Fig. 3.12).

  AIVR usually does not require treatment. If it is accompanied by evidence of hypoperfusion, atropine, 0.8 to 1.0 mg IV, should be administered in an attempt to accelerate the sinus rate. If this treatment fails, temporary pacing with a transvenous pacemaker should be considered.

7. Torsades de pointes. This term refers to a characteristic morphologic pattern of VT occurring at rates between 200 and 250 beats per minute in which the complexes seem to rotate about a point. The pattern was described originally as part of a syndrome that also involves a prolonged Q–T interval. It often occurs after administration of a variety of antiarrhythmic drugs such as procainamide, sotalol, or propafenone. An attack of torsades de pointes may be self-terminating or followed by a brief period of ventricular standstill. Syncope may occur if the attack is prolonged, although VF is rare (Fig. 3.13).

  Antiarrhythmic drugs are contraindicated in treating this disturbance and will often exacerbate the problem. The treatment of choice is withdrawal of antiarrhythmic medication and temporary atrial or ventricular pacing at rates of approximately 110 beats per minute, which will typically abolish the rhythm disorder. Some authorities administer IV magnesium sulfate (2 to 6 g IV over several minutes) to assist in abolishing

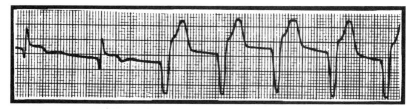

FIG. 3-12. Two junctional beats (note the absence of P waves) initiate this rhythm strip and are followed by an episode of accelerated idioventricular rhythm at a heart rate of 80 beats per minute.

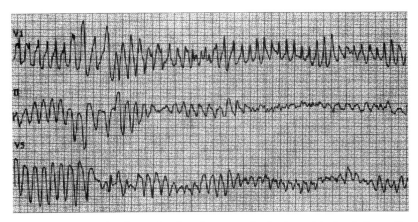

FIG. 3-13. An episode of torsades de pointes or polyphasic ventricular tachycardia. Note the changing QRS axis.

this rhythm disturbance. Whether this is of therapeutic benefit is not definitively known, but it is unlikely that it does any harm.

8. AV dissociation. In AV dissociation, the atria and ventricles are controlled by two separate and independent pacemakers, with the pacemaker in the AV node or ventricles firing faster than the supraventricular pacemaker. This arrhythmia may accompany various degrees of AV block and VT. Treatment may not be required if the patient tolerates the rhythm. Correction of underlying disease or coexisting rhythm disturbance will often terminate AV dissociation.

9. VF. No effective ventricular contractions occur during VF. Its appearance is a medical emergency demanding immediate therapy. VF complicates high-grade AV block, unstable ischemic heart disease, and/or MI. Rarely, it is seen in patients with mitral valve prolapse, digitalis or antiarrhythmic drug toxicity, hypothermia, phenothiazine toxicity, and the long Q–T syndrome. Therapy is urgent electrical countershock, although even this modality may not succeed. Time should not be wasted applying ECG leads or attempting to intubate the pulseless patient. Even a delay of 2 minutes may make VF more difficult to convert to sinus rhythm. So-called blind countershock is justified in pulseless adult patients. For any patient weighing more than 50 kg, 400 J is the recommended countershock setting; in smaller patients, 5 J/kg should be used. Once effective rhythm has been reestablished, a 100-mg IV bolus of lidocaine should be administered, followed by a drip of 2 mg per minute for the next 24 hours (for more details on the treatment of cardiac arrest, see Chapter 8).

C. Conduction disturbances. In addition to the rhythm disturbances already discussed, a variety of abnormalities of conduction can occur. His bundle recording has been used extensively in the analysis of cardiac conduction. In the normal conduction system, three deflections are recorded: the atrial wave (A wave), which represents atrial depolarization near the catheter; the ventricular wave (V wave), formed by depolarization of ventricular tissue near the catheter; and the H deflection, which is formed by rapid passage of the electrical signal through the bundle of His. Two intervals are of clinical importance: (i) the A–H interval represents the conduction time from the lower right atrium to the bundle of His; and (ii) the H–V interval is the time from the beginning of depolarization of the bundle of His to depolarization of the ventricular myocardium. Prolongation of the A–H interval generally indicates abnormalities in conduction through the AV node. Prolongation of the H–V interval suggests an infranodal block. Prolongation of the AH interval is considered to be a more benign rhythm disturbance compared with prolongation of the HV interval.

1. AV block. AV block has traditionally been divided into three categories based on ECG criteria. First-degree AV block is identified by prolongation of the P–R interval. Second-degree AV block is characterized by intermittent failure of the supraventricular impulse to reach the ventricle, with resultant dropped ventricular beats. In third-degree AV block, no AV conduction occurs and the ventricles are driven by a nodal or ventricular pacemaker. Atrial electrical activity represented by the P wave of the ECG has no relationship to ventricular depolarization represented by the QRS on the ECG recording.

   a. First-degree AV block. First-degree AV block generally indicates conduction impairment at the AV junction proximal to the His bundle (Fig. 3.14). Possible underlying etiologies for this block include drug toxicity (verapamil, diltiazem, beta-blockers, digoxin, antiarrhythmic agents); inflammatory, degenerative, or toxic processes; and a variant of normal. In the absence of other accompanying heart disease, no treatment is necessary.

   b. Second-degree AV block. Two forms exist: Mobitz type I and Mobitz type II. In Mobitz type I block (also known as Wenckebach block) the P–R interval progressively increases until an atrial impulse is blocked and a ventricular beat is dropped. His bundle recordings usually show that impaired conduction occurs proximal to the bundle of His in this type of block (prolonged AH interval). The number of atrial beats between dropped ventricular beats may vary considerably. Mobitz type I block with 2:1 conduction is sometimes difficult to distinguish from 2:1 Mobitz type II block, which carries a more ominous prognosis. Underlying etiologies for Mobitz type I block include drug toxicity (verapamil, diltiazem, beta-blockers, digoxin, and antiarrhythmic agents), ischemic heart disease, and increased vagal tone (for example in a highly trained athlete). Mobitz type I AV block is often a transient phenomenon that generally needs no treatment unless hemodynamic compromise ensues. In the latter situation, IV atropine or pacemaker therapy may be required.

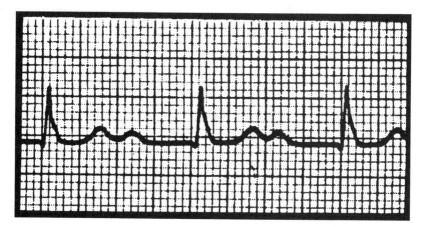

FIG. 3-14. First-degree atrioventricular block with a heart rate of 75 beats per minute and a P–R interval of 0.36 seconds.

Mobitz type II block is recognized by a fixed P–R interval, with repetitively dropped beats. Beats may be dropped irregularly or in a regular pattern, ordinarily 2:1, 3:1, or 4:1. His bundle recordings indicate that this type of block is the result of a conduction disturbance in or below the bundle of His (prolonged HV interval). The most common etiologies for Mobitz type II AV block are anterior MI, myocarditis, fibrocalcific degeneration of the myocardium that involves the conduction system (Lev's disease), and idiopathic sclerosis of the myocardium also involving the conduction system (Lenegre's disease). Mobitz type II block may be transient, or it may progress suddenly to complete heart block. It is often seen in patients with Stokes-Adams attacks (syncopal episodes caused by inadequate cerebral perfusion). Patients with chronic Mobitz type II block usually require treatment with a permanent-demand pacemaker. (Figs. 3.15 and 3.16).

   c. Third-degree AV block (complete heart block). The conduction defect known as third-degree AV block is characterized by atrial depolarizations that are never transmitted to the ventricle. The ventricles are depolarized by an independent pacemaker, generally nodal or infranodal. The ventricular rate is usually 30 to 50 beats per minute. Underlying etiologies for chronic third-degree AV block include acute anterior wall MI, degeneration of the myocardium and conduction system (Lev's disease, Lenegre's disease; see Section **III.C.1.b**, drug toxicity [verapamil, diltiazem, beta-blockers, digoxin, antiarrhythmic agents]), congenital anomalies, and occasionally surgical trauma. Third-degree AV block may be a transient complication of inferior/posterior MI, in which setting, disease of the right coronary artery reduces blood flow to the AV node. This situation is almost always temporary. The prognosis is more grave if complete heart block accompanies anterior MI. This complication suggests a large infarction with ischemic damage to both the right and left bundles with resultant high mortality. In the setting of acute MI, Mobitz type II block or new bifascicular block warrants the insertion of a temporary transvenous pacemaker (see Chapter 15). This dreaded complication of anterior MI has become much less common in the era of early reperfusion therapy.

2. Bundle branch block. Bundle branch blocks reflect conduction disturbances in specific portions of the right or left bundle branch, the anterior or posterior division of the left bundle, or both. The diagnosis is made by ECG criteria of QRS prolongation and axis shift (see Selected Readings). Chronic bundle branch blocks are caused by the same diseases and toxicities that are responsible for third-degree AV block. Acute bundle branch block may occur in the setting of MI or ischemia. Patients with chronic bundle branch block or bifascicular block are treated if third-degree AV block is documented or strongly suspected. Treatment

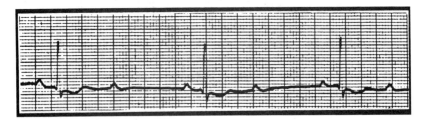

FIG. 3-15. Second-degree atrioventricular block with 2:1 atrial to ventricular conduction. Note two P waves to each QRS complex.

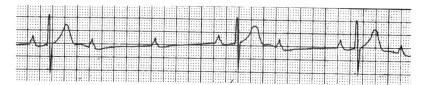

FIG. 3-16. High-grade atrioventricular (AV) block but not yet third-degree (complete) heart block. Note the fixed regular P–R interval (0.30 seconds) before each QRS complex. There is one cycle with 3:1 AV block and one cycle with 2:1 AV block.

consists of implantation of a permanent pacemaker. In some individuals, right or left bundle branch block are not associated with underlying structural heart disease. This is more commonly the case with right bundle branch block (Figs. 3.17 and 3.18).

3. Preexcitation syndromes. Preexcitation syndromes are characterized by premature depolarization of a portion of ventricular muscle. A small bypass tract enables the wave of electrical depolarization to reach the ventricular muscle without going through the AV node. Preexcitation syndromes are usually recognized from specific ECG changes in the QRS complex that result from premature ventricular depolarization. Occasionally, preexcitation is suspected because of recurrent supraventricular arrhythmias. In Wolff-Parkinson-White syndrome, ECG criteria include normal P waves, P–R interval of 0.11 second or less, initial slurring of the QRS (delta wave), and prolongation of the QRS (Fig. 3.19). Lown-Ganong-Levine syndrome is characterized by a shortened P–R interval only. His bundle and anatomic studies have shown that these syndromes reflect the presence of anomalous conduction pathways that bypass the AV node.

The occurrence of various supraventricular tachyarrhythmias in these disorders reflects anomalous reentrant electrical conduction that involves the bypass tract and the AV node. Preexcitation syndromes generally occur as isolated entities but have also been reported in conjunction with congenital anomalies, hyperthyroidism, hypertrophic cardiomyopathy,

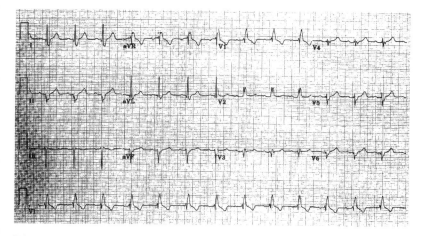

FIG. 3-17. Right bundle branch block and normal sinus rhythm with a heart rate of 80 beats per minute.

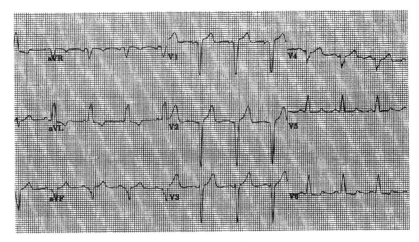

FIG. 3-18. Left bundle branch block and normal sinus rhythm with a heart rate of 80 beats per minute.

and mitral valve prolapse. Patients may be either asymptomatic or troubled by palpitations and syncopal episodes. Sudden death occurs on occasion. Pharmacologic treatment involves beta-blockers and other antiarrhythmic agents. Electrophysiologic ablation of the bypass tract is usually performed and permanently cures this condition in the overwhelming majority of patients.

IV. Pharmacologic treatment of arrhythmias
  A. General comments. The rational choice of an antiarrhythmic agent is based on three considerations: (i) correct clinical diagnosis of the arrhythmia, (ii) an understanding of the electrophysiology of the rhythm disturbance, and (iii) an understanding of the mechanism of action and side effects of antiarrhythmic

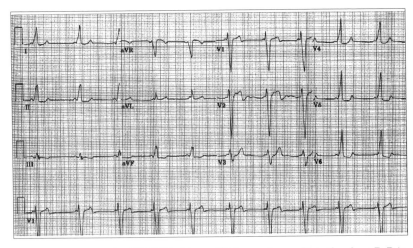

FIG. 3-19. An example of Wolff-Parkinson-White syndrome. Note the short P–R interval and slurred upstroke of the QRS (the delta wave) in leads I, II, V$_4$, V$_5$, and V$_6$.

agents. Antiarrhythmic drugs are divided up into different classes based on their membrane actions. The classification system most widely used is the Vaughn-Williams classification. In this system, there are four categories of drugs: type I (a, b, and c subclasses; traditional antiarrhythmics), type II (beta-blockers), type III (newer antiarrhythmics), and type IV (calcium blockers such as verapamil and diltiazem).

B. Commonly used antiarrhythmic agents
  1. Type Ia agents: sodium channel blockers
    a. Procainamide (Pronestyl)
      (1) Electrophysiologic properties. Procainamide raises the threshold of ventricular muscle to electrical stimulation. It increases the effective refractory period and decreases conduction velocity and automaticity. The major metabolite of procainamide is N-acetylprocainamide (NAPA), which has different electrophysiologic properties compared with those of the parent compound. NAPA does not prolong the effective refractory period but does prolong the action potential of ventricular muscle and Purkinje fibers.
      (2) Absorption, excretion, and plasma levels. GI absorption of oral procainamide is approximately 95%. Peak plasma levels are achieved between 15 minutes and 2 hours after ingestion. Its half-life is approximately 3.5 hours. Therapeutic plasma levels are 4 to 8 mcg/ml. Excretion is 100% renal (60% excreted unchanged, 40% metabolized to NAPA and then excreted by kidneys).
      (3) Clinical uses and dosages. Procainamide can be effective in treatment of both ventricular and supraventricular arrhythmias. Because of its short half-life and many untoward effects (drug-induced lupus erythematosus, rashes, nausea, agranulocytosis), procainamide is infrequently used orally. Procainamide can be given intramuscularly or intravenously to achieve serum concentrations of 4 to 10 g/ml. It is used intravenously to terminate and prevent further episodes of VT and AF. Blood pressure and ECG must be monitored continuously during IV administration. Intravenous dosage is 20 to 50 mg per minute to a total dose of 1 g, followed by a constant infusion of 2 to 4 mg per minute.
      (4) Toxicity. Procainamide can cause GI upset (nausea, vomiting, anorexia), immunologic disturbances (positive antinuclear antibody titer and lupus erythematosus cell preparation develop in 50% to 70% of patients on the drug), rash, drug fever, and agranulocytosis (rare). Procainamide has direct myocardial depressant action; it is also a vasodilator. It is contraindicated in patients with second- or third-degree block and should be used with caution in patients with intraventricular conduction defect. Hypotension may occur with IV administration. Torsades de pointes can develop in patients receiving procainamide.
    b. Quinidine
      (1) Electrophysiologic properties. The electrophysiologic properties of quinidine are similar to those of procainamide. Its major effect is to depress the rate of spontaneous depolarization. It increases the effective refractory period and decreases conduction velocity and automaticity.
      (2) Absorption, excretion, and plasma levels. The GI absorption of oral quinidine is greater than 95%; 60% of the drug is bound to serum albumin. Peak concentrations occur 1 to 3 hours after dosage. Therapeutic plasma levels are 2 to 7 mcg/ml. Biologic half-life is 5 to 7 hours. The drug is metabolized in the liver and excreted in the urine.

(3) Clinical uses and dosages. Quinidine can be used to suppress both ventricular and supraventricular arrhythmias. The drug increases both the atrial and the VF threshold.

Two preparations of quinidine are available: quinidine sulfate and quinidine gluconate (Quinaglute). Quinaglute is said to allow doses to be given less frequently by sustaining adequate blood levels longer. Recommended oral doses are quinidine sulfate 300 to 600 mg q6h or quinidine gluconate 660 mg q6–8h. Using maintenance dosages, steady state is achieved in 24 to 36 hours. Quinidine may be given intravenously. This route is hazardous and must be closely monitored. Severe hypotension secondary to vasodilatation is the most frequent and dangerous adverse reaction. Because of its adverse effects, including torsades de pointes, quinidine is rarely used today.

(4) Toxic effects and contraindications. Quinidine should not be administered to patients with second- or third-degree AV block. Intraventricular block is a relative contraindication. Quinidine should be avoided in individuals with prolonged Q–T interval. Torsades de pointes can develop in patients taking quinidine, leading to syncope or even cardiac arrest. GI side effects (nausea, vomiting, diarrhea) are common. When mild, they may be symptomatically controlled if quinidine is essential. Symptoms of cinchonism may occur (tinnitus, vertigo, visual disturbances). Allergic responses (rash, thrombocytopenia, hemolytic anemia) are less common. Idiosyncratic central nervous system reactions (respiratory arrest, convulsions) have been reported but are rare. Quinidine also has direct myocardial toxicity. Depressed myocardial contractility and peripheral vasodilatation can occur. Specific signs of myocardial toxicity include a greater than 50% widening of the QRS, AV block, and ventricular arrhythmias. Often toxicity is preceded by widening of the QRS, but any of the above reactions can occur without prior ECG changes. Any signs of toxicity (with the possible exception of mild GI symptoms) are indication for cessation of the drug.

c. Disopyramide (Norpace)

(1) Electrophysiologic properties. Disopyramide has electrophysiologic effects resembling those of quinidine and procainamide, although its chemical structure is quite different. It prolongs the refractory period and action potential duration and slows conduction time in the Purkinje fibers.

(2) Absorption, excretion and plasma levels. Disopyramide is absorbed 80% to 90% following oral ingestion. The half-life of disopyramide is 6 to 7 hours in healthy volunteers and is prolonged to almost 10 hours in heart failure patients. Renal, hepatic, or cardiac insufficiency all prolong elimination time and require that loading and maintenance doses be adjusted downward. Peak blood levels after oral administration occur within approximately 2 hours. Bioavailability is greater than 80%. Metabolism is both hepatic and renal. Therapeutic blood levels are 2 to 5 mcg/ml.

(3) Clinical uses and dosages. Typical doses are 100 to 200 mg orally every 6 hours. A controlled release form of the drug exists that can be given twice a day. Daily dosages range from 400 to 1200 mg.

Disopyramide is effective against both ventricular and supraventricular arrhythmias. In both AF and atrial flutter, the ventricular rate must be controlled before administration to prevent 1:1 conduction that results from the vagolytic effects of disopyramide. This drug terminates and prevents recurrent episodes of PSVT and is particularly effective in Wolff-Parkinson-White, in which it prolongs the anterograde and retrograde refractory periods of the accessory pathway.

(4) Toxicity. Disopyramide has potent parasympatholytic effects that can lead to urinary retention, constipation, blurred vision, and dry mouth. It is a myocardial depressant and should be used with extreme caution in patients with preexisting left ventricular dysfunction. It may provoke torsades de pointes by prolonging the Q–T interval. It is contraindicated in patients who have had previous torsades de pointes. AV block may develop during disopyramide administration.

2. Type Ib agents: shorten repolarization
   a. Lidocaine (Xylocaine)
      (1) Electrophysiologic properties. Lidocaine shortens the effective refractory period and decreases the duration of the action potential. It depresses the rate of spontaneous depolarization, decreases automaticity (particularly in the bundle of His and Purkinje system), and speeds conduction at Purkinje fiber-myocardial junctions. Lidocaine slows conduction through ischemic myocardium. Lidocaine raises the threshold for VF.
      (2) Absorption, excretion, and plasma levels. Lidocaine is poorly absorbed through the GI tract. Ninety percent of orally administered lidocaine is metabolized rapidly by the liver. In most instances, the preferred route of administration is IV, although the intramuscular route also is acceptable. There are two phases of lidocaine washout from the circulation.

      Half-life for the first phase is less than 10 minutes and for the second phase is approximately 2 hours (thus, toxic levels may accumulate with repeated bolus dosages). The usual effective plasma concentration is 1.5 to 6 mcg/ml. Initial effective levels are achieved within 20 to 60 minutes after IV administration. More than 90% of lidocaine metabolism occurs in the liver, and the agent should be administered cautiously in the presence of liver disease.
      (3) Clinical uses and dosages. Lidocaine has widespread utility in the treatment of ventricular arrhythmias. It is the drug of choice for acute treatment of VT and/or frequent VPCs in the setting of unstable ischemic heart disease. Recommended dosages are as follows: IV, 75 to 100 mg, followed by a constant infusion of 1 to 4 mg per minute; intramuscularly, 300 mg (yields therapeutic levels for up to 2 hours).
      (4) Toxic effects and contraindications. Lidocaine offers the advantage of essentially no cardiac toxicity at therapeutic levels. Hypotension may occur at high serum levels. At toxic levels there may be central nervous system disturbances, including numbness, paresthesias, tremors, confusion, and occasionally coma or respiratory arrest. Seizures may result from high serum concentrations. GI adverse effects include nausea and vomiting. The treatment for symptoms of toxicity is discontinuance of the drug. Seizures are controlled with diazepam, 5 to 10 mg IV.
   b. Mexiletine (Mexitil). Mexiletine is an oral form of lidocaine. The molecular structure is similar to lidocaine, but the molecule has been altered in a way that markedly slows hepatic metabolism, thereby making the drug more appropriate for oral dosing.
      (1) Electrophysiologic properties. Many of the electrophysiologic properties of mexiletine are similar to lidocaine. It shortens the duration of the refractory period and action potential of Purkinje fibers and depresses the automaticity of these fibers. It does not appear to alter the refractory period of either atrial or ventricular muscle.

(2) Absorption, excretion, and plasma levels. Peak plasma levels occur 2 to 4 hours after oral administration. The bioavailability of the drug is approximately 85% to 90%. Mexiletine is metabolized in the liver. Less than 10% is excreted unchanged in the urine. Therapeutic plasma levels are 0.5 to 2 mcg/ml.

(3) Clinical uses and dosages. Recommended starting dose is 200 mg orally every 8 hours. Dosage may be increased or decreased 50 to 100 mg every 2 to 3 days. Typical dosages are 200 to 300 mg every 6 to 8 hours. Total daily dose should not exceed 1200 mg. Mexiletine is effective for both acute and chronic ventricular tachyarrhythmias. It has a reported success rate of approximately 50% to 60%. Its most important role may be as an adjunct to other antiarrhythmics, for example, quinidine or procainamide. It may also be an excellent choice for controlling ventricular arrhythmias in patients with baseline prolonged Q–T intervals. Mexiletine is infrequently used today.

(4) Toxicity. Adverse effects severe enough to warrant discontinuation of the drug may occur in 30% to 40% of patients. Most troublesome noncardiac effects are tremors, paresthesias, dizziness, and dysarthria. Cardiac side effects include hypotension, bradycardia, and exacerbation of ventricular arrhythmias (proarrhythmia).

c. Tocainide (Tonocard)

(1) Electrophysiologic properties. Tocainide is a primary amine analog of lidocaine with electrophysiologic properties almost identical to lidocaine and mexiletine.

(2) Absorption, excretion, and plasma levels. Peak plasma concentrations occur between 0.5 to 2.0 hours after oral administration. It is nearly 100% bioavailable. Approximately 40% of the drug is excreted unchanged in the urine. There is also substantial hepatic metabolism. The half-life is 11 to 19 hours. Therapeutic blood levels range between 4 and 10 mcg/ml.

(3) Clinical usages and dosages. The fact that tocainide is an amine analog of lidocaine protects it from first-pass elimination in the liver, making it an effective oral medication. It is slightly less effective than quinidine in suppressing ventricular ectopy. The response to IV lidocaine helps predict the response to tocainide. If lidocaine has been ineffective, tocainide will be effective in only 15% of patients. If lidocaine was effective, the success rate of tocainide is approximately 60%. Metabolism is both renal and hepatic. Consequently, dosages should be decreased in patients with renal, hepatic, or cardiac insufficiency.

Tocainide, like lidocaine and mexiletine is effective against ventricular arrhythmias. It is slightly less effective than quinidine. Tocainide is often combined with type Ia antiarrhythmic agents such as quinidine and procainamide. Oral dosing is generally in the range of 300 to 400 mg two or three times a day.

(4) Toxicity. Side effects are similar to those of lidocaine, with GI upset, memory impairment, and tremors most prominent. Pulmonary fibrosis and aggravation of arrhythmia (proarrhythmia) have been reported in a small number of patients. Serious hematologic side effects, including agranulocytosis and bone marrow suppression, have been reported in a small number of patients.

3. Type Ic agents: marked slowing of conduction

a. Propafenone (Rythmol)

(1) Electrophysiologic properties. Propafenone has strong membrane stabilizing effects. It also has weak beta-blocking properties. Conduction velocity is markedly slowed after administration of this agent.

(2) Absorption, excretion and plasma levels. Propafenone is essentially 100% absorbed. It undergoes extensive hepatic metabolism that may be rapid or slow, depending on the genetics of the patient's hepatic P450 system. The half-life ranges from 2 to 12 hours (mean, 6 hours). Steady state may take as much as 72 hours to achieve.

(3) Clinical uses and dosages. Propafenone is effective for both atrial and ventricular arrhythmias. It has been widely used as prophylaxis against AF; it is effective in approximately 50% of patients. The recommended starting dose is 150 mg three times a day. The dose may be increased to 300 mg three times a day if needed, although the higher dose is associated with considerably more toxicity.

(4) Toxicity. Adverse effects include nausea, vomiting, a bitter taste in the mouth, dizziness, constipation, rashes, and tremor. Torsades de pointes can occur in approximately 3% to 10% of patients. A rare patient develops drug-induced lupus erythematosus or neutropenia. Propafenone raises serum digoxin levels when the two drugs are combined. Warfarin effect is also accentuated by propafenone.

b. Moricizine (Ethmozine)

(1) Electrophysiologic properties. Moricizine is a phenothiazine derivative with antiarrhythmic properties. The drug has membrane-stabilizing properties and resembles a type Ic antiarrhythmic agent most closely. The drug slows conduction velocity in the His Purkinje system.

(2) Absorption, excretion, and plasma levels. Moricizine is absorbed readily through the GI tract. Its systemic bioavailability is reduced to 30% to 40% because of significant first-pass metabolism in the liver. Peak plasma concentrations are achieved within 1 to 2 hours after an oral dose. It is almost completely biotransformed by the liver. Less than 1% of moricizine is excreted unchanged in the urine. Approximately 39% of moricizine and its metabolites are eliminated in the urine, and 56% is excreted in the feces. Initially, the half-life is 6 hours, but with long-term administration, the half-life extends to 12 hours.

(3) Clinical uses and dosages. Moricizine is predominantly used to treat ventricular arrhythmias, although it has shown some efficacy against paroxysmal AF. Most patients can be adequately treated with 200 to 300 mg q8h. Initial dosage is 200 mg q8h, and this may be gradually increased over 3-day intervals to 250 mg and then 300 mg q8h.

(4) Toxicity. Moricizine may worsen cardiac performance in patients with preexisting left ventricular dysfunction or a history of congestive heart failure. Moricizine exacerbates ventricular arrhythmias (proarrhythmia) in 3% to 4% of treated patients. Other adverse effects include nausea, paresthesias, vertigo, dry mouth, dizziness, headache, fatigue, dyspnea, diarrhea, and excessive sweating.

c. Flecainide (Tambocor)

(1) Electrophysiologic properties. Flecainide prolongs refractoriness and slows conduction in the atria, the AV node, the His Purkinje system, and the ventricles.

(2) Absorption, excretion, and plasma levels. Flecainide has excellent bioavailability (90% to 95%) after ingestion. The drug's half-life ranges from 12 to 27 hours (mean, 20 hours). Metabolism is primarily performed by the liver, although 30% of absorbed flecainide is excreted by the kidney. Peak blood levels are achieved within 2 to 4 hours after oral ingestion. Therapeutic blood levels range from 0.4 to 1.0 mcg/ml.

(3) Clinical uses. Flecainide is active against both ventricular and supraventricular arrhythmias. Because this agent was associated with considerable proarrhythmia during CAST (Cardiac Arrhythmia Suppression Trial), it is only used today for control of paroxysmal AF or refractory supraventricular arrhythmias in patients with normal left ventricular function.

(4) Toxicity. As already noted, flecainide is strongly proarrhythmic. In CAST, many episodes of torsades de pointes and cardiac arrest were attributed to this drug. The patients who developed proarrhythmia had ischemic heart disease with reduced left ventricular function. Hence, the agent is not recommended for this group of patients. Other adverse effects include dizziness, visual disturbances, headache, and depression of left ventricular function. Flecainide can worsen preexisting sinus or AV nodal dysfunction.

4. Class II agents: beta-blockers
   a. Electrophysiologic properties. Beta-blocking agents shorten the effective refractory period and the action potential. They decrease automaticity. Beta-blockers have little effect on the His-Purkinje system or ventricular conduction, although they slow conduction through the AV node.
   b. Absorption, excretion, and plasma levels. GI absorption of beta-blockers is generally good, although considerable differences exist among individuals and among the different preparations. Intravenous formulations are available for atenolol, metoprolol, propranolol, and esmolol. Most beta-blockers are predominantly metabolized in the liver (greater than 90%), and metabolites are excreted in the urine.
   c. Clinical uses and dosages. All beta-blockers are effective against both ventricular and supraventricular arrhythmias. In the setting of acute, unstable ischemic heart disease, beta-blockage diminishes VT and VF. Propranolol is the only beta-blocker specifically approved by the Food and Drug Administration for the treatment of supraventricular arrhythmias. However, all beta-blockers are potentially effective in the treatment of both supraventricular and ventricular arrhythmias. Beta-blockade is also used as prophylaxis against atrial arrhythmias and particularly against paroxysmal AF.

      Beta-blockade is also useful for slowing the ventricular response to AF. In this latter setting, beta-blockade is often combined with digoxin. Beta-blockers are effective in managing ventricular arrhythmias caused by digitalis toxicity (second choice after lidocaine).
   d. Toxic effects and contraindications. Beta-blockade may precipitate excessive sinus bradycardia. These drugs also have direct depressant effects on the myocardium and may precipitate or exacerbate congestive heart failure. However, long-term beta-blockade reduces mortality in patients with congestive heart failure (see Chapter 4) when used judiciously. Beta-blockers are contraindicated in patients with bronchial asthma because of the tendency of the drugs to exacerbate bronchospasm in these individuals. Other manifestations of beta-blocker toxicity include GI distress (nausea, vomiting), rash, drowsiness, fatigue, impotence, lightheadedness, and mental depression.

3. Type III agents: prolongation of repolarization
   a. Bretylium tosylate (Bretylol)
      (1) Electrophysiologic properties. Bretylium causes an initial release of norepinephrine followed by subsequent prevention of norepinephrine release. It causes significant increase in VF thresholds and lengthens the action potential of proximal cells in the myocardial conduction system.
      (2) Absorption, excretion, and plasma levels. Bretylium is approved only for parenteral use. GI absorption is erratic, and bioavail-

ability is less than 50%. Elimination is 100% by renal excretion; elimination half-life is 5 to 10 hours.

(3) Clinical uses and dosages. Bretylium is the fourth-line drug for life-threatening recurrent tachyarrhythmias in the intensive care setting that do not respond to lidocaine, procainamide, or quinidine. It may be more useful than lidocaine in helping to restore rhythm in VF, but this remains controversial. It is approved for parenteral use only. Bretylium is administered in doses of 5 to 10 mg/kg diluted in 50 to 100 ml of 5% dextrose in water and administered slowly over 10 to 20 minutes. During a cardiac arrest, this dosage may be administered as an IV bolus over 2 to 3 minutes in an attempt to convert VF. Maintenance infusion is 0.5 to 2.0 mg per minute.

(4) Toxic effects and contraindications. Hypotension (either orthostatic or in the supine patient) is the most serious side effect. Transient hypertension caused by initial norepinephrine release may occur. Nausea, vomiting, and parotid pain and swelling have been reported.

b. Amiodarone (Cordarone)

(1) Electrophysiologic properties. Amiodarone, when given orally, prolongs the refractory period and action potential of all cardiac fibers. It prolongs the Q–T interval and may change the contour of the T wave and produce U waves. Sinus rate is typically slowed 20% to 30%. IV administration results in less prolongation of conduction time (except in AV node) and less prolongation of refractory periods.

(2) Absorption, excretion, and plasma levels. Amiodarone is metabolized almost exclusively by the liver, with minimal plasma clearance and renal excretion. It is absorbed slowly and incompletely with a bioavailability of 35% to 65%. It is accumulated in liver, fat, and lungs. Onset of action after IV administration is typically 1 to 2 hours; after oral administration, onset of action may not occur until 2 to 3 days or even 1 to 2 weeks. Loading doses may decrease the period to onset of action. Because there is considerable variability among patients in these pharmacokinetic parameters, close patient monitoring is essential.

(3) Clinical uses and dosages. Some debate remains concerning optimal dosing schedules. One commonly used oral loading regimen starts with 800 to 1600 mg daily (in divided doses) for 1 to 3 weeks followed by 800 mg daily for 2 to 4 weeks, then 600 mg daily for 4 to 8 weeks followed by a maintenance dose of 400 mg per day. Intravenous loading and dosage regimens are under investigation and often involve a loading dose of 5 to 10 mg/kg over 20 to 30 minutes followed by 1 g every 24 hours for several days. Amiodarone has been used to treat a wide spectrum of supraventricular and ventricular tachyarrhythmias. It is typically successful in 60% to 80% of PSVTs and 40% to 60% of VTs. Because of its long half-life, unpredictable absorption, and the difficulty in starting another drug, amiodarone should be one of the last antiarrhythmic agents tried for suppression of arrhythmias. It is often the final antiarrhythmic tried when others have failed to control life-threatening ventricular arrhythmias.

(4) Toxicity. Adverse effects occur in about 75% of patients receiving chronic amiodarone therapy and require its discontinuance in 10% to 20% of patients.

Pulmonary toxicity is the most serious noncardiac toxicity and typically occurs within 30 months of initiation of therapy. It is manifested by dyspnea, nonproductive cough, and infiltrates on chest radiography. It requires cessation of the drug.

The incidence of pulmonary toxicity is 5% to 15%. Asymptomatic elevations in liver enzymes occur in most patients.

The drug should be stopped if these elevations exceed three times normal. Photosensitivity, hyperthyroidism and hypothyroidism, and corneal microdeposits may also occur. Cardiac side effects include symptomatic bradycardias in about 2% of patients and exacerbation of ventricular tachyarrhythmias in about 2% to 3%. Drug interactions of amiodarone with other antiarrhythmics, warfarin, and digoxin require monitoring and adjustment of doses of these other drugs.

c. Sotalol (Betapace)

   (1) Electrophysiologic properties. Sotalol hydrochloride has unique electrophysiologic properties. It is indicated for treatment of a wide spectrum of ventricular arrhythmias. It also has been shown to be of benefit in the treatment of supraventricular arrhythmias, although it lacks official indication for this use. It possesses two distinct properties—a combination of class II and class III antiarrhythmic activity, which distinguishes it from other antiarrhythmic agents. Its class II activity is characterized by beta-blocking properties. Its class III activity is characterized by selective lengthening of the effective refractory period and action potential duration.

   (2) Absorption, excretion, and plasma levels. Sotalol is absorbed rapidly (2 to 3 hours) and completely (greater than 90%) through the GI tract and has an oral bioavailability of almost 100%. It is eliminated primarily through the kidney. Approximately 75% of a single dose is detected unchanged in the urine within 72 hours.

   (3) Clinical usage and dosages. Sotalol is effective against both atrial and ventricular arrhythmias. No loading dose is necessary. Therapy is begun with 80 mg twice a day. Most patients require maintenance doses of 240 to 300 mg per day. Occasional patients require dosages as high as 480 to 640 mg per day. Maximum dose should not exceed 640 mg per day.

   (4) Toxicity. Sotalol may worsen preexisting diminished cardiovascular performance. It may also prolong the acute Q–T interval and result in torsades de pointes.

d. Dofetilide (Tikosyn)

   (1) Electrophysiologic properties. Dofetilide prolongs the action potential and the effective refractory period of atrial and ventricular muscle. The Q–T interval is prolonged after administration of this agent.

   (2) Absorption and excretion. Dofetilide is well absorbed and has a bioavailability in excess of 90%. Peak plasma concentrations are achieved 2 hours after ingestion. The elimination half-life averages 9.5 hours. Sixty percent of the drug is excreted unchanged in the urine, and the rest is metabolized in the liver.

   (3) Clinical usage and dosage. Dofetilide is very effective in converting AF to sinus rhythm. Approximately 50% of patients with AF will convert to sinus rhythm with dofetilide therapy. It appears to be the most effective antiarrhythmic agent for this indication. Dofetilide has no effect on long-term survival in patients with heart failure. The drug is capable of suppressing ventricular arrhythmias but is not approved for this indication. Only physicians who have successfully completed a special training course in the use of dofetilide are allowed to use this agent. Dofetilide dosing depends on the patient's creatinine clearance with dosages ranging from 125 mcg to 500 mcg every 12 hours based on renal function.

   (4) Toxicity. This agent is associated with proarrhythmia: 1.3% of patients given dofetilide can be expected to develop torsades de

pointes. Other adverse effects include headache, chest and/or abdominal pain, dizziness, dyspnea, nausea, flulike symptoms, insomnia, back pain, rash, and diarrhea.

e. Ibutilide (Corvert)

   (1) Electrophysiologic properties. Ibutilide prolongs the action potential and Q–T interval. There are negligible effects on heart rate and AV nodal conduction. The agent also lowers the defibrillation threshold of the myocardium.

   (2) Absorption and excretion. The drug is well absorbed, with a half-life of 3–6 hours. It is metabolized in the liver to eight different inactive metabolites.

   (3) Clinical usage and dosage. This drug is very effective in terminating AF and atrial flutter. The efficacy is about the same as that of Dofetilide. The drug is given intravenously, 1 mg over 10 minutes followed by a second dose if the first dose was ineffective.

   (4) Adverse effects. This agent can be proarrhythmic. It prolongs the Q–T interval and leads to torsades de pointes in 2% of treated patients. Other adverse reactions include orthostatic hypotension, AV block, bradycardia, nausea, headache, and tachycardia.

6. Type IV agents: calcium channel blockers. Verapamil (Calan, Isoptin) and diltiazem (Cardizem)

   a. Electrophysiologic properties. Verapamil and diltiazem are the only calcium channel blockers approved for control of arrhythmias. Verapamil and diltiazem block the slow inward current of depolarization which is calcium mediated. They suppress normal sinus and AV node activity by depressing the slope of diastolic depolarization. In most clinical settings, this action will not slow sinus rhythm because it is counterbalanced by sympathetic stimulation caused by peripheral dilatation.

   b. Absorption, excretion, and plasma levels. After IV administration, both drugs produce effects on AV nodal conduction within 1 to 2 minutes. Both agents are well absorbed after oral ingestion, and both undergo extensive hepatic metabolism. Verapamil bioavailability is only 35%, suggesting extensive first-pass metabolism in the liver. After oral dosing, measurable effects on AV conduction begin to occur in 30 minutes and last as long as 6 hours. Effective plasma concentrations are approximately 0.1 to 0.4 mcg/ml for verapamil. The elimination half-life for verapamil is 3 to 8 hours.

   c. Clinical uses and dosages. Verapamil and diltiazem are highly effective in terminating supraventricular tachycardias if vagal maneuvers fail. More than 90% of supraventricular tachycardias will be terminated in 2 minutes. Verapamil/diltiazem will occasionally terminate AF or atrial flutter; they also slow the ventricular response in these rhythms. Neither drug is indicated for control of ventricular arrhythmias. Verapamil is administered at a IV dose of 0.1 mg/kg over 1 to 2 minutes. A second dose may be given in 30 minutes. If a constant infusion is required, it is administered at 0.005 mg/kg per minute. Oral dosage is 80 to 120 mg given three or four times a day, or 120 to 240 mg once per day in a long-acting preparation. Diltiazem is given as an IV bolus of 0.25 mg/kg. Continuous infusion is administered at a dose of 0.15 mg/kg per minute. Oral diltiazem is given as a daily dose of 90 to 360 mg, either as a single dose with long-acting preparations or three times a day using the routine preparation.

   d. Toxic effects and contraindications. Verapamil/diltiazem should be used cautiously in patients with left ventricular dysfunction or sinus node disease and in patients being treated with beta-blockers. Contraindications include advanced heart failure, significant sinus node dysfunction, cardiogenic shock, or second- or third-degree AV block. Verapamil may decrease digoxin excretion by as much as 30%. Less serious adverse consequences include constipation, nausea, headache, dizziness, hypotension, fatigue, and peripheral edema. Diltiazem is generally better tolerated than is verapamil. Less serious adverse effects associated with diltiazem include headache, hypotension, fatigue, and peripheral edema.

V. Electrical therapy of arrhythmias

A. Cardioversion

1. Theory and technique. The use of electrical cardioversion for the treatment of cardiac arrhythmias is based on several theoretical considerations. First, although a variety of mechanisms may be responsible for initiating a rhythm disturbance, once the disorder has begun, it is frequently self-sustaining.

Second, if the abnormal rhythm can be temporarily interrupted, the sinus node, which has the highest intrinsic automaticity in the cardiac conduction system, will have the opportunity to recapture the depolarization process. Initial trials of electrical cardioversion in animals were attempted with alternating current. Although this technique often successfully terminated arrhythmias, it resulted in an unacceptably high risk of VF and cardiac arrest. Modern defibrillation equipment consists of a capacitor-discharge unit that delivers a direct-current electrical pulse synchronized with the ECG at the most efficacious and least dangerous time during the cardiac cycle.

Various protocols exist for performing cardioversion. It is usually performed as an outpatient procedure. If cardioversion is being performed on a patient with AF or flutter, an antiarrhythmic medication such as a beta-blocker, sotalol, or propafenone, is administered 24 to 48 hours before the procedure. The patient is anesthetized with a short-acting agent, for example, a benzodiazepine or barbiturate. The electrical discharge is delivered by means of two paddles applied to the patient's chest. The initial electrical setting depends on the arrhythmia to be converted, for example, 100 J for AF. If reversion is not accomplished at this setting, progressively higher energy levels are used (200, 300, and 400 J).

2. Clinical uses

a. AF. AF is the most common indication for cardioversion. Successful reversion to sinus rhythm (at least temporarily) can be expected in more than 90% of cases. Patients who cannot be reverted generally have mitral valvular disease and massively dilated atria. A left atrial diameter greater than 50 mm suggests that reversion to sinus rhythm after cardioversion is less likely. The longer a patient remains in AF, the more difficult it will be to cardiovert that individual to sinus rhythm. Patients who have been in AF for more than 1 year usually will not remain in sinus rhythm. Only one third to one half of all patients converted from AF to sinus rhythm will remain in sinus rhythm as long as 1 year.

b. VT. VT is a medical emergency. Electrical cardioversion is the treatment of choice and should be undertaken immediately, particularly if the arrhythmia is accompanied by hypotension or pulmonary edema. The patient may be given a 75- to 100-mg bolus of IV lidocaine while preparations for cardioversion are being made. Occasionally sinus rhythm is restored by administration of this drug. Cardioversion is not indicated for short repetitive bursts of VT, which respond better to treatment with lidocaine or other antiarrhythmic agents. Patients who have been resuscitated from VT may be candidates for an ICD.

c. Atrial flutter. Cardioversion is highly effective in the treatment of atrial flutter. This arrhythmia is easy to convert, often requiring less than 50 J. A 24-hour trial of an antiarrhythmic agent, for example, sotalol, a beta-blocker, or propafenone, is often performed before attempted cardioversion; this frequently results in reversion to sinus rhythm.

d. Supraventricular tachycardia. Supraventricular tachycardias require electrical conversion only if they produce hemodynamic compromise. Otherwise, pharmacologic treatment should be initially attempted. Arrhythmias resulting from digitalis toxicity generally do not respond to cardioversion, and its application may be potentially dangerous in this setting. If the possibility of digitalis toxicity exists, low-energy (5 W per second) cardioversion should be tried first, with subsequent cautious increases in energy.

Some authors recommend pretreatment with a bolus of lidocaine (75 to 100 mg IV) followed by a continuous infusion (2 to 3 mg per minute) when attempting to cardiovert rhythm disturbances thought to be caused by digitalis toxicity.

3. Complications and contraindications. Although the incidence of serious complications resulting from cardioversion is low (3%), a variety of complications have been described, and some well-defined contraindications to cardioversion exist. Difficulties with the technique can be minimized by careful patient selection and cautious application of the technique. Electrolyte abnormalities should be corrected before cardioversion. Patients suspected of having digitalis toxicity should not be subjected to cardioversion. Patients should be euthyroid. Cardioversion is contraindicated in the presence of third-degree AV block. Intolerance to multiple antiarrhythmic agents and failure to remain in sinus rhythm after a previous cardioversion are also contraindications. Some arrhythmias, including sinus tachycardia and multifocal atrial tachycardia, should not be treated with cardioversion. These arrhythmias will not revert to sinus rhythm with cardioversion because they are the result of comorbid conditions, for example, sepsis and respiratory failure.

The incidence of arterial embolism after cardioversion from AF is estimated at 1% to 2%. All patients who have been in AF for more than 36 to 48 hours should be anticoagulated with warfarin for 3 to 4 weeks before cardioversion **unless** a transesophageal echo has shown that the left atrial appendage and the left atrium are free of clot. Most cardiologists anticoagulate patients with new onset AF with unfractionated or fractionated heparin until cardioversion can be performed or until warfarin anticoagulation is successfully implemented.

B. Pacemaker therapy. Pacemaker therapy has assumed increasing importance since its introduction in 1960. Technologic advances have occurred both in power sources and in electronic circuitry. Long-lasting lithium batteries (6 years or more) are now used routinely in current pacemakers. Demand pacemakers have universally supplanted earlier fixed-rate models. Dual chamber (sense and pace in both the atria and the ventricle) allows for nearly physiologic heart rate control that is usually considerably better tolerated than that of single-chamber ventricular pacing. A number of the dual-chamber pacemakers in common use today also track the patient's activity level and automatically increase the heart rate when the patient performs exertion of any type. Patients with AF require only a single-chamber ventricular pacemaker. The indications for permanent pacemaker therapy differ somewhat from those for temporary pacing, and the two topics are discussed separately.

1. Permanent pacing

a. Clinical uses. The criteria for implantation of a permanent pacemaker are not rigid and should be individualized. Symptoms such as syncope and hypotension accompanying certain arrhythmias and conduction disturbances generally indicate the need for pacing therapy. Permanent pacing may be indicated with third-degree AV block, second-degree AV block with slow ventricular response, marked sinus bradycardia (if symptomatic), sick sinus syndrome with alternating episodes of bradycardia and tachycardia, AF with slow ventricular response, and persistent bifascicular or trifascicular block after MI (see Chapters 15 and 24).

Dual-chamber pacing is preferable to single-chamber pacing in any condition in which ventricular compliance is diminished. Such conditions include hypertension, hypertrophic obstructive cardiomyopathy, acute MI, and right ventricular infarction.

b. Complications. The most common complication of permanent pacing is power source failure. This is often heralded by slowing of the pacemaker rate of 3 to 5 beats per minute. Other complications include broken pacing wires, infection, electrode displacement, and myocardial perforation.

2. Temporary pacing

a. Clinical uses. Temporary pacing may be indicated until a permanent pacemaker can be implanted in any of the settings discussed in the previous section. Temporary pacing may also be indicated (and lifesaving in an occasional patient) in acute MI. In anterior MI, emergency temporary pacing may be indicated in a variety of conditions (see Chapter 15). In inferior MI, AV block generally reflects temporary ischemia of the AV node. Temporary pacing may be indicated for extreme bradycardia or hypotension, since AV block in this setting is likely to be transient (see Chapter 15). Temporary pacing can be performed in an emergency by electrical energy delivered to the chest wall by a device known as the external pacemaker.

C. ICD therapy. The ICD is a small self-contained device resembling a large pacemaker. It is placed in a subcutaneous pocket overlying the pectoralis major muscle, similar to the deployment of a pacemaker. The ICD is connected to two electrode catheters, one in the superior vena cava and one in the apex of the right ventricle. The ICD is inserted under local anesthesia usually in the EPS laboratory. The device detects VT and/or VF and administers a small shock that nearly always restores the heart to normal sinus rhythm. The device can also perform a variety of pacing protocols that can often terminate VT without the need for the defibrillator component of the ICD to discharge and shock the heart. As noted earlier (Section **III.B.5.a.**), ICD therapy has revolutionized the management of patients with resuscitated sudden death and malignant ventricular arrhythmias such as VT. For many of these patients, the preferred therapy is implantation of an ICD and oral antiarrhythmic drug therapy.

SELECTED READINGS

Bryce M, Spielman SR, Greenspan AM, et al. Evolving indications for permanent pacemakers. *Ann Intern Med* 2001;134:1130–1141.
Up-to-date review and future directions for use of pacemakers
Connolly SJ, Hallstrom AP, Cappato R, et al. Meta-analysis of the implantable cardioverter defibrillator secondary prevention trials. *Eur Heart J* 2000;21:2071–2078.
Benefit of cardioverter-defibrillators confirmed in selected patients.
Connolly SJ, Kerr CR, Gent M, et al. Effects of physiologic pacing versus ventricular pacing on the risk of stroke and death due to cardiovascular causes. *N Engl J Med* 2000;342:1385–1391.
Dual-chamber pacing is no better than single-chamber pacing with death and stroke as the measured end point.
Exner DV, Klein GJ, Prystowsky EN. Primary prevention of sudden death with implantable defibrillator therapy in patients with cardiac disease. *Circulation* 2001;104: 1564–1570.
ICDs prevent sudden death.
Fuster V, Ryden LE, Asinger, RW, et al. ACC/AHA/ESC guidelines for the management of patients with atrial fibrillation: executive summary: a report of the American

College of Cardiology/American Heart Association Task Force on Practice Guidelines and the European Society of Cardiology Committee for Practice Guidelines and Policy Conferences (Committee to Develop Guidelines for the Management of Patients With Atrial Fibrillation): developed in collaboration with the North American Society of Pacing and Electrophysiology. *J Am Coll Cardiol* 2001;38:1231–1265.
Extensive review of the mechanisms, diagnosis, and management of AF.
Goldschlager N, Epstein AD, Naccarelli, G, et al. Practical guidelines for clinicians who treat patients with amiodarone. *Arch Intern Med* 2000;160:1741–1748.
Helpful hints for the clinician who uses amiodarone.
Gollob MH, Seger JJ. Current status of the implantable cardioverter-defibrillator. *Chest* 2001;119:1210–1221.
Excellent current review of ICDs, the indications and results.
Gregoratos G, Cheitlin MD, Conill A, et al. ACC/AHA guidelines for implantation of cardiac pacemakers and antiarrhythmia devices: a report of the American College of Cardiology/American Heart Association Task Force on Practice Guidelines (Committee on Pacemaker Implantation). *J Am Coll Cardiol* 1998;31:1175–1209.
Standard guidelines for use of pacemakers and ICDs.
Kowey PR. Pharmacological effects of antiarrhythmic drugs. *Arch Intern Med* 1998;158: 325–332.
A complete and knowledgeable review of mechanisms and indications of antiarrhythmic drugs.
Lown B. Electrical reversion of cardiac arrhythmias. *Br Heart J* 1967;29:469–489.
Classic paper on cardioversion.
Mason JW. Amiodarone. *N Engl J Med* 1987;316:455–466.
Good summary of pharmacology and clinical use of this drug.
Naccarelli GV. Antiarrhythmic drugs In: Willerson JT, Cohn JN, eds. *Cardiovascular medicine.* Philadelphia: Churchill Livingstone, 2000.
A thorough, well-organized review of antiarrhythmic drugs.
Roden DM. Mechanisms and management of proarrhythmia. *Am. J. Cardiol.* 1998;82: 49I–57I.
Proarrhythmia defined and mechanisms reviewed.
Sheldon R, Connolly S, Krahn A, et al. Identification of patients most likely to benefit from implantable cardioverter-defibrillator therapy: the Canadian Implantable Defibrillator Study. *Circulation* 2000;101:1660–1664.
A multicenter trial that helps to define who benefits the most from an ICD.
Straka RJ, et al. Antiarrhythmic agents. In: Rippe JM, Irwin RS, Fink MP, et al., eds. *Intensive care medicine.* Boston: Little, Brown and Company, 1995.
A comprehensive discussion of available antiarrhythmic agents.
Zipes DP. Genesis of cardiac arrhythmias: electrophysiological consideration, management of cardiac arrhythmias, specific arrhythmias: diagnosis and treatment. In: Braunwald E, ed. *The heart,* 4th ed. Philadelphia: Saunders, 1992.
An exhaustive, up-to-date review of all clinical aspects of arrhythmias.

4. HEART FAILURE

I. Introduction
   A. Definition and background. During the past two decades, new fundamental knowledge and a number of new therapies have become available that have changed the way congestive heart failure (CHF) is approached. For example, a number of multicenter trials have shown that the addition of vasodilator therapy to digoxin and diuretics significantly improves 1-year survival in patients with CHF. Despite these new modalities, mortality from CHF remains high. Moreover, CHF is often a disease of older individuals who represent the most rapidly growing segment of the American population. Consequently, CHF has become one of the most common admission diagnoses for acute care hospitals.

   On the most fundamental level, heart failure represents the failure of the heart to supply adequate blood flow and, hence, nutrients and oxygen to metabolizing tissues. The underlying reasons for heart failure are often complex, and the physiologic basis is incompletely understood; however, all forms of heart failure can ultimately be traced to the relative or absolute failure of the heart as a pump. This inadequate cardiac function sets off a series of compensatory actions that eventually do more harm than good; that is, they "overcompensate" by causing the body to retain salt and water, thereby leading to edema formation. The abnormally active compensatory actions involve the sympathetic nervous system, the renin-angiotensin system, and antidiuretic hormone released from the pituitary gland. Decreased cardiac output combined with pulmonary and peripheral edema results in effort intolerance. As heart failure progresses, various cytokines are activated. Tumor necrosis factor appears to play an important role in the fatigue, skeletal muscle atrophy, and eventual cachexia that affects patients with severe CHF.

   A patient with heart failure usually has one or more symptoms (e.g., fatigue, dyspnea, orthopnea, paroxysmal nocturnal dyspnea [PND]) and a variety of physical signs (e.g., pulmonary rales, gallop rhythms, peripheral edema). The problems faced by the clinician in the diagnosis of heart failure are three-fold: (i) differentiating heart failure from other conditions that may mimic it, (ii) identifying underlying cardiac disease, and (iii) determining any precipitating cause. True cardiac failure always implies some form of underlying heart disease. Although almost any type of cardiac disease can lead to cardiac failure, the most common cardiac etiologies are listed in Table 4-1. The diagnostic problem is complicated by the fact that many forms of cardiac disease present as cardiac failure without prior symptoms.

   Major precipitating causes of cardiac failure are shown in Table 4-2. A careful and systematic search for these precipitants should be undertaken in all patients presenting with cardiac failure. The search for precipitating causes assumes particular importance in patients whose initial presentation is one of cardiac failure, in patients with known cardiac disease who suffer acute deterioration, and in patients who fail to respond to conventional therapies.

   B. Types of heart failure. Various terms have been used to describe subsets of patients with heart failure. Many of these terms are either self-explanatory (acute heart failure vs. CHF) or disputed (forward vs. backward heart failure). Two frameworks for categorizing heart failure, however, should be noted:
      1. High-output versus low-output heart failure. Although the range of "normal" cardiac output is large, certain types of heart failure tend to involve higher output states, whereas others display low cardiac outputs. High output is associated with arteriovenous fistula, Paget's disease, anemia, and hyperthyroidism. Although the term *high output* is often used to describe these conditions, a more correct term should be *high, but not high enough, cardiac output*. This latter statement emphasizes

TABLE 4-1. MAJOR CARDIAC DISEASE UNDERLYING HEART FAILURE

A. Direct myocardial damage
  1. Atherosclerotic heart disease
  2. Cardiomyopathies and/or myocarditis
  3. Vitamin deficiency states (e.g., beriberi)
B. Ventricular overload
  1. Volume overload
    a. Atrial septal defect
    b. Ventricular septal defect
    c. Aortic regurgitation
    d. Mitral regurgitation
    e. Patent ductus arteriosus
  2. Pressure overload
    a. Aortic stenosis
    b. Systemic hypertension
    c. Pulmonic stenosis
    d. Coarctation of the aorta
C. Restriction of ventricular filling
  1. Mitral stenosis
  2. Constrictive pericarditis
  3. Restrictive cardiomyopathies

the fact that the cardiac output may be surprisingly normal in patients with arteriovenous fistula, Paget's disease, anemia, or hyperthyroidism, but it is not sufficient to supply the peripheral demand for blood flow given the marked decrease in peripheral vascular resistance and/or increased metabolic demand of the peripheral tissues.

Typical low-output states include hypertension, coronary artery disease, and the cardiomyopathies.

  2. Right-sided versus left-sided heart failure. The clinical presentation of heart failure may vary depending on which ventricle is more affected. Pressure increases behind the more affected chamber result in transudation of fluid. In right-sided failure, hepatic congestion and its attendant symptoms occur; when left-sided failure predominates, pulmonary congestion and its attendant symptoms assume more prominence. In long-standing or severe heart failure, both ventricles are dysfunctional, and these distinctions become blurred.

C. Pathophysiology. The underlying pathophysiology of heart failure remains the object of intense research. It appears that abnormal release and reuptake of intracellular calcium from the sarcoplasmic reticulum is one of the central pathophysiologic mechanisms operating in CHF. For the clinician, one aspect of the pathophysiology of heart failure remains foremost: Is the observed episode of CHF based on a primary failure of the contractile function of the heart muscle itself (e.g., ischemia or infarction), or is it the result of the myocardium's inability to respond to an altered external condition (such as valve rupture or acute hypertensive crisis)? This fundamental distinction dramatically alters the therapy that is selected.

II. Diagnosis
  A. History. Significant items in the history of patients with heart failure are presented in Table 4-3. The most commonly quoted symptoms in patients with heart failure are the triad of respiratory complaints: dyspnea, orthopnea, and PND.
    1. Dyspnea. Dyspnea represents the most prevalent and often the earliest symptom of heart failure. The sense of shortness of breath arises from the increased effort of breathing that accompanies heart failure. It is partic-

TABLE 4-2. PRECIPITATING CAUSES OF HEART FAILURE

Precipitating cause	Comment
Systemic hypertension	Particularly when rise in arterial pressure is rapid
Myocardial infarction	Particularly a fresh infarct in a patient with a previously compromised ventricle
Pulmonary embolism	Patients with low cardiac output at high risk for pulmonary embolism, which may further reduce cardiac output
Infection	Inability of compromised ventricle to keep up with increased metabolic demand
Arrhythmias	Inability of patients with already dysfunctioning ventricles to compensate for unfavorable hemodynamic effects of many arrhythmias
Thyrotoxicosis	Inability to keep up with increased metabolic demand
Anemia	Inability of compromised ventricle to supply increased cardiac output obligated by decreased oxygen-carrying capacity
Myocarditis	Primary dysfunction of the myocardium
Bacterial endocarditis	Inability of heart to meet increased needs caused by fever, possible valve damage, and myocarditis
Dietary or environmental excess	Increased sodium intake in compensated heart failure; overexertion in heat or humidity
Development of an unrelated illness	Worsening of renal dysfunction may cause fluid retention in a patient with compensated congestive heart failure
Administration of salt-retaining or cardiac-depressant medication	Both steroids and nonsteroidal antiinflammatory agents can cause salt and water retention; many medications can depress myocardial function (e.g., many antiarrhythmics, beta-adrenergic blocking agents, and some anti-neoplastic agents)

ularly common when left ventricular failure predominates: Left atrial and ultimately pulmonary venous pressures rise, and fluid transudes into the pulmonary interstitium, thereby reducing pulmonary compliance. A history of the activities that provoke dyspnea is important. Typically, dyspnea occurs with progressively smaller amounts of exercise and finally develops at rest as CHF worsens. Patients often unconsciously restrict their activity to avoid this unpleasant sensation, and they should be questioned closely concerning effort intolerance.

2. Orthopnea. Orthopnea is said to be present when the patient breathes more comfortably with the upper part of the body elevated rather than in recumbent position. In severe heart failure, patients may spend the entire night sleeping in a chair to maintain this elevation.

3. PND. PND refers to episodes of severe shortness of breath, often occurring at night and, in contrast to orthopnea, frequently not relieved by sit-

TABLE 4-3. IMPORTANT HISTORICAL ITEMS IN PATIENTS WITH HEART FAILURE

Category	Item	Comment
History of present illness (HPI)	Respiratory symptoms	Orthopnea, dyspnea on exertion, paroxysmal nocturnal dyspnea, cardiac asthma, Cheyne-Stokes respiration
	History of cardiac disease	Direct myocardial damage, ventricular overload, restriction of ventricular filling (see Table 4-1)
Past medical history (PMH)	History of disease that might produce symptoms mimicking heart failure	Particularly pulmonary disease; also liver disease
Family history	Familial forms of heart disease	Idiopathic hypertrophic subaortic stenosis, cardiomyopathy
Current medications	Medications for heart failure	Check for understanding and compliance
	Other medications	Check for salt-retaining or myocardial-depressant properties
	Diet	Salt excess
Review of systems	Constitutional	? Weight gain (edema), weight loss (cardiac cachexia)
	Cardiovascular	See HPI
	Pulmonary	See PMH
	Gastrointestinal	See PMH
	Genitourinary	Symptoms underlying renal disease if hypertensive
	Endocrine	Symptoms of thyroid disease
	Hematologic	Symptoms of anemia

ting upright. PND is one of the most specific symptoms of left-sided heart failure.

Other respiratory symptoms that can accompany heart failure include cardiac asthma and Cheyne-Stokes respiration. Wheezing from cardiac asthma results, at least in part, from bronchial edema caused by transudated fluid. Patients who have bronchospasm for other reasons appear more susceptible to cardiac asthma. The symptoms of cardiac asthma are sometimes difficult to distinguish from those arising secondary to bronchial asthma or bronchitis. Cheyne-Stokes respiration (also called cyclic respiration) is recognized as periods of hyperpnea followed by periods of apnea. This abnormal pattern of breathing often occurs in patients with cerebral atherosclerosis and low cardiac output. Other items to emphasize in the history of the present illness deal directly with possible acute precipitating events. The ten most common precipitating events that lead to heart failure are listed in Table 4-2. These events should be considered in any patient with heart failure of unknown etiology. All patients who present with heart failure should have a complete cardiac history to uncover possible underlying cardiac disease. Current medications and diet should also be discussed. Patients frequently are confused concerning medication schedules and dietary restrictions, and compliance with medication regimens and/or dietary restrictions (e.g., salt) is often a problem.

B. **Physical examination.** Physical findings of heart failure are listed in Table 4-4. The overall condition of a patient in heart failure varies according to the degree of cardiac dysfunction present. Physical findings may be divided into two large categories: (i) findings within the cardiovascular system itself and (ii) findings in other organ systems resulting from heart failure.

1. **Cardiovascular findings in heart failure.** Gallop sounds are common in heart failure. A ventricular gallop (S3), which may be normal in some populations (children and young adults), is the result of a marked compliance change in the left ventricle. Left ventricular gallops are best heard at the apex with the bell of the stethoscope; right ventricular gallops are best heard in the subxiphoid region or over the right ventricle. Atrial gallops (S4) may also be heard in heart failure, although this finding is much less specific. A sustained left ventricular lift or evidence of cardiac enlargement (dilatation) may be discovered by palpation. A brisk

TABLE 4-4. PHYSICAL FINDINGS ASSOCIATED WITH HEART FAILURE

System	Finding	Significance
General	Patient position, level of distress	Can the patient comfortably lie flat?
Vital signs	Heart rate	? Anemia or thyrotoxicosis
	Blood pressure	? Hypertension
	Temperature	? Subacute bacterial endocarditis or other infection
	Respiratory rate	? Degree of pulmonary compromise
Skin	Peripheral cyanosis	Peripheral vasoconstriction
Cardiac/chest	Increased heart size	Ventricular dilatation
	Third heart sound (S3)	Hallmark of ventricular failure (except under age 35)
	Fourth heart sound (S4)	Frequently present but nonspecific
	Murmurs	Underlying valvular disease or acute valvular lesion
	Rales	Pulmonary edema
Peripheral vascular	Pulsus alternans	
	Elevated neck veins	Systemic venous hypertension
	Bruits	Evidence of atherosclerosis
Abdominal examination	Enlarged liver with hepatojugular reflux	Right-sided failure, elevated left ventricular filling pressures
	Ascites	? Cardiac or hepatic origin
Extremities	Peripheral edema	Check for symmetry (if unilateral, is peripheral venous disease present?)
Neuromuscular	Focal signs	Evidence of previous cerebrovascular accident or of atherosclerosis

but unsustained left ventricular lift is characteristic of patients with high-output failure (e.g., hyperthyroidism anemia). A more sustained lift is associated with hypertensive heart disease and aortic stenosis. Both systolic and diastolic murmurs can be heard in specific conditions. Neck veins should be examined for evidence of elevated central venous pressure. The presence of hepatojugular reflux should be ascertained because this finding has excellent correlation with elevation of the pulmonary capillary wedge (PCW) pressure.

2. Findings caused by the effect of heart failure on other organ systems. Pulmonary rales may be found at varying levels in both lung fields. Bronchial wheezing may be present on the basis of heart failure alone. Liver engorgement from right-sided heart failure may lead to tender hepatomegaly. Resultant liver dysfunction can eventually lead to jaundice and ascites. Transudation of fluid into the extracellular space may produce peripheral edema (particularly in dependent extremities) or pleural effusions. A patient who has been bedridden should be checked for sacral edema.

C. Laboratory tests. The diagnosis of heart failure is usually based on clinical criteria. Recently, elevated levels of brain natruretic peptide (BNP) have been observed in patients with CHF. The degree of elevation of plasma BNP levels correlates well with the severity of CHF. Because of these observations, some authorities have argued that a diagnosis of CHF should not be made unless the patient has an elevated plasma BNP level. Much work remains to be done in this arena, and consequently, most cardiologists are not ready to accept BNP determination as the gold standard for the diagnosis of CHF. Certain basic laboratory work should be performed in all patients with heart failure; other laboratory studies are made when specific diagnoses are suspected. All patients should have the following blood tests: complete blood cell count, electrolytes, blood urea nitrogen (BUN), creatinine, and urinalysis. Liver function tests may be added when hepatomegaly is present on examination, although the pattern of abnormality is likely to be nonspecific in hepatic congestion.

D. ECG. No ECG findings are specific for heart failure. An ECG should be obtained, however, to look for both signs of possible underlying cardiac disease (signs of ischemia, left ventricular hypertrophy, right ventricular hypertrophy, rhythm disturbances) and signs of acute precipitating events (QRS evidence of myocardial infarction; S1,Q3,T3 of pulmonary embolism). An initial ECG also provides baseline data for comparison with future ECGs.

E. Chest x-ray examination. Radiologic signs of heart failure are important, often subtle, and, in the early stages of CHF, frequently missed. The earliest radiographic sign of heart failure may be pulmonary venous hypertension caused by elevated left-sided filling pressures (pulmonary vascular redistribution, dilatation of the pulmonary artery). As pulmonary vascular pressure continues to rise, interstitial edema develops with thickening of interlobar fissures (in the lower lung fields, these are called Kerley B lines; similar longer lines in the upper and mid lung fields are termed Kerley A lines). Subpleural fluid and free pleural fluid also may accumulate at this stage. Any or all of these findings may precede the classic x-ray finding of the "butterfly" pattern of alveolar pulmonary edema.

F. Echocardiography. An echocardiographic study does make the diagnosis of CHF, despite the fact that ventricular dysfunction is observed. Clinical signs and symptoms must be present to make the clinical diagnosis of CHF. However, echocardiographic studies are extremely useful in patients with CHF because these studies help to establish the diagnosis of any underlying form of heart disease. Thus, echocardiography is helpful if valvular, congenital, or ischemic heart disease is thought to underlie heart failure. In addition, echocardiographic evaluation of left ventricular function may be determined serially to assess the effect of therapy.

G. Radionuclide studies. Radionuclide studies are often useful for detecting congenital defects, left ventricular wall motion abnormalities, and ventricular aneurysms, all of which may underlie heart failure (see Chapter 2).

H. Catheterization and angiography. Cardiac catheterization can aid in the diagnosis of heart failure. Hemodynamic measurements reveal elevated left and/or right ventricular filling pressures in patients with CHF. Angiography helps in defining heart disease that may be the cause of CHF, for example, critical coronary artery disease. Catheterization may also be used to help assess the therapeutic efficacy of various pharmacological agents used in patients with severe forms of heart failure.

I. Protocol for the diagnosis of heart failure

1. Confirmatory tests needed to make the diagnosis. The diagnosis is suggested by observation of a combination of the symptoms and signs previously discussed. Further support for the diagnosis of heart failure is derived from the demonstration of an underlying cardiac disease (Table 4-1). The protocol for establishing the diagnosis in each of the underlying cardiac diseases is outlined in appropriate chapters in this book. A general protocol for establishing the diagnosis of heart failure is outlined in Table 4-5.

2. Differential diagnosis. Other diseases that present with signs or symptoms mimicking those of heart failure are listed in Table 4-6.

a. Pulmonary disease. In some situations, the distinction between underlying cardiac or pulmonary disease in a dyspneic patient may be difficult to make. Diagnostic problems are further complicated when the diseases coexist. In general, dyspnea secondary to pulmonary disease develops more gradually than does dyspnea based on cardiac dysfunction. An important exception occurs when a patient with underlying pulmonary disease develops an acute pulmonary infection in which onset of dyspnea may be extremely rapid. Quantity and characteristics of sputum production must be assessed. Other signs of infection (fever, elevated white blood cell count, and left-shifted differential) should be sought. Patients with long-standing asthma or chronic bronchitis are more susceptible to wheezing and bronchoconstriction if left ventricular failure occurs (so-called cardiac asthma)

TABLE 4-5. PROTOCOL FOR ESTABLISHING THE DIAGNOSIS OF HEART FAILURE

A. All patients
1. History focuses on effort intolerance secondary to dyspnea/fatigue and on any previous manifestations of heart disease (see Table 4-3)
2. Physical examination, with emphasis on cardiovascular system and lungs (see Table 4-4)
3. Laboratory studies
   a. Initial blood tests CBC, electrolytes, BUN, creatinine, liver function studies
   b. Urinalysis
   c. PA and lateral chest x-ray examination
   d. 12-lead ECG (look for signs of underlying disease)

B. Selected patients (based on results of initial laboratory and clinical suspicion of specific underlying cardiac diseases)
1. Echocardiography (valvular disease, cardiomyopathy, congenital heart disease)
2. Blood cultures (subacute bacterial endocarditis)
3. Exercise test (coronary artery disease)
4. Lung scan (pulmonary embolism)
5. Cardiac catheterization (valvular disease; coronary artery disease)
6. Pulmonary angiography (pulmonary embolism)

CBC, complete blood cell count; BUN, blood urea nitrogen.

TABLE 4-6. CONDITIONS IN WHICH SIGNS AND SYMPTOMS MAY MIMIC THOSE OF HEART FAILURE

1. Noncardiac diseases presenting with dyspnea
   a. Chronic obstructive pulmonary disease
   b. Bronchial asthma
   c. Pulmonary infection

2. Noncardiac diseases presenting with peripheral edema
   a. Cyclic edema
   b. Peripheral venous disease
   c. Leg trauma
   d. Renal disease
   e. Cirrhosis
   f. Drug-induced edema, e.g., dihydroperidine calcium channel blockers

compared with patients without pulmonary disease. Cardiac asthma generally produces more diaphoresis and cyanosis than does a primary asthmatic attacks; however, the distinction is often hard to draw. After resolution of the acute process, pulmonary function studies may help define the extent of underlying lung dysfunction.

 b. Noncardiac causes of peripheral edema. Occasionally, confusion arises over the etiology of ankle edema. Although cyclic edema and peripheral venous disease may cause ankle swelling, dyspnea and increased systemic venous pressure will be absent. Careful chest and neck vein examination should resolve any question. It is important to check for peripheral edema bilaterally to rule out unilateral edema from venous blockage or trauma.

 c. Other noncardiac causes of edema. The possibility of renal dysfunction as the cause of underlying edema may be suggested by a history of renal disease.

  Initial blood studies (BUN, creatinine, calcium, phosphate, and total protein) and urinalysis (proteinuria, hematuria, casts) will help confirm or exclude renal disease. Edema from cirrhosis may be suggested by history (alcoholism), physical examination (jaundice, spider angiomas, other peripheral stigmata of liver disease), and laboratory studies (total and direct bilirubin, serum glutamic oxaloacetic transaminase, lactic acid dehydrogenase, alkaline phosphatase levels).

III. Therapy. There are three major aspects of the treatment of heart failure: (i) management of the acute or chronic condition, (ii) treatment of any underlying cardiac disease, and (iii) treatment of any precipitating factor. The treatment of cardiac diseases that can cause heart failure (Table 4-1) is discussed in chapters on each disease. Precipitating causes of heart failure (Table 4-2) should be corrected. For example, patients with hematocrits less than 30% should receive blood transfusions of packed red blood cells and diuretics; individuals with pneumonia should receive appropriate antibiotics, etc.

 A. Medical therapy. Medical modalities for the treatment of heart failure seek to improve overall cardiac function while removing excess salt and water that has accumulated. The classic view of ventricular function is summarized in the Frank-Starling relationship between cardiac muscle fiber length and strength of contraction (Fig. 4.1).

  The hearts of patients with heart failure operate on depressed ventricular function curves or from a disadvantageous position on a normal function curve. A number of interventions can improve ventricular function.

  Inotropic agents augment myocardial contractility and establish a more favorable function curve. Sympathomimetic agents such as dopamine and

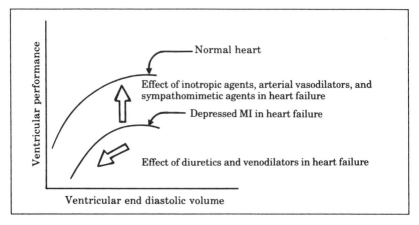

FIG. 4-1. Schematic Frank-Starling curves for patients with heart failure indicating the effect of therapy.

dobutamine may act through both inotropic augmentation and afterload reduction. Arterial vasodilators allow the dysfunctioning heart to operate on a more normal Starling curve. Diuretics and venodilators (e.g., nitrates) act by reducing central blood volume and hence cardiac dilatation, thus achieving a more favorable position on the same ventricular function curve. Three basic types of pharmacologic therapy are available to improve ventricular function in heart failure: (i) agents that decrease excessive retention of fluid (move to the left on the Frank-Starling curve), (ii) agents that augment myocardial contraction (establishment of new Starling curve), and (iii) agents that decrease cardiac work load.

1. Decrease of excessive fluid retention. Diuretics are the main treatment for fluid retention. In general, these agents should be used in conjunction with vasodilators and, at times, digitalis along with modifications in dietary salt intake and activity.

    The choice of diuretic or combination of diuretics used in heart failure depends largely on the severity of the clinical situation. If fluid retention is mild, no treatment or an oral diuretic is used. When used alone, potassium-sparing diuretics (spironolactone and triamterene) generally are less effective than are thiazides; however, these two agents potentiate other diuretics (furosemide and ethacrynic acid) and are thus effective when used in combination with other agents. Spironolactone is particularly advantageous in this regard because it has been shown to reduce mortality in patients with CHF. The loop diuretics (furosemide and ethacrynic acid) are the agents of choice in severe heart failure. A general approach to the use of diuretics in heart failure is outlined in Table 4-7. Dietary and activity recommendations are discussed in later sections.

    a. Spironolactone (Aldactone). The addition of spironolactone to thiazide or loop diuretics has been a long-standing recommendation for patients with severe CHF. In recent years, multicenter trials have demonstrated decreased morbidity and mortality when spironolactone is used in patients with CHF. Consequently, 25 to 50 mg of spironolactone once or twice per day is now commonly prescribed for patients with moderate or severe CHF. Careful monitoring of renal function and electrolytes is required since these patients are commonly also treated with angiotensin-converting enzyme (ACE) inhibition or angiotensin receptor blockade. The combination of blockade of the renin angiotensin system together with spironolactone can result in renal insufficiency and/or life-threatening hyperkalemia.

TABLE 4-7. APPROACH TO DIURETIC THERAPY IN HEART FAILURE

| Degree of heart failure | Drug | | Dosage | Route of administration | Possible supplemental therapy | Side effects/ contraindications |
	Generic name	Trade name				
Mild (NYHA class I)	Chlorothiazide	Diuril	500 mg qd	PO	KCl or high-potassium diet	Potassium depletion Arrhythmias (with or without digitalis)
	or Hydrochlorothiazide	Hydrodiuril	500 mg qd	PO	KCl or high-potassium diet	Potassium depletion
	or Chlorthalidone	Hygroton	50–100 mg qod or 5 days/wk	PO	KCl or high-potassium diet	Arrhythmias (with or without digitalis)
	or Indapamide	Lozol	2.5–5 mg qd	PO	KCl or high-potassium diet	Same as chlorothiazide
	or Metolazone	Zaroxolyn	5–20 mg qd	PO	KCl or high-potassium diet	Same as chlorothiazide; also pancreatitis, aplastic anemia
Moderate (NYHA class II)	Chlorthalidone	Hygroton	100 mg/day	PO	KCl or high-potassium diet	Potassium depletion
	or Hydrochlorothiazide	Hydrodiuril	50 mg bid	PO	KCl or high-potassium diet	Arrhythmias (with or without digitalis)
	or Furosemide	Lasix	40–80 mg qd	PO	KCl or high-potassium diet	Potassium depletion Arrhythmias (with or without digitalis)

(continued)

TABLE 4-7. *(Continued)*

Degree of heart failure	Drug		Dosage	Route of administration	Possible supplemental therapy	Side effects/contraindications
	Generic name	Trade name				
	or Bumetanide	Bumex	0.5–2 mg qd	PO	KCl or high-potassium diet	Same as furosemide
	or Torsemide	Demadex	10–20 mg qd	PO	KCl or high-potassium diet	Same as furosemide
	or Indapamide	Lozol	2.5–5 mg qd	PO	KCl or high-potassium diet	Same as chlorothiazide
	or Metolazone	Zaroxolyn	5–20 mg qd	PO	KCl or high-potassium diet	Same as chlorothiazide; also pancreatitis, aplastic anemia
Severe (NYHA class III or IV)	Furosemide	Lasix	40–120 mg qd or bid	PO	Potassium supplementation (as above)	Hypokalemia Hypovolemia with or without hypertension
	or Ethacrynic acid	Edecrin	50–100 mg qd	PO	Hydrochlorothiazide Chlorothiazide	Hypokalemia Hypovolemia with or without hypotension
	or Bumetanide	Bumex	0.5–2 mg qd	PO	KCl or high-potassium diet	Same as furosemide

Condition	Drug	Brand	Dose	Route	Add-on	Side effects
	or Bumetanide	Bumex	0.5–1.0 mg (up to 10 mg per day)	IV, IM	Thiazide diuretic	Same as furosemide
	or Torsemide	Demadex	10–20 mg (up to 200 mg per day)	IV	Thiazide diuretic	Same as furosemide
Cor pulmonale	Furosemide	Lasix	40–120 mg qd	PO	KCl	Contraction alkalosis Potassium depletion
Refractory heart failure	Furosemide	Lasix	40–120 mg qd or more	IV	Chlorothiazide, 500 mg IV, may be added if needed	Hypovolemia with or without hypotension Hypokalemia
	or Bumetanide	Bumex	0.5–1.0 mg (up to 10 mg per day)	IV, IM	Thiazide diuretic	Same as furosemide
	or Torsemide	Demadex	10–20 mg (up to 200 mg per day)	IV	Thiazide diuretic	Same as furosemide
	Spironolactone	Aldactone	25–50 mg bid	PO	—	Renal failure, agranulocytosis, gynecomastia

NYHA, New York Heart Association.

2. Decrease of cardiac workload. Vasodilators reduce the impedance (resistance) against which the heart must pump. Although diuretics reduce the preload of the heart and digitalis augments contractility, vasodilators reduce afterload by direct action on the peripheral vascular bed. These agents have been demonstrated to reduce mortality and morbidity in a variety of acute heart failure and CHF states. Specific drugs, dosages, side effects, and contraindications are given in Table 4-8. Vasodilator therapy can be lifesaving in patients with severe, acute heart failure and pulmonary edema secondary to cardiomyopathy or ischemic heart disease. Improvement in cardiac output and relief of congestion may ameliorate dyspnea and cause significant diuresis. Careful monitoring to avoid hypotension is essential in these fragile patients.

Beta-blockers (see below) also decrease cardiac work and can lead to remarkable clinical improvement. Patients with CHF who are treated with long-term beta-blockade often demonstrate remarkable improvement in measured left ventricular function. A number of multicenter trials have demonstrated decreased mortality and morbidity in patients with CHF who are treated with beta-blockers.

a. Vasodilator therapy in chronic heart failure. In many patients with CHF, a diagnostic workup including cardiac catheterization demonstrates underlying or precipitating conditions that are not remediable by either specific medical or surgical intervention. These patients can often derive substantial benefit (reduced mortality and morbidity) from therapy that includes vasodilatation with ACE inhibitors or angiotensin receptor blockers, as well as weight loss, sodium-restricted diets, diuretics, beta-blockers, and, at times, digitalis. The combination of nitrates and hydralazine is also effective in this setting, but it is not as efficacious as ACE inhibition or angiotensin receptor blockade (Table 4-8).

b. Vasodilator therapy in acute heart failure. A variety of vasodilators have been shown to have beneficial effects in patients with acute heart failure. Both arterial and venous vasodilators are effective. Intravenous vasodilatation with nitroprusside is particularly beneficial in patients with volume overload states, for example, mitral and/or aortic regurgitation. Intravenous forms of ACE inhibitors are also available for this indication. Nitroglycerin and other nitrates fall into the general class of drugs that dilate small venules and thereby increase venous capacitance (venodilators). This reduces central blood volume and cardiac dilatation and results in a reduction in preload and a fall in PCW pressure and left ventricular end diastolic pressure. This is, in effect, an anatomic "diuresis," that allows the ventricle to function on a more favorable point on the Starling curve. Because nitrates also dilate coronary collateral blood vessels, they are particularly useful in patients with acute heart failure secondary to ischemic heart disease. Intravenous nitroglycerin is frequently used in this setting.

c. Beta-blockade. Beta-blockers have been shown to reduce mortality and morbidity in patients with CHF. Even patients with severe CHF can benefit from these agents. Patients treated with long-term beta-blockade demonstrate improvement in left ventricular ejection fraction after a number of months of therapy. It is essential that beta-blocker therapy commence with very small doses, for example, 12.5 mg of metoprolol twice a day or 3.25 mg of carvedilol twice a day. Dosage is slowly advanced as tolerated over a number of weeks, aiming for 50 mg of metoprolol bid or 25 mg of carvedilol twice a day. During this up-titration, it may be necessary to increase the dose of diuretics because some patients experience increased fluid retention at this time.

3. Augmentation of myocardial contraction. Three types of medication are available to augment myocardial contraction: digitalis preparations,

TABLE 4-8. VASODILATOR THERAPY IN HEART FAILURE

Drug					
Generic name	Trade name	Mechanism of action	Route of administration	Average dose	Side Effects/contraindications	Comments
Isosorbide dinitrate	Isordil	Primarily venodilation	SL PO	5–10 mg q4–6h 20–40 mg q6h	Severe postural hypotension, severe anemia, headache, dizziness, weakness	Particularly efficacious for extending inpatient vasodilator therapy into outpatient setting
Nitroglycerin ointment	Nitropaste, Nitrobid ointment		Cutaneous	1–2 in. q6h	Postural hypotension	
Isosorbide mononitrate	Ismo, Imdur Monoket	Same as isosorbide dinitrate	PO	20 mg bid	Same as isosorbide dinitrate	Same as isosorbide dinitrate
Nitroglycerin (slow release)	Nitro-Bid	Same as isosorbide dinitrate	PO	2.5–9 mg bid	Same as isosorbide dinitrate	Same as isosorbide dinitrate
Hydralazine	Apresoline	Arterial wall relaxation	PO	25–100 mg tid or qid	Headache, tachycardia, dose-dependent SLE (dosage >50 mg qid)	Carefully monitor heart rate, blood pressure, and baseline ANA
Nitroprusside	Nitropress	Primarily arteriolar vasodilation	IV infusion	0.5–8 µ/kg	Nausea, vomiting, restlessness, headache, palpitations, hypotension, thiocyanate toxicity (dose dependent)	Must be diluted in 5% D/W and administered through an infusion pump
Captopril	Capoten	Blocks conversion of angiotensin I to angiotensin II causing arteriolar vasodilation	PO	25–150 mg q8h	Hypotension, impaired renal function, occasionally nephrotic syndrome	Initial doses should be 12.5 mg q8h; may cause favorable redistribution of blood as well as vasodilation *(continued)*

TABLE 4-8. (*Continued*)

Drug						
Generic name	Trade name	Mechanism of action	Route of administration	Average dose	Side Effects/ contraindications	Comments
Enalapril	Vasotec	Same as captopril	PO	5–20 mg q12h or qd	Same as captopril	Initial dosage is 2.5 mg PO bid or 5 mg PO qd
Quinipril	Accupril	Same as captopril	PO	5–20 mg bid	Same as captopril	Start with low dose and increase gradually
Perindopril	Aceon	Same as captopril	PO	4–16 mg qd	Same as captopril	Start with low dose and increase gradually
Ramipril	Altace	Same as captopril	PO	5 mg bid	Same as captopril	Start with low dose and increase gradually
Benazepril	Lotensin	Same as captopril	PO	5–20 mg qd	Same as captopril	Start with low dose and increase gradually
Trandolapril	Mavik	Same as captopril	PO	1–4 mg po qd	Same as captopril	Start with low dose and increase gradually
Fosinopril	Monopril	Same as captopril	PO	10–40 mg qd	Same as captopril	Start with low dose and increase gradually

Lisinopril	Zestril, Prinivil	Same as captopril	PO	5–40 mg qd	Same as captopril	Start with low dose and increase gradually
Moexipril	Univasc	Same as captopril	PO	7.5–30 mg qd	Same as captopril	Start with low dose and increase gradually
Losartan	Cozaar	Blocks angiotensin receptor	PO	25–100 mg qd	Angioedema, hypotension, renal failure	Start with low dose and increase dose gradually
Candesartan	Atacand	Same as losartan	PO	2–32 mg qd	Same as losartan	Same as losartan
Irbesartan	Avapro	Same as losartan	PO	75–300 mg qd	Same as losartan	Same as losartan
Valsartan	Diovan	Same as losartan	PO	80–320 mg qd	Same as losartan	Same as losartan
Telmisartan	Micardis	Same as losartan	PO	20–80 mg qd	Same as losartan	Same as losartan
Eprosartan	Teveten	Same as losartan	PO	600–800 mg qd	Same as losartan	Same as losartan

SL, sublingual; SLE, systematic lupus erythematosus; ANA, antinuclear antibody titer; D/W, dextrose in water.

other inotropic agents (amrinone, milrinone), and certain sympatho-mimetic agents (dopamine, dobutamine). Although amrinone, milrinone, and the sympathomimetic agents also have some vasodilating properties, their primary role is to augment myocardial contraction, and they will be discussed in this section.

  a. Digitalis. Digitalis increases the contractility of the failing heart (establishes a more advantageous Frank-Starling curve) and increases cardiac output. The multicenter DIG trial (The Digitalis Investigation Group; see Suggested Reading) found that digoxin therapy did not increase or decrease mortality during long-term follow-up in patients with CHF. Hospitalization for heart failure was reduced by digoxin therapy. Digoxin is not as efficacious as vasodilators and diuretics, and hence, it has become a third-line drug for the management of CHF.

  The following precautions should be observed before digitalis is administered to a patient: (i) a detailed history should be sought. In addition to the history of cardiac disease and possible precipitating events already discussed, a history of previous use of digitalis is important. Any adverse reaction to previous administration should be carefully explored. History of any renal, pulmonary, hepatic, or thyroid disease also should be ascertained. Knowledge of other current medications is essential, because many medicines interfere with gastrointestinal absorption of digitalis (e.g., antacids, cholestyramine). Concomitant administration of amiodarone or verapamil and digitalis results in higher serum levels (and increased evidence of toxicity) of digitalis than when glycoside is administered alone. (ii) Certain laboratory procedures should be undertaken. Serum electrolytes, creatinine, and BUN should be drawn before digitalis is administered, and electrolyte abnormalities should be corrected. A 12-lead control ECG is essential, because once digitalis has been administered, ischemic changes may be impossible to distinguish from digitalis effects. Serum digitalis levels may be helpful; low levels suggest poor compliance or inadequate gastrointestinal absorption.

  (1) Protocol for administration of digitalis. Various methods have been developed for determining the proper initial dose of digitalis and the appropriate ongoing maintenance dosage. The following general considerations apply: (i) modern physicians only use one digitalis preparation, digoxin. (ii) When rapid digitalization is desired, in an average-sized patient with no body stores of digitalis and normal renal function, 1 mg of oral digoxin over 24 hours in divided doses is recommended. Maintenance dosage for this patient would be 0.125 mg per day by mouth. (iii) When it is not essential to achieve rapid digitalization, the process can be accomplished by a daily maintenance dose without a loading dose. In average-sized patients with normal renal function, 0.125 mg of digoxin per day will allow digitalization within 1 week. (iv) In patients with impaired renal function, the amount of digitalis administered must be appropriately reduced. Calculating creatinine clearance in addition to obtaining serum creatinine may be helpful in this situation.

  It is important to remember that other medications may influence the pharmacokinetics of digitalis preparations. Cholestyramine, neomycin, nonabsorbable antacids, and Kaopectate may all decrease absorption of oral digoxin. Quinidine has been shown to decrease both renal and nonrenal elimination of digoxin and to decrease its apparent volume of distribution. When conventional dosages of quinidine are administered, serum digoxin concentrations average a two-fold increase. Thus, digoxin dosage must be reduced appropriately if quinidine is added. Amiodarone, flecainide, and verapamil administration can also raise serum digoxin levels. Thus, when any of these antiarrhythmic agents is introduced, digoxin levels must be closely monitored and dosages adjusted accordingly.

Numerous ECG changes can occur during therapy with digitalis: lengthening of the P–R interval, shortening of the Q–T interval, depression or "scooping" of the S–T segment (or both), and flattening or inversion of T waves.

(a) Digitalis intoxication. Both noncardiac and cardiac signs of digitalis toxicity may occur. Early noncardiac symptoms include visual changes (yellow vision, blurred vision, diplopia), gastrointestinal complaints (anorexia, nausea, vomiting), and neurologic manifestations (headache, lethargy).

Cardiac evidence of digitalis toxicity may precede noncardiac symptoms. The chief cardiac manifestation is arrhythmia. Almost every cardiac arrhythmia may be provoked by digitalis intoxication except for atrial flutter. Digitalis levels, when available, may assist in the diagnosis of digitalis toxicity. The diagnosis, however, remains clinical and electrocardiographic.

To treat digitalis-induced arrhythmias one should (i) stop digitalis, (ii) measure serum electrolyte levels and correct any abnormalities (particularly hypokalemia), and (iii) if the arrhythmias associated with an episode of digitalis toxicity are serious, administer specific antiarrhythmic drug therapy, for example, intravenous (IV) lidocaine or betablockers for malignant ventricular arrhythmias (see Chapter 3 on arrhythmias). When large doses of digoxin are ingested during a suicide attempt, severe digitalis toxicity and life-threatening hyperkalemia often develops. The appropriate therapy in this situation is IV monoclonal antidigitalis antibodies (e.g., Digibind). Clinical information on digoxin is found in Table 4-9.

b. Other inotropic agents. IV amrinone and milrinone are positive inotropes and peripheral vasodilators. They cause dose-dependent reductions in both left- and right-heart filling pressures and increases in cardiac output. Systemic and pulmonary vascular resistance are decreased. Amrinone's hemodynamic effects are similar to a combination of dobutamine and nitroprusside. The drug acts synergistically with digoxin and sympathomimetics. Amrinone is useful in patients with heart failure that has been refractory to digoxin, diuretics, and vasodilators. Amrinone is administered with an initial IV bolus of 0.75 mg/kg followed by a continuous infusion of 5 to 10 mcg/kg per minute. Hypotension may be a limiting factor in patients already on a vasodilator. Amrinone is particularly effective in patients with reversible myocardial depression after cardiac surgery and after acute myocardial infarction. Tolerance, a potential problem with combination therapy with dobutamine and nitroprusside, does not appear to occur with amrinone.

c. Sympathomimetic amines. A variety of investigations has assessed the utility of sympathomimetic amines and catecholamines in the treatment of heart failure. Investigations using isoproterenol, epinephrine, and norepinephrine have largely failed because of adverse hemodynamic consequences associated with these medicines, such as tachycardia and peripheral vasodilatation or vasoconstriction. Two other sympathomimetic amines—dopamine and dobutamine—have fewer undesirable hemodynamic side effects and are useful in the management of heart failure.

(1) Dopamine (Intropin). Dopamine is an endogenous catecholamine that is the precursor of norepinephrine. It has beta$_1$ (cardiac

TABLE 4-9. DIGOXIN

| Agent | Gastrointestinal absorption | Onset of action[a] | Peak effect | Average half-life[b] | Principal metabolic route (excretory pathway) | Average digitalizing dose | | Usual daily oral maintenance dose[e] |
						Oral[c]	Intravenous[d]	
Digoxin	60%–85%	15–30 min	1.5–5 hr	36 hr	Renal; some gastrointestinal excretion	1.25–1.5 mg	0.75–1.0 mg	0.25–0.5 mg

[a]For intravenous dose.
[b]For healthy subjects (prolonged by renal impairment).
[c]Divided doses over 12–24 hr q6–8h.
[d]Given in increments for initial subcomplete digitalization to be supplemented by further small increments as necessary.
[e]Average for adult patients without renal or hepatic impairment; will vary widely among individual patients and requires close medical supervision.

stimulatory) activity, alpha activity (peripheral vasoconstricting), and an independent vasodilatory effect (at low dosages) on the renal and mesenteric vascular beds. At low dosages (less than 5 mcg/kg per minute) the $beta_1$ and renal vasodilatory effects predominate. At dosages between 5 and 10 mcg/kg per minute, both alpha and beta stimulation occur. At dosages greater than 10 mcg/kg per minute, alpha peripheral constriction predominates. In decompensated or acute heart failure, dopamine in low dosages (less than 5 mcg/kg per minute) may exert favorable hemodynamic actions by increasing both cardiac output and renal blood flow, thereby promoting a diuresis.

(2) Dobutamine (Dobutrex). Dobutamine is a synthetic sympathomimetic amine with $beta_1$ (cardiac stimulatory), $beta_2$ (peripheral vasodilatory), and minimal $alpha_1$ (vasoconstricting) effects.

In decompensated heart failure, dobutamine in IV dosages up to 10 mcg/kg per minute exerts favorable hemodynamic effects by improving cardiac output and decreasing PCW pressure and congestive symptoms. Dobutamine is particularly valuable in patients with severe heart failure and an elevated PCW and normal systemic blood pressure.

(3) Dobutamine versus dopamine. A number of trials have compared dopamine and dobutamine in severe or acutely decompensated heart failure. Both medications will successfully improve cardiac output; however, dobutamine appears more effective in lowering filling pressures and in reducing congestive symptoms. Dopamine may be more effective when the patient is hypotensive or when its independent renal effects are desired. The choice between these two medications ultimately will hinge on the clinical situation in each patient. These medications have been successfully used together with vasodilators for refractory heart failure.

(4) Combination sympathomimetic amine and vasodilator therapy for refractory heart failure. Refractory heart failure is said to be present when deterioration in the patient's condition occurs despite intensive therapy (see Section **III.C.3.d.**).

Some individuals with such severe heart failure will benefit from hospitalization in the intensive or coronary care unit and from therapy with a combination of a sympathomimetic amine and a vasodilator. A typical combination is IV dobutamine and nitroprusside, although the combination of dopamine and nitroprusside has been used as well.

4. Long-term pharmacologic treatment of severe heart failure. As noted earlier, patients with heart failure should receive ACE inhibitors and beta-blockers if tolerated. Other vasodilators such as angiotensin receptor blockers or hydralazine/nitrate combinations can be used if the patient does not tolerate ACE inhibitors, for example, because of chronic cough.

A number of large trials have demonstrated that daily aspirin decreases long-term morbidity and mortality in patients with CHF. The exact dose of aspirin has not been well studied, but most investigators use 160 to 325 mg per day.

5. Activity. Appropriate restriction of physical activity remains a central therapeutic tool in heart failure. For the patient with mild heart failure, slight reduction in cardiac work load (such as resting on weekends, taking a nap in the middle of the day, or slightly reducing the work week) may allow continued gainful employment. In the patient with severe heart failure, periods of bed rest and an overall diminution in activity are essential to lessen cardiac work. In the acute setting of symptomatic heart failure, 1 to 2 weeks of significantly reduced activity is often necessary.

Note that bed rest, particularly in elderly patients, increases the risk of venous thrombosis and pulmonary embolism. Patients are allowed up two or three times daily and are encouraged to remain ambulatory. Once medical therapy has stabilized the patient with CHF, a gentle and progressive exercise program can be beneficial. Such exercise programs are most successful when careful supervision (i.e., a formal cardiac rehabilitation program) is available.

6. Diet. Dietary therapy has two aims in the treatment of heart failure. First, any patient who is overweight should be encouraged to lose weight and is given specific advice and guidance on caloric restriction. Weight reduction lowers the demand on the heart and often results in significant symptomatic relief. Second, sodium restriction remains an important component of therapy in heart failure. For the patient with severe heart failure, rigid sodium restriction is essential.

The average daily American diet in the absence of sodium restriction contains 8 to 15 g of salt (1 level teaspoon contains 6 g of salt). A reduction to 4 to 7 g per day can be accomplished by removing the salt shaker from the table. A further reduction to 3 to 4 g can be achieved by restricting salt addition during cooking. Reduction in sodium intake is further accomplished by eliminating high-salt–containing foods from the diet. Foods to be avoided include canned vegetables and soups, as well as processed cheeses, breads, and cereals. Allowable foods include fresh produce, specially processed bread, low-sodium milk, and salt substitutes. Because it is difficult to make a severely sodium-restricted diet palatable, compliance with these regimens is frequently a problem.

7. Environment and psychological support. Emotional rest is as important as reduced physical activity for the heart failure patient. Both lessen cardiac work load. Efforts should be made to lower the patient's level of anxiety. In the setting of acute heart failure, mild sedation with a benzodiazepine may be helpful in addition to calm reassurance. The use of morphine in acute pulmonary edema is important not only as a pulmonary vasodilator but also as a sedative to relieve anxiety (see Chapter 5). Long-term psychological support is essential to the patient with heart failure who must face the issues of reduced activity, chronic medication, and a restricted, often unpalatable, diet.

B. Surgical treatment. The treatment of CHF can often be managed with medicines, diet, and limitation of activity. In certain situations, however, surgical intervention and/or device implantation is the treatment of choice.

1. Cardiac transplantation. The technical capability to perform cardiac transplantation has been available since the late 1960s. High mortality caused by rejection of grafted hearts caused this option to fall into disfavor in the 1970s.

Major advances in the immunologic management of the cardiac transplantation patient has made this a very viable option for some patients with intractable heart failure. At Stanford University after its first 250 heart transplantations, a 1-year survival rate of 82% was reported. Over half the patients operated on at Stanford had myocardial dysfunction based on coronary artery disease; most of the rest had cardiomyopathy from other causes. At the University of Arizona, 1-year survival rates of 90% have been observed. The most important pharmacologic agent for suppressing rejection in transplant patients appears to be cyclosporin A. The transplanted heart lacks normal autonomic innervation; however, it will respond to circulating catecholamines that allow cardiac output to rise during exercise. A small percentage of patients develop reinnervation of the heart with time. These individuals will have a normal increase in heart rate during exercise. Functional rehabilitation is possible in more than 90% of patients successfully transplanted. Currently, cardiac transplantation is performed in many United States centers with considerable success.

2. Circulatory assist devices. The intraaortic balloon pump is the most commonly used mechanical circulatory assist device. The intraaortic balloon pump is often successful in stabilizing patients with acute CHF while appropriate medical and/or surgical therapy is instituted. In addition, both temporary and permanent left and/or right ventricular assist devices are being implanted in many cardiac surgical centers in the United States. The power source for these pumps is external to the patient, requiring a chronic transthoracic connection. These indwelling power connections can be a site for serious infections. Some technical problems remain, for example, embolized thrombus from the pump itself, but advances continue in this area. Completely self-sustaining, implantable devices are available, and early clinical work with these high technology instruments has been encouraging.

3. Other indications for surgical intervention in heart failure. Pulmonary embolism can be treated by means of embolectomy and/or inferior vena caval interruption or filtration (see Chapter 22). Surgical treatment may be lifesaving when heart failure is precipitated by acute dysfunction of a cardiac valve (ruptured chordae tendineae or acute bacterial endocarditis).

   When coronary artery disease with acute ischemic myocardial dysfunction underlies heart failure, coronary bypass surgery is beneficial. Surgical correction is also the treatment of choice in most forms of congenital heart disease complicated by CHF. When left ventricular aneurysm causes heart failure, aneurysmectomy may be necessary. Finally, for patients with chronic CHF caused by an underlying cardiomyopathy, cardiac transplantation should be considered (see above).

4. Biventricular pacing. Patient with severe heart failure and left bundle branch block or intraventricular conduction delay with a very wide QRS complex (greater than 0.12 second) should be considered for biventricular pacing therapy. These patients have dis-coordinated ventricular contraction as a result of the marked conduction disturbance. A pacing catheter is placed in the distal coronary sinus. Pacing from this site captures the left ventricle. A second pacing catheter is placed at the apex of the right ventricle. A special biventricular pacemaker induces a more coordinated contraction of the left and right ventricles. This has been shown to increase cardiac output and decrease symptoms in patients with severe CHF.

C. Protocols for treatment of heart failure
   1. Medical management of mild heart failure
      a. Perform initial history, physical examination, and screening laboratory tests with particular emphasis on the cardiovascular system. Look for possible underlying cardiac disease or precipitating causes of heart failure (Tables 4-1 and 4-2).
      b. Perform additional laboratory investigations to establish the diagnosis of a specific underlying or precipitating cause of heart failure, for example, echocardiography and/or coronary angiography.
      c. While the diagnostic workup is in progress, begin symptomatic treatment:
         (1) Diuresis. Initiate a gentle diuresis with oral diuretics at modest dosages, for example, furosemide 20 mg every day in the morning. Monitor electrolytes and renal function.
         (2) ACE inhibitors. Place the patient on modest to moderate doses of an ACE inhibitor if tolerated (Table 4-8). If side effects are a problem with ACE inhibition, for example, chronic cough, try modest to moderate doses of an angiotensin receptor blocker (Table 4-8).
         (3) Beta-blockers. Consider starting the patient on beta-blockade, using small doses initially.

(4) Diet. Remove salt from table and eliminate foods with high sodium content from diet. Advise weight reduction if obesity is present.

(5) Activity. Establish a plan with the patient for appropriate temporary reduction in activity. Suggest that the patient purchase a scale and record daily weights and that the patient inform you of sudden weight gain of 3 lbs or more.

(6) At follow-up appointment in 2 to 4 weeks, check blood pressure, signs of CHF, renal function, and electrolyte levels; obtain an ECG if ischemic heart disease was the underlying cause for CHF.

2. Medical management of moderate heart failure

   a. History, physical examination, initial screening, and additional laboratory investigations looking for underlying and precipitating causes of heart failure; similar to evaluation for mild CHF.

   b. Treat symptoms of heart failure while diagnostic workup is in progress.

      (1) Vasodilators. Place patient on an ACE inhibitor. Gradually increase the dose; monitor blood pressure, electrolytes, and renal function. If the patient cannot tolerate ACE inhibition, try an angiotensin receptor blocker, for example, losartan 50 mg every day. Place the patient on **aspirin**, 325 mg per day (Table 4-8).

      (2) Diuresis. Administer full dose furosemide orally (40 mg every day in the morning). A single IV dose may be given to the patient in the office setting to initiate therapy. Daily oral potassium supplementation is often required; however, care must be taken if ACE inhibitors or spironolactone are also prescribed since hyperkalemia may result if excess potassium supplementation is given in the face of ACE inhibition/spironolactone.

      (3) Beta-blockers. Initiate beta-blockade with small doses. Increase the dose slowly. Increased diuresis may be required when beta-blockade is initiated.

      (4) Digitalis. If the patient remains symptomatic, add 0.125 mg PO of digoxin per day.

      (5) Aldactone. If the patient remains symptomatic, add spironolactone 25 once or twice per day. Follow renal function and electrolytes carefully, particularly if ACE inhibitors and/or potassium supplementation have already been prescribed.

      (6) Diet. Specify no table salt, no high—sodium-content foods, and no salt in cooking. Advise weight reduction if obesity is present.

      (7) Activity. Make clear that definite activity reduction is needed, with periodic time for rest. Control work stress and avoid strenuous lifting or other forms of isometric exercise. Suggest that the patient purchase a scale and record daily weights. Inform the physician of any sudden weight gain of 3 lbs or more.

      (8) At return appointment in 2 weeks, check blood pressure, electrolytes, BUN, and creatinine levels and examine the patient for signs of CHF. Obtain an ECG if ischemic left ventricular dysfunction was the cause of CHF. If no symptomatic improvement is found, consider increase of ACE inhibitor and diuretic doses. Monitor renal function and electrolytes following the increase in therapy. Beware of hyperkalemia and renal insufficiency that may result from the combination of ACE inhibitors, potassium supplements, and spironolactone. Slowly increase the dose of beta-blocker over many weeks.

3. Medical management of severe heart failure

   a. Acute heart failure

      (1) Hospitalize.

      (2) Institute investigative efforts to **determine precipitating cause**.

(3) Treat symptomatically while diagnostic workup is in progress. Symptomatic treatment must be based on the best available evidence of the precipitating cause of acute heart failure: (i) diuretic, IV furosemide (Table 4-7); (ii) vasodilator therapy (e.g., IV nitroprusside, Table 4-8 for details; administration of IV vasodilators **may** require admission to the intensive care unit for arterial blood pressure monitoring); and (iii) sympathomimetic amines (dopamine or dobutamine). Consider addition of amrinone if the combination of diuretic, positive inotrope (dobutamine or dopamine), and vasodilator does not achieve the desired result.

(4) Diet. Nothing by mouth during acute episode.

(5) Activity. Bed rest with head of bed elevated.

b. Acute pulmonary edema. See Chapter 5 on pulmonary edema.

c. Chronic severe heart failure. Search for underlying etiology as in mild and moderate CHF protocol. Institute symptomatic treatment with IV furosemide and oral ACE inhibition, beta-blockade, and spironolactone. Monitor renal function and electrolytes frequently. Add oral digoxin 0.125 mg every day if the patient remains symptomatic.

(1) Diuretics. If the patient remains symptomatic despite therapy with IV furosemide, add a daily dose of a thiazide diuretic to the already prescribed dose of furosemide. Increase furosemide dosage to 80 or more mg once or even twice per day as needed to control symptoms and weight gain. (Table 4-7; monitor electrolyte levels closely.) Add spironolactone 25 mg once or twice a day if not already initiated. Note that monitoring of potassium is essential when this regimen is used concurrently with digitalis.

(2) Vasodilator therapy. Monitor blood pressure carefully while titrating upward on ACE inhibitor dosage. Unless contraindicated, place patients on one **aspirin** (325 mg) per day

(3) Diet. Restrict sodium as severely as the patient can tolerate. Advise weight reduction as needed in obese patients.

(4) Activity. Call for significant reduction, with daily rest periods. Suggest a formal exercise program with supervision (e.g., a cardiac rehabilitation program). Suggest that the patient purchase a scale and record daily weights. Inform the physician of any sudden weight gain of 3 lbs or more.

d. Refractory heart failure. If heart failure persists despite an intensive search for remediable underlying or precipitating cause and intensive symptomatic therapy, refractory heart failure is said to exist.

(1) Carefully review treatment to date. Have any possible precipitants been overlooked? Is patient complying with the therapeutic regimen?

(2) Repeat selected tests, for example, echocardiography and catheterization.

(3) Hospitalize the patient in an intensive or coronary care unit for IV therapy with nitroprusside alone or in combination with dopamine or dobutamine.

(4) Consider a trial of amrinone therapy if therapy with vasodilators and IV dobutamine fails.

(5) If combination therapy is successful, devise an outpatient regimen with maximum tolerated doses of diuretics, spironolactone, beta-blockers, and vasodilators (see Section **III.A.4.d.**).

(6) Consider biventricular pacing.

(7) In carefully selected patients, consider cardiac transplantation.

SELECTED READINGS

Barold SS. What is cardiac resynchronization therapy? *Am J Med* 2001; 111: 224–232. *Biventricular pacing is effective therapy in patients with CHF.*

Braunwald E. Congestive heart failure: a half century perspective. *Eur Heart J* 2001;22:825–836.
An extensive review of the pathophysiology, clinical manifestation, and therapy of CHF.

Brophy JM, Joseph L, Rouleau JL. Beta-blockers in congestive heart failure: a Bayesian meta-analysis. *Ann Intern Med* 2001;134:550–560.
Beta-blocker therapy is associated with clinically meaningful reductions in morbidity and mortality in patients with stable CHF.

Caputo R, Laham R. Acute heart failure in the intensive care setting. In: Rippe JM, Irwin RS, Fink MP, et al., eds. *Intensive care medicine.* Boston: Little, Brown and Company, 1995.
A comprehensive review of acute heart failure and its management in the coronary care unit.

Cazeau S, Leclercq C, Lavergne T, et al. Effects of multisite biventricular pacing in patients with heart failure and intraventricular conduction delay. *N Engl J Med* 2001;344:873–880.
Atrioventricular pacing improves exercise tolerance in CHF patients with intraventricular conduction delay on the ECG.

Drazner MH, Rame JE, Stevenson LW, et al. Prognostic importance of elevated jugular venous pressure and a third heart sound in patients with heart failure. *N Engl J Med* 2001;345:574–581.
In patients with CHF, both elevated jugular venous pressure and a third heart sound are associated with adverse outcomes.

The effect of digoxin on mortality and morbidity in patients with heart failure: the Digitalis Investigation Group. *N Engl J Med* 1997;336:525–533.
Digoxin decreases heart failure admissions to hospital but not mortality in patients with CHF.

Effects of enalapril on mortality in severe congestive heart failure: results of the Cooperative North Scandinavian Enalapril Survival Study (CONSENSUS): the CONSENSUS Trial Study Group. *N Engl J Med* 1987;316:1429–1435.
This study showed that the addition of an ACE inhibitor to digoxin and diuretic improved 6-month survival in patients with severe heart failure.

Feldman AM, Combes A, Wagner D, et al. The role of tumor necrosis factor in the pathophysiology of heart failure. *J Am Coll Cardiol* 2000;35:537–544.
A review of the role of tumor necrosis factor and other cytokines in the pathophysiologic sequence of heart failure.

Francis GS. Pathophysiology of chronic heart failure. *Am J Med* 2001;110(7A):37S–46S.
A concise review of current knowledge of the pathophysiology of CHF.

Gomberg-Maitland M, Baran DA, Fuster V. Treatment of congestive heart failure: guidelines for the primary care physician and the heart failure specialist. *Ann Intern Med* 2001;161:342–352.
A concise review of modern therapy for patients with CHF.

Krumholz HM, Chen YT, Radford MJ. Aspirin and the treatment of heart failure in the elderly. *Ann Intern Med* 2001;161: 577–582.
Daily aspirin decreases mortality in older patients with CHF.

Leier CV, Alvarez RJ, Binkley PF. The problem of ventricular dysrhythmias and sudden death mortality in heart failure: the impact of current therapy. *Cardiology* 2000;93:56–69.
Advances in the management of patients with CHF have decreased sudden death in the heart failure population.

Mosterd A, Cost B, Hoes AW, et al. The prognosis of heart failure in the general population: the Rotterdam Study. *Eur Heart J* 2001;22:1318–1327.
Heart failure is a disease of older individuals and carries a poor prognosis. Sudden death is markedly increased in this population.

Packer M. Current role of beta adrenergic blockers in the management of chronic heart failure. *Am J Med* 2001;110(7A): 81S–94S.
A review of the use of beta-blockers in the management of heart failure.

Packer M, Coats AJS, Fowler MB, et al. Effect of carvedilol on survival in severe chronic heart failure. *N Engl J Med* 2001;344:1651–1658.

The beta-blocker carvedilol decreased morbidity and mortality in patients with severe CHF.

Packer M, Poole-Wilson PA, Armstrong PW, et al. Comparative effects of low and high doses of the angiotensin-converting enzyme inhibitor, lisinopril, on morbidity and mortality in chronic heart failure: Atlas Study Group. *Circulation* 1999;100:2312–2318.

Higher doses of lisinopril were better than lower doses in decreasing morbidity in patients with heart failure.

Recommendations for exercise training in chronic heart failure patients. *Eur Heart J* 2001;22:125–135.

Specially designed exercise training programs benefit patients with chronic CHF.

Remme WJ, Swedberg K. Guidelines for the diagnosis and treatment of chronic heart failure: task force for the diagnosis and treatment of chronic heart failure. *Eur Heart J* 2001;22:1527–1560.

Current guidelines for understanding, diagnosing, and treating patients with heart failure.

Rich MW, McSherry F, Williford, WO, et al. Effect of age on mortality, hospitalizations and response to digoxin in patients with heart failure: the DIG study. *J Am Coll Cardiol* 2001;38:806–813.

Increasing age is associated with progressively worse outcomes for patients with CHF; however, the benefit of digoxin was maintained despite advancing age.

A trial of the beta-blocker bucindolol in patients with advanced chronic heart failure. *N Engl J Med* 2001;344:1659–1667.

The beta-blocker bucindolol decreased morbidity but not mortality in patients with severe heart failure.

5. PULMONARY EDEMA

I. Introduction. Patients with either acute or chronic cardiac disease may develop pulmonary edema. The recognition and prompt treatment of acute pulmonary edema can be lifesaving. Because both cardiac and noncardiac disease can produce pulmonary edema, the physician must be aware of possible underlying conditions so that treatment can be directed toward the cause and the symptoms of pulmonary edema. The clinical problem is complicated by the fact that patients may have cardiac and pulmonary disease concurrently.

The **pathophysiology** for the formation of pulmonary edema is similar to that of edema formation in the subcutaneous tissues. Although much recent work has been performed on the mechanism of pulmonary edema formation, large gaps in our knowledge remain. Elaborate mechanisms function to keep the interstitial tissue of the lung interstitium dry: (i) plasma oncotic pressure is held higher than pulmonary capillary hydrostatic pressure, (ii) connective tissue and cellular barriers are relatively impermeable to plasma proteins, and (iii) an extensive lymphatic system exists in the lung to carry off any interstitial fluid that is generated.

The basic opposing hemodynamic forces are the pulmonary capillary pressure and the plasma oncotic pressure. In normal individuals, the pulmonary capillary pressure ("wedge" pressure) is between 7 and 12 mm Hg. Because normal plasma oncotic pressure is approximately 25 mm Hg, this force tends to pull fluid back into the capillaries. The hydrostatic pressure operates across connective tissue and cellular barriers, which under normal circumstances are relatively impermeable to plasma proteins. Finally, the lung has an extensive lymphatic system that can increase its flow five or six times when faced with excess water in the interstitial tissue of the lung. When normal mechanisms to keep the lung dry malfunction or are overwhelmed by excess fluid, edema tends to accumulate through a predictable sequence of steps. This process has been divided into three stages. During **stage 1**, fluid transfer is increased into the interstitial tissue of the lung; because lymphatic flow also increases, no net increase in interstitial volume occurs. During **stage 2**, the capacity of the lymphatics to drain excess fluid is exceeded, and liquid begins to accumulate in the interstitial spaces that surround the bronchioles and lung vasculature (which yields the roentgenographic pattern of interstitial pulmonary edema). As fluid continues to build up, increased pressure causes it to track into the interstitial space around the alveoli and finally to disrupt the tight junctions of the alveolar membranes. Fluid first builds up in the periphery of the alveolar capillary membranes (stage 3a) and finally floods the alveoli (stage 3b). During **stage 3**, the roentgenographic picture of alveolar pulmonary edema is generated, and gas exchange becomes impaired.

In addition to the processes occurring at the level of each alveolus, gravity also exerts an important influence on the fluid mechanics of the lung. Because blood is much denser than air and air-containing tissue, the effect of gravity on it is most pronounced in the lung. Under normal circumstances, more perfusion occurs at the lung bases than at the apices; however, when pulmonary venous pressure rises and when fluid begins to accumulate at the lung bases, the blood flow in the lung is redistributed toward the apices. Apical redistribution of pulmonary blood flow is apparently the result of increased pressure from accumulated fluid within the walls of the basilar pulmonary blood vessels and from hypoxia-mediated vasoconstriction. This process results in the roentgenographic finding of pulmonary vascular redistribution, an important early sign of pulmonary edema.

When any disease process alters the capillary hydrostatic pressure, plasma oncotic pressure, lung permeability, or lymphatic function, pulmonary edema can occur. Most cardiac causes of pulmonary edema ultimately can be traced to increased capillary hydrostatic pressure. A partial list of conditions causing pulmonary edema is found in Table 5-1.

II. Diagnosis

    A. History. A careful history of previous cardiac or pulmonary disease should be elicited. Pulmonary edema can result from an exacerbation of previously known cardiac disease. It can also be the presenting symptom in previously undiagnosed cardiac disease. In acute pulmonary edema, the patient may be extremely fearful or agitated. Breathlessness, dizziness, and faintness are common complaints. Because pulmonary edema frequently arises from left ventricular failure, questions concerning underlying causes for heart failure of left ventricular origin should be asked: Has the patient had chest pain? Is there any history of congenital or valvular disease? Has the patient ever been treated for hypertension? All the questions concerning left ventricular failure outlined in Chapter 4 are relevant and should be asked to determine

TABLE 5-1. CAUSES OF PULMONARY EDEMA (BY UNDERLYING MECHANISM)

I. Altered capillary permeability
    A. Infectious pulmonary edema (viral or bacterial)
    B. Inhaled toxins
    C. Circulating toxins
    D. Vasoactive substances (histamine, kinins)
    E. Disseminated intravascular coagulation
    F. Immunologic reactions
    G. Radiation pneumonia
    H. Uremia
    I. Near-drowning
    J. Aspiration pneumonia
    K. Smoke inhalation
    L. Adult respiratory distress syndrome

II. Increased pulmonary capillary pressure
    A. Cardiac causes
        1. Left ventricular failure from any cause (see Chapter 4)
        2. Mitral stenosis
        3. Subacute bacterial endocarditis
    B. Noncardiac causes
        1. Pulmonary venous fibrosis
        2. Congenital stenosis of the origin of the pulmonary veins
        3. Pulmonary venoocclusive disease
    C. Excessive infusion of intravenous fluids

III. Decreased oncotic pressure
    A. Hypoalbuminemia from any cause (renal, hepatic, nutritional, or protein-losing enteropathy)

IV. Lymphatic insufficiency

V. Mixed or unknown mechanisms
    A. High-altitude pulmonary edema
    B. Neurogenic pulmonary edema (central nervous system trauma, subarachnoid bleeding)
    C. Heroin overdose (also other narcotics)
    D. Pulmonary embolism (very rare)
    E. Pulmonary parenchymal disease
    F. Eclampsia
    G. Cardioversion
    H. Postanesthetic
    I. Cardiopulmonary bypass

Source: Adapted from Robin ED, Cross CE, Zelis R. Pulmonary edema. *N Engl J Med* 1973;288:292.

extent and duration of symptoms (e.g., shortness of breath, dyspnea on exertion, paroxysmal nocturnal dyspnea). The possibility of recent infection should be explored, and any history of pulmonary disease should be obtained. Specific questions should be addressed concerning exposure to toxic inhalants, smoke, or possible aspiration.

In some situations, the cause of pulmonary edema will be apparent or suspected (smoke inhalation, near-drowning, excess infusion of intravenous (IV) fluids, heroin or other narcotic overdose), or the history may be brief or not obtainable. When none of the foregoing lines of questioning are fruitful, it is helpful to resort to a detailed differential diagnosis of possible underlying etiologies for pulmonary edema (Table 5-1). Specific questions may then be directed to the possibility of unusual etiologies (e.g., radiation pneumonia, uremia). In acute pulmonary edema, prompt treatment is essential, and it is often not be possible to elicit a detailed history before some form of treatment is undertaken. Once the clinical situation has stabilized, however, a detailed history is required to plan rational long-term therapy. An approach to history taking in pulmonary edema is outlined in Table 5-2.

B. Physical examination. The patient may be terrified. Frequently, he or she will have difficulty talking because of respiratory distress. The patient is usually sitting, standing, or occasionally pacing in an agitated manner. Respirations are rapid and shallow (often reaching 30 to 40 respirations per minute in the adult, and higher in children). The heart rate is rapid (often more than 100 beats per minute), and the pulse is thready (if the heart rate is slow, heart block must be considered). Both systolic and diastolic blood pressures may be elevated, but this should not be confused with true, chronic, systemic hypertension. An elevated body temperature should raise a suspicion of underlying or concurrent infection (rectal temperatures are preferable because the patient is often breathing rapidly). The skin is often cold and clammy, and peripheral cyanosis may be present. The alae nasi may be dilated or flaring with the increased respiratory effort. Chest examination is likely to reveal retraction of intercostal muscles and extensive use of accessory muscles of respiration. The patient will often grasp the side rails of a hospital bed or stretcher to provide extra mechanical advantage to allow the use of these accessory muscles. Moist rales are present (starting at the

TABLE 5-2. IMPORTANT HISTORICAL ITEMS IN PATIENTS WITH PULMONARY EDEMA

Category	Item	Comment
History of present illness	Symptoms of heart failure History of cardiac disease Exposure to toxic inhalants or smoke	See Chapter 4
	Recent event that might have precipitated pulmonary edema Recent infection High altitude exposure	See Table 5-1 for differential diagnosis
Past history	History of pulmonary disease History of radiation to the chest	
Current medications	Antihypertensive medications Heart failure medications	
Review of systems	Constitutional (weight gain), cardiovascular, pulmonary	

lung bases and extending to various levels of the lung, depending on the severity of the edema). Coughing may be present and, in fulminant cases, productive of pink frothy sputum. Wheezing and a prolonged expiratory phase may also be observed. The cardiac examination usually is difficult because of respiratory noise. An third heart sound (S3) gallop is frequently present. Careful auscultation for murmurs is necessary because of possible valvular or congenital etiologies of pulmonary edema. Peripheral edema should be looked for as evidence of right ventricular failure accompanying pulmonary edema. The finding of peripheral edema suggests that chronic heart failure has been present. A neurologic examination helps to rule out neurogenic causes of pulmonary edema (central nervous system [CNS] trauma, epilepsy, subarachnoid hemorrhage). An approach to the physical examination in patients with pulmonary edema is given in Table 5-3.

C. Laboratory tests. Serum electrolyte values must be obtained in all patients with pulmonary edema. These values assume particular importance in patients who are being treated with diuretics for hypertension or heart failure, or in whom diuretic or digitalis treatment (or both) is contemplated. Blood urea nitrogen and creatinine readings are needed to assess renal function. Serum protein levels should be ascertained because of possible hypo-

TABLE 5-3. PHYSICAL FINDINGS THAT MAY BE ASSOCIATED WITH
PULMONARY EDEMA

System	Finding	Significance
General	Patient agitated, frightened	Respiratory distress
Vital signs	Elevated temperature	Consider infection
	Tachycardia, bradycardia	Supraventricular tachycardia, heart block
	Elevated blood pressure	Chronic vs. acute hypertension
Skin	Cold and clammy	High sympathetic nervous tone
HEENT	Dilated alae nasi	Respiratory distress
	Signs of trauma	? CNS etiology for pulmonary edema
Cardiac/chest	Third heart sound (S3)	Left ventricular failure
	Murmurs	Valvular lesion
	Moist rales	Pulmonary edema
	Use of accessory muscles of respiration; wheezing	Cardiac asthma
Peripheral vascular	Bruits	Atherosclerotic peripheral vascular disease
Abdominal	Pulsatile mass	Aortic aneurysm
Extremities	Edema	Biventricular or right ventricular failure
	Cyanosis	Hypoxemia
Neurologic	Focal signs	? Neurogenic causes for pulmonary edema (subarachnoid hemorrhage, CNS trauma)

HEENT, head, ears, eyes, nose, and throat; CNS, central nervous system.

albuminemia. A urinalysis and microscopic examination of the urine should be performed routinely to assess the patient for possible underlying renal disease. A complete blood cell count with differential should be obtained. This is particularly important in patients in whom pulmonary infection or endocarditis is suspected.

Room-air arterial blood gas concentrations are essential to assess the patient's level of oxygenation and acid-base status. In the past, it was commonly taught that patients with pulmonary edema were hypocapnic and alkalotic because of hyperventilation. However, approximately 50% of such patients are eucapnic or retain carbon dioxide, whereas 80% of these patients are at least mildly acidemic.

Pulmonary function tests are difficult or impossible to interpret in the acute setting. They may be obtained after respiratory stabilization to establish baseline pulmonary function. A typical pattern of respiratory mechanics for a patient with residual pulmonary edema includes decreases in vital capacity and total lung capacity. Vital capacity provides a simple bedside parameter that can be followed serially as the patient recovers.

D. Chest x-ray examination. As outlined in Chapter 4, the chest x-ray film often yields valuable and early information about the presence of excess fluid in the pulmonary interstitium. Assuming normal capillary permeability and normal plasma oncotic pressure, transudation of fluid in the lung begins to occur when capillary hydrostatic pressure approaches the oncotic pressure of plasma proteins (approximately 25 mm Hg). The roentgenographic pattern of pulmonary edema reflects the anatomic location of collected fluid. Initially, **interstitial edema** is seen as fluid gathers in tissues immediately surrounding the capillary membrane. Early roentgenographic signs of interstitial edema include thickening and loss of definition of the shadows of the pulmonary vasculature. Fluid then accumulates in septal planes and interlobular fissures, resulting in Kerley A and B lines. Subpleural or free pleural fluid (recognized as blunting of the costophrenic angles) also may be seen at this juncture. Finally, as transudated fluid collects in the parenchymal space, roentgenographic signs of alveolar edema become apparent. These roentgenographic changes may be diffuse, may be confined to the lower portion of one or both lungs, or may surround the hilus ("butterfly pattern").

E. ECG. The ECG in pulmonary edema should be examined to aid in defining the underlying etiology. Evidence of myocardial infarction (MI) and arrhythmias should be sought. ECG evidence of left ventricular hypertrophy suggesting aortic stenosis, systemic hypertension, or cardiomyopathy may be present.

F. Echocardiography. Echocardiography is not essential to recognize pulmonary edema. It does help identify underlying disease that may lead to pulmonary edema. For example, echocardiography can assist the physician in recognizing established valvular disease, which may lead to pulmonary edema. Echocardiograms are often successful in demonstrating valvular vegetations in patients with endocarditis. Abnormalities of left ventricular wall motion after MI, and poor left ventricular function in patients with cardiomyopathy can easily be documented by echocardiography.

G. Radionuclide studies. Radionuclide studies can be of value in quantitating left ventricular function in patients with pulmonary edema. Moreover, radionuclide angiocardiography can demonstrate a left-to-right shunt in patients with ventricular septal rupture secondary to MI.

H. Catheterization and angiography. The use of cardiac catheterization to document underlying etiologies for pulmonary edema is well established and discussed elsewhere in this book under specific disease entities. In addition to the traditional diagnostic use of catheterization, Swan-Ganz (balloon-tipped) catheters, inserted at the patient's bedside, may provide important information, although their use is not mandatory. Measurement of pulmonary capillary wedge (PCW) pressure can distinguish cardiogenic from noncardiogenic pulmonary edema. Other hemodynamic parameters such as cardiac output, oxygen saturation in various cardiac chambers, and the presence of giant V waves in the PCW tracing are also available from right-sided heart catheterization. Recent reports have demonstrated that giant V waves may be present in a variety of conditions other than acute mitral regurgitation, including mitral stenosis, coronary artery disease, mitral valve prosthesis, and ventricular septic defect. Moreover, in long-standing mitral regurgitation (MR) the large, compliant left atrium may prevent generation of V waves. Despite these limitations, mitral regurgitation remains the most common cause of V waves, and this finding in the PCW position tracing during pulmonary artery catheterization provides useful diagnostic information. Finally, the catheter may be left in the pulmonary artery for several days and can continue to provide hemodynamic information while therapy for pulmonary edema is administered. Such serial measurements of pulmonary pressures are particularly important when pulmonary edema and diminished cardiac output occur together. In this situation, left ventricular filling pressures should be monitored to produce maximum cardiac output with minimum elevation in pulmonary pressure.

I. Protocol for the diagnosis of pulmonary edema

1. Confirmatory tests. The diagnosis of pulmonary edema is a clinical one. Patients generally present with a history of underlying cardiac or pulmonary disease but sometimes with pulmonary edema as the initial manifestation of underlying disease. The diagnosis is made by a combination of history, physical examination, and chest x-ray studies that reveal excess fluid in the lung. Other confirmatory tests are not needed for diagnosis.

2. Differential diagnosis. The major differential diagnostic problem in pulmonary edema resides not in establishing the diagnosis but in distinguishing among the possible underlying causes. Table 5-1 lists cardiogenic and noncardiogenic causes of pulmonary edema.

3. How to distinguish among underlying causes

   a. Pulmonary edema caused by altered permeability of endothelial barriers. The group of disorders that alter either alveolar or pulmonary capillary membrane permeability comprises the largest group of causes of noncardiogenic pulmonary edema. Distinction among these entities (Table 5-1) and cardiogenic causes of pulmonary edema may be very difficult. The problem is complicated by the fact that elevated pulmonary capillary pressure itself can increase capillary permeability. Furthermore, increased lung fluid from any cause makes the lung more susceptible to secondary infection, and patients with pulmonary edema of cardiac origin may have intercurrent bacterial pneumonia. It is important to consider altered permeability as a cause of pulmonary edema in any patient who has an underlying disease capable of damaging pulmonary capillary or alveolar endothelium. In this category are patients with bacterial or viral pneumonia, patients exposed to toxins (including the administration of high concentrations of oxygen), patients with smoke inhalation, and patients with radiation pneumonitis (generally secondary to radiation therapy for chest tumors). A more complete listing is found in Table 5-1. Even with this list in mind, the picture may be confusing. The most direct diagnostic procedure in this case is the insertion of a balloon-tipped catheter to measure PCWP, which is normal or low in patients with noncardiogenic pulmonary edema.

   b. Pulmonary edema caused by decreased oncotic pressure. Lowered oncotic pressure should be considered in all patients with hepatic or renal disease who present in pulmonary edema. Nutritional deficits and protein-losing enteropathy are the more two unusual causes of decreased oncotic pressure pulmonary edema.

   c. Pulmonary edema caused by increased pulmonary capillary pressure

(1) Cardiac causes. Any cardiac disease that causes (or simulates, e.g., mitral stenosis) left ventricular dysfunction can lead to pulmonary edema. Although this category encompasses almost every major form of cardiac disease, the most common cardiac etiologies of pulmonary edema are systemic hypertension and MI. The diagnosis of specific underlying cardiac disorders is covered in depth in other chapters in this manual. The level of PCW pressure does not always correlate with the degree of pulmonary edema. Furthermore, it is important to understand that the roentgenographic picture of pulmonary edema may lag behind the clinical syndrome. The oncotic pressure, status of the pulmonary lymphatics, presence of intercurrent diseases that alter capillary and alveolar endothelial permeabilities, and individual patient differences all influence the pressures at which transudation of fluid begins.

(2) Noncardiac causes. A number of rare conditions that involve abnormalities of the pulmonary vasculature may give rise to increased pulmonary capillary pressure. Included in this category are pulmonary venoocclusive disease, congenital stenosis of the origin of the pulmonary veins, and pulmonary venous fibrosis. Although these conditions are rare, they should be considered in young patients with chronic pulmonary edema.

d. Miscellaneous and unusual causes of pulmonary edema. A variety of rare conditions that involve either direct damage to the lung or indirect alterations in pulmonary function may cause pulmonary edema: disorders of the pulmonary lymphatics (silicosis, lymphangitic carcinomatosis), CNS disturbances (CNS trauma, subarachnoid hemorrhage), cardioversion, eclampsia, heroin overdose, and high-altitude pulmonary edema. The diagnosis of these conditions usually rests on a careful history.

Summary. Despite the varied underlying etiologies of pulmonary edema, it is possible to develop an overall diagnostic approach to the clinical problem. Such an approach is outlined in Table 5-4.

III. Therapy

A. Medical treatment. The treatment of pulmonary edema involves two types of action: (i) general measures for the acute symptoms and (ii) measures to correct specific underlying abnormalities.

1. General measures and drugs

a. Oxygen and other measures designed to improve respiratory gas exchange. Oxygen should be a first priority in the patient with respiratory distress. If possible, a room-air arterial blood gas level should be obtained before institution of therapy. For most patients, adequate oxygenation is achieved with a nasal catheter or face mask; however, patients with severe hypoxia often require further measures. Endotracheal intubation with controlled, mechanical ventilation will be required in such patients. At times, intermittent positive pressure breathing (IPPB) through a specially adapted mask will be sufficient to correct hypoxia in such patients. If, however, arterial Po_2 levels cannot be maintained above 80 mm Hg with either IPPB alone or after endotracheal intubation, or if an Fio_2 of 60% or more is required to maintain Po_2 above this level, positive end-expiratory pressure (PEEP) should be used.

Various criteria have been developed for determining when a patient requires intubation and controlled ventilation. Controlled ventilation via an endotracheal tube should usually be instituted when high flows of approximately 100% oxygen through a rebreathing apparatus are unsuccessful in maintaining arterial Po_2 levels at or above 80 mm Hg. **Important exceptions to this rule are patients with chronic obstructive pulmonary disease, who**

TABLE 5-4. PROTOCOL FOR ESTABLISHING THE DIAGNOSIS OF PULMONARY EDEMA

I. All patients
  A. History. Focus on previous history of cardiac or pulmonary disease, any previous episodes of pulmonary edema or heart failure, any cardiac medicines; keep differential diagnosis in mind
  B. Physical examination. See Table 5-3; most items of importance on physical examination involve signs of ventricular failure, manifestations of dyspnea, signs of fluid in the lungs, or signs of hypoxia
  C. Laboratory studies
    1. Initial blood studies: CBC with differential; electrolyte, BUN, creatinine, and serum protein concentrations
    2. Urinalysis and microscopic examination of the urine; particularly note presence of protein on urinalysis
    3. Posteroanterior and lateral chest x-ray films; particularly note early signs of pulmonary edema
    4. ECG. Note signs of myocardial infarction or long-standing pressure overload (left ventricular hypertrophy)
    5. Room air arterial blood gas concentration

II. Selected patients or patients in whom the underlying etiology of pulmonary edema is in question
  A. Catheterization: insertion of balloon-tipped catheter to measure pulmonary capillary wedge pressure
  B. Echocardiography (valvular lesion, cardiomyopathy)
  C. Blood cultures
  D. Pulmonary function tests, obtained several days after clinical situation has stabilized

CBC, complete blood cell count; BUN, blood urea nitrogen.

often have a baseline Po_2 of around 50 mm Hg. Intubation of such patients should be attempted only in critical situations, because it can be difficult to wean them from the respirator.

As noted earlier, when controlled ventilation does not provide adequate oxygenation, PEEP may be added. End-expiratory pressures from 5 to 20 mm Hg generally are used. In severe degrees of pulmonary edema, the respiratory management is identical to ventilatory management of the adult respiratory distress syndrome. The primary effect of PEEP seems to be that of increasing functional residual capacity, thereby preventing premature closure of small airways during expiration.

It should be remembered that the amount of oxygen delivered to the tissues is a function of both cardiac output and the level of arterial oxygen. Controlled ventilation with and without PEEP may have the adverse side effect of decreasing cardiac output through restriction of venous return. The most accurate way of determining the effect of mechanical ventilation on cardiac output is by monitoring the cardiac output with a thermodilution balloon-tipped catheter or by measuring the mixed venous oxygen content in the pulmonary artery by means of a right-heart catheterization. The lower the cardiac output, the lower will be the mixed venous oxygen content.

  b. Other general measures. Measures to ensure patient comfort should be instituted; for example, the head of the bed should be elevated to at least 30 degrees.

Fluid management will be dictated by clinical condition and blood pressure. If the patient is hypotensive, diuresis should be done with great caution to prevent worsening hypotension secondary to dehydration. In this event, the clinician walks the fine line between inadequate fluid depletion and exacerbation of pulmonary edema. Measurement of PCW pressure is often important in this setting to make this distinction. Central venous pressure does not adequately reflect filling of the left side of the heart. Treatment of hypotension is discussed together with shock in Chapter 6. If the patient is hypertensive, measures should be taken to lower arterial pressure, as outlined in Chapter 12.

  c. Drugs

    (1) Furosemide and other diuretics. Parenteral furosemide (Lasix) has become standard in the management of acute pulmonary edema, although patients can, at times, be managed adequately without this drug. The initial dose is generally 10 to 20 mg IV for patients who have never been treated with furosemide before, although doses of 40 to 80 mg by slow IV bolus (over 1 to 2 minutes) are common in patients who have been treated with diuretics as outpatients. Continuous IV infusion of furosemide may produce a diuresis in patients who have been previously refractory to bolus infusions of furosemide. The dosage here ranges from 10 to 40 mg per hour, depending on the level of renal function. Patients with decreased renal function require higher dosage of IV furosemide. Ethacrynic acid (Edecrin) is an alternative loop diuretic to furosemide. Initial doses of 20 to 60 mg IV bolus are typically used. Occasionally, a diuresis can be achieved by combination of furosemide (100 mg IV slow bolus) and chlorothiazide(500 mg IV slow bolus) when neither furosemide nor ethacrynic acid alone is successful. There are at least three mechanisms of action of furosemide: (i) rapid peripheral, vasodilative effect; (ii) diuretic effect; and (iii) mild afterload reduction.

    (2) Digitalis. The use of digitalis glycosides has virtually disappeared in recent years as a therapeutic intervention for patients with acute pulmonary edema. Digitalis is still used in the management of chronic heart failure (Chapter 4).

    Digitalis may be used in patients whose pulmonary edema is secondary to a supraventricular arrhythmia. For example, digitalis may be used to control ventricular response in atrial fibrillation. However, there are drugs that are more effective for this indication (Chapter 3). A control ECG and serum potassium level should be obtained before digitalis preparations are administered.

    (3) Morphine. Morphine is an important drug in the treatment of acute pulmonary edema. It is thought to have both a direct venodilating effect and a CNS effect (allaying anxiety). Morphine may be administered either intramuscularly (5 to 10 mg repeated in 2 to 4 hours) or intravenously (1 to 4 mg).

    In patients in whom MI is a possibility, the IV route is preferred, because intramuscular injections increase serum creatine phosphokinase levels. Caution must be exercised in the administration of morphine to patients with obstructive pulmonary disease, because morphine blunts respiratory drive and may result in respiratory arrest.

    (4) Aminophylline. If bronchospasm is present, aminophylline may be beneficial. In addition, aminophylline provides inotropic stimulation to the heart. Standard dosage is a loading dose of 6 mg/kg followed by a constant infusion of 0.5 to 1.0 mg/kg per hour. Aminophylline also exerts a mild diuretic effect.

    (5) Vasodilators. A variety of vasodilators are available that reduce left ventricular work. The dosages and clinical characteristics

TABLE 5-5. PROTOCOL FOR TREATMENT OF PULMONARY EDEMA

I. Brief history, physical examination, and laboratory tests as outlined in diagnosis protocol, seeking to establish underlying etiology of pulmonary edema

II. Treat any underlying etiology discovered with specific measures

III. As diagnostic workup is initiated, simultaneously begin symptomatic treatment
   A. Morphine
   B. Furosemide
   C. Aminophylline
   D. Vasodilators
   E. Intravenous inotropic agents

IV. Diet: restrict salt to 2000 mg/d

V. Activity: bed rest with head of bed elevated

of these medications are summarized in Chapter 4. Both nitroglycerin (IV, sublingual, or oral) and IV nitroprusside have been used for this purpose. When nitroprusside is used, a common starting dose is 20 to 40 mcg per minute, with increments of 5 mcg per minute every 5 to 10 minutes until the desired effects (lowering pulmonary artery pressure or initiating a diuresis) are achieved. Therapy with nitroprusside should be monitored carefully to prevent hypotension.

Vasodilators are used most commonly for pulmonary edema secondary to chronic, intractable left ventricular failure, or for acute pulmonary edema secondary to MI (see Chapter 15).

(6) IV inotropic agents. IV inotropes such as dobutamine or dopamine are occasionally used in patients with severe and/or refractory pulmonary edema, particularly if hypotension is present (see Chapter 6).

(7) Miscellaneous medicines used to treat pulmonary edema. IV albumin may be indicated when hypoproteinemia contributes to pulmonary edema.

2. Activity. The activity recommendations outlined in Chapter 4 also apply to patients with pulmonary edema. Initially, patients should be kept at bed rest until they stabilize and much of their pulmonary edema has resolved. At this point, they may be rapidly and progressively mobilized.

3. Diet. The dietary recommendations outlined for patients with moderate to severe heart failure also apply to patients with pulmonary edema. Salt restriction is advised.

B. Surgery. Surgical intervention for patients with pulmonary edema may be helpful in a number of different situations, including correction of surgically remediable causes such as acute mitral regurgitation. Surgery may also be used for and insertion of an intraaortic balloon pump (IABP).

Surgically remediable causes of pulmonary edema include valvular lesions and ventricular septal rupture after MI. The IABP may be lifesaving in severe left ventricular failure. The use of the IABP is discussed in greater detail in Chapter 15. A general protocol for the treatment of pulmonary edema is found in Table 5-5.

SELECTED READINGS

Bersten AD, Holt AW, Vedig AE, et al. Treatment of severe cardiogenic pulmonary edema with continuous positive airway pressure delivered by face mask. *N Engl J Med* 1991;325:1825–1830.

Continuous positive airway pressure therapy reduces the need for intubation in patients with pulmonary edema.

Brater DC. Diuretic therapy. *N Engl J Med* 1998;339:387–395.

An extensive review of the indications for and correct usage of diuretics.

Brown NJ, Vaughan DE. Angiotensin-converting enzyme inhibitors. *Circulation* 1998;97:1411–1420.

An authoritative review of angiotensin-converting enzyme inhibitors and their use in acute and chronic heart failure.

Fedullo AJ, Swinburne AJ, Wahl GW, et al. Acute cardiogenic pulmonary edema treated with mechanical ventilation: factors determining in-hospital mortality. *Chest* 1991;99:1220–1226.

Mortality in patients with pulmonary edema depends on the severity of left ventricular dysfunction. Variables related to the degree of respiratory failure were not predictive of mortality.

Goodfriend TL, Elliott ME, Catt KJ. Angiotensin receptors and their antagonists. *N Engl J Med* 1996;334:1649–1654.

A review of the underlying mechanisms for the efficacy of angiotensin receptor blocking agents.

Lin M, Yang YF, Chiang HT, et al. Reappraisal of continuous positive airway pressure therapy in acute cardiogenic pulmonary edema: short-term results and long-term follow-up. *Chest* 1995;107:1379–1386.

Continuous positive airway pressure therapy results in physiologic cardiovascular and pulmonary function improvement in patients with pulmonary edema.

Pang D, Keenan SP, Cook DJ, et al. The effect of positive pressure airway support on mortality and the need for intubation in cardiogenic pulmonary edema: a systematic review. *Chest* 1998;114:1185–1192.

Positive pressure airway support decreases the need for intubation and may decrease mortality in patients with pulmonary edema.

Robin ED, Cross CE, Felix R. Pulmonary edema. *N Engl J Med* 1973;288:239–246.

The classic paper on pulmonary edema; an excellent review, particularly of pathophysiology of pulmonary edema formation.

Schuster DP. Pulmonary edema: etiology and pathogenesis. In: Rippe JM, Irwin RS, Fink MP, et al., eds. *Intensive care medicine.* Boston: Little, Brown and Company, 1995.

A good recent summary with particular emphasis on the underlying pathophysiology of pulmonary edema.

Sharon A, Shpirer I, Kaluski E, et al. High dose intravenous isosorbide dinitrate is safer and better than bilevel positive airway ventilation combined with conventional treatment for severe pulmonary edema. *J Am Coll Cardiol* 2000;36:832–837.

Long-acting nitrate therapy is safe and highly effective therapy for patients with severe pulmonary edema.

6. SHOCK

I. **Introduction.** Shock is a medical emergency that demands rapid action and constant attention on the part of physicians and nurses to prevent irreversible cell damage and death. Although the most frequent cause of shock in cardiac patients is massive myocardial infarction (MI), shock can be caused by a wide variety of disturbances, either cardiac or noncardiac in origin.

A. **Definition.** Early definitions of shock emphasized a precipitous drop in systemic arterial blood pressure. It is now recognized that blood pressure varies considerably in shock, depending on the underlying etiology, duration, and adequacy of compensatory mechanisms. The essential concept to understand is that the major hemodynamic problem in shock is not inadequate **pressure** (although hypotension is often present) but inadequate tissue **perfusion**. The modern definition of shock is a circulatory state in which inadequate tissue perfusion occurs, thereby leading to progressive organ dysfunction that, unless rapidly reversed, results in irreversible organ damage and death. The early stage of organ hypoperfusion has been termed **preshock**. The cardinal signs of preshock and shock are manifestations of progressive dysfunction of vital organs—brain, heart, and kidneys. These signs are listed in Table 6-1.

Despite advances in antibiotic therapy, blood-product separation, parenteral therapy, circulatory assistance devices, and hemodynamic monitoring, the mortality from shock remains distressingly high. Mortality from bacteremic shock may range as high as 40% to 80%, depending on the patient's age and a variety of comorbid predictors. Cardiogenic shock after MI is associated with a fatality rate that ranges from 45% to 90%. With these grim statistics in mind, considerable emphasis has been placed on early recognition and treatment of decreased perfusion (preshock or low-flow state) rather than waiting for the occurrence of true shock. In preshock or early shock, subtle signs of activated compensatory mechanisms substitute for the cardinal signs of shock as clues to the diagnosis (Table 6-1).

B. **Etiology.** A wide variety of disease states can produce shock. Table 6-2 lists the major causes of shock. Although the list is lengthy and the clinical presentation varies depending on the underlying etiology, arterial hypotension, signs of organ hypoperfusion, and metabolic acidosis are common to most etiologies of shock.

In the vast majority of patients with shock, the underlying etiology lies within one of the following three categories: cardiovascular shock, hypovolemic shock, or septic shock. The clinical recognition and treatment of these three entities are emphasized in this chapter. Although separated for discussion, in practice the categories often overlap.

C. **Pathophysiology.** The clinical syndrome of shock is not a single entity but a dynamic state with many gradations. Patients who develop shock may be viewed as passing through the following three stages:

1. **Stage I.** In the initial phase, the patient may be asymptomatic. Blood pressure may be either normal or slightly depressed. Compensatory mechanisms include sympathetic discharge that causes mild peripheral vasoconstriction (cool skin) and tachycardia. This stage may be viewed as equivalent to preshock. A previously healthy individual can compensate for approximately a 10% reduction in blood volume (about 1 U of blood) by means of these mechanisms.

2. **Stage II.** Despite intense activity of compensatory mechanisms, in stage II blood pressure declines and organ hypoperfusion begins. Clinically, the patient often demonstrates declining blood pressure, tachycardia, and restlessness.

   If coronary artery disease is present, angina may occur. These signs develop after a 20% to 25% reduction in effective circulating blood volume.

TABLE 6-1. CLINICAL SIGNS OF SHOCK AND PRESHOCK

I. Signs of shock (organ hypoperfusion)
   A. Metabolic acidosis
   B. Systolic blood pressure <90 mm Hg
   C. Urine output <20 ml/hr
   D. Cold, clammy skin
   E. Mental confusion

II. Signs of preshock or low-flow state
   Any of the following unexplained findings in a patient clinically suspected of being at risk for developing shock:
   A. Fall in urine output
   B. Rise in heart rate
   C. Fall in systolic blood pressure
   D. Fall in skin temperature

TABLE 6-2. UNDERLYING ETIOLOGIES IN SHOCK

I. Cardiovascular shock
   A. Myocardial infarction
   B. Critical aortic stenosis
   C. Arrhythmia
   D. Ruptured aortic aneurysm
   E. Obstruction to flow between cardiac chambers (atrial myxoma)
   F. Severe congestive heart failure
   G. Massive pulmonary embolism
   H. Cardiac tamponade
   I. Acute aortic insufficiency
   J. Acute mitral insufficiency
      1. Ruptured papillary muscle
      2. Ruptured chordae tendineae
   K. Acute ventricular septic defect

II. Hypovolemia
   A. Hemorrhage
   B. Burns
   C. Insensible water loss without adequate replacement
   D. Diarrhea
   E. Vomiting
   F. Intestinal obstruction
   G. Fractures

III. Septicemia
   A. Gram-negative sepsis
   B. Other infections

IV. Other
   A. Anaphylactic shock
   B. Neuropathic shock
      1. Spinal cord transection
      2. Anesthesia
      3. Drug overdose
   C. Abuse of diuretics
   D. Addisonian crisis
   E. Myxedema

3. Stage III. As the patient progresses into stage III, organ dysfunction becomes evident. Cardiac output declines, urine production falls or ceases, and mental status proceeds from restlessness to agitation, followed by somnolence and coma. Unless circulating blood volume is restored rapidly, compensatory mechanisms contribute to the deteriorating clinical picture in a vicious circle (e.g., intense vasoconstriction increases afterload, thereby causing a further decline in cardiac output).

Shock can have deleterious effects on a variety of vital organs. Arterial mean pressures below 70 to 80 mm Hg are inadequate to maintain adequate coronary arterial blood flow, myocardial oxygen, and nutrient supply. Pressures below 60 mm Hg are insufficient to maintain adequate cerebral blood flow. Even brief periods of severe hypotension are thought to contribute to the pulmonary vascular injury that is characteristic of adult respiratory distress syndrome. Hypovolemic damage to the liver can compromise its role in detoxification and thereby exacerbate the shock state as metabolic wastes accumulate in the blood. Renal function deteriorates, and the patient progresses from oliguria to anuria. If hypovolemia persists for several hours, irreversible tubular necrosis may occur.

II. Diagnosis. Patients often arrive in the emergency department in shock. In this event, it is imperative to initiate therapy promptly, using general measures to support respiration and circulation (see Section **III.**). Once the clinical situation has stabilized, the important issues are (i) determining the etiology of the shock state and (ii) instituting specific measures to correct the underlying problem

A. History. Evidence of underlying disease should be sought. Of particular importance is a history of cardiac disease and/or hypertension.

Episodes of chest pain, shortness of breath, exercise intolerance, or palpitations should be explored. Recent trauma or burns should be considered. The possibility of recent infection or reasons for hypovolemia must be taken into account (hemorrhage, gastrointestinal fluid or blood loss, renal disease). In the elderly or very young, insensible losses without adequate replacement have to be considered. History of neurologic disease (spinal cord injury, previous problems with orthostatic hypotension) should also be considered. A history of drug ingestion is important (both prescribed and nonprescribed drugs) because of the myocardial-depressant effects of some drugs (particularly antiarrhythmics) and the volume-depleting effect of others (diuretics). In addition, anaphylactic shock can arise from drug ingestion. Historical items of diagnostic relevance in shock are shown in Table 6-3.

B. Physical examination. Physical findings in shock vary considerably, depending on the clinical stage and the underlying etiology of the shock state. Many of the physical findings relate either to compensatory mechanisms that have been activated or to the extent of organ hypoperfusion. The patient's general appearance can vary from normal to moribund. Skin is often cool, and peripheral cyanosis may be present; however, the skin may be warm in terminal stages of shock because blood vessels are unable to constrict. The skin also may be warm in septic shock because of the local effects of bacterial endotoxins that cause inappropriate dilatation of peripheral vessels. Beads of perspiration reflect heightened sympathetic tone. The level of the arterial blood pressure often indicates the degree of shock (numerous exceptions, however, preclude complete reliance on this sign). Heart rate usually reflects the adequacy of compensatory mechanisms, with tachycardia the rule.

Respiratory rate and temperature reflect underlying hypoxia, acid-base imbalance, or possible infection. Chest examination can provide secondary evidence of high left ventricular filling pressures (rales). The cardiac examination should focus on findings compatible with complications of MI (ventricular septal rupture, aneurysm, papillary muscle dysfunction; see Chapter 15). It is important to remember that a murmur will be soft or absent in up to 50% of patients with papillary muscle rupture, leading to torrential mitral regurgitation and shock. Abdominal examination may reveal evidence of trauma or bowel obstruction. A rectal examination is essential to rule out

TABLE 6-3. HISTORICAL ITEMS IN THE DIAGNOSIS OF SHOCK

Category	Item	Comment
History of present illness (HPI)	Symptoms of myocardial infarction or any significant heart disease	? Cardiogenic shock
	Recent infection	? Septic shock
	Recent trauma of any kind	? Hypovolemic shock
	History of hypotensive episodes	
	Recent GI surgery	? Intestinal obstruction
	Recent drug ingestion	? Anaphylactic shock
Past medical history	History of heart disease	
	History of renal disease	Hypovolemia from renal disease
Medications	All current medicines	Possibility of diuretic abuse
		Ganglionic blocking, antihypertensive medications
Review of systems	Constitutional	Weight gain (? edema from heart failure)
	Cardiovascular	See HPI
	Pulmonary	? Pulmonary embolus or tension pneumothorax
	GI	? GI hemorrhage
		? GI obstruction
	Genitourinary	Renal disease (hypovolemia)
	Endocrine	? Addison's disease (addisonian crisis)
		? Myxedema
	Neurologic	? Spinal cord injury
		? Anesthesia

GI, gastrointestinal.

gastrointestinal bleeding. Serial examination of adequacy of peripheral pulses provides one way of monitoring therapeutic progress. A neurologic examination is also important. Physical findings that may be present in shock are found in Table 6-4.

C. Laboratory tests. Various laboratory tests are helpful in defining the underlying cause of shock and in monitoring therapy. Many of them will be needed daily or more frequently. Suggested tests are listed in Table 6-5. Evidence of disseminated intravascular coagulation is a frequent and ominous sign in shock of any cause. Insertion of a pulmonary arterial and peripheral arterial catheter often is necessary in cases of shock and facilitates necessary blood sampling without undue patient discomfort. A guide for the use of laboratory tests in shock is given in Table 6-5.

D. Chest x-ray examination. Chest x-ray films should be obtained on a daily basis during the acute phase of shock. They are particularly important in demonstrating subtle signs of left ventricular failure, thereby aiding in monitoring fluid therapy. The chest x-ray film may reveal widening of the mediastinum in cases of aortic dissection. The chest x-ray examination may also reveal pulmonary edema or the picture of adult respiratory distress syndrome, improper placement of central venous pressure (CVP) and pulmonary

TABLE 6-4. PHYSICAL FINDINGS THAT MAY BE PRESENT IN SHOCK

System	Finding	Significance
General	Agitation, somnolence	Diminished cerebral blood flow
Vital signs	Blood pressure <90 mm Hg systolic	Blood pressure not always a good sign because of compensatory mechanisms
	Heart rate >100 beats/min	An early sign of preshock if unexplained
	Increased respiratory rate	May be sign of respiratory compensation for metabolic acidosis
	Elevated temperature	? Septic shock
Skin	Cool, moist skin	Sign of compensatory peripheral vasoconstriction; skin may be warm in final stages when compensatory mechanisms fail
Neck	Position of neck veins	Low neck veins, hypovolemia; elevated neck veins, heart failure or restricted filling
Chest and lungs	Rales	? Left ventricular failure with pulmonary edema ? Hemothorax
Cardiac	Abnormally fast, slow, or irregular heart rate	Arrhythmias may cause shock
	Dyskinetic impulse	? Ventricular aneurysm after myocardial infarction
	Murmurs	Critical aortic stenosis, papillary muscle dysfunction, ventricular septal rupture after myocardial infarction
Abdominal	High-pitched bowel sounds	? Intestinal obstruction
	Evidence of trauma	? Hemorrhage
Genital/rectal	Blood on rectal examination	? Gastrointestinal bleeding
Neurologic	Abnormal motor, sensory, reflex findings	? Spinal cord injury ? Peripheral neuropathies

arterial catheters, or incorrect placement of an endotracheal tube. Calcium should be sought in the aortic or mitral valves as well as in the coronary arteries.

E. Echocardiography. Echocardiography may be useful in the initial diagnosis of shock if a cardiovascular etiology is suspected. Cardiovascular causes of shock include MI and its complications, dissection of the aorta, critical aortic stenosis, cardiac tamponade, and massive pulmonary embolism. Other cardiovascular causes of shock are listed in Table 6-2.

F. Catheterization and angiography. Knowledge of cardiac filling pressures and cardiac output is often helpful in preshock patients and is essential in individuals with severe or progressive shock. Although it is possible to perform retrograde catheterization of the left ventricle to measure these parameters, this exposes the patient to the risks of cardiac catheterization. If

TABLE 6-5. LABORATORY TESTS IN THE DIAGNOSIS AND MONITORING OF SHOCK AND PRESHOCK

I. Diagnostic tests
  A. All patients
    1. Blood work: electrolytes, BUN, and creatinine levels, CBC with differential
    2. Urine: urinalysis
    3. Serial arterial blood gases: PO_2, PCO_2, pH
    4. Chest x-ray examination
    5. Serial ECGs
  B. Selected patients
    1. Blood cultures
    2. Platelets, fibrin split products, protime, activated partial thromboplastin time, and other tests to identify disseminated intravascular coagulation

II. Monitoring tests
  A. All patients
    1. Flow charts: monitoring vital signs, blood gases, urine output, all fluids and drugs, hematocrit, electrolytes, BUN, and creatinine
    2. Central venous pressure
  B. Selected patients
    1. PCWP and cardiac output: balloon-tipped pulmonary artery catheter
    2. Direct arterial monitoring of blood pressure: arterial cannula

BUN, blood urea nitrogen; CBC, complete blood cell count; PCWP, pulmonary capillary wedge pressure.

catheterization is elected, use of a balloon-tipped catheter for measuring pulmonary artery pressures and cardiac output is preferred. If a thermodilution catheter is used, serial cardiac outputs can be measured.

G. Protocol for the diagnosis of shock
  1. Confirmatory tests needed to make the diagnosis. The diagnosis of shock or preshock rests on the demonstration of organ hypoperfusion or signs of early compensatory mechanisms outlined in Table 6-1. It is important to distinguish among the various underlying etiologies that can lead to shock, so that therapy can be aimed at the specific disease process.
  2. Differential diagnosis of shock. A differential diagnostic list of conditions that cause shock is provided in Table 6-2. The most common underlying etiologies are cardiac disease, hypovolemia, and sepsis.
    a. Cardiogenic shock. A severe complication of acute MI, cardiogenic shock, is discussed in Chapter 13. Several items should be emphasized: (i) shock occurs in approximately 5% to 10% of patients hospitalized with the diagnosis of acute MI; (ii) shock usually occurs in patients in whom more than 40% of the left ventricle has been damaged; and (iii) mortality is high in these patients, ranging from 50% to 90% or more.

       Cardiogenic shock usually can be distinguished from septic and hypovolemic shock by history. Cardiogenic shock may involve an element of hypovolemia. The measurement of pulmonary capillary wedge pressure (PCWP) may be important to make this distinction in selected patients. Because the mortality from cardiogenic shock is high, it is also important to make the diagnosis as early as possible, for example, during the preshock period, so that appropriate therapy can be instituted. Urine output should be monitored carefully. Patients with large MIs who have trouble urinating, or whose urine output falls below 20 ml per hour, should have a Foley catheter placed in the bladder. Although direct damage to the left ventricular myocardium is by far the most common cause of cardiogenic shock, a variety of other cardiovascular conditions can also lead to the shock state. Used in the broadest sense, **cardiogenic shock** implies a pathophysiologic state in which the pumping function of the heart is so impaired that it is unable to provide for adequate tissue perfusion.

A number of mechanical problems may accompany MI and lead to shock (see Chapter 15). Acute ventricular septal results from myocardial necrosis of the septum and usually occurs 1 to 7 days after MI. It is an equally common complication of inferior and anterior MI. Acute mitral regurgitation may result from papillary muscle dysfunction caused by ischemia, change in geometry or dilatation of the left ventricle, ruptured chordae tendineae, or ruptured papillary muscle. It is particularly important to recognize rupture of the papillary muscle because 75% of individuals with this lesion will expire within 24 hours unless surgical intervention is undertaken on an emergency basis.

Acute valvular disruption may occur in settings other than MI and result in cardiogenic shock. Aortic dissection may lead to acute aortic insufficiency or may extend into the pericardium, thereby producing cardiac tamponade. Acute aortic insufficiency also may result from infectious endocarditis or disruption of the suture ring in a prosthetic aortic valve. Shock in a patient with a prosthetic valve should be considered prosthetic valve disruption until proven otherwise. Patients with long-standing mitral valve disease (on the basis of either rheumatic valvulitis or myxomatous degeneration) may suffer acute decompensation that leads to cardiogenic shock. Patients in both of these groups are susceptible to ruptured chordae tendineae and acute mitral regurgitation. Infectious endocarditis may also result in acute mitral regurgitation.

Obstructive valvular lesions can also produce cardiogenic shock. Critical aortic stenosis or severe mitral stenosis can significantly impair cardiac output. Left atrial myxoma can severely compromise left ventricular filling, thereby markedly decreasing cardiac output. All these lesions should be considered when one assesses a patient with unexplained shock.

Nonvalvular outflow obstruction from supravalvular or subvalvular aortic stenosis or hypertrophic obstructive cardiomyopathy also may result in cardiogenic shock. Rhythm disturbances such as the onset of atrial fibrillation can lead to acute decompensation in these patients. Cardiogenic shock caused by left ventricular outflow obstruction is an important entity to recognize because conventional therapy such as vasopressors or afterload reduction may lead to further deterioration. Cardiac lesions that restrict ventricular filling, such as constrictive pericarditis or tamponade, may result in cardiogenic shock. These lesions are also important to recognize, because specific therapies are available and may be lifesaving.

Right ventricular infarction can also be a cause of cardiogenic shock. Some degree of right ventricular damage occurs in more than 40% of acute inferior MIs. Elevated CVPs, clear lung fields, and hypotension in the setting of an acute inferior MI should suggest right ventricular infarction. Right ventricular infarction usually responds to volume repletion, although occasionally atrioventricular sequential pacing is required to stabilize the patient.

Finally, some degree of myocardial depression may be present in shock states that are not based on underlying cardiac pathologic conditions. The pathophysiology of this decrease in myocardial function may involve myocardial depressant substances such as tumor necrosis factor, nitric oxide, and altered acid-base status.

b. **Hypovolemic shock.** Hypovolemia is present in many forms of shock. It is the main cause of shock in burns, hemorrhage, and trauma;

however, enough volume depletion to result in shock may occur in patients with severe volume losses secondary to diabetic ketoacidosis, vomiting, diarrhea, and intestinal obstruction. Generally, intravascular volume loss in excess of 1 L is necessary before compensatory mechanisms fail and shock ensues.

The diagnosis of hypovolemic shock is suggested by history. Insertion of a CVP catheter may provide information on the patient's volume status (patients with hypovolemia often have very low CVP readings). It is important to recognize, however, that compensatory mechanisms may allow CVP to remain relatively normal in the presence of significant hypovolemia. The most important evidence in the diagnosis of hypovolemic shock is whether the patient's condition improves after a volume challenge (for details, see Section **III.**).

c. Septic shock. Septic shock is a state of organ hypoperfusion that may accompany severe infection. It is caused either by the circulatory spread of bacteria or by their metabolic products. Although a wide variety of pathogens may induce septic shock, it is most commonly seen with gram-negative bacterial infections. The mechanism of shock in this setting is the release of endotoxin (a component of the bacterial wall) into the bloodstream.

Endotoxin interacts with vasoactive substances in the bloodstream and may cause syndromes that range from increased vascular permeability to disseminated intravascular coagulation. The diagnosis is suggested by a history of infection plus physical examination and laboratory studies consistent with an infective focus. Metabolic (lactic) acidosis is common in this form of shock. A progressively increasing anion gap carries grave implications and should prompt a reassessment of the therapeutic regimen.

III. Therapy
   A. Medical treatment
      1. Monitoring the patient with shock. Probably no other entity demands more constant and skillful monitoring than shock. The potential for rapid deterioration demands that the physician expand clinical impressions with monitoring equipment that can provide accurate hemodynamic data. Four types of monitoring are commonly used in patients with shock: (i) CVP, (ii) pulmonary arterial pressure, (iii) systemic arterial pressure, and (iv) urine output (bladder catheterization). The combination of monitoring used is dictated by the clinical situation and the type of data needed. Pulmonary arterial hemodynamic monitoring is said by some authorities to be essential in these sick patients. However, data to support this contention are lacking, and many clinicians manage these patients without the use of invasive hemodynamic monitoring.
         a. CVP. A large-bore (no. 14 or no. 16) needle is used to introduce a cannula into a large vein that empties into the right side of the heart. Mean right ventricular filling (right atrial) pressures are measured (normal is 0 to 7 mm Hg). In the setting of significant pulmonary disease or left ventricular disease, CVP does not accurately reflect left-heart filling pressures, and a pulmonary arterial catheter must be used. In addition to monitoring pressure, the central venous line can be used to assess the response to initial fluid challenge (see Section **III.A.1.b.2.a.**). Right ventricular filling pressures as high as 15 mm Hg may be necessary to provide adequate cardiac output in the acute phase of shock.
         b. Pulmonary arterial pressure. The preferred instrument for monitoring left ventricular filling pressures is a balloon-tipped pulmonary arterial catheter (Swan-Ganz catheter) that may be introduced percutaneously and allowed to "float" out into the pulmonary artery. With the balloon deflated, the catheter is advanced to a small branch of the pulmonary arterial tree.

When the balloon is reinflated, the small pulmonary artery is occluded and an approximation of PCWP is obtained. Utilization of the pulmonary arterial catheter is important when (i) the patient's blood pressure does not respond to an initial fluid challenge, or (ii) MI is suspected or known to underlie shock, and accurate left ventricular filling pressures may be useful in selecting and monitoring therapy. Normal PCWPs range from 2 to 12 mm Hg. In patients with cardiogenic shock, however, the heart is operating on a depressed Starling curve, and wedge pressures of 15 to 18 mm Hg usually are required to provide maximum cardiac output. As noted earlier, many physicians prefer to manage their patients in shock without invasive hemodynamic monitoring because no data exist that confirm the usefulness of pulmonary arterial hemodynamic monitoring in these patients.

Thermodilution pulmonary arterial catheters can be used to monitor serial cardiac output. When pharmacologic agents such as inotropic drugs or vasodilators are used, a pulmonary arterial catheter provides useful hemodynamic data on the efficacy of treatment.

c. Systemic arterial pressure. An arterial cannula is advisable in patients with overt shock. There are three major reasons: (i) in shock, the auscultatory blood pressure may not accurately reflect the true systemic arterial pressure, particularly in the patient who is peripherally vasoconstricted and has thready pulses. Because adequate blood pressure is essential to survival, accurate blood pressure determination by means of an arterial catheter is desirable. (ii) The vasoactive agents used to treat shock (both vasodilators and sympathomimetic agents) require continuous monitoring that is best achieved by an arterial catheter. (iii) Numerous blood samples (both arterial blood gases and blood chemistry samples) are necessary to monitor the therapy of shock. Patient comfort is maximized if blood is drawn through an indwelling arterial cannula.

d. Urine output. Patients in shock or preshock should have a Foley catheter placed in the bladder to assist in monitoring hourly urine output.

2. General measures. Shock is an acute situation that can rapidly deteriorate. Certain general measures should be instituted immediately for **any** patient in shock.

a. Intravenous access. At least one and preferably two large-bore (no. 14 or no. 16) intravenous cannulas ensure adequate vascular access. Unless the patient has signs of fluid overload (rales, elevated neck veins), an initial fluid challenge of 500 ml over 30 minutes should be given. The choice of fluid remains controversial (normal saline, albumin, and dextran are all acceptable). The goal of fluid replacement is to establish a systolic pressure of 90 to 100 mm Hg, not the previous level of systemic blood pressure.

b. Oxygen. An arterial PO_2 of 70 mm Hg should be established by increasing inspiratory oxygen with nasal cannulas or a face mask, except in patients with obstructive pulmonary disease. Many patients with chronic obstructive pulmonary disease have an arterial PO_2 in the 55 to 60 mm Hg range. Adequate respiratory function in these individuals is based on central nervous system hypoxic drive, and increasing arterial PO_2 above 70 mm Hg can lead to respiratory arrest.

c. Position. Patients with shock should be supine or in reverse Trendelenburg position.

d. Pain relief. Careful administration of an analgesic (morphine, 2 to 4 mg intravenously, may be administered to relieve pain) is frequently necessary.

e. Flow charts. Flow charts should be established to follow volume replacement, drugs administered, acid-base status, arterial PO_2, pulmonary wedge pressure, systemic blood pressure, and urine output.

3. Drugs. A wide variety of agents are available to treat shock. Two large classes of drugs commonly used are vasopressors and vasodilators. The use of any specific drug or class of drug is dictated by the clinical setting and suspected underlying etiology.

a. Vasopressors. Often vasopressors are used incorrectly in the therapy of shock. Remember that shock indicates inadequate tissue perfusion rather than any absolute level of blood pressure. With this caveat in mind, vasopressors can serve as a valuable component of an overall plan to support adequate tissue perfusion. In general, vasopressors should not be used until an adequate fluid challenge has been attempted. If appropriate fluid has been given, and signs of inadequate organ perfusion persist, a trial of vasopressors is indicated.

Which vasopressor should be used? The decision is based on two parameters: (i) the underlying pathophysiology of the shock state and (ii) a knowledge of the pharmacology of each vasopressor.

Assessment of the pathophysiology of the compromised circulation is accomplished in the fashion outlined in Section **III**. This is combined with hemodynamic information derived from appropriate monitoring. Several classifications for vasopressors exist. The most rational classification is based on the type of sympathetic receptor affected by a given vasopressor. There are two types of sympathetic receptors: alpha and beta. Alpha-receptor stimulation causes arteriolar vasoconstriction, whereas beta stimulation augments cardiac performance and causes arteriolar vasodilatation. An example of a pure alpha-receptor stimulator is methoxamine; isoproterenol is a pure beta-receptor stimulator. Most vasopressors have both alpha and beta effects. In addition to alpha and beta effects, dopamine in low doses (2 to 10 g/kg per minute) has a dilative effect on the renal vascular bed, independent of beta effects. The choice of agent is dictated by the combination of myocardial stimulation and vasoconstriction/vasodilatation required for a particular patient's hemodynamic status. In general, the larger the dose of vasopressor required to support the circulation, the less likely are the patient's chances of recovery.

A list of the various vasopressors available and their modes of action, dosages, and side effects is found in Table 6-6. Practical guidelines for mixing solutions of vasopressors are shown in Table 6-7. Some of the more frequently used vasopressors are discussed briefly here.

(1) Levarterenol (Levophed, norepinephrine). Levarterenol stimulates both alpha- and beta-receptors. It has some stimulatory effect on the myocardium, although its principal action is through arteriolar vasoconstriction. It is most effective if used to raise blood pressure to 90 to 100 mm Hg (above this number, reflex bradycardia occurs with concomitant decreases in cardiac output).

(2) Dopamine (Intropin). Dopamine has primarily beta effects, with some alpha effects. In addition, low-dose dopamine has a direct vasodilative effect on the renal and mesenteric vascular beds.

(3) Dobutamine (Dobutrex). Dobutamine, a synthetic congener of isoproterenol, is effective in the treatment of severe left ventricular failure and cardiogenic shock. It possesses primarily beta$_1$ (cardiac stimulation) activity. It does possess some beta$_2$ (peripheral vasodilatation) activity, but much less than that of isoproterenol, and some alpha-adrenergic activity, although less than that of dopamine and much less than that of levarterenol. It does not possess the independent renal dilatation properties of dopamine. It is probably most useful when PCWP is markedly elevated and hypotension is not severe. If hypotension is the

TABLE 6-6. VASOPRESSORS AVAILABLE FOR USE IN SHOCK

Drug				Effects					
Generic name	Trade name	Dose (IV)	Action (type of receptor)	Cardiac stimula-tion	Vaso-constric-tion	Vaso-dilatation	Cardiac output	Side Effects	Comments
Dopamine	Intropin	2–50 µg/kg/min	Alpha- and beta-dopami-nergic	++	++	++	Usually elevated	Ventricular arrhythmias, nausea, vomiting, angina pectoris	Type of stimulation that predominates depends on infusion rate: >10 µg/kg/min alpha-vasocon-striction pre-dominates; <10 µg/kg/min has independent vasodilative effect on renal vasculature
Levarterenol	Levophed	2–8 µg/min	Primarily alpha, some beta-1 (cardiac)	++	++++	0	Usually slightly decreased	Dose-related hyper-tension, reflex bradycardia	Must avoid reflex bradycardia; therapeutic goal is systolic blood pressure ~90 mm Hg; primary effect is vasoconstric-tion; useful when loss of venous tone predomi-nates; not useful in hypovolemic shock

(continued)

TABLE 6-6. (Continued)

| Drug | | | | Effects | | | | | |
Generic name	Trade name	Dose (IV)	Action (type of receptor)	Cardiac stimulation	Vasoconstriction	Vasodilatation	Cardiac output	Side Effects	Comments
Dobutamine	Dobutrex	2.5–20.0 µg/kg/min	Primarily beta-1, some beta-2, some alpha	++++	+	++	Increased	Tachycardia, ventricular arrhythmias, occasional gastrointestinal distress	A synthetic derivative of isoproterenol that causes less peripheral dilatation and tachycardia. Particularly useful in low-output congestive heart failure; less peripheral vasoconstriction than that of dopamine; causes fewer arrhythmias than does isoproterenol
Isoproterenol	Isuprel	2–4 µg/min	Beta	++++	0	++++	Increased	Tachycardia, angina pectoris, facial flushing, sweating	A pure beta stimulator; has both inotropic and chronotropic effects; causes cardiac stimulation and vasodilatation; cardiac output goes up;

myocardial oxygen consumption increases

Metaraminol	Aramine	0.5–5.0 mg	Alpha and beta	+	+++	++	Reduced	Dose-related hypertension, reflex bradycardia	Indirect-acting alpha and beta stimulator; same effects as those of Levophed, but less potent
Phenylephrine	Neo-Synephrine	40–180 µg/min	Alpha	0	++++	0	Reduced		Pure alpha stimulator; uses in shock limited to neurogenic causes or to reflex inhibition of supraventricular tachyarrhythmias
Ephedrine		5–25 mg	Alpha and beta	+++	++	+	Elevated		An indirect-acting central nervous system stimulant; limited value in shock therapy
Epinephrine		0.1–0.25 mg	Alpha and beta	++++	++++	+++	Elevated	Palpitations, hypertension, angina pectoris, cardiac arrhythmias	Specific therapy for anaphylactic shock

0, no effect; +, modest effect; ++, moderate effect; +++, marked effect; ++++, very marked effect.

TABLE 6-7. COMMON MIXTURES AND CONCENTRATIONS OF VASOPRESSORS USED IN SHOCK

Drug	Standard solution	Concentration (μg/ml)	Comments
Dopamine (single-strength)	400 mg/500 ml 5% D/W	800	Ampules are 200 mg each
Dopamine (double-strength)	800 mg/500 ml 5% D/W	1600	
Dobutamine (single-strength)	250 mg/1000 ml 5% D/W	250	Ampules are 20 mg each
Dobutamine (double-strength)	500 mg/1000 ml 5% D/W	500	
Levarterenol (Levophed)	8 mg/500 ml 5% D/W	16	Check label of Levophed ampule for concentration
Metaraminol (Aramine)	100 mg/500 ml 5% D/W	200	Ampules are 10 mg each
Isoproterenol (Isuprel)	2 mg/500 ml 5% D/W	4	Ampules are both 1 and 2 mg; check label
Epinephrine	2 mg/500 ml 5% D/W	4	Add 2 ml of 1:1,000 (2 ampules; each contains 1 ml or 1 mg)

General comments: (a) Administer all solutions through constant infusion pump; (b) pediatric infusion set should be used (1 ml = 60 drops); and (c) all drugs should be remixed every 24 hours.
5% D/W, 5% dextrose in water.

major problem, dopamine or levarterenol probably represent better choices. Dobutamine has the advantage over isoproterenol of causing less peripheral vasodilation and thus is less likely to provoke a compensatory tachycardia.

   (4) Isoproterenol (Isuprel). Isoproterenol activates beta-receptors, which stimulate the myocardium; peripheral arteriolar vasodilatation and tachycardia also occurs.

  b. Vasodilators. Vasodilators have been used in patients with cardiogenic shock, elevated left ventricular filling pressures, systemic arterial pressures around 100 mm Hg, and low cardiac output. Vasodilator therapy has even been of benefit in occasional patients with systemic arterial pressures of 80 to 90 mm Hg. Pulmonary arterial and systemic arterial catheters should be inserted before vasodilator therapy is initiated. The patient must be monitored in an intensive care unit to prevent hypotension. Specific drugs and dosages of vasodilators are outlined in Chapter 4.

  4. Myocardial reperfusion. Improved cardiac function and outcome occur after myocardial reperfusion, whether brought about by pharmacologic thrombolysis, percutaneous transluminal coronary angioplasty, or emergency coronary artery bypass grafting. Recent multicenter trial data support early mechanical reperfusion by angioplasty or coronary bypass surgery as the best approach for the critically ill patient with cardiogenic shock after MI.

B. Surgery

  1. General measures. Surgical intervention is indicated to remedy a number of the underlying disorders that cause shock (see Table 6-2). In some in-

stances, such as hemorrhage, intestinal obstruction, and hemothorax, emergency surgery can be lifesaving and must be undertaken without delay. In other settings, as with burns, initial management is primarily medical, with subsequent surgical intervention. Shock can be compounded by surgery and general anesthesia. Fluid balance, oxygenation, electrolyte levels, and acid-base balance must be adjusted before an acutely ill patient is sent to surgery.

2. Intraaortic balloon pump (IABP). In recent years, a number of mechanical methods have been used to support the circulation. The most commonly used mechanical device is the IABP. It is used for a variety of conditions, including intractable left ventricular failure after cardiopulmonary bypass, cardiogenic shock after MI, and refractory angina pectoris. The IABP is effective, at least temporarily, in reversing the shock state in patients with cardiogenic shock secondary to MI or its complications. Because IABP is not definitive therapy by itself, this intervention should be combined with angioplasty or cardiac surgery if mortality is to be avoided. Improvements of 15% to 20% in cardiac output can predictably be expected in such patients, and hemodynamic stability often will be achieved with the IABP in place. In the absence of any reversible lesion, however, such patients are almost impossible to wean from the IABP.

In contrast, patients who experience the mechanical complications that accompany MI (e.g., acute mitral regurgitation, acute ventricular septic defect) may often be salvaged after IABP insertion, which allows them to be stabilized for cardiac catheterization and definitive surgical intervention. Patients with unstable angina refractory to maximal pharmacologic therapy may also benefit from IABP insertion, which allows them to undergo cardiac catheterization and surgical or catheter revascularization.

The IABP is a helium-filled, sausage-shaped balloon, which is introduced into the thoracic aorta from the femoral artery. Balloon filling is electronically synchronized with the patient's ECG so that the balloon inflates during diastole and deflates during systole. The balloon influences the physiology of the heart in two ways: (i) it augments coronary blood flow through increased aortic diastolic pressure, and (ii) it decreases left ventricular afterload by deflation early in systole. Most centers report hemodynamic improvement in 80% to 90% of patients with shock following treatment with IABP.

SELECTED READINGS

Chou TM, Amidon TM, Ports TA, et al. Cardiogenic shock: thrombolysis or angioplasty? *J Intensive Care Med* 1995;11:37–48.
An up-to-date discussion of the benefits and limitations of these reperfusion techniques in cardiogenic shock.
Fink MP. Shock: An overview. In: Rippe JM, Irwin RS, Fink MP, et al., eds. *Intensive care medicine.* oston: Little, Brown and Company, 1995.
A comprehensive and up-to-date chapter by one of the leading investigators in the field.
Flesch M, Kilter H, Cremers B, et al. Effects of endotoxin on human myocardial contractility: involvement of nitric oxide and peroxynitrite. *J Am Coll Cardiol* 1999;33: 1062–1070.
Endotoxin exposure to the human myocardium leads to release of nitric oxide and subsequent myocardial depression.
Goldberg RJ, Samad NA, Yarzebski J, et al. Temporal trends in cardiogenic shock complicating acute myocardial infarction. *N Engl J Med* 1999;340:1162–1168.
Short-term survival rates have improved in recent years for patients with cardiogenic shock after MI. This would appear to be the result of more aggressive reperfusion therapy in these patients.

Hochman JS, Sleeper LA, Webb JG, et al. Early revascularization in acute myocardial infarction complicated by cardiogenic shock. *N Engl J Med* 1999;341:625–634.
Early revascularization improves the outlook for patients who develop cardiogenic shock after MI.
Hochman JS, Sleeper LA, White HD, et al. One-year survival following early revascularization for cardiogenic shock. *JAMA* 2001;285:190–192.
Early revascularization results in improved 1-year survival for patients with acute MI and cardiogenic shock.
Price S, Anning PB, Mitchell JA, et al. Myocardial dysfunction in sepsis: mechanisms and therapeutic implications. *Eur Heart J* 1999;20:715–724.
An excellent review of the underlying mechanisms operating in septic shock.
White HD. Cardiogenic shock: a more aggressive approach is now warranted. *Eur Heart J* 2000;21:1897–1901.
Early reperfusion therapy is clearly warranted in patients with cardiogenic shock after MI.

7. SYNCOPE

I. **Introduction.** Syncope, faintness, and light-headedness are frequent problems in patients with cardiac disease. The physician caring for patients with known cardiac dysfunction often faces the difficult problem of determining the etiology of such episodes. Many episodes of syncope have a cardiac basis, and a careful cardiovascular examination is therefore necessary in patients with a history of syncope or light-headedness.

    A. **Definitions.** The clinical entities of syncope and faintness are difficult to distinguish from each other. As used in this chapter, syncope refers to a transient loss of consciousness and inability to retain an upright posture. A temporary decrease in cerebral blood flow is generally implied. Faintness, in contrast, refers to a sense of weakness and impending loss of consciousness without actual loss of consciousness. True syncope is a serious, perhaps even life-threatening, illness and may require hospital admission to a monitored bed. Patients whose syncopal episodes are based on underlying cardiac disease have an increased 1-year mortality of 18% to 25% compared with that of comparably aged healthy individuals. Syncope based on noncardiac causes does not appear to carry significantly increased 1-year mortality.

    B. **Pathophysiology.** The final common pathway leading to cardiovascular syncope is usually a decrease in blood flow to the brain that is below the critical level required to support the metabolic activity of the brain at a level ensuring maintenance of consciousness.

        The circulation and metabolism of the brain are unique. The brain has a relatively stable oxygen consumption and hence requirement (around 3.6 ml of oxygen per 100 g brain tissue per minute). Moreover, the brain is unable to store energy substrates. It therefore depends on continuous cerebral blood flow to resupply needed glucose. When cerebral blood flow is interrupted, consciousness is lost within 10 seconds.

    C. **Etiologies.** A wide variety of conditions can lead to syncope and faintness (Table 7-1). Despite many underlying etiologies, most syncopal episodes are caused by disturbances in circulatory, metabolic, or neurophysiologic function. This chapter focuses on circulatory derangements that cause syncope and faintness, as contrasted with metabolic and neurophysiologic mechanisms.

II. **Diagnosis.** Syncope or the feeling of faintness complicates a wide spectrum of cardiac diseases. Cerebral blood flow depends on cardiac output and systemic blood pressure. Any lesion, therefore, that either impairs cardiac pump function or greatly diminishes peripheral vascular resistance can create a transient state of inadequate cerebral blood flow. Furthermore, underlying cardiac or vascular disease can impair the ability of the circulatory system to increase cardiac output to meet the changing physiologic conditions of daily living such as rising from a recumbent position or exercising, thereby leading to syncope. Finally, a number of medications routinely prescribed for cardiac disease can inhibit normal compensatory mechanisms needed to support adequate blood pressure and hence cerebral blood flow.

    A. **History: syncope as a complication of cardiac disease.** A complete history of cardiac disease or cardiovascular symptoms, together with any current medication, should be obtained from every patient with a syncopal episode. Information obtained from history and screening laboratory alone will pinpoint the etiology underlying cardiovascular syncope in 50% of patients. When data obtained from physical examination are added, an accurate diagnosis is possible in approximately three fourths of patients.

        Arrhythmias are the principal cardiac cause of syncope. Patients should be questioned concerning palpitations or sensations of rapid heart rate. Bradycardia or tachycardia can produce syncope. Atrioventricular block is a common cause of syncope (Adams-Stokes disease). Runs of ventricular

117

TABLE 7-1. CAUSES OF SYNCOPE AND FAINTNESS

I. Cardiac diseases
   A. Arrhythmias
      1. Bradyarrhythmias
         a. Sinus bradycardia
         b. Sinus arrest
         c. Sinoatrial block
         d. Ventricular asystole
         e. Pacemaker malfunction
         f. AV block with Adams-Stokes attacks
      2. Tachyarrhythmias
         a. Supraventricular tachycardias, including paroxysmal atrial tachycardia, atrial flutter, and atrial fibrillation
         b. Ventricular tachycardia
         c. Episodic ventricular fibrillation
         d. Familial episodic ventricular fibrillation (long Q–T syndrome)
   B. Myocardial infarction
   C. Valvular lesions (particularly aortic stenosis)
   D. Congenital lesions (particularly tetralogy of Fallot with or without repair)
   E. Mitral valve prolapse (rare)
   F. Pericardial disease (cardiac tamponade)
   G. Atrial myxoma, ball-valve thrombus with transient obstruction of a cardiac valve orifice
   H. Treatment of cardiac disease with sympathetic blocking agents (alpha or beta sympathetic receptor blocking medications)

II. Other cardiovascular diseases
   A. Orthostatic hypotension
   B. Vasovagal attacks
   C. Carotid sinus syncope
   D. Cerebrovascular disease in the vertebral or basilar arteries
   E. Vascular obstruction (pulmonary embolism, acute aortic dissection)
   F. Vasodepressor syncope

III. Noncardiac diseases
   A. Neurologic causes of syncope
      1. Hysterical syncope
      2. Vertigo
      3. Syncope accompanying migraine headaches
      4. Seizure disorder
   B. Metabolic causes of syncope
      1. Hyperventilation
      2. Hypoglycemia (rare)
   C. Other causes of syncope
      1. Prolonged coughing spells
      2. Micturition
      3. Emotional disorders (particularly anxiety attacks)
      4. Anemia
      5. Fluid loss (diarrhea, ascites, burns, excessive diuresis)
      6. Drugs (particularly antiarrhythmic medications)

tachycardia or bursts of ventricular fibrillation may also underlie syncopal episodes. A history of previously documented arrhythmias, together with current treatment, should be sought. Some individuals have syncope secondary to a familial form of episodic ventricular fibrillation, with a prolonged Q–T interval on the ECG. Therefore, any family history of syncopal episodes should be noted. Syncope may accompany attacks of supraventricular tachyarrhythmia such as atrial flutter or paroxysmal atrial tachycardia. Patients with supraventricular arrhythmias often recall the sensation of rapid heartbeat before their syncopal episode. Cardiac diseases that may be complicated by syncope include myocardial infarction (MI), valvular lesions (particularly aortic stenosis [AS]), congenital lesions (particularly tetralogy of Fallot), and, rarely, mitral valve prolapse. Symptoms that might arise from any of these conditions should be explored. Important historical items relevant to patients with syncope are found in Table 7-2.

B. Physical examination. Physical examination in a patient with syncope should focus on the cardiovascular and neurologic systems. Often the physician is asked to assess a patient who gives a history of syncopal episodes but is currently asymptomatic. In this setting, in addition to a complete physical examination, some provocative tests may be cautiously undertaken in an attempt to duplicate the conditions under which syncope occurred. The physician may

TABLE 7-2. HISTORICAL ITEMS IN PATIENTS WITH SYNCOPE AND FAINTNESS

Category	Item	Significance
History of present illness	Detailed history of syncopal episodes (Any premonitory signs, unusual feelings, or aura? Was patient sitting or standing? Any palpitations? Did anyone observe episode?)	Cardiac vs. cardiovascular or noncardiovascular etiology of syncope
	Is syncope associated with head turning or tight collars?	? Carotid sinus syncope
Past medical history	History of past cardiac disease	Particularly arrhythmias, aortic stenosis, or myocardial infarction
	History of neurologic disease	Particularly headaches or dizziness
	History of metabolic disease	Is patient being treated for diabetes?
	History of emotional problems	Hyperventilation, anxiety
Current medications	Any medication for hypertension?	? Orthostatic hypotension ? Vasovagal episode
Family history	Family history of syncopal episodes or cardiac disease	Familial episodic ventricular fibrillation (long Q–T syndrome)
Social/personal history	Evaluate sources of stress in individual, particularly if syncopal episodes are associated with particular settings	? Vasovagal syncope ? Anxiety ? Emotional stability

be called to assess the patient during a syncopal episode or immediately after a syncopal episode. In that event, concern for treatment supersedes diagnostic maneuvers, although certain physical findings are important in this acute situation.

1. Physical examination of the patient with a history of syncopal episodes who is asymptomatic at the time of examination. A general assessment of the patient's emotional status should be made. Vital signs are important. Blood pressure and pulse rate should be recorded in both arms, when the patient is lying and immediately after the patient rises from a supine to a standing position. The resting pulse should be felt for at least a minute, and any abnormalities in rate or rhythm noted. A tendency toward hyperventilation should be noted. Skin color, moisture, and temperature are observed. Gentle palpation of the carotid pulse is followed by auscultation for bruits. Supraorbital pulses are palpated bilaterally. Auscultation for bruits over both subclavian arteries also is indicated. Cardiac examination emphasizes rate, rhythm, and the presence of any murmurs. Peripheral pulses are judged for strength and regularity. Focal neurologic deficits are sought. Physical findings in patients with a history of syncopal episodes who are asymptomatic at the time of examination are summarized in Table 7-3.

2. Physical examination of a patient in the midst of or immediately after a syncopal episode. The patient should be placed in a position with legs higher than head (reverse Trendelenburg). Adequacy of airway, breathing, and circulation are assessed. Pulse rate and regularity are noted, as is any seizure activity.

3. Provocative maneuvers in the patient with a history of syncope. In the asymptomatic patient being evaluated for syncopal episodes, a variety of provocative maneuvers may be undertaken in an attempt to elucidate the mechanisms of syncope. A complete history and physical examination must be undertaken before any of these procedures are tried because, in certain patients, maneuvers such as carotid sinus pressure may be dan-

TABLE 7-3. PHYSICAL FINDINGS IN PATIENTS WITH A HISTORY OF SYNCOPE

System	Finding	Comment/significance
General	Patient's emotional status	? Anxiety-induced syncope
Vital signs	Resting pulse (rate and rhythm)	? Arrhythmia or heart block
	Blood pressure (both supine and after standing)	? Orthostatic hypotension
	Respiratory rate and depth	? Hyperventilation syndrome
Head, eyes, ears, nose, throat	Palpation of supraorbital pulses	? Retrograde flow because of unilateral carotid occlusion
Neck	Palpation and auscultation Auscultation of subclavian arteries	? Carotid atherosclerotic narrowing ? Subclavian steal syndrome
Cardiac	Murmurs	? Aortic stenosis ? Mitral valve prolapse
Peripheral vasculature	Bruits, strength of pulses	Peripheral vascular disease
Neurologic	Thorough examination	? Neurologic basis of syncope

gerous. For example, carotid sinus pressure should not be performed in a patient with significant carotid atherosclerosis. Table 7-4 lists provocative maneuvers that may be undertaken in a patient with syncope.

C. Laboratory tests. All patients with syncope should have blood drawn for hematocrit, electrolytes, and blood sugar, particularly in the acute setting.

D. ECG. All patients with syncope should have a 12-lead ECG and a rhythm strip recorded. Items of particular interest on the ECG include evidence of prolonged Q–T interval; evidence of acute ischemia; S1,Q3,T3 pattern (sometimes seen in massive acute pulmonary embolism); and any disturbance in rate or rhythm. Pacing and sensing should be evaluated in patients with permanent pacemakers. Patients with syncope in whom an arrhythmia is suspected, or in whom the cause of syncope remains in question, should undergo a period of ambulatory ECG monitoring. One method of performing this is Holter monitoring. The Holter monitor is a device worn by the patient over a 24-hour period, during which time a diary of activities is kept. The monitor records the ECG during this time on electromagnetic tape that is subsequently scanned for arrhythmias. Because patients frequently have no symptoms when arrhythmias are occurring, the Holter monitor provides important clinical information about the etiology of syncopal episodes. It is important to correlate any symptoms that the patient might record in their diary with the presence or absence of arrhythmias at that moment in time.

E. Echocardiography. Echocardiography can demonstrate the presence of AS. Noninvasive investigation of the cerebral circulation is often helpful. Doppler flow studies of the carotid and vertebral circulation may provide useful information. An electroencephalogram may help distinguish cardiac syncope from seizure disorders.

F. Catheterization and angiography. Cardiac catheterization has a well-defined role in many of the cardiac diseases that can cause syncope. For example, the presence and severity of AS may be examined, or alternatively, an acute aortic dissection may be discovered. Patients with possible carotid or vertebral arterial atherosclerosis underlying syncope may require cerebral angiography.

G. Electrophysiologic studies. Programmed atrial or ventricular stimulation in the electrophysiology laboratory may help establish a conduction system abnormality that underlies syncope and may uncover supraventricular or ventricular arrhythmias. Corrected sinus node recovery-time abnormalities indicate sinus node disease (this test is very specific, but it is not very sensitive). The ability to induce ventricular tachycardia makes this a likely cause of syncope, although induction of supraventricular tachycardias is much more common and less useful. If the H–V interval (His bundle to ventricular conduction time) is prolonged on bundle of His recordings in a patient with

TABLE 7-4. PROVOCATIVE MANEUVERS THAT MAY BE PERFORMED IN A PATIENT WITH A HISTORY OF SYNCOPAL EPISODES

Maneuver	Comment
Voluntary hyperventilation	? Hyperventilation syndrome
Carotid sinus pressure	? Carotid sinus syncope
Rapid rising from a supine position	? Orthostatic hypotension
Upper extremity exercises	? Subclavian steal syndrome
Hyperelevation of the arm	? Subclavian steal syndrome
Tilt table	? Reproduces the syncopal episode and defines the pathophysiology: orthostatic hypotension, vasodepressor syncope

unifascicular or bifascicular block, and the patient has experienced syncope, a strong case can be made for insertion of a permanent pacemaker. Despite the types of specific information available, electrophysiologic studies are of limited usefulness in establishing the underlying cause in most patients with syncope. Therefore, these specialized studies are reserved for patients in whom clinical information strongly points to occult supraventricular or ventricular arrhythmias as the cause for syncope.

H. Tilt Table. The tilt table test is a laboratory method for identifying patients with neurally mediated (e.g., vasovagal) syncope. Patients are held in a head-up position without muscular activity for a predetermined period of time to see they will inappropriately vasodilate and drop their arterial blood pressure. Often, patients develop presyncope or frank syncope. This test has many false-positive and false-negative responses, and its use remains controversial.

I. Protocol for the diagnosis of syncope
1. Making the diagnosis. The diagnosis of syncope is a clinical one. The distinction between syncope and feelings of faintness usually can be made by a careful history. The difficult diagnostic problems in syncope lie not in recognizing the entity itself but in determining which of many possible underlying causes is responsible for the transient loss of consciousness.
2. Differential diagnosis. A detailed differential diagnosis for syncope is provided in Table 7-1. Neurologic and metabolic abnormalities can coexist with cardiac disease and must be considered. Successful determination of the etiology of syncope frequently hinges on taking an accurate history and performing simple diagnostic maneuvers. Laboratory tests support clinical suspicions.
   a. Syncope due to cardiac diseases. Each of the cardiac diseases that may cause syncope is discussed in a separate chapter in this manual; however, it is useful to consider some of the more common cardiovascular problems that may underlie a syncopal episode.
      (1) Arrhythmias. Syncope is the first manifestation of ventricular asystole or fibrillation. Obviously, this constitutes a medical emergency. Loss of consciousness occurs within 10 seconds of loss of cerebral perfusion, and unless effective cardiopulmonary resuscitation is initiated, ischemic seizures may occur within 30 to 40 seconds. Both bradyarrhythmias and tachyarrhythmias can lead to syncope, particularly in patients with underlying cardiovascular disease and diminished cardiac reserve.
         Antiarrhythmic medications occasionally exacerbate arrhythmias and lead to syncope. This is particularly common with type Ia, Ic, and III antiarrhythmic medications, for example, quinidine, procainamide, propafenone, flecainide, and sotalol, which can prolong the Q–T interval and result in torsades de pointes—a special form of ventricular tachycardia in which the ECG axis of the QRS complexes appears to "rotate around a point." Antianginal medications such as beta-blockers and verapamil may result in conduction system abnormalities that can lead to syncope. This is particularly common if the two drugs are used together. Pacemaker failure to sense or capture can also result in syncope.
      (2) Syncope accompanying cardiovascular disease
         (a) Valvular heart disease. Syncope is a common and worrisome symptom in patients with AS. Because it often signifies critical narrowing of the valve, patients with AS who have a syncopal episode should undergo a careful echocardiographic study and/or cardiac catheterization. Syncope rarely can complicate pulmonic stenosis or mitral valve prolapse, although in these settings it does not appear to carry adverse prognostic consequences. Positional syncope suggests left atrial myxoma with obstruction of the mitral

valve orifice by the pedunculated mass of the myxoma in certain positions. Dysfunction of a prosthetic valve (particularly the ball-cage valves) may lead to syncope. Immediate surgery is indicated in this setting.

(b) Myocardial disorders. Patients with hypertrophic obstructive cardiomyopathy may experience syncope in a variety of settings. Decreased preload from the Valsalva maneuver (e.g., straining at stool) can lead to syncope, as can decreased afterload (e.g., nitrate therapy) or change in rhythm (atrial fibrillation, ventricular tachycardia). Syncope may accompany angina, MI, or Prinzmetal's angina. In all of these cases, syncope implies a worsened prognosis for the patient and should trigger a careful evaluation of the underlying disease.

(c) Vascular obstruction. Between 15% and 20% of patients with pulmonary embolism experience syncope as an early presenting symptom. Syncope in acute pulmonary embolism implies obstruction of more than 50% of the pulmonary circulation. Effort-related syncope may accompany pulmonary hypertension. Twenty percent of patients with acute aortic dissection present with syncope. Patients with pericardial tamponade or constrictive pericarditis may experience syncope.

b. Other cardiovascular etiologies of syncope

(1) Orthostatic hypotension. Orthostatic hypotension is caused by failure of the normal compensatory mechanisms that are responsible for maintenance of arterial blood pressure on assumption of the upright posture. Orthostatic hypotension is usually the result of a failure of autonomic function. Although a number of different neurologic deficits can produce this syndrome (e.g., diabetic or alcoholic neuropathies, tabes dorsalis), orthostatic hypotension occurs most often in cardiac patients who have either (i) been subjected to a period of prolonged bed rest or (ii) been treated with medications that alter autonomic function or decrease intravascular volume. Patients with orthostatic hypotension have a variable time of onset of syncope after assuming an upright position (varying from seconds to minutes, depending on the degree of autonomic dysfunction). Often these patients have few, if any, premonitory signs of impending syncope (e.g., pallor, sweating, or change in pulse rate). Family history is important, because there is a familial syndrome of orthostatic hypotension, tachycardia, and syncope. Tilt table testing may help in the diagnosis of this entity.

(2) Vasovagal syncope (vasodepressor syncope). Vasovagal syncope is the most common form of syncope in healthy individuals. Typically, it occurs when a person is placed in a stressful or an uncomfortable situation.

Studies have demonstrated that cardiac output remains essentially unchanged during such episodes. Peripheral resistance, however, drops precipitously, which results in a fall in blood pressure. Patients with cardiac disease are particularly susceptible to this form of syncope because cardiac output may already be compromised. Cardiac diseases that are frequently complicated by vasovagal syncope include AS and MI. Nitrate therapy in patients with angina pectoris, especially elderly patients, can result in a pharmacologic form of vasodepressor syncope. Patients taking cardiovascular medications that may lower blood pressure or slow heart rate, who have a previous history of vasovagal syncope, appear particularly susceptible to exacerbation of this problem. Tilt table testing may also help in the diagnosis of this entity.

(3) Carotid sinus syncope. When carotid sinus pressure is applied to a healthy individual, the typical response is mild hypotension and transient cardiac slowing. In patients who have a particularly sensitive carotid sinus reflex, these responses may be exaggerated to the point of syncope, which may be caused by even mild carotid sinus pressure. For example, wearing a shirt with a collar that fits tightly may provoke a syncopal episode. Patients with cardiac disease are more susceptible to carotid sinus syncope than are healthy individuals. The clinical syndrome ordinarily is seen in elderly patients with diffuse atherosclerotic disease that involves both carotid arteries and is associated with an abnormal conduction system in the heart. The syndrome may also occur in patients with AS or in the aftermath of MI. Carotid bruits are common. Patients with carotid sinus syncope may give a history of premonitory signs before syncope occurs. Some patients experience a sensation of slowing of the heart; others have few or no premonitory sensations.

Extreme caution must be exercised in performing carotid sinus pressure in patients suspected of having carotid atherosclerotic disease.

(4) Cerebral-occlusive syncope. Cerebral-occlusive syncope may occasionally result from many diseases that compromise blood flow to the brain, such as diffuse atherosclerotic disease (often difficult to distinguish from carotid sinus syncope), pulseless disease (Takayasu's arteritis; see Chapter 30), and subclavian steal syndrome. Patients with this form of syncope will recount a variety of symptoms depending on the type of disease and the extent to which cerebral blood flow is impaired.

Patients with diffuse atherosclerosis that involves the carotid and vertebral arteries (often elderly patients with hypertension) may give a history of episodes of light-headedness and dizziness on arising from bed. Sometimes the attacks are severe enough to cause short episodes of "blanking out" (transient ischemic attacks) that may be accompanied by transient focal neurologic signs such as altered speech or sensory deficits. These symptoms and signs are ominous indicators that the patient may be at risk for a cerebrovascular accident, and prompt investigation of the carotid and vertebral-basilar circulation is indicated. Carotid sinus pressure should not be attempted. Patients with subclavian steal syndrome often give a history of syncope after upper-extremity exercise.

c. Syncope from neurologic causes. In addition to the etiologies for syncope based on cardiac and vascular diseases, certain neurologic conditions can cause syncope in patients with a normal cardiovascular system (Table 7-1). These should be considered in patients with suspected cardiovascular disease because the conditions may coexist. Included in this category are hysterical syncope, vertigo, and syncope accompanying migraine headaches. Although detailed description of these entities is beyond the scope of this book, their existence is noted. The presence of an aura suggests a seizure disorder. Observers who witnessed the patient's syncopal episode should be questioned with attention to abnormal movements, eye rolling, etc. A history of previous seizures or migraine headaches should be elicited. The patient who complains of "dizziness" before syncope should be questioned in detail about the exact nature of the symptoms experienced.

d. Metabolic causes of syncope. Anxious patients can provoke a syncopal episode by hyperventilating. Hypoglycemia can also lead to syncope. These metabolic etiologies should be considered in patients who have emotional disorders or who are under treatment for diabetes mellitus.

   e. Other causes of syncope. Syncope can be provoked by a prolonged paroxysm of coughing, micturition, emotional disorders, and anemia. These etiologies also should be considered in any unexplained syncopal episode.
   f. Summary. A general approach to the patient with syncope of undetermined etiology is as follows:
      (1) History: focus on the exact nature of the episode, particularly any history of cardiac or neurologic disease.
      (2) Physical examination: emphasis on heart, peripheral vasculature, neurologic examination.
      (3) Provocative testing: when appropriate, attempt to duplicate conditions under which syncope occurred.
      (4) Routine laboratory tests: initial blood work, 12-lead ECG, and rhythm strip.
      (5) Specialized laboratory work: echocardiography, Holter monitor, Doppler flow studies, tilt table testing, and cerebral angiography as dictated by clinical setting.

III. Therapy. Therapy of syncopal episodes can be divided into three general categories: (i) general measures undertaken during the acute phase of a syncopal episode, (ii) specific measures to counteract underlying etiologies of syncope, and (iii) measures to prevent complications resulting from transient loss of consciousness.
   A. General measures to be undertaken during a syncopal episode. When confronted with a patient in the midst of a syncopal episode, the physician must be concerned both with managing the event and with ascertaining if any life-threatening problem underlies the episode. The following points should be kept in mind:
      1. The patient should be placed with the head lower than the feet to maximize cerebral blood flow.
      2. Adequacy of airway, breathing, and pulse should be assessed immediately.
      3. Tight clothing should be loosened.
      4. If the patient recovers consciousness rapidly, he or she should be prevented from rising for several minutes, and then observed for several minutes after rising.
      5. If the syncopal episode occurs in the hospital setting, blood should be drawn for hematocrit, electrolytes, and blood sugar evaluation. A 12-lead ECG should be obtained, and one ampule of 50% dextrose in water should be administered intravenously.
      6. The patient should be checked for signs of trauma occurring during any fall that accompanied the syncopal episode.
      7. The possibility of life-threatening underlying illness, such as acute hemorrhage or MI, should be assessed and treated appropriately.
   B. Therapy of syncope presenting as a complication of cardiac disease. In most instances, therapy is directed toward the specific underlying disease. If an arrhythmia has been documented, pharmacologic therapy, cardioversion, or pacemaker/internal cardioverter-defibrillator therapy is undertaken. Pacemaker therapy is preferred in a variety of conduction or rhythm disturbances, such as atrioventricular block, chronic bradycardia, or severe carotid sinus syncope. Pharmacologic and electrical (external or internal cardioversion) therapy of arrhythmias, as well as pacemaker therapy, are discussed in more detail in Chapter 3. Syncope-complicating AS is managed with valve replacement. Beta-blockade is often useful in patients with paroxysmal tachyarrhythmias.
   C. Therapy of syncope presenting as the major symptom of diseases of the heart or vasculature

1. Orthostatic hypotension. Therapy of orthostatic hypotension varies according to the underlying cause. Treatment may include combinations of the following: elastic stockings, high-salt diet, mineralocorticoids, beta-blockade (e.g., propranolol 20 to 40 mg per day in divided doses), alpha-agonists (e.g., midodrine 2.5 to 10 mg three times a day), caffeine, and a variety of experimental medications. Patients should be encouraged to rise slowly from bed. Drugs that inhibit the autonomic nervous system (guanethidine, reserpine, certain tranquilizers) should be avoided in these individuals.
2. Vasovagal syncope. Treatment of vasovagal syncope involves both avoidance of stressful settings that provoke this response and attempts at improving any underlying cardiac disease that may make the patient more susceptible to vasovagal episodes. Beta-blockade or alpha-agonism may be given as a therapeutic trial.
3. Carotid sinus syncope. There are several ways to treat carotid sinus syncope. Prevention is emphasized by encouraging the patient to wear loose collars and to avoid rapid head movements. During an acute attack, persistent bradycardia is treated with intravenous atropine. Severe, recurrent carotid sinus syncope may require insertion of a pacemaker.
4. Cerebral-occlusive syncope. Once occlusive cerebrovascular disease has been demonstrated, a variety of surgical procedures may be undertaken to relieve the obstruction. Carotid endarterectomy or a bypass graft may be used, depending on the location of the vascular lesions.

D. General measures to prevent complications from syncopal episodes. In many patients, syncopal episodes recur despite vigorous efforts to determine and eradicate their cause. These patients should be instructed to avoid activities or settings that seem to provoke such episodes. Implantation of a cardiac pacemaker should be considered. In addition, environmental modifications may help to minimize possible complications from syncopal episodes. For example, thick carpeting might be placed in the patient's bedroom, if this is the most frequent site of syncopal episodes. Driving should be avoided.

SELECTED READINGS

Alboni P, Brignole M, Menozzi C, et al. Diagnostic value of history in patients with syncope with or without heart disease. *J Am Coll Cardiol* 2001;37:1921–1928.
The presence of suspected or definite heart disease after an initial clinical evaluation is a strong predictor of a cardiac cause for syncope.

Benditt DG, Fahy GJ, Lurie KG, et al. Pharmacotherapy of neurally mediated syncope. *Circulation* 1999;100:1242–1248.
A review of the various drugs that can be used in the management of neurally mediated syncope.

Brignole M, Alboni P, Benditt D, et al. Guidelines on management (diagnosis and treatment) of syncope. *Eur Heart J* 2001;22:1256–1306.
Complete and thorough discussion of diagnosis and management of syncope from the Task Force on Syncope of the European Society of Cardiology.

Connolly SJ, Sheldon R, Roberts RS, et al. The North American Vasovagal Pacemaker Study (VPS): a randomized trial of permanent cardiac pacing for the prevention of vasovagal syncope. *J Am Coll Cardiol* 1999;33:16–20.
Dual-chamber pacing reduces the likelihood of syncope in patients with recurrent vasovagal syncope.

Cuello C, Bonavita G, Wagshal A, et al. Syncope. In: Rippe JM, Irwin RS, Fink MP, et al., eds. *Intensive care medicine.* Boston: Little, Brown and Company, 1995.
A detailed discussion of circulatory and other causes of syncope.

Fenton AM, Hammill SC, Rea RF, et al. Vasovagal syncope. *Ann Intern Med* 2000;133:714–725.
A review of the pathophysiology, diagnosis, and therapy of vasovagal syncope.

Grimm W, Degenhardt M, Hoffmann J, et al. Syncope recurrence can better be predicted by history than by head-up tilt testing in untreated patients with suspected neurally mediated syncope. *Eur Heart J* 1997;18:1465–1469.
Clinical history was more useful than tilt table testing in the diagnosis of patients with neurally mediated syncope.
Kapoor WN. Syncope. *N Engl J Med* 2000;343:1856–1862.
A thorough review of the clinical diagnosis and therapy of syncope.
Linzer M, Yang EH, Estes NAM, et al. Diagnosing syncope, part I: value of history, physical examination, and electrocardiography. *Ann Intern Med* 1997;126:989–996.
A careful history, physical examination, and ECG will provide a diagnosis or determine whether diagnostic testing is necessary in most patients with syncope.
Linzer M, Yang EH, Estes NAM, et al. Diagnosing syncope, part 2: unexplained syncope. *Ann Intern Med* 1997;127:76–86.
Diagnostic testing strategy in patients with unexplained syncope.
Mosqueda-Garcia R, Furlan R, Tank J, et al. The elusive pathophysiology of neurally mediated syncope. *Circulation* 2000;102:2898–2906.
An interesting review of the various theories and the evidence supporting them surrounding the pathophysiology of neurally mediated syncope.
Sarasin FP, Louis-Simonet M, Carballo D, et al. Prospective evaluation of patients with syncope: a population-based study. *Am J Med* 2001;111:177–184.
Seventy-six percent of patients with syncope had the etiology defined with a standardized clinical evaluation protocol.
Silver KH, Alpert JS. Syncope. *J Intensive Care Med* 1992;7:138.
A good recent review of the various causes of syncope.

8. SUDDEN CARDIAC DEATH AND CARDIOPULMONARY RESUSCITATION

I. Introduction. Sudden cardiac death (SCD) is a worldwide health concern. It results in a significant number of all-natural fatalities in industrially developed countries. By far, the most common cause of sudden death is a recent or remote myocardial infarction (MI). Although the syndrome may arise in a wide variety of settings, such as a ruptured aortic aneurysm, an underlying cardiac disease is most often found.

Sudden death is common in the United States, where it is estimated that one American dies each minute, or where there are more than 400,000 sudden deaths each year.

Many lives could be saved if patients at very high risk were provided automatic implantable defibrillators (see Chapter 3). Likewise, many lives could be saved if basic cardiac life support was instituted rapidly after unexpected cardiac arrest and if basic cardiac life support was followed by prompt defibrillation. This chapter provides not only an update on SCD but also reviews the major changes of the new 2000 International Guidelines for Cardiopulmonary Resuscitation and Emergency Cardiac Care.

II. Sudden cardiac death
   A. Definition. A number of definitions have been offered for SCD. Perhaps the one most widely accepted is that of the World Health Organization, which classifies sudden death as nontraumatic, unexpected, non–self-inflicted death in an individual with or without underlying, preexisting disease who dies within 6 hours of the terminal event. If the death is not witnessed, the victim must have been observed to be healthy within the 24 hours preceding the terminal event.
   B. Etiology. A wide variety of underlying etiologies, both cardiac and noncardiac, have been linked to SCD. Some of these are listed in Table 8-1.
      1. SCD and coronary artery disease (CAD). Epidemiological studies have demonstrated a strong linkage between SCD and the presence of CAD.

         In one study, more than 70% of patients resuscitated for out-of-hospital ventricular fibrillation (VF) had a history of cardiovascular disease, and more than 90% were found to have significant narrowing of at least one coronary artery. The presence or absence of a new "Q-wave" MI as the cause of VF carries important prognostic significance. Patients successfully resuscitated from VF without a new Q-wave MI have a 1-year mortality of 26 %; patients who suffered VF as a complication of an acute Q-wave MI and were resuscitated had a 1-year mortality of only 4%.

         Patients with an open infarct-related artery after MI are less likely to develop SCD.
      2. SCD and nonischemic cardiovascular disease. SCD may complicate a variety of cardiovascular diseases. It has been estimated that hypertrophic cardiomyopathy is present in one in 200 instances of SCD. In one series of 29 young athletes who suffered SCD, hypertrophic cardiomyopathy that had been overlooked during life was present in 14 of the athletes. SCD is a well-recognized complication of severe aortic stenosis. Patients with symptomatic aortic stenosis have a significantly increased risk of SCD. Symptomatic aortic stenosis is an indication that valve replacement surgery should be considered. SCD is a very rare but reported complication of mitral valve prolapse. The etiology of SCD in mitral valve prolapse is in dispute but may relate to the increased incidence of arrhythmias that often accompany the condition. SCD may complicate the numerous causes of the prolonged Q–T syndrome, preexcitation syn-

TABLE 8-1. ETIOLOGIES OF SUDDEN DEATH—CARDIOVASCULAR COLLAPSE

Cardiac factors	Noncardiac factors
Coronary artery disease	Respiratory arrest
Myocardial infarction	Foreign body
Cardiogenic shock	Edema of upper airway (burns, smoke
Rapidly progressive congestive heart	inhalation)
failure	Drowning
Arrhythmias	Pulmonary embolism
Ventricular tachycardia	Sudden infant death syndrome
Supraventricular tachyarrhythmias	Asphyxiation
Bradyarrhythmias	Volatile hydrocarbon exposure ("sniffing
Ventricular fibrillation	death")
Asystole	Central nervous system events
Aortic dissection	Head trauma
Ventricular or septal rupture	Stroke
Subacute bacterial endocarditis	Epilepsy
Cardiac tumors	Drug overdose
Aortic stenosis	Metabolic factors
Mitral stenosis	Hypoglycemia
Mitral valve prolapse	Hypoxia
Prolonged Q–T interval	Hypercalcemia
Pericardial tamponade	Anaphylaxis
Drugs	Poisoning
Digitalis	Electrical shock
Quinidine	Overwhelming sepsis
	Sudden death in the setting of strong
	emotion
	Hemorrhage
	Poisoning
	Trauma

Source: Adapted from Rippe JM, Csete ME, eds., *Manual of intensive care medicine.* Boston: Little, Brown and Company 1983:53.

dromes (presumably on the basis of rapid conduction of atrial fibrillation down the bypass tract), and cardiac tamponade. Rarely, SCD occurs in an individual with an apparently healthy heart.

Unfortunately, SCD can be provoked by antiarrhythmic therapy. SCD presumable secondary to *torsades de point* or other forms of ventricular tachycardia (VT) has been reported not only with antiarrhythmic drugs (particularly with quinidine, procainamide, encainide, and flecainide) but also with other drugs or drug combinations. SCD is a well-recognized complication of heart failure of any cause, including cardiomyopathy. It is estimated that over one third of patients with heart failure die of sudden death. Other causes of SCD include right ventricular dysplasia and right ventricular outflow tract tachycardia.

3. SCD in the absence of cardiovascular diseases. SCD may occur in the absence of recognizable cardiac disease, the so-called idiopathic VF. It is probable that many of these deaths are caused by genetic mutations of the cardiac ion channels, such as the long Q–T syndrome or Brugada's syndrome.

C. Treatment. Approaches to the treatment of SCD may be divided into four general categories: (i) specific measures to terminate VF, (ii) treatment of underlying conditions that may predispose to SCD, (iii) treatment of cardiac electrical instability, and (iv) screening and prophylaxis in populations at increased risk for SCD.

1. Specific measures to terminate VF. Protocols for basic cardiac life support (BCLS) and advanced cardiac life support (ACLS) have been developed by the American Heart Association (AHA) International Guidelines of 2000 and are discussed in detail in Section **III**. The specific therapy of VF or pulseless VT is prompt defibrillation. Although a blow to the chest with one's fist (chest thump) is recommended in witnessed sudden collapse, this is rarely effective. Immediate defibrillation is now available via implantable cardioverter-defibrillators (ICDs). Patients with depressed ejection fraction and nonsustained VT with inducible VT are at high risk for SCD secondary to VT. These patients have enhanced survival when treated with automatic ICDs.

   The availability of automatic external defibrillators (AEDs; see below) placed in the hands of nontraditional providers has improved survival.

   The use of ICDs and AEDs are an important improvement in our armamentarium, as survival from VF decreases 10% for each minute delay in the application of defibrillation.

2. Treatment of underlying conditions that may predispose individuals to SCD. Evidence for any of the entities listed in Table 8-1 should be carefully sought and treated. Because most SCDs are caused by CAD, obviously the ideal is to prevent CAD. In fact, the incidence of SCD is slowly decreasing in the United States.

   Often rhythm strips are available from around the time of the episode of SCD, which may help elucidate its etiology. Once the patient has been stabilized, a thorough history and physical examination and echocardiogram are of obvious importance. Often cardiac catheterization and electrophysiologic studies (EPSs) are necessary.

3. Treatment of cardiac electrical instability
   a. Conventional antiarrhythmic therapy. Conventional antiarrhythmic therapy, including amiodarone, for survivors of sudden cardiac arrest has been disappointing. Most studies have shown that ICDs are the most effective therapy.
   b. Acute drug testing and multidrug regimens. Acute drug testing and multidrug regimens were pioneered by Lown and co-workers and involve administering an acute drug-loading dose intravenously in a monitored setting followed by 72-hour continuous ambulatory monitoring and exercise stress testing. This approach, although somewhat better than empiric drug therapy, is no longer recommended, as even with suppression of all high-grade ventricular ectopy, survival was still poor.
   c. Antiarrhythmic therapy guided by EPS. Over the past two decades, programmed electrical stimulation has played a role in the diagnosis of cardiac rhythm disturbances and as an aid to selection of antiarrhythmic drug therapy. A number of studies have demonstrated the efficacy of EPS in guiding therapy in individuals who have suffered out-of-hospital cardiac arrest. Initially EPSs, such as that used in the ESVEM (Electrophysiologic Study Versus Electrocardiographic Monitoring) trial, were used to identify patients at high risk of sudden death and to test the effectiveness of a variety of antiarrhythmic drugs. Now, EPS is most often used to identify patients with depressed ejection fraction and nonsustained VT who might benefit from ICD implantation.

4. Screening and prophylaxis against SCD in populations at increased risk. It is now well known that patients with depressed left ventricular ejection fractions (below 40%) and nonsustained VT are at increased risk of SCD. Patients with depressed left ventricular ejection fraction and nonsustained VT who have inducible monomorphic VT on EPS, or a positive signal averaged ECG are at high risk of SCD and benefit from ICDs. Studies are now underway to determine if just the presence of a decreased left ventricular ejection fraction and nonsustained VT on

ambulatory ECG monitoring is enough to identify a higher risk group that would benefit from ICDs.

III. Cardiopulmonary resuscitation. Considerable advances have been made in the past 40 years in techniques for resuscitating victims of cardiac arrest.

Major advances have been made in our understanding of the importance of uninterrupted chest compression during basic cardiopulmonary resuscitation (CPR) and the importance of early defibrillation, often available via the use of AEDs.

A. Etiology. Fortunately, cardiac arrest is most often secondary to VF, a condition that is curable if treated early enough. Unfortunately, a significant number of patients have cardiac arrest secondary to asystole. As noted above, the most common predisposing condition in patients with cardiac arrest is CAD. Nevertheless, uncommon conditions need to be ruled out to prevent recurrence. Severe electrolyte abnormalities may provoke cardiac arrest. And as noted above, a variety of other conditions, including the long Q–T syndromes may be the cause. Cardiac arrest also may also occur secondary to respiratory arrest.

Respiratory arrest is the most common cause of arrest in children and young adults. Respiratory arrest results from either inadequate oxygenation of blood or inadequate flow of blood to the brain. In the nonhospital setting, the chief cause of respiratory arrest is upper airway obstruction (UAO). UAO may be caused by any structure blocking the upper airway. The tongue is a common cause of UAO, especially in patients with drug or alcohol overdose or an accident in which the victim has been knocked unconscious. UAO also can result from a foreign body (particularly in children), edema of the tissues of the airway (burns, smoke inhalation, and drug allergy), drowning, or strangulation.

A major cause of UAO leading to respiratory arrest is foreign body obstruction by a piece of food. This emergency can be mistaken for primary cardiac arrest and has been called "the café coronary." Factors that contribute to UAO include (i) large, poorly chewed pieces of food; (ii) dentures; and (iii) elevated blood alcohol levels.

B. Pathophysiology. Regardless of the underlying etiology, cardiac arrest invariably results from one of the following five rhythms: (i) VF, (ii) pulseless VT, (iii) pulseless electrical activity, (iv) agonal rhythm, or (v) ventricular standstill (asystole).

C. Diagnosis

1. Cardiac arrest. The sudden collapse of any patient must be considered a cardiac arrest until proved otherwise. Speed of diagnosis is critical, because the chance of resuscitation is adversely affected by as little as 1 minute of elapsed time. Within 4 minutes of cardiac arrest, some cerebral damage is likely.

The patient with cardiac arrest rapidly loses consciousness. In the absence of ECG monitoring, the diagnosis of cardiac arrest is based on the absence of heart sounds and pulses. However, because most out-of-hospital cardiac arrests are initially attended to by nonmedical professionals, and because such individuals have difficulty discerning the presence of absence of a pulse, the latest AHA International Guidelines for Emergency Cardiac Care no longer recommend that the rescuer tries to determine the presence or absence of an arterial pulse. Emergency CPR should be instituted.

2. Respiratory arrest. The diagnosis of UAO as the cause of respiratory arrest is particularly important because its treatment differs from that used with other causes of respiratory arrest. A foreign body may result in either partial or total airway obstruction. When partial airway obstruction with adequate air exchange occurs, the victim is able to cough forcefully.

There may be wheezing between coughs. The rescuer should not interfere with the victim's own attempts to dislodge the foreign body. Total airway obstruction is diagnosed when the conscious victim (who often either is eating or has just finished eating) is suddenly *unable to speak or cough*. The rescuer should ask, "Can you speak?" The victim may grasp his or her throat, giving the "distress signal for choking." Their skin color may rapidly turn dusky, breathing efforts may become exaggerated, and the victim may collapse. Rapid action is essential.

D. Treatment of cardiac arrest

The major determinants of survival from witnessed out-of-hospital cardiac arrest owing to VF include the presence or absence of bystander-initiated CPR and the speed with which defibrillation is accomplished.

The now classic observations of Eisenberg, Bergner, and Hallstrom were that in patients with out-of-hospital cardiac arrest owing to VF, 43% of these individuals survived to leave the hospital if bystander CPR was initiated within 4 minutes and definitive therapy was delivered within 8 minutes. Survival decreased to less than 7% if basic CPR was not initiated until after 8 minutes, and none survived after 16 minutes of untreated VF.

Although bystander-initiated CPR is critical to survival of out-of-hospital cardiac arrest, the incidence of bystander-initiated CPR throughout the world is extremely low. In a survey of 975 laypersons told to assume that they knew how to do basic CPR, only 15% would "definitely" do CPR that required mouth-to-mouth assisted ventilation on a stranger. In contrast, 68% would "definitely" provide CPR on a stranger if chest compression only were required. The vast majority had an aversion to or a fear of infection from mouth-to-mouth breathing.

An often espoused, but impractical, approach to improve the incidence of bystander CPR would be for everyone to carry barrier masks. Another approach has been to investigate the actual need for assisted ventilation during the early phases of cardiac arrest owing to VF. It must be emphasized that both experience and experimental studies have clearly shown that in respiratory arrest, assisted ventilation is essential (see above). In the pediatric and young adult age groups, cardiac arrest is frequently secondary to respiratory arrest. However, at the time of sudden cardiac arrest owing to VF in adults, the pulmonary veins, the left atrium, the left ventricle, and the entire arterial system are filled with oxygenated blood. To waste time by performing assisted ventilation before initiating chest compression does not make physiologic sense. The most reasonable approach is prompt, rapid, forceful chest compressions.

The major determinant of the effectiveness of basic CPR in subjects with recent onset VF is myocardial and cerebral perfusion, as the brain and the fibrillating heart continue to consume adenosine triphosphate and other energy sources. Without adequate perfusion, they become dysfunctional and eventually cease to function. For example, electrical shocks of subjects with prolonged VF result in defibrillation to pulseless electrical activity or asystole.

Because the coronary and cerebral vessels are maximally dilated early in cardiac arrest, the major determinant of myocardial perfusion during basic CPR is the coronary perfusion pressure, for example, the aortic "diastolic" (the release phase of chest compression) pressure minus the coronary sinus or right atrial "diastolic" pressure. The cerebral perfusion pressure is related to the "systolic" or the chest compression phase of CPR.

Myocardial and cerebral perfusion pressure falls every time chest compressions are interrupted for assisted ventilation, and it takes time to build the coronary perfusion pressure up again once chest compressions are re-initiated. As a result, with a 15:2 compression/ventilation ratio, the highest perfusion pressures are present for less than one half of the time. More importantly, it takes laypersons trained in CPR about 15 seconds to stop chest compression, tilt the head, pinch the nostrils, make a seal with their mouth over the victims, and deliver two full breaths! Thus, trained laypersons providing bystander CPR compress the chest (the vital portion of resuscitation) for less than half of the time!

Our CPR research laboratory became interested in chest-compression-only CPR (CC-CPR) several years ago. One impetus to our interest was a recording that I heard from the Seattle group during its early experience with telephone-directed CPR. After performing telephone-instructed CPR for several minutes, the women asked the dispatcher, "Why is it every time I press on his chest, he opens his eyes, and every time I stop to breathe for him, he goes back to sleep?" This simple observation was in accord with our experimental findings. Over the past decade, our CPR research laboratory has studied VF-induced cardiac arrest using swine and has repeatedly shown that 24-hour survival is similar with CC-CPR and with the now standard airway, breathing, and chest compression CPR (ABC-CPR). More importantly, survival with CC-CPR is dramatically better than no bystander CPR, that is, delaying attempts until the simulation of paramedic arrival 8 to 12 minutes later.

The recent but classic study by Hallstrom and associates from Seattle is of immense importance and will have worldwide implication. It and their previous report are the most elegant studies to date to confirm the experimental laboratory findings in humans that with witnessed nonrespiratory sudden cardiac arrest, CC-CPR is as good as, and possibly better than, the now standard ABC-CPR. The setting of the trial reported by Hallstrom, Cobb, Johnson, and Copass was an urban, fire department–based, two-tiered emergency medical care system with central dispatching and a receptive citizenry. In a randomized manner, telephone dispatchers gave bystanders at the scene of cardiac arrest instructions in either CC-CPR or the now standard ABC-CPR. The primary end point was survival to hospital discharge. A total of 241 patients were randomized to receive CC-CPR and 279 to receive ABC-CPR. The survival rate to hospital discharge was greater among patients randomized to the CC-CPR arm than those in the ABC-CPR arm (14.6% vs. 10.4%) but was not statistically significant ($P = 0.18$). They concluded that CC-CPR resulted in a similar outcome to chest compression with mouth-to-mouth ventilation, and may be the preferred approach for inexperienced bystanders.

The only other study that compared a significant number of cardiac arrests in man was an observational study from Belgium. Paramedics observed the type and quality of layperson CPR when they arrived on the scene. They found survival of patients receiving good CC-CPR was the same as those receiving good ABC-CPR.

Finally, recent studies from our CPR laboratory have shown that uninterrupted chest compression without ventilation results in dramatically better survival than does the standard ABC-CPR performed in the manner that laypersons perform CPR, for example, taking 15 seconds to deliver two breaths by mouth-to-mouth rescue breathing.

For in-hospital cardiac arrest, the importance of these observations is that to be most effective, chest compression must be uninterrupted until defibrillation. Every second that chest compression is interrupted for intubation, starting intravenous lines, or checking the patient's status, compromises the patient's chance for survival.

E. Defibrillation essential

Although slight improvements in basic CPR will save many lives, CC-CPR, ABC-CPR, and improved compression/ventilation ratios can not sustain life—they only slow the process of dying, buying precious minutes for definitive therapy, early defibrillation. An analysis of many studies has shown that survival from out-of-hospital cardiac arrest owing to VF decreases 10% for each minute defibrillation is delayed. The observations with the AED parallel these findings. The use of the AEDs in locations where there are significant numbers of a population at risk and where paramedic response times are inappropriately long will improve survival. Long paramedic response times are the rule in airplanes, airports, ships, and in some if not most large cities, high-rise office buildings or apartments, gated communities, golf courses, and gaming establishments.

It is clear that the weakest links in the chain of survival of out-of-hospital cardiac arrest owing to VF is the lack of bystander-initiated basic CPR and the delay in defibrillation. We can strengthen these two critical links by encouraging the prompt application of bystander uninterrupted CC-CPR and by encouraging the appropriate use of AEDs.

1. BCLS. BCLS involves the recognition of a cardiac or respiratory arrest, a call for help (e.g., ACLS by activating the 911 emergency care system for out-of-hospital cardiac arrest, or a "code" for in-hospital cardiac arrest) and rapid initiation of life support. BCLS is continued until personnel trained and equipped for ACLS arrive, the victim can maintain basic life functions on his or her own, or it is obvious that continued BCLS efforts are futile. The resuscitation effort of BCLS for respiratory arrest rests on steps that can be remembered by the mnemonic **A, B, C,** which stands for **A**irway, **B**reathing, **C**irculation. These aspects of CPR are discussed in the following paragraphs. On the other hand, when an adult witnesses cardiac arrest, the most important first step (if a defibrillator is not readily available) is the prompt initiation of uninterrupted chest compression.

   a. Airway and breathing. Assessment of a victim's ventilatory status constitutes the first step in all unconscious individuals. In the situation of respiratory arrest without accompanying cardiac arrest, clearing the airway and assisting respiration for several cycles may be sufficient treatment to resuscitate the victim.

      (1) Airway. The first maneuver during resuscitation is establishing an open airway. An unconscious victim who has collapsed forward and is lying face down must be rotated quickly into the supine position. In most instances, a patent airway can be established by the "head tilt" maneuver, in which the rescuer places one hand behind the victim's neck and lifts while pressing down on the victim's forehead.

      As a rule, the head tilt is an effective method of establishing an open airway. If this maneuver fails, additional forward displacement of the jaw can be accomplished by (i) placing one or two fingers behind the angle of the victim's jaw and displacing the mandible forward, (ii) tilting the head back, and (iii) forcing the mouth open with both thumbs ("jaw thrust").

      (2) Breathing. In some patients with respiratory arrest, establishing an open airway enables the victim to resume spontaneous respiration. If this does not occur, artificial ventilation should begin immediately. The most effective and certain method of artificial ventilation is either mouth-to-mouth or mouth-to nose ventilation.

      Two breaths are recommended, each lasting 1 to 1.5 seconds to fully inflate the lungs. Thereafter, in respiratory arrest, a breath should be delivered once every 5 seconds in the adult or once every 3 seconds in the child. Adequate ventilation is assessed by (i) observing the chest rise and fall, (ii) hearing or feeling the air escape during exhalation, or (iii) sensing in one's own airway, the compliance/resistance of the victim's lungs as they expand.

      (3) Foreign bodies. Foreign bodies in the upper airway should be sought only if the maneuvers just described fail to establish an open airway and if adequate ventilation cannot be accomplished. In this setting, an attempt should be made to clear the victim's mouth. The victim is rotated onto his or her side. The mouth is forced open with the thumb and crossed index finger technique. The rescuer then sweeps his fingers across the back of the victim's throat. If this technique does not work (e.g., when the foreign body is lodged below the epiglottis), the victim should be rolled onto his side toward the rescuer, who delivers several sharp blows between the shoulder blades. Mouth-to-mouth

ventilation is then attempted again. If these maneuvers initially fail, they should be rapidly repeated.

If all maneuvers fail, emergency tracheostomy is indicated. However, this procedure carries significant risk and preferably is performed by a trained individual with appropriate instruments.

(4) Accident cases. In the setting of a motor vehicle accident, extreme caution must be observed in extending a victim's neck, as neck fracture may have occurred. The presence of facial lacerations often provides a valuable clue. A modification of the jaw thrust should be used with the rescuer's hands holding either side of the victim's head to pull the mandible forward with minimum neck extension.

b. Circulation. The **C** in the **A,B,C** of CPR stands for "circulation." In a victim of cardiac arrest, artificial circulation is maintained by external cardiac compression (ECC). A cardiac output of one fourth to one third of normal can be achieved through ECC. Even these flow rates maintain adequate perfusion to the brain and other vital organs, thus preventing irreversible damage.

(1) ECC. The rescuer kneels on a firm surface at the side of the victim. The heel of one hand is placed parallel to and over the lower half of the sternum. The other hand is placed on top of this hand, and the fingers are interlocked. ECC is accomplished by rhythmically depressing the sternum a minimum of 2 in. in an adult at a rate of 100 compressions per minute.

(2) ECC in infants and children. The basic technique of ECC in children is the same as that for adults; however, pressure should be exerted slightly higher over the sternum (midsternum). For infants, sternal compression is applied with the thumbs with the fingers encircling the infant's chest.

c. Complications. Numerous complications from ECC have been reported because of improper technique. These include lacerations of the heart, lungs, and liver; multiple rib fractures; and internal hemorrhage. The worse complication is failing to attempt BCLS or inadequate perfusion from timid performance of ECC. One should not be concerned about fracturing ribs, a result of appropriate chest compression force.

2. ACLS. ACLS, as defined by the National Conference on Standards for Cardiopulmonary Resuscitation and Emergency Cardiac Care, consists of seven elements: (i) BCLS, (ii) use of adjunctive equipment and special techniques (e.g., endotracheal intubation), (iii) cardiac monitoring for arrhythmias, (iv) defibrillation, (v) intravenous therapy, (vi) use of drug therapy, and (vii) stabilization of the patient after resuscitation. For details of these therapeutic modalities, the reader is referred to International Guidelines for Emergency Cardiac Care.

The guidelines for CPR and emergency cardiac care are well known to most physicians. The development of the 2000 guidelines was a truly international effort. A real effort was made for the recommendations to be culturally neutral and thus adaptable throughout the world. One consequences of this international effort is that some of the drugs and devices recommended are not presently approved or available in the United States.

The most heavily discussed and debated ACLS changes were defibrillation, techniques of ventilation, circulatory adjuncts, medications, and when to discontinue CPR efforts. Because most of these areas related to the VF/pulseless VT algorithm, it is useful to review the "Primary **ABCD** Survey," or basic CPR and defibrillation algorithm.

The recommendations are to check responsiveness; activate the emergency response system; and call for a defibrillator and then **A** (airway), open the airway; **B** (breathing), provide positive-pressure ventilation; **C** (circulation), give chest compressions; and **D** (defibrillation), assess for and shock VF/pulseless VT up to three times using 200-J, 200- to 300-J, and 360-J monophasic or equivalent biphasic shocks.

The guidelines state that all health professionals with duty to perform CPR should be trained, equipped, and authorized to perform defibrillation. The goal of out-of-hospital defibrillation is early defibrillation by 5 minutes. To reach this goal, AEDs will have to be placed and non-traditional providers (e.g., police officers, firefighters, security personnel sports marshals, airline flight attendants) trained in their use. The goal of in-hospital or ambulatory care areas is the application of defibrillator shock within 3 minutes. This means that AEDs will have to be placed in some area of large facilities.

The secondary **ABCD** survey for more advanced assessment and treatments has the same mnemonic, but they stand for different approaches: **A** (airway), place airway device as soon as possible; **B** (breathing), confirm airway device placement by examination and by confirmation devices, secure airway (purpose-made tube holders preferred), and confirm effective oxygenation and ventilation; **C** (circulation), establish intravenous access, identify rhythm and monitor, and administer drugs appropriate for rhythm and condition; and **D** (differential diagnosis), search for and treat identified reversible causes.

Tracheal intubation is strongly recommended if performed by an experienced provider, for example, six or more intubations per year. If an experienced provider is not available, placement of a laryngeal mask airway or an esophageal-tracheal Combitube is recommended over continued bag-mask devices. Once intubated, it is recommended that one confirm that the tube is in the trachea by use of an end-tidal CO_2 detector or esophageal detector device. The use of commercially available tracheal tube holder is recommended.

For patients with continued cardiac arrest, circulatory adjuncts such as interposed abdominal pressure CPR, active compression decompression CPR, and or an inspiratory impedance device are available in some institutions. The latter two devices are currently not approved for use in the United States.

Another controversial recommendation is the use of either 1 mg of epinephrine intravenously, repeated every 3 to 5 minutes, or 40 U of vasopressin intravenously (single dose, once only). The use of vasopressin is controversial. Although there are a number of animal studies that support its use, not all do so, and there is no data in humans that survival to hospital discharge in improved.

The next major change involves the use of antiarrhythmics before resuming attempts at defibrillation. The guidelines state that amiodarone is recommended for persistent or recurrent VF or pulseless VT. This was a class IIb recommendation, which is possibly useful and has fair supporting data. Lidocaine and procainamide were mentioned as a indeterminate drugs for persistent or recurrent VF or pulseless VT. Magnesium is recommended if there is a known hypomagnesemic state. After these therapies, one should resume attempts to defibrillate.

Finally, cessation of resuscitation efforts is recommended if asystole persists for at least 10 minutes of ACLS, except for arrests owing to drowning and those in children, in hypothermia, or in patients with suspected or known drug overdose.

SELECTED READINGS

American Heart Association. Guidelines 2000 for cardiopulmonary resuscitation and emergency cardiovascular care. *Circulation* 2000;102(Suppl 1):1–1384.

Berg RA, Kern KB, Hilwig RW, et al. Assisted ventilation does not improve outcome in a porcine model of single-rescuer bystander cardiopulmonary resuscitation *Circulation* 1997;95:1635–1641.

Eisenberg MS, Bergner L, Hallstrom A. Cardiac resuscitation in the community: importance of rapid provision and implication of program planning *JAMA* 1979;241: 1905–1907.

The ESVEM Trial: electrophysiology study versus electrocardiographic monitoring for selection of antiarrhythmic therapy of ventricular tachyarrhythmias. *Circulation* 1989;79:1354–1360.

Higano ST, Oh JK, Ewy GA, et al. The mechanism of blood flow during closed chest cardiac massage in humans: transesophageal echocardiographic observations. *Mayo Clin Proc* 1990;65:1432–1440.

Kern KB, Ewy GA, Voorhees WD, et al. Myocardial perfusion pressure: a predictor of 24-hour survival during prolonged cardiac arrest in dogs. *Resuscitation* 1988;16: 241–250.

Kern KB, Sanders AB, Raife J, et al. A study of chest compression rates during cardiopulmonary resuscitation in humans. *Arch Intern Med* 1992;152:145–149.

Kudenchuk PJ, Cobb LA, Copass MK, et al. Amiodarone for resuscitation after out-of-hospital cardiac arrest due to ventricular fibrillation. *N Engl J Med* 1999;341:871–878.

Moss AJ, Hall WJ, Cannom DS, et al. Improved survival with an implanted defibrillator in patients with coronary disease at high risk for ventricular arrhythmia. *N Engl J Med* 1996;335:1933–1940.

Sanders AB, Kern KB, Atlas M, et al. Importance of the duration of inadequate coronary perfusion pressure on resuscitation from cardiac arrest. *J Am Coll Cardiol* 1985;6, 1:113–118.

Sanders AB, Kern KB, Otto CW, et al. End-tidal carbon dioxide monitoring during cardiopulmonary resuscitation: a prognostic indicator for survival. *JAMA* 1989;262: 1347–1351.

9. HEMODYNAMIC MONITORING

I. Introduction. The performance of hemodynamic monitoring entails a small but definite risk for the patient. Morbidity and occasionally a rare mortality are directly attributable to the procedure associated with the initiation or maintenance of hemodynamic monitoring. Therefore, these procedures should only be performed by a medical team thoroughly familiar with the equipment and procedures used. In addition, the results of hemodynamic monitoring are used to guide therapy. If inaccurate or incorrect measurements are obtained, then incorrect or inappropriate therapy may well be administered. A number of studies, retrospective and observational in design, have failed to document benefit from hemodynamic monitoring. Consequently, physicians should be conservative in their use of this modality.

Hemodynamic monitoring should not be undertaken lightly: Certain indications must be present before hemodynamic monitoring is initiated. Hemodynamic monitoring has four central objectives: (i) to access left or right ventricular function; (ii) to monitor changes in hemodynamic status as convalescence progresses; (iii) to guide therapy with a variety of vasoactive, positively inotropic, or antiarrhythmic medications; and (iv) to provide diagnostic information (Table 9-1). Hemodynamic monitoring is often appropriate in a critically ill patient admitted to an intensive care unit (e.g., coronary, medical, surgical, pediatric, neurologic). Table 9-2 lists the most common indications for hemodynamic monitoring.

II. Management of complicated myocardial infarction (MI). One of the most common indications for hemodynamic monitoring is management of patients with complicated MI. Patients with hypotension may be dehydrated because of overly aggressive diuretic therapy, vomiting, diarrhea, or profuse diaphoresis. On the other hand, hypotension may be the first manifestation of cardiogenic shock. Individuals with severe left ventricular failure and a loud systolic murmur may have suffered one of the life-threatening mechanical complications of MI: ventricular septal rupture or acute mitral regurgitation. Other individuals develop marked signs and symptoms of severe left ventricular failure secondary to extensive infarction without mechanical disruption of the ventricular septum or papillary muscles.

Right ventricular infarction occurs in approximately one third of patients with inferoposterior MI. Extensive necrosis of right ventricular myocardium produces a syndrome characterized by hypotension and elevated right ventricular filling pressures. At times, it may be difficult to differentiate right ventricular infarction from pericardial tamponade.

Patients with refractory ventricular tachycardia or unstable angina after infarction have often sustained extensive infarction. The physician's attention may be focused on the episodes of unstable angina or ventricular tachycardia without recognition of the underlying left ventricular failure secondary to extensive infarction. Hemodynamic monitoring is one measure of the severity of left ventricular dysfunction and can aid in its management.

III. Determining the cause of dyspnea and hypoxia. Patients with coexisting pulmonary and cardiac disease often represent difficult diagnostic and therapeutic dilemmas.

Hemodynamic monitoring enables the physician to determine the severity of the respective cardiac and pulmonary conditions. The patient's response to therapy can be monitored with hemodynamic monitoring.

IV. Assessment of afterload reduction therapy. Individuals with left ventricular failure secondary to MI or other cardiac disease may benefit when a vasodilator drug is added to their therapeutic regimen. However, some patients become hypotensive during vasodilator therapy or fail to respond to these agents. Hemodynamic monitoring enables the physician to monitor patients' responses to therapy and to prevent potentially dangerous hypotension.

TABLE 9-1. INFORMATION THAT CAN BE OBTAINED FROM HEMODYNAMIC MONITORING

Depressed left ventricular systolic/diastolic function
Depressed right ventricular systolic/diastolic function
Acute mitral regurgitation
Ventricular septal rupture
Right ventricular infarction
Cardiac tamponade

V. Differential diagnosis of shock. A variety of conditions can produce the shock syndrome. A number of these entities are associated with a reasonably specific abnormal hemodynamic pattern (Table 9-3). Thus, hemodynamic monitoring can aid in differentiating the different etiologic agents that might cause shock. In addition, the patient's response to therapy can be monitored by hemodynamic monitoring.

VI. Assessment of possible cardiac tamponade. Patients with pericardial effusion may be totally unaffected by the presence of large quantities of pericardial fluid. Conversely, life-threatening pericardial tamponade may result from a moderate volume of pericardial effusion. Hemodynamic measurements determine the degree of tamponade present (if any). The response to therapy can also be monitored in these patients by hemodynamic monitoring.

VII. Management of postoperative open-heart surgery patients. Transient left ventricular failure, hypovolemia, and hypoxemia are common during the first 24 to 48 hours after open-heart surgery. Hemodynamic monitoring is essential in these patients to monitor the administration of fluids, pressors, and antiarrhythmic medications.

VIII. Management of critically ill medical patients with associated cardiovascular disease. Individuals with concomitant cardiac and noncardiac disease who are critically ill frequently benefit from hemodynamic monitoring. For example, patients with coronary or valvular heart disease have maximum cardiac output

TABLE 9-2. MOST COMMON INDICATIONS FOR HEMODYNAMIC MONITORING

Management of complicated myocardial infarction
    Hypovolemia vs. cardiogenic shock
    Ventricular septal rupture vs. acute mitral regurgitation
    Severe left ventricular failure, including cardiogenic shock
    Right ventricular infarction
    Severe and refractory unstable angina
    Refractory ventricular tachycardia
Determining the cause of dyspnea and hypoxia
    Severe pulmonary disease vs. left ventricular failure
Assessment of afterload reduction therapy in patients with left ventricular failure
Differential diagnosis of shock (e.g., pulmonary embolism, heart failure, sepsis, hemorrhage, dehydration)
Assessment of possible cardiac tamponade—measurement of right ventricular function and filling pressures
Management of postoperative open heart surgical patients
Management of critically ill medical patients with associated cardiovascular diseases
    Gastrointestinal hemorrhage
    Sepsis
    Respiratory failure
    Renal failure
Management of critically ill surgical patients with associated cardiovascular disease during noncardiac surgery

TABLE 9-3. TYPICAL HEMODYNAMIC MONITORING PATTERNS IN VARIOUS CLINICAL ENTITIES

Clinical setting	RA	RV	PA	PCW	Saturation (%)			CI L/min/min
					RA	PA	Art	
Normal	0–6	25/0–6	25/6–12	6–12	60	60	98	2.1
Cardiac tamponade	18	30/18	30/18	18	60	62	98	2.0
Chronic obstructive lung disease	10	70/10	70/35	<12	60	60	88	2.1
Cardiogenic shock (myocardial infarction)	8	50/8	50/35	35	50	50	98	1.5
Ventricular septal defect	6	60/8	60/35	30	55	75	92	1.9
Left ventricular failure	4–6	45/4–6	45/>18	>18	60	60	98	1.8
Acute pulmonary embolism	8–12	50/12	50/12–15	<12	60	60	88	1.9
Congestive heart failure (biventricular)	6–8	65/6	65/25	25	55	55	98	1.9
Hypovolemic shock	0–2	15–20/0–2	15–20/2–6	2–6	65	65	98	2.5
Septic shock								
Warm	0–2	20–25/0–2	20–25/0–6	0–6	65	65	98	2.5
Cold	0–4	25/0–4	25/4–10	4–10	50	50	98	1.5

RA, right atrial; RV, right ventricle; PA, pulmonary artery; PCW, pulmonary capillary wedge; Art, arterial; CI, cardiac index.

at a certain limited range of ventricular filling pressures. If such patients sustain a gastrointestinal hemorrhage, they will become hypovolemic and possibly hypotensive. On the other hand, an excessive volume of transfused blood could result in hypervolemia with attendant signs and symptoms of left ventricular failure. Hemodynamic monitoring enables the physician to maintain ventricular filling pressures in a range that leads to optimum cardiac output.

IX. Management of critically ill patients with associated cardiovascular disease during noncardiac surgery. Surgery is associated with a variety of stresses for the heart: Loss of blood, fever, catabolism, transfusion, and administration of a number of intravenous fluids all conspire to place a burden on the myocardium. Hemodynamic monitoring may be essential for shepherding patients with a variety of cardiovascular diseases through such stresses. Pulmonary arterial and systemic arterial catheters are often placed before surgery. Hemodynamic monitoring is used before, during, and after surgery.

SELECTED READINGS

Alia I, Esteban A, Gordo R, et al. A randomized and controlled trial of the effect of treatment aimed at maximizing oxygen delivery in patients with severe sepsis or septic shock. *Chest* 1999;115:453–461.
Treatment for these critically ill patients was directed by measurements made in a variety of ways, including hemodynamic monitoring. Treatment effect was observed.
Connors AF, Speroff T, Dawson NV, et al. The effectiveness of right heart catheterization in the initial care of critically ill patients. *JAMA* 1996;276:889–897.
An observational study of critically ill patients that demonstrates that bedside right heart catheterization was associated with increased mortality and utilization of resources.
Dalen JE, Bone RC. Is it time to pull the pulmonary artery catheter? *JAMA* 1996;276: 916–918.
The case against widespread use of bedside hemodynamic monitoring.
Gardner RM, Schwartz R, Wong HC, et al. Percutaneous indwelling radial-artery catheters for monitoring cardiovascular function: prospective study of the risk of thrombus and infection. *N Engl J Med* 1974;290:1227–1331.
One of the earliest studies of complications secondary to bedside hemodynamic monitoring.
Gattinoni L, Brazzi L, Pelosi P, et al. A trial of goal-oriented hemodynamic therapy in critically ill patients. *N Engl J Med* 1995;333:1025–1032.
Hemodynamic therapy aimed at achieving supranormal values for the cardiac index or normal values for mixed venous oxygen saturation does not reduce morbidity or mortality among critically ill patients.
Gore JM, Goldberg RJ, Spodick DH, et al. A community-wide assessment of the use of pulmonary artery catheters in patients with acute myocardial infarction. *Chest* 1987;92:721–727.
The first paper to call into question the widespread use of hemodynamic monitoring.
Kearney TJ, Shabot MM. Pulmonary artery rupture associated with the Swan-Ganz catheter. *Chest* 1995;108:1349–1352.
An extensive review of this often fatal complication of bedside right heart catheterization.
Layton AJ. The pulmonary artery catheter: nonexistential entity or occasionally useful tool? *Chest* 1999;115:859–862.
A carefully worded editorial that supports occasional and conservative use of bedside hemodynamic monitoring.
Merrer J, DeJonghe B, Golliot F, et al. Complications of femoral and subclavian venous catheterization in critically ill patients: a randomized trial. *JAMA* 2001;286:700–707.
Femoral venous catheterization is associated with a greater risk of infection and thrombosis than is subclavian catheterization in intensive care unit patients.
Mueller HS, Chatterjee K, Davis KB, et al. ACC expert consensus document: present use of bedside right heart catheterization in patients with cardiac disease. American College of Cardiology. *J Am Coll Cardiol* 1998;32:840–864.
A careful analysis and series of recommendations for the use of hemodynamic monitoring.

Polanczyak CA, Rohde LE, Goldman L, et al. Right heart catheterization and cardiac complications in patients undergoing noncardiac surgery: an observational study. *JAMA* 2001;286:309–314.
There was no benefit associated with the use of right heart catheterization in this population of patients.
Robinson JF, Robinson WA, Cohn A, et al. Perforation of the great vessels during central venous line placement. *Arch Intern Med* 1995;155:1225–1228.
Perforation of a great vessel is an uncommon but often fatal complication of central venous cannulation.
Shoemaker WC, Appel PL, Kram HB, et al. Prospective trial of supranormal values of survivors as therapeutic goals in high-risk surgical patients. *Chest* 1988;94:1176–1186.
Bedside hemodynamic monitoring was used to direct therapy in critically ill patients with good results.
Swan HJC, Ganz W, Forrester J, et al. Catheterization of the heart in man with the use of a flow-directed balloon-tipped catheter. *N Engl J Med* 1970;283:447–451.
The original report of bedside hemodynamic monitoring.
Weil MH. The assault on the Swan-Ganz catheter: a case history of constrained technology, constrained bedside clinicians, and constrained monetary expenditures. *Chest* 1998;113:1379–1386.
The case in favor of bedside hemodynamic monitoring.
Wiedemann HP, Matthay MA, Matthay RA. Cardiovascular-pulmonary monitoring in the intensive care unit: part 1. *Chest* 1984;85:537–549.
Wiedemann HP, Matthay MA, Matthay RA. Cardiovascular-pulmonary monitoring in the intensive care unit: part 2. *Chest* 1984;85:656–668.
Yarzebski J, Goldbert RJ, Gore JM., et al. Temporal trends and factors associated with pulmonary artery catheterization in patients with acute myocardial infarction. *Chest* 1994;105:1003–1008.

10. EXERCISE AND THE CARDIOVASCULAR SYSTEM

I. Introduction. The effects of exercise on the cardiovascular system have interested physiologists and cardiologists for many years. There is clear evidence that a sedentary lifestyle increases the risk of coronary artery disease (CAD), a fact recognized and incorporated into many American Heart Association's (AHA) statements on exercise. Conversely, individuals who remain active throughout their life significantly lower their risk of CAD. Millions of Americans are engaged in physical exercise programs, many with the express purpose of improving their cardiovascular health.

Others engage in supervised exercise as part of postmyocardial infarction (post-MI) rehabilitation. Exercise testing plays an important role in assessing cardiovascular disease and monitoring therapy or prevention. Data from the Harvard Alumni Health Study, the Multiple Risk Factor Intervention Trial (MRFIT), and many other studies strongly support the concept that consistent lifelong activity decreases the likelihood of developing CAD. In an analysis performed by the Centers for Disease Control in Atlanta, Georgia, it was noted that compared with the most active group, the least active adults were 1.9 times more likely to develop CAD. Knowledge of the effects of exercise on the heart has become important for every physician. This chapter briefly discusses the physiologic effects of exercise on the heart, and the epidemiologic studies that have attempted to assess the role of exercise either in preventing atherosclerosis or in preventing reinfarction in patients who have already suffered an MI. In addition, this chapter reviews clinical aspects of exercise testing and prescription.

Significant information has accumulated through structured cardiac rehabilitation programs concerning the effects of exercise on the cardiovascular system in individuals who have suffered an MI. Levels of physiologic functioning previously thought unattainable in post-MI patients are now prescribed routinely.

II. Biochemistry and physiology of exercise
   A. Biochemical aspects. A detailed discussion of the biochemistry of energy metabolism during exercise is beyond the scope of this manual; however, a basic understanding of the biochemistry involved is essential to explain the clinical effects of exercise.

   The basic biochemical problem in exercise is the conversion of stored energy contained in ingested food into the mechanical energy of muscular contraction. This transformation occurs intracellularly by two processes: (i) anaerobic metabolism and (ii) aerobic metabolism.

   When oxygen is used in the biochemical reactions, the process is called *aerobic metabolism;* it occurs within the mitochondria of the cell, using the Krebs cycle.

   Under normal conditions, anaerobic metabolism and aerobic metabolism are linked. Under conditions of severe stress, a disproportionate amount of energy production occurs anaerobically. Lactic acid accumulates in the bloodstream, which causes muscles to ache and creates the sensation of fatigue. Aerobic metabolism is more efficient than is anaerobic metabolism and yields significantly more high-energy compounds for cellular use. Endurance training (e.g., running, swimming, or bicycling) augments the capacity for aerobic metabolism, whereas training for brief bursts of intense exercise increases anaerobic capacity (e.g., heavy weight lifting).
   B. Physiologic aspects
      1. The interface between cardiology and exercise physiology. The use of high-intensity exercise in cardiac rehabilitation programs has led to the deployment of a number of concepts developed in the exercise physiology laboratory. Familiarity with some of the terms commonly used by the exercise physiologist is useful to the clinician (Table 10-1).

TABLE 10-1. USEFUL TERMS AND CONCEPTS IN CARDIOVASCULAR PHYSIOLOGY

Term	Abbreviation	Definition	Comment
Aerobic		Exercise occurring at a level at which the body can supply adequate oxygen to allow energy production through the Krebs cycle	Pulmonary patients are more likely to maintain a normal aerobic capacity than are patients with cardiac disease and impaired left ventricular function
Anaerobic		Strenuous exercise that requires recruitment of glycosides to meet energy demands; lactic acid is produced	Typically occurs in bursts of sudden strenuous exercise or at high levels of exertion; can be maintained only for short periods
Anaerobic threshold		That amount of work beyond which anaerobic metabolism begins to contribute significantly to energy production	The body will attempt to buffer lactic acidemia with the bicarbonate system; VO_2 will rise slowly or level off while CO_2 production (VCO_2) and minute ventilation (VE) will increase sharply
Total body oxygen consumption	VO_2	The amount of oxygen consumed by the cells of the body at any level of activity	VO_2 measurement is the best basis for exercise prescription
Maximum total body oxygen consumption	max VO_2	The point at which the individual has attained the maximum capacity to deliver and utilize oxygen to exercising muscles	Measures a combination of cardiac output and peripheral oxygen extraction under maximum exertion
Metabolic equivalent	MET	The metabolic cost of a 70-kg person sitting quietly at rest (3–5 ml/kg/min VO_2)	MET classifications are available for most leisure and work activities
Isometric exercise		Occurs when a muscle attempts to shorten but is unable to; force is generated, but muscle shortening does not occur	In practice, most forms of exercise combine some isometric and isotonic aspects; shot-putting and heavy weightlifting are primarily isometric
Isotonic exercise		Exercise that allows the muscle to contract throughout its full range in a repetitive fashion	The best form of exercise for cardiovascular conditioning; examples include jogging, bicycling, and swimming

Source: Adapted from Rippe JM, Maher P, Ockene J. Care and rehabilitation of the patient following myocardial infarction. In: Rippe JM et al., eds. *Intensive care medicine.* Boston:Little, Brown and Company, 1985.

Automated systems are available that can rapidly measure total body oxygen consumption (VO_2), CO_2 production, respiratory quotient (RQ), and a variety of other physiologic parameters.

2. Cardiovascular effects

   a. Response to immediate exertion. Cardiovascular adaptation to the increased demands of exercise involves complex interactions between the heart and the peripheral vasculature. Early investigators such as Starling believed that cardiac output in healthy individuals increased during exercise primarily because of cardiac dilatation with resultant increased stroke volume (Starling's law of the heart). Subsequent investigators have shown that increased heart rate secondary to sympathetic nerve stimulation is more important than cardiac dilatation in the cardiovascular response to exercise. Less important contributions come from the Starling mechanism and increased myocardial contractility. Highly trained athletes achieve very large cardiac outputs through increases in both heart rate and stroke volume during exercise.

   In contrast, most of the cardiovascular adaptations that occur in individuals involved in training programs after MI are peripheral in nature. High-intensity exercise in such individuals does result in some improvement in myocardial performance; however, the major effect is still increased efficiency of peripheral muscle oxygen extraction.

   The peripheral vasculature responds to exercise with dilatation of arterioles in the involved muscles. Blood flow may increase 20-fold in these muscles during severe exertion. Compensatory vasoconstriction occurs in the viscera and skin.

   b. Training effects. Training effects occur in sedentary individuals who begin exercise training. These effects are observed as early as 2 weeks after a person begins to train, provided that the training is on a daily basis. If exercise training is performed three times a week (preferably on nonconsecutive days), training effects may occur as early as 1 month after training is begun.

   The most important physiologic parameter that improves during training is the ability to use oxygen. This variable, also written as VO_2, differs considerably among individuals. An average-sized, normally active man will have a VO_2 of 3 to 4 liters per minute during maximal exercise (women have slightly lower values). Average values of maximum VO_2 decline predictably with age, as does maximum heart rate. A champion athlete may have a VO_2 in excess of 7 liters per minute. The ability to use oxygen is determined by the entire oxygen transport system, which includes cardiac output and the efficiency of peripheral oxygen extraction. To achieve an optimal training effect in normal persons, the cardiovascular system must be stressed to at least 70% of maximum for 20 to 30 minutes three times a week. In the past, stress on the cardiovascular system during exercise was estimated by monitoring heart rate. With the availability of automated equipment to analyze oxygen consumption, clinicians are increasingly performing direct measurements of maximum VO_2. Individuals who perform prescribed exercise, however, must still rely on monitoring their own heart rate to determine if they are exercising at the appropriate intensity. A good rule of thumb for a normal individual to achieve 70% maximum exercise is to maintain a heart rate of 195 beats per minute minus the individual's age during exertion. For sedentary individuals, those participating in post-MI rehabilitation, and those receiving beta-blockers, heart rates during exercise should and will be considerably lower. Specific training programs are discussed in Section IV.

Clinical manifestations of the training effect include a decrease in resting heart rates, an increase in heart size, and greater ability to perform physical work. Weight loss and improvement in blood lipid and glucose values frequently accompany regular training, and subjective feelings of improved health and increased joie de vivre are often described.

c. Long-term adaptations to exercise. In normal persons, increases in maximum oxygen utilization from 25% to 40% are commonly reported after training. Sedentary individuals may achieve even greater increases.

Most of the improvement occurs within the first 6 months of exercise, after which a plateau is reached. An additional increase of 10% to 15% in oxygen utilization can be achieved by exercising at more strenuous levels. The long-term effects of exercise are also positive. A trained athlete who continues to exercise after retiring from competition continues to exhibit higher Vo_2, greater work capacity, larger heart volume, and lower resting heart rate than does a healthy, active, age-matched control. Former athletes who lead sedentary lives after retiring from competition revert to physiologic measurements that are indistinguishable from those of age-matched controls. Thus, it appears that to maintain a training effect, continued regular exercise is required.

d. General considerations. It should be emphasized that the training effects on the cardiovascular system already discussed are responses to endurance exercise that involves large muscle groups (particularly leg muscles) performed in a regular, repetitive fashion to evoke a training response (e.g., walking, running, bicycling, or swimming). It has been shown that periods of exercise at 70% maximum capacity for 3 to 5 minutes, followed by an equivalent rest period, will confer a training effect, provided that the exercise periods total more than 20 minutes three times a week. Such exercise is frequently referred to as *aerobic*. A summary of the cardiovascular effects of training is found in Table 10-2.

3. Noncardiac effects. Regular exercise exerts effects on a variety of organ systems in addition to the cardiovascular system. Some of these effects are summarized in Table 10-3.

C. Epidemiologic considerations
1. Exercise in primary prevention of CAD. A number of epidemiologic studies have addressed the question of whether regular exercise reduces the likelihood of developing CAD. Early studies of London bus drivers and conductors suggested that the conductors had a lower incidence of CAD than did the more sedentary drivers. Similar results were shown comparing letter carriers with more sedentary postal clerks. Both of these studies, however, were retrospective and did not control for the fact that healthier individuals might have selected the more active job. The classic studies of Paffenbarger and colleagues and of others (see Selected

TABLE 10-2. CARDIOVASCULAR EFFECTS OF TRAINING

Parameter	Effect
Resting heart rate	Decreased
Maximum oxygen utilization	Increased
Heart rate at submaximal work loads	Decreased
Maximum heart rate	Increased
Heart volume	Increased
Heart weight	Increased

TABLE 10-3. NONCARDIAC EFFECTS OF EXERCISE TRAINING

Organ system	Effect
I. Locomotive organs	
A. Strength of bones and ligaments	Increased
B. Thickness of articular cartilage	Increased
C. Muscle mass	Increased
II. Respiration	
A. Lung volumes, adults	No effect
B. Pulmonary ventilation, maximal work	Increased
C. Respiratory rate, resting	No effect
D. Respiratory rate, maximal work	Increased
III. Other	
A. Body density	Increased
B. Serum cholesterol	Decreased or no effect

Readings) provide strong epidemiologic evidence for a decreased incidence of CAD in individuals who engage in regular exercise programs.

One problem in demonstrating a direct linkage between exercise and decreased CAD has been the lack of a suitable animal model. Recently, however, it has been shown that monkeys fed an atherogenic diet and exercised regularly on a treadmill were less likely to develop CAD than was a control group kept at rest (see Selected Readings).

2. Exercise in the prevention of reinfarction. A number of studies have examined exercise in patients recovering from MI. In general, most of these studies have shown beneficial effects in these patients.

III. Clinical testing of exercise. A number of exercise tests are used in the evaluation of the cardiovascular system. The exercise tolerance test (ETT) and hemodynamic monitoring of exercise during cardiac catheterization may yield valuable diagnostic information.

A. Exercise tolerance test

1. Procedure. The ETT is used most commonly to diagnose CAD and to determine prognosis for patients already known to have CAD. It may also be used, however, to provide serial monitoring in cases of established CAD, judge progress in post-MI rehabilitation, provide baseline data before recommendation of an exercise program, or document cardiovascular disability.

The main aspects of cardiovascular function judged by ETT are (i) adequacy of cardiac output, (ii) adequacy of cardiac conduction, (iii) presence of exercise-provoked arrhythmias, and (iv) heart rate response. The initial protocol for the ETT was developed by Masters and involved repetitive ascent and descent of two steps of different heights. The current protocol used in most hospitals involves walking, running, or both on a treadmill at a gradually progressive speed and a gradually increased incline (see Chapter 15). At the University of Arizona Health Science Center, we use both a progressive walk-run treadmill protocol and an exclusively walking protocol to perform ETTs. Published equations exist for estimating Vo_2 max from a standardized walking protocol (see Selected Readings). The safety record for centers that perform ETTs has been excellent and reflects careful screening of patients before testing and careful monitoring during and after the procedure. Contraindications for performing an ETT and precautions during the procedure are listed in Tables 10-4 and 10-5.

2. Clinical information derived from ETT

a. Myocardial ischemia. S–T segment depression on the ETT is usually caused by an imbalance between myocardial oxygen supply and

TABLE 10-4. PRECAUTIONS TO BE OBSERVED DURING EXERCISE TESTING

I. Absolute indications to stop exercise tolerance test
   A. Ventricular tachycardia
   B. Staggering or ataxic gait
   C. Decrease in blood pressure below usual resting level
   D. Exhaustion

II. Relative indications to stop exercise tolerance test
   A. S-T depression >3 mm
   B. Development of bundle branch block
   C. Failure of blood pressure to rise

TABLE 10-5. CONTRAINDICATIONS TO EXERCISE AND EXERCISE TESTING

I. Absolute contraindications
   A. Congestive heart failure, uncompensated
   B. Acute myocardial infarction with evidence of instability
   C. Active myocarditis
   D. Highly unstable angina pectoris
   E. Recent embolism, either systemic or pulmonary
   F. Dissecting aneurysm
   G. Acute infectious diseases of major proportion, e.g., pneumonia
   H. Thrombophlebitis, deep

II. Relative contraindications[a]
   A. Uncontrolled or high-rate supraventricular dysrhythmias
   B. Repetitive or frequent ventricular ectopic activity
   C. Untreated severe systemic or pulmonary hypertension
   D. Ventricular aneurysm
   E. Aortic stenosis greater than moderate severity
   F. Uncontrolled metabolic diseases (diabetes, thyrotoxicosis, myxedema)
   G. Severe hypertrophic obstructive cardiomyopathy (subaortic stenosis)
   H. Marked cardiac enlargement
   I. Toxemia of pregnancy

III. Conditions requiring special consideration or precautions
   A. Conduction disturbances
      1. Complete AV block
      2. Left bundle branch block
      3. Wolff-Parkinson-White syndrome
   B. Pacemakers
   C. Other arrhythmias with marked tachycardia or bradycardia
   D. Electrolyte disturbances, uncorrected
   E. Certain cardiac medications, for example, digitalis
   F. Severe hypertension (diastolic pressure >110 mm Hg)
   G. Angina pectoris, unstable and untreated
   H. Cyanotic heart disease
   I. Intermittent or fixed right-to-left shunts
   J. Severe anemia
   K. Marked obesity
   L. Renal, hepatic, and other metabolic insufficiency of greater than moderate severity
   M. Overt psychoneurotic disturbances uncompensated and requiring therapy
   N. Neuromuscular, musculoskeletal, and arthritic disorders that prevent activity

[a]The value of testing may exceed the risk in patients with these relative contraindications.

demand. This may be owing to either inadequate supply (CAD) or to markedly increased demand (left ventricular hypertrophy, hypertension). The most common cause of S–T depression on the ETT is atherosclerosis of the coronary arteries.

False-positive S–T depression is said to be more common in women, although this contention is debatable. ST depression may also be observed in hypokalemia and a variety of other situations, for example, during digoxin therapy. False-negative ETTs are also possible (e.g., no evidence of S–T depression despite significant CAD). ETTs may be negative in as many as 45% of patients with significant (greater than 70% narrowing) single-vessel disease. False-negative results can occur too in patients who have had a previous MI. A major consideration in the interpretation of ETTs is the issue of sensitivity versus specificity. These terms are defined as:

$$\text{Sensitivity} = \frac{\text{true positive} \times 100}{\text{true positives} + \text{false negatives}}$$

$$\text{Specificity} = \frac{\text{true negatives} \times 100}{\text{false positives} + \text{true negatives}}$$

Assuming an adequate heart rate during the test and requiring S–T segment depression of greater than 2 mm in any lead, together with downsloping of the S–T segment for a positive result, specificity for CAD is very high. This specificity, however, is achieved at the expense of sensitivity.

A positive ETT carries important prognostic value. In one study, individuals with greater than 2 mm of exercise-induced S–T depression were 16 times more likely to die of cardiac events than were individuals with normal ETTs. Patients who are symptomatic and have a positive ETT are at greatest risk. A low-level (modified) ETT is commonly administered to patients 3 to 10 days after an uncomplicated MI. The safety of performing such a test so soon after MI has been clearly demonstrated. The purpose of performing an early modified ETT is to provide prognostic information. The most useful finding on the modified ETT is the presence or absence of exercise-induced S–T segment depression. If significant S–T segment depression is present on a low-level ETT before discharge, the patient has a 19% to 60% chance of another MI or sudden cardiac death within the next year. Such patients should be scheduled for early cardiac catheterization. The findings of chest pain or ventricular arrhythmias on low-level ETT are much less specific.

b. Heart rate. Individuals with CAD develop faster heart rates at submaximal exercise than do healthy individuals. Furthermore, patients with CAD reach significantly lower maximum heart rates for symptom-limited maximum exercise.

c. Arrhythmias. Ventricular premature beats (VPBs) are a frequent occurrence during exercise in men and women over 50 years of age. In one study, VPBs were provoked in more than 50% of men over age 55 during stair climbing. Exercise-induced VPBs increase with age in both men and women and are more prevalent in patients with CAD than in healthy individuals. VPBs also increase with increasing heart rates. The risk of a dangerous arrhythmia during or immediately after an ETT is 0.05%. Continuous ECG monitoring for at least 5 minutes after an ETT is essential. The ETT is a much less useful test than 24-hour ambulatory monitoring for quantitating VPBs, and it should be reserved for individuals whose symptoms suggest ischemic or exercise-related ventricular ectopy.

    d. Conduction defects. In a small number of patients, conduction defects may be provoked by exercise (2% of ETTs). Conduction defects observed include (i) right or left bundle branch block (most frequent) and (ii) left anterior or posterior hemiblock.

  B. Exercise during cardiac catheterization. Exercise may be used during cardiac catheterization to assess whether ventricular dysfunction, which is not apparent under basal conditions, is present. Most commonly, a bicycle ergometer is used, and the patient pedals in the supine position. Isometric handgrip exercises may also be used.

      The normal hemodynamic response to exercise is an increase in cardiac output. Catheterization studies have shown that in many individuals with cardiac disease, pulmonary capillary wedge pressure rises during exercise, followed by increases in right atrial pressure and eventually a decline in cardiac output. Various indexes have been proposed to assess ventricular function during exercise. Maximum cardiac output and maximum oxygen extraction (Vo_2) both appear insensitive to *mild* impairment in ventricular function. The ratio of cardiac output to oxygen consumption has also been proposed but appears to suffer from the same difficulty.

IV. Clinical aspects of exercise training

  A. Exercise training in CAD. Exercise training has become an important aspect of the overall management of individuals with CAD. Specific exercise programs must be cautiously designed and implemented (see Section **V**). Patients with CAD often achieve higher levels of work performance after training than do comparably aged sedentary individuals without CAD; however, although a training effect usually occurs in healthy persons in response to exercise, in patients with CAD the response is more variable.

    1. Angina. After exercise training, individuals generally are able to achieve higher levels of work performance (as measured by oxygen consumption) before the onset of angina. This improvement appears to involve both myocardial and peripheral effects. Comparable levels of submaximal work can be accomplished at lower heart rates after exercise training. Because increase in heart rate is a major contributor to increased myocardial oxygen consumption, exercise becomes less "oxygen expensive" after training. Moreover, exercise training improves peripheral oxygen extraction, further diminishing demands on the heart.

    2. After MI. Exercise training as part of post-MI rehabilitation generally enables individuals to achieve work capacity comparable with that of age-matched sedentary individuals. Without exercise training, post-MI patients have been shown to have higher resting heart rates than that of normal individuals. Resting heart rates decrease in patients who train. Even after exercise training, however, people who have suffered an MI are unable to achieve the same maximum heart rates as those noted in healthy sedentary individuals, probably because ventricular dysfunction after infarction is irreversible.

      Individuals involved in high-intensity exercise programs after MI are often able to achieve exercise capacities comparable to those of healthy individuals. In one study, post-MI patients ran a 6-km race in times similar to those of individuals who had never suffered a coronary event. The healthy individuals had, on average, higher maximum Vo_2, but the post-MI patients were able to exercise at higher percentages of their aerobic capacity. This provides further evidence that peripheral effects of exercise are particularly prominent in post-MI patients involved in regular exercise programs.

  B. Exercise training in healthy sedentary individuals. The training effects described in Section **II.B.2.b.** can be elicited in healthy individuals who enter exercise training programs. The more sedentary the individual, the greater the potential training effect. Training programs, however, may pose some danger to previously inactive persons, who should commence exercising cautiously, with gradual increases in intensity of exercise (see Section **V**).

Middle-aged individuals commonly stop exercising because of a musculo-skeletal injury (e.g., general aching of muscles, muscle strain). This is another reason for gradually increasing the intensity of exercise. Training three times a week for 20 minutes per session appears to be the minimum exercise required to induce and maintain a training effect.

V. Prescribing exercise

A. General considerations. Individuals who wish to begin an exercise program frequently consult physicians for advice. Patients recovering from MI or suffering from CAD require careful supervision to derive maximum benefit and safety during participation in exercise programs.

In general, any individual over age 40 years who has lived a sedentary life should be examined by a physician before beginning an exercise program. Examination should focus on blood pressure measurement and auscultation of the heart. A 12-lead ECG should be performed. Individuals over the age of 45 years, even if they have been moderately active, should also be examined before beginning a more strenuous exercise program. Examination should include the items just mentioned and an ETT.

Any abnormalities found on examination or ETT must be weighed before a specific exercise program is prescribed. In addition, the physician should ascertain whether symptoms or conditions that might be either relative or absolute contraindications to an exercise program are present. A partial listing of these conditions is found in Table 10-4. Exercise programs must be geared to the individual's specific needs. A sedentary person without heart disease may derive the most benefit from a program that builds toward periods of exercise at heart rates of 75% to 85% maximum, whereas individuals with CAD or healed MI may require slower progression to a lower percentage of maximum heart rate. Three general parameters should be considered in formulating any exercise program: intensity, duration, and frequency.

1. Intensity. A general sense for the intensity at which an individual can safely exercise may be obtained from the ETT. In individuals with a history of MI or suspected CAD, particular attention should be paid to symptoms that may occur at levels of exercise well below predicted maximum heart rates. Individuals are taught to monitor their respiratory rate during effort and to exercise to a particular respiratory rate that correlates with a measured heart rate. In the absence of an ETT, maximum heart rate for an individual may be estimated from the formula: maximum heart rate = 220 minus age in years.

Precautions to be emphasized in sedentary individuals who are hard-driving and competitive, or in patients with CAD, are as follows: (i) competitive athletics should be avoided, and (ii) the appropriate intensity of exercise for rehabilitation after MI may be monitored by treadmill testing 6 weeks or less after infarction (if no complications have occurred during recovery).

2. Duration and frequency. As already indicated, three periods a week of 20 minutes of exercise at 70% to 80% maximum heart rate are required to evoke a reasonable training response. Exercise sessions should not be on consecutive days. Exercise need not be continuous for 20 minutes. Periods of 3 to 5 minutes of exercise followed by a comparable period of rest, which is then repeated until a total of 20 minutes of exercise is achieved, will confer similar effects. The level of exercise should increase gradually. In addition to the 20 minutes of exertion, 3 to 5 minutes should be allowed for stretching and warm-up and for cooling down to minimize muscle strain and decrease cardiovascular stress.

B. Types of exercise. Most cardiovascular benefit is derived from continuous, repetitive forms of physical exertion. Studies have repeatedly shown that participants in various competitive games (e.g., football, baseball, tennis) achieve much lower aerobic capacities than do endurance athletes. Forms of exercise that use large muscle groups such as leg or back muscles appear most beneficial. Exercise involving leg muscles elevates systemic arterial pressures less than does exercise using arm muscles.

Types of exercise that provide maximum cardiovascular benefit include walking, jogging, swimming, bicycling, and calisthenics. Once a stable aerobic exercise program has been established, many cardiac rehabilitation programs allow gradual introduction of weight training in addition to continued aerobic exercise.

C. Recommending increased activity. As the benefits of an active lifestyle for reducing risk of chronic diseases in general and cardiovascular disease in particular have become increasingly apparent, recommendations have been established to promote regular physical activity. The Centers for Disease Control and the American College of Sports Medicine have recommended that all adults be counseled to accumulate 30 minutes of moderate intensity physical activity on most or preferably all days as a way of lowering their risk of heart disease, decreasing obesity, and increasing general well-being.

SELECTED READINGS

Blair SN, Kohl HW, Paffenbarger RS, et al. Physical fitness and all-cause mortality: a prospective study of healthy men and women. *JAMA* 1989;262:2395–2401.
This study established that even a small amount of exercise significantly lowers the risk of CAD.
Blumenthal JA, Babyak MA, Moore KA, et al. Effects of exercise training on older patients with major depression. *Arch Intern Med* 1999;159:2349–2356.
Exercise training was as effective as antidepressant medication in relieving depression in older patients.
Fagard R, Van den Broeke C, Amery A. Left ventricular dynamics during exercise in elite marathon runners. *J Am. Coll Cardiol* 1989;14:112–118.
Elite athletes have left ventricular adaptations to exercise that are not present in more sedentary individuals.
Fletcher GF, Blair SN, Blumenthal J, et al. AHA medical/scientific statement: benefits and recommendations for physical activity programs for all Americans: AHA Scientific Council. *Circulation* 1992;86:340–344.
Major statement by the AHA recommending regular physical exercise as an excellent modality for lowering the risk of heart disease. This statement also supplies the rationale for why the AHA cites a sedentary lifestyle as one of the four major risk factors for CAD.
Hambrecht R, Wolf A, Gielen S, et al. Effect of exercise on coronary endothelial function in patients with coronary artery disease. *N Engl J Med* 2000;342:454–460.
Exercise training improves myocardial collateral blood flow in patients with CAD.
Kramsch DM, Aspen AJ, Abramowitz BM, et al. Reduction of coronary atherosclerosis by moderate conditioning exercises in monkeys on an atherogenic diet. *N Engl J Med* 1981;305:1483–1489.
Monkeys on an atherogenic diet who exercised regularly had less CAD than did sedentary controls.
LaPorte RE, Dearwater S, Cauley JA, et al. Physical activity or cardiovascular fitness: which is more important for health? *Phys Sports Med* 1985;13:145.
Good summary of the case for consistent activity as the key to lowering the incidence of CAD.
Lee IM, Hsieh CC, Paffenbarger RS. Exercise intensity and longevity in men: the Harvard Alumni Health Study. *JAMA* 1995;273:1179–1184.
An inverse relationship is demonstrated between total physical activity and mortality.
Levine BD, Zuckerman JH, Pawelczyk JA. Cardiac atrophy after bed-rest deconditioning: a non-neural mechanism for orthostatic intolerance. *Circulation* 1997;96:517–525.
Two weeks of bed rest causes deterioration in left ventricular size and function.

Paffenbarger RS Jr, Laughlin ME, Gima AS, et al. Work activity of longshoremen as related to death from coronary heart disease and stroke. *N. Engl. J. Med.* 1970;282: 1109–1114.
The classic epidemiologic study relating physical activity at work to the prevalence of CAD.
Paffenbarger RS Jr, Wing AL, and Hyde RT. Physical activity as an index of heart risk in college alumni. *Am J Epidemiol* 1978;108:161–175.
Important epidemiologic study linking leisure time physical exertion to the prevalence of CAD.
Paffenbarger RS Jr, Hyde RT, Wing AL, et al. Physical activity, all-cause mortality and longevity of college alumni. *N Engl J Med* 1986;314:605–613.
Results of major epidemiologic study showing consistent activity reduces the incidence of CAD.
Pate RR, Pratt M, Blair SN, et al. Physical activity and public health: a recommendation from the Centers for Disease Control and Prevention and the American College of Sports Medicine. *JAMA* 1995;273:402–407.
Standardized advice for regular exercise in the American population.
Rippe JM, Ward A, Porcari J, et al. Walking for health and fitness. *JAMA* 1988;259: 2720–2724.
A comprehensive summary of the known cardiovascular and other benefits of walking.

11. PSYCHOLOGICAL ASPECTS OF HEART DISEASE

I. Introduction. Links between heart and mind have long been known. The familiar symptoms of tachycardia, palpitations, and even chest pain during anxious moments attest to the influence of emotion on cardiovascular events. In literature, lovers scorned by the object of their affection are often said to "die of a broken heart." This suggestion of a catastrophic influence of the mind on the heart also exists in folklore concerning sudden death. Victims of voodoo hexes, it has been suggested, are literally "frightened to death," succumbing to a fatal arrhythmia.

Recent interest in links between emotion and the cardiovascular system have focused on the relation between psychological states and common diseases such as hypertension and coronary artery disease (CAD). New technologies introduced into the care of patients with heart disease have resulted in new psychological hazards. The emotional status of patients in coronary care units (CCUs) and the psychological issues of rehabilitation after myocardial infarction (MI) have concerned both physicians and nurses. Moreover, postoperative delirium after open-heart surgery is not infrequent. A number of psychiatric and emotional disorders may present with symptoms related to the cardiovascular system. It has been estimated that 10% to 20% or more of patients seen by cardiologists have primarily a psychiatric basis for their symptoms. Individuals with anxiety states and depressive disorders comprise the largest segment of these patients.

The number of individuals being treated with psychotropic medications has risen dramatically over the recent years. The antianxiety benzodiazepine drugs are among the most commonly prescribed medications in the United States. New psychotropic medicines are constantly appearing with different adverse reactions, many of them related to the cardiovascular system. Frequently, psychotropic medication is considered in patients with known cardiac disease. Cardiovascular effects of these medicines and potential interactions with other medications must be considered carefully. Finally, the availability of psychotropic medications creates opportunities for their abuse. Overdoses of psychotropic agents (particularly tricyclic antidepressants [TCAs]) may have a profound influence on the cardiovascular system. The patient's psychological status may exert an important influence on individual compliance with prescribed drug regimens. Each of these topics is discussed in this chapter.

II. Relation between psychological stress and cardiovascular disease

    A. CAD. The connection between emotional stress and CAD has been reviewed in detail (see Selected Readings). Attempts to link stress to CAD are traced in part to the frequent clinical observation that angina pectoris may be provoked by emotional stimuli. Although the pathophysiology of angina is complex, evidence has accumulated over the past 20 years that suggests a link does exist between chronic stress and CAD.

        Rosenman and Friedman have developed the concept of the "type A" personality, linking certain kinds of overt behavior to an increased incidence of MI. The concept of type A behavior has often been loosely and incorrectly applied. Rosenman and Friedman described type A behavior during a specific, highly structured interview as a "characteristic action-emotion complex." According to these investigators, type A individuals tend to possess excessive aggression, competitiveness, and hostility. These individuals are likely to evidence a sense of urgency as they attempt to accomplish poorly defined goals in the shortest amount of time. Other investigators have assessed type A behavior by questionnaire rather than structured interview and have documented a higher incidence of morbid cardiac events in type A patients. Both the general concept of type A behavior and the methods for assessing it remain controversial. Recent studies combining coronary angiography with personality assessment have yielded results that are at odds. One study showed more atherosclerotic lesions in patients with type A behavior as measured by questionnaire. Another failed to corroborate this result.

Almost from its inception, the role of type A personality as a risk factor for CAD has been controversial. Although a 1981 expert panel listed it as an independent risk factor, the American Heart Association (AHA) does not list it as such. Further confusion developed when it was shown that patients with type A personality who survived an initial MI were significantly less likely than type B individuals to suffer reinfarction. Recent studies have suggested that hostility may be a more important factor in the development of CAD than is the cluster of emotions associated with the type A personality. In one study of 255 physicians, men who had a high hostility index when they were 25 years old had four to five times the likelihood of developing CAD by the age of 50 when they were compared with men with low hostility.

Although the debate on the role of type A personality and CAD is likely to continue, a general consensus has arisen that there are multiple, if ill-defined, links between personality and heart disease. For example, some of the behavior modifications required to lower other risk factors such as cigarette smoking cessation and consumption of lower fat diets, may be impossible for some patients to achieve who perceive their lives to be filled with stress. Numerous epidemiologic investigations have tried to link job-related stress to CAD, with conflicting results. Some studies have focused on life changes as precipitants of MI. Events such as divorce, financial setback, or the death of a spouse or close relative have been shown to be more prevalent in the 6 months before the onset of MI than in the prior six month period.

Most of the evidence that links stress to CAD is only suggestive; direct proof is lacking. This situation is not surprising in a disease that has been demonstrated to be multifactorial. Most investigators agree that stress has some link to CAD. That it is as strong a risk factor as elevated cholesterol, smoking, or hypertension remains to be demonstrated.

B. Hypertension. Since Cannon coined the phrase "fight, fright, or flight" to describe the physiologic changes that occur during stress, physiologists have known that emotional stimuli can cause transient elevations of blood pressure. This observation, coupled with the knowledge that sustained hypertension frequently develops in individuals who initially exhibit transient blood pressure elevation, has served as the basis for research on emotional components in hypertension.

Epidemiologic studies reveal elevated blood pressures in soldiers in time of war, civilians faced with natural disasters (e.g., floods, explosions), and whole societies in which the social order is unstable. Some data in experimental animals suggest that constant stress leads to elevated blood pressure. In one study involving rats, overcrowding and an environment that forced frequent confrontations led to significant increases in arterial diastolic blood pressure.

Establishing links between personality traits and hypertension has proved more difficult. According to some reports, patients with repressed hostility often have hypertension secondary to increased cardiac output (similar to borderline or labile hypertension); however, subsequent hemodynamic studies have not corroborated this finding. Some studies have sought to link sustained hypertension to life changes, but results are conflicting. A number of studies have shown that blood pressure in patients with hypertension can be further elevated by emotional stress. Moreover, these increases in blood pressure tend to be greater in magnitude and longer lasting than similar episodes in normotensive patients. There is no evidence that stress changes the natural history of hypertension. In summary, although some link between stress and hypertension probably exists, the evidence is far from conclusive. The various psychological and behavioral modalities that have been used in the treatment of hypertension are discussed in Chapter 12.

C. Psychological bases of arrhythmias and sudden death. Palpitations and tachycardia are often the result of emotional stress. These common cardiac symptoms provided early evidence that emotional stimuli could alter cardiac rhythm.

Anecdotal evidence suggests that individuals may collapse and die when faced with a sudden, overwhelming emotional stress. Death in these instances has been assumed to be the result of cardiac arrhythmia. Engel has reviewed a number of cases in which psychological stress appeared to cause sudden death. Common settings for the occurrence of sudden death included (i) hearing of the death of a friend or relative, (ii) an acute episode of grief, (iii) mourning or the anniversary of a sad event, (iv) loss of status or self-esteem, (v) personal threat or danger, and (vi) reunion or triumph. The assumption in most of these instances is that sudden death results from a transient arrhythmia. Specific evidence, however, is generally lacking. The advent of continuous monitoring in CCUs and continuous 24-hour monitoring in outpatient settings has provided some data concerning the types of arrhythmias provoked by emotional stimuli.

Individuals most susceptible to arrhythmias provoked by emotion are those with underlying cardiac disease, particularly CAD. A high percentage of patients monitored while driving in busy city traffic developed sinus tachycardia, often to heartbeats greater than 140 beats per minute. Evidence of ischemia occurred in less than 10% of persons with normal coronary arteries, but more than 50% of those with CAD developed ECG evidence of ischemia. More than 20% of the patients with CAD had multifocal ventricular premature contractions accompanying sinus tachycardia.

Another study was performed monitoring 23 healthy subjects and seven individuals with CAD who were delivering public speeches. Heart rates as high as 180 beats per minute were observed in both groups, and six of the seven individuals with CAD exhibited ischemic S–T segment depression. Although individuals with CAD appear most at risk, those with normal coronary vasculature can also develop emotion-provoked arrhythmias. There are reports of patients with normal coronary arteries who developed recurrent ventricular fibrillation in stressful settings.

In summary, at least some arrhythmias are caused by emotion. Although the feelings of joy, anger, or depression may be complex functions, the body has a limited vocabulary of physiologic responses to them. Sympathetic nervous stimulation is common to many of these emotions, causing inotropic and chronotropic cardiac activation with resultant increased myocardial oxygen consumption. The threshold for arrhythmia may thus be lowered, particularly in patients with CAD with limited myocardial oxygen supply.

Parasympathetic stimulation such as that which occurs during vasovagal syncope may have equally deleterious effects. Bradycardia and peripheral vasodilatation can lower coronary arterial perfusion pressure and hence myocardial blood flow, thus provoking ischemia and a fatal arrhythmia. The diagnosis of emotion-provoked arrhythmias may be facilitated by psychological stress testing during ECG monitoring. Twenty-four—hour outpatient ECG monitoring is also likely to prove helpful. Treatment may include attempts to avoid situations in which arrhythmias are likely to develop and/or beta-blockade. Detailed discussion of the treatment of specific arrhythmias is found in Chapter 3.

III. Psychological issues in coronary care. Many studies have outlined typical psychological responses to MI and to the atmosphere and hazards of the emergency room, the CCU, and—during the recuperation phase—the cardiac step-down unit or general medical ward.

A. Psychological issues during the acute phase of MI. The most common psychological response in the early stages of MI is denial of the event. Studies have estimated that the typical delay between first symptoms and arrival at the emergency ward is approximately 4 to 5 hours. This statistic is particularly alarming because more than 50% of deaths due to MI occur within the first 4 hours after onset of infarction. Delay is not related to occupation, socioeconomic status, or educational background. Patients who correctly attributed the source of their symptoms to the heart tended to delay for a shorter time. The shortest delays occurred in individuals who were strongly advised or ordered to report to the hospital. Here, employers were significantly more successful than were spouses.

Once the individual has arrived at the hospital, a variety of stressful settings are encountered. Most patients recall only portions of their stopover in the emergency ward. Several studies have emphasized the importance of perceived competence, reassurance, and speed. Although the time spent in the emergency ward should be brief, the patient may be extremely frightened. Because much of the anxiety is based on uncertainty, attempts should be made to explain procedures and medical facts with as much reassurance as possible. That the patient is about to be transferred to the CCU, why the transfer is occurring, and what to expect once there should be discussed. One study showed that Catholic patients were not alarmed by the administration of last rites as long as the priest emphasized the routine nature of the blessing. The psychological response to the CCU has also been studied. The predominant emotion most patients experience during the first few days in a CCU is anxiety, coupled with gratitude for surviving. Although the presence and sounds of cardiac monitors were initially thought to pose a psychological hazard, patients usually felt reassured by the presence of monitors, provided that their purpose was explained.

Surprisingly, a majority of patients denied being frightened by witnessing a cardiac arrest and resuscitation in another patient. When questioned about the event, most patients who had witnessed a cardiac arrest emphasized how rapidly physicians and nurses had responded. However, denial is a central adaptive mechanism for many patients in the CCU. Paradoxically, the same denial response that may harm the patient by causing excessive delay in seeking treatment may become an asset during the initial period in the CCU. Often during the second and third day in the unit, anxiety gives way to reactive depression. Patients are likely to worry about their future lives and mourn the sense of loss associated with their heart attack. Some investigators have termed this process "ego infarction." Many patients will deny that they have had a MI during this period.

A second period of anxiety often occurs when the patient is transferred from the CCU to the step-down unit or medical ward. Treatment of the psychological aspects of MI is discussed in Chapter 15. An antianxiety agent should be regularly prescribed. Diazepam (2 to 10 mg by mouth four times a day) or alprazolam (0.25 mg three times a day) are commonly used. Chlordiazepoxide (5 to 25 mg by mouth four times a day) is an acceptable substitute. Flurazepam may be prescribed at night as a soporific. Medications should be prescribed on a regular dosage schedule rather than as needed, because many patients will view requesting them as a sign of weakness. The depression typically experienced in the CCU rarely requires pharmacologic treatment. A listening ear is, of course, very important. Calm reassurance and education from physicians and nurses provide an essential aspect of the psychological management of the acute phase of MI.

B. Psychological aspects of convalescence and rehabilitation. Specific activity schedules for rehabilitation after MI are discussed in Chapter 15. Rehabilitation must involve both psychic and physical mending. Many patients experience "homecoming depression." This syndrome typically consists of a sensation of weakness coupled with a strong sense of loss. Even walking from one room to another may cause fatigue. The patient may be consumed by apprehension about the ability to lead a productive and vigorous life. Often family arguments occur as the patient struggles to adjust.

Problems of homecoming depression can be mitigated with sensitive treatment by the physician and the cardiac rehabilitation team. Specific feelings experienced by the patient should be thoroughly discussed at discharge and during subsequent visits. The patient's participation in his own rehabilitation should be encouraged by formulation of a specific plan of gradually increasing activity (see Chapter 15).

If homecoming depression is particularly severe or lasts more than several months, a short course of supportive psychotherapy may be considered. Major advances in the treatment of the psychological problems after MI have been achieved through cardiac rehabilitation programs. Many hospitals now have rehabilitation teams consisting of cardiologists, nurses, psychologists, social workers, dietitians, and physical therapists. Patient education and active participation in cardiac rehabilitation may greatly reduce the adverse psychological impact of an MI.

The environment into which the post-MI patient is discharged can have a profound impact on both emotional state and clinical outcome. In one study, individuals who lived alone after MI were significantly more likely to suffer morbidity and mortality than those who lived with a significant other.

IV. Psychological aspects of cardiac surgery: postoperative delirium. Early studies of the psychological sequelae of open-heart surgery showed a high incidence of postoperative confusional states. Most investigators found that more than half the patients who had cardiac surgery underwent periods of delirium during postoperative recovery. Some estimates have ranged as high as 80% of patients having open-heart surgery (in contrast, less than 5% of CCU patients experience delirium).

Delirium is defined as a confusional state characterized by excitement and hyperactivity. *Delirium* and *clouded sensorium* frequently are used interchangeably. Delirium in the patient after cardiac surgery generally occurs 2 to 6 days postoperatively and typically lasts less than 24 hours. During a period of delirium, the patient may appear alternately somnolent and agitated. In a period of agitation, the patient may become confused or belligerent, pulling out intravenous lines or even attempting to get out of bed and leave the hospital. Various factors have been postulated as provoking delirium: (i) administration of drugs (narcotics, anticholinergics, steroids), (ii) electrolyte imbalance, (iii) psychodynamic factors in the patient's personality, (iv) hypoxemia, and (v) amount of time on cardiopulmonary bypass. Very young patients and elderly patients appear most susceptible. Clinical signs of postoperative delirium may include mental status changes (disorientation, diminished attention span), hallucinations, and somnolence and lethargy alternating with agitation. Blood pressure, pulse, and respiratory rate may all increase, and pupils may become dilated. Fluctuations in both mental status and vital signs are common.

Precautions can be taken to reduce the incidence of delirium. In recent years, the incidence of delirium has declined attributable to two factors: (i) more complete preoperative discussions with patients outlining what to expect, often including a preoperative visit to the intensive care unit, and (ii) shortened periods of cardiopulmonary bypass.

In managing the delirious patient, one must first review medications, eliminating unnecessary narcotics and sedatives that may cloud the sensorium. A calm, reassuring manner on the part of the CCU staff is also helpful. Concrete explanations that detail their location and what is happening should be repeatedly given to the patients. Environmental stimulation such as a light in the room or a radio may be beneficial.

If the delirium is thought to be secondary to anticholinergic medications, physostigmine should be administered. If sedation is required, haloperidol is the agent of choice.

V. Emotional disorders presenting with cardiovascular symptoms. As already indicated, 10% to 20% of cardiac patients may have symptoms that are primarily the result of emotional disorders. The most common emotional disorders with symptoms referred to the cardiovascular system are anxiety states, panic disorder, and depression.

    A. Anxiety states. Anxiety states are conditions of overconcern that often contain elements of edginess, worry, or dread. A spectrum of anxiety states extends from chronic anxiety, through attacks of anxiety in specific settings, to attacks of overt panic. Anxiety states are likely to be accompanied by somatic symptoms that include tachycardia, palpitations, chest pain or tightness, and shortness of breath. The anxious patient is frequently referred for cardiovascular examination because of these symptoms. Terms coined to describe such a cluster of symptoms include *soldier's heart, Da Costa's syndrome, cardiac neurosis,* and *neurocirculatory asthenia.*

Symptoms associated with anxiety are probably related to increased activity of the sympathetic nervous system. The exact mechanisms involved are controversial.

The physical examination is often normal, although the patient may have cold, moist skin, tachycardia, anxious facies, and brisk tendon reflexes. Laboratory tests are characteristically normal. Symptoms may be severe and recurrent, leading to cardiac catheterization in some patients. Some individuals with "angina and normal coronaries" probably have symptoms based in an anxiety state.

The differential diagnosis of diseases that produce symptoms similar to those resulting from an anxiety state include (i) a variety of acute and chronic cardiac diseases (MI, arrhythmias, pulmonary embolism) and (ii) any condition that stimulates the sympathetic nervous system, including metabolic, neurologic, and respiratory diseases.

Therapy of an anxiety state begins with support and reassurance. The patient should derive some reassurance from the understanding that organic disease has been considered and ruled out. The physician should emphasize the favorable long-term prognosis. In patients whose primary manifestations of anxiety are tachycardia, palpitations, or both, a trial of beta-blockade is often indicated. Beta-blockers may also be effective in diminishing panic attacks. Relaxation techniques and psychotherapy may also be beneficial in selected patients.

B. Panic disorder. Although panic disorder is one of the anxiety states, its presentation may be so dramatic and so similar to cardiovascular disease that it merits separate discussion. Patients with panic disorder experience sudden sympathetic outpourings accompanied by feelings of terror and impending doom.

Somatic complaints during an episode often include chest pain, dyspnea, and palpitations, which may resemble angina or MI. Attacks may occur in predictable settings (crowded rooms, theaters, or other public places where exit may be somewhat restricted). The typical response is to flee. After several panic attacks, a generalized anxiety state may set in (which should be distinguished from the panic attack), and the patient will try to avoid settings that provoke attacks. Often patients will consume alcohol or barbiturates to calm their nerves. The pathophysiology of panic disorder is poorly understood, although it has been observed that infusion of sodium lactate will often provoke an attack in an individual with the disorder. The diagnosis is largely made by a careful history. It is an important diagnosis for the cardiologist to be able to make, because it can prevent an expensive and invasive cardiovascular workup in a patient with this disorder. Effective treatment for panic disorder is available with imipramine (Tofranil), alprazolam, or both.

C. Depression. The cardiologist or general internist usually sees a depressed patient under one of the following circumstances: (i) because antidepressant medication or electroconvulsive therapy (ECT) is being contemplated in a patient with depression and suspicion of underlying heart disease, and the cardiovascular system needs to be evaluated, or (ii) because depression has resulted from treatment of cardiovascular disease. The first situation will be discussed in Section **VI;** the latter is considered here.

Two types of depression commonly exist: (i) **reactive (neurotic) depression** usually results from grief over a loss. It is rarely accompanied by somatic complaints, is not genetically transmitted, and frequently responds to supportive psychotherapy; (ii) **endogenous depression** is generally more severe, is often accompanied by somatic complaints and vegetative signs, and seldom responds to supportive psychotherapy. TCAs, fluoxetine (Prozac) or other selective serotonin reuptake inhibitors (SSRIs), or ECT may be beneficial in this setting. Endogenous depression is more likely to progress to psychotic depression, in which feelings of worthlessness and guilt become overwhelming. Auditory hallucinations often accompany psychotic depression.

Symptoms experienced by the depressed patient may include early morning awakening, loss of appetite, loss of interest in pleasurable activity, psychomotor retardation, and constipation. Symptoms referred to the cardiovascular system include palpitations, tachycardia, and a sensation of chest pressure and fatigue. The differential diagnosis includes consideration of organic heart disease and neurologic or neoplastic disease. A patient's current medications should be reviewed, with the physician being alert for drugs that cause depression (particularly antihypertensive medications).

Treatment of depressive disorders varies according to the suspected etiology. Reactive depression may be treated with support or psychotherapy. Drugs of choice for endogenous depression are TCAs and SSRIs. Dosages and possible side effects are discussed in Section **VI.** ECT is often effective in refractory depression and may be used in some patients with cardiac disease (see Section **VI.E.**).

VI. Psychotropic medications and the cardiovascular system. A list of cardiovascular side effects from psychotropic medications is found in Table 11-1.

   A. Antipsychotic agents. A variety of compounds have clinically useful antipsychotic properties. The phenothiazines are probably most frequently prescribed. Phenothiazines likely to be encountered by the general internist or cardiologist include chlorpromazine (Thorazine), thioridazine (Mellaril), fluphenazine (Prolixin), and trifluoperazine (Stelazine). Another commonly prescribed antipsychotic is the butyrophenone haloperidol (Haldol). Although antipsychotic medications generally possess less cardiac toxicity than do TCAs, cardiovascular complications and side effects have been reported.

    Antipsychotic medicines are thought to exert their beneficial effects by lessening the severity of psychotic episodes through blockade of central dopamine receptors. In addition, most antipsychotic agents are central and peripheral alpha-adrenergic blockers and thus may lead to troublesome orthostatic hypotension. Chlorpromazine and thioridazine frequently cause orthostatic symptoms.

TABLE 11-1. CARDIOVASCULAR SIDE EFFECTS FROM PSYCHOTROPIC MEDICATIONS

Class of drug or treatment	Generic name	Trade name	Complications
Antipsychotics: phenothiazines	Thioridazine	Mellaril	Arrhythmias, sudden death
	Chlorpromazine	Thorazine	Arrhythmias, sudden death, myocardial depression
Antianxiety drugs: benzodiazepines	Diazepam	Valium	Rare cardiac arrest with IV administration
Antidepressants: tricyclics	Amitryptiline	Elavil	Most have anticholinergic properties, cause arrhythmias
	Imipramine Doxepin Desipramine	Tofranil Sinequan Norpramin	All tricyclic antidepressants possess cardiac toxicity to various degrees; see text
Lithium	Lithium		Myocarditis, congestive heart failure
Electroconvulsive therapy	Electroconvulsive therapy		Hypertension, arrhythmias, myocardial infarction

Most antipsychotic agents have anticholinergic properties that may provoke tachycardia. Thioridazine possesses particularly strong anticholinergic properties. It is often chosen for elderly patients because of its low incidence of extrapyramidal side effects; however, its anticholinergic actions can produce cardiac arrhythmias.

On occasion, sudden death in an apparently healthy individual has been attributed to antipsychotic agents. Myocardial depression has sometimes been linked to phenothiazine administration as well. ECG changes may occur in patients taking phenothiazines. T wave changes are most commonly reported. These changes are reversible on withdrawal of the antipsychotic agent. Other ECG abnormalities reported include QRS widening and prolongation of P–R and Q–T intervals. Q–T prolongation made lead to dangerous arrhythmias such as polymorphic ventricular tachycardia. The choice of antipsychotic agent hinges both on its efficacy in controlling psychotic episodes and on its potentially dangerous side effects. In elderly patients or patients with significant heart disease, chlorpromazine and thioridazine are probably best avoided. Haloperidol appears to be the agent of choice for most of these individuals. Haloperidol possesses potent antipsychotic action and minimal alpha-blocking or anticholinergic properties.

B. Antianxiety agents. The most commonly prescribed antianxiety agents are the benzodiazepines. Drugs ordinarily encountered in this class are diazepam (Valium), chlordiazepoxide (Librium), oxazepam (Serax) alprazolam (Xanax), and flurazepam (Dalmane). These drugs are often prescribed in the CCU. Reasons for their popularity include predictable efficacy in anxiety relief, and relative absence of cardiovascular toxicity. Intravenous diazepam, frequently used to control seizures, has been linked to isolated cases of cardiac arrest.

C. TCAs. Many drugs have been used in the treatment of depression. For most patients, the drug of first choice for endogenous depression is one of the TCAs. TCAs commonly used include imipramine (Tofranil), desipramine (Norpramin), amitriptyline (Elavil), and doxepin (Sinequan).

Many of the cardiovascular side effects already mentioned for phenothiazine medications also occur with TCAs. In contrast to phenothiazines, however, TCAs exert regular and powerful influences on the cardiovascular system. These agents should be used cautiously in the elderly or in patients with significant cardiac disease.

The antidepressant action of TCAs arises from their ability to block reuptake of catecholamines at the synaptic cleft of central neurons. This property also extends to the myocardium and peripheral vasculature. Alpha-blockade leads to the regularly observed side effect of postural hypotension. Alpha-blockade is greatest with amitriptyline and doxepin and least with desipramine and protriptyline (Vivactil). TCAs have strong anticholinergic properties that may provoke tachycardia and other rhythm disturbances. Amitriptyline possesses the strongest anticholinergic properties, followed by those of doxepin, nortriptyline (Pamelor), imipramine, and desipramine. TCAs also have a direct myocardial depressant action and a quinidine-like effect on electrical conduction. Indeed, some TCAs have been demonstrated to have mild antiarrhythmic properties. Patients taking any TCA should have dosages of any type I antiarrhythmic (e.g., quinidine, procainamide, disopyramide) reduced. TCAs interact with certain cardiac medications. Vasopressor effects of catecholamines may be attenuated and the antihypertensive action of guanethidine blocked. Synergism with other myocardial depressants may occur. A number of cardiovascular complications have been attributed to TCAs, including sudden death, arrhythmias, MI, hypertension, and congestive heart failure. Postural hypotension is a common side effect. More than two thirds of patients with cardiovascular disease who receive imipramine have a measurable drop in systemic diastolic pressure.

ECG changes take place regularly after administration of TCAs. Reversible T wave changes are common. Tachycardia (sinus) may occur in up to 30% of patients. Other ECG alterations include widened QRS and prolonged P–R, Q–T, and S–T segment changes. Atrioventricular and intraventricular conduction defects also have been reported.

The cardiovascular side effects of TCAs are major limiting factors in their administration. They are effective agents for 60% to 80% of patients with depression. The choice of a particular TCA should be based on the clinical setting and its known side effects. When arrhythmias are a primary concern, amitriptyline is a poor choice; desipramine is a better selection. When postural hypotension is a problem, a switch from amitriptyline or doxepin to desipramine or protriptyline may be beneficial. In some instances, postural hypotension occurs with any TCA. If the medication is essential, the patient should be encouraged to rise from bed slowly. Elastic stockings may be helpful. The TCA dosage can be reduced.

TCAs should be administered with caution in elderly patients; however, depressive disorders carry morbidity and mortality, and the risk of cardiovascular side effects may be more acceptable than untreated depression. Patients receiving TCAs should be monitored with serial ECGs. Recent reports have focused attention on the cardiovascular sequelae of TCA overdose. A variety of cardiovascular complications may occur in TCA overdose, including arrhythmias, bundle branch block, hypotension, cardiac arrest, and sudden death. Arrhythmias are the most common serious sequelae. Almost any arrhythmia may be provoked, including sinus bradycardia or tachycardia (more common), complete atrioventricular block, bundle branch block, supraventricular and ventricular tachycardia, ventricular premature contractions, and asystole. Most reports indicate that the vast majority of cardiovascular side effects occur within the first 24 hours after ingestion; however, toxic levels (greater than 1000 ng/ml) of TCA may remain in the bloodstream for as long as 4 days after overdose. Initial treatment of suspected TCA overdose is the same as in any other type of poisoning. Emesis should be provoked, gastric lavage begun, or both. Supportive measures for respiratory depression and shock should be undertaken. Intravenous physostigmine has been advocated for control of both central nervous system and cardiac complications (adult dosage of intravenous physostigmine in this setting is 1 to 4 mg q30–60min as needed). Once the patient's clinical status has stabilized, he or she should be admitted to an intensive care unit. Cardiac monitoring should be continued for at least 48 hours.

D. SSRI antidepressants. These agents are the newest agents in the pharmacological management of depression. They are well tolerated with few cardiovascular side effects. Q–T prolongation has been observed, and the physician should monitor this interval by ECG during SSRI therapy. Commonly prescribed SSRIs are fluoxetine (Prozac), citalopram (Celexa), paroxetine (Paxil), and sertraline (Zoloft). Although these drugs are very popular antidepressants, they have not been shown to be more effective than TCAs.

E. Lithium. Lithium carbonate is the agent of choice for many patients with bipolar mood disorders, particularly manic-depressive illness. Initial reports of lithium cardiotoxicity probably overestimated this problem. Reports document that cardiac side effects are rare. Myocarditis occasionally occurs. Congestive heart failure has been reported and is probably a function of decreased renal lithium clearance. ECG changes occur regularly in patients receiving lithium. T wave flattening is most common. Conduction defects and increased extrasystoles have also been reported.

F. ECT. ECT may provide an alternative to TCAs or SSRIs in severely depressed cardiac patients. Although the mortality with this therapy is low (less than 0.01%), it does have cardiovascular effects that should be considered. The sympathetic nervous system stimulation that follows an electrically induced seizure may cause transient hypertension or arrhythmias. Several reports of MI after ECT have appeared.

ECT should be avoided in patients with previous MI or serious arrhythmia.

SELECTED READINGS

Angerer P, Siebert U, Kothny W, et al. Impact of social support, cynical hostility and anger expression on progression of coronary atherosclerosis. *J Am Coll Cardiol* 2000;36:1781–1788.
Patients with CAD and low emotional social support who express anger outwardly are at increased risk for atherosclerotic disease progression.
Ariyo AA, Haan M, Tangen CM, et al. Depressive symptoms and risks of coronary heart disease and mortality in elderly Americans. *Circulation* 2000;102:1773–1779.
Depressive symptoms represent an independent risk factor for the development of CAD in elderly Americans.
Case RB, Moss AJ, Case N, et al. Living alone after myocardial infarction: impact on prognosis. *JAMA* 1992;267:515–519.
This study showed that individuals who live in loving relationships lower their risk of subsequent cardiac events after an MI.
Engel GL. Sudden and rapid death during psychological stress: folklore or folk wisdom? *Ann Intern Med* 1971;74:771–782.
Fascinating review of psychological aspects of sudden death; most evidence is anecdotal.
Hackett TP, Cassem NH, Wishnie, HA. The coronary-care unit: an appraisal of its psychologic hazards. *N Engl J Med* 1968;279:1365–1370.
The classic paper on the psychological hazards of the CCU.
Iribarren C, Sidney S, Bild DE, et al. Association of hostility with coronary artery calcification in young adults: the CARDIA Study. *JAMA* 2000;283:2546–2551.
High hostility levels may predispose to CAD.
Januzzi JL, Stern TA, Pasternak RC, et al. The influence of anxiety and depression on outcomes of patients with coronary artery disease. *Arch Intern Med* 2000;160: 1913–1921.
A concise review of the relationship between anxiety and depression and CAD.
Krantz DS, Sheps DS, Carney RM, et al. Effects of mental stress in patients with coronary artery disease: evidence and clinical implications. *JAMA* 2000;283:1800–1802.
A summary of the data linking mental stress to coronary heart disease.
Ornish D. *Reversing heart disease.* New York: Random House, 1990.
Comprehensive summary of a program that achieved significant results in reducing heart disease. Stress reduction is a key component.
Orth-Gomer K, Wamala SP, Horsten M, et al. Marital stress worsens prognosis in women with coronary heart disease: the Stockholm Female Coronary Risk Study. *JAMA* 2000;284:3008–3014.
Marital stress predicts poor prognosis in women with CAD.
Ragland DR, Brand RJ. Type A behavior and mortality from coronary heart disease. *N Engl J Med* 1988;318:65–69.
Individuals with type A personality were significantly less likely to suffer reinfarction than were patients with type B personality.
Rosenman RH, Brand RJ, Jenkins CD, et al. Coronary heart disease in the Western Collaborative Group Study: final follow-up experience of 8 1/2 years. *JAMA* 1975; 233:872–875.
The original prospective study showing that individuals with type A personality had twice the incidence of CAD as did individuals with type B.
Rozanski A, Blumenthal JA, Kaplan J. Impact of psychological factors on the pathogenesis of cardiovascular disease and implications for therapy. *Circulation* 1999;99: 2192–2217.
A thorough review of the relationship between psychological factors and cardiovascular disease.
Williams R. *Anger kills.* New York: Random House, 1992.
Comprehensive summary of research stating that the hostility component of type A behavior is particularly dangerous as a risk factor for CAD.

II. SPECIFIC DISORDERS

12. HYPERTENSION

I. Introduction
   A. Definition. Systemic arterial pressure in the adult represents a continuum. Although no sharp dividing line exists between elevated and normal blood pressure, it is generally agreed that arterial pressure of 140/90 mm Hg on three consecutive visits establishes the diagnosis of hypertension. The diagnosis of hypertension is complicated by the fact that a patient's blood pressure may vary considerably from visit to visit and that the stress of visiting the physician sometimes leads to falsely elevated readings. An ideal blood pressure is one that is closer to 120/80 mm Hg rather than to 140/90 mm Hg.
      The general definition of hypertension has more clinical applicability and prognostic value if subdivided into more specific categories. The categories are based on either the etiology or the degree of pressure elevation.
   B. Hypertension classified by etiology
      1. Primary hypertension. There is no demonstrable underlying cause (greater than 94% of all people with hypertension).
      2. Secondary hypertension. Hypertension is associated with and secondary to an underlying disease (for list of diseases with hypertension as a complication, see Table 12-1).
   C. Hypertension classified by degree or type
      1. Borderline hypertension (also referred to as labile hypertension). Blood pressure readings average between 135 to 140/90 mm Hg and 150/100 mm Hg, together with some normal readings and no evidence of end organ damage.
      2. Mild hypertension. Diastolic blood pressure is persistently elevated above 90 mm Hg but below 105 mm Hg (at least three readings). Systolic blood pressure is persistently in the range of 140 to 150 mm Hg.
      3. Moderate hypertension. Average diastolic pressure is persistently between 105 and 114 mm Hg (at least three readings).
      4. Moderately severe to severe hypertension. Diastolic blood pressure is persistently between 115 and 129 mm Hg. This hypertension is associated with severe complications over a relatively short period of time. Three separate readings are not needed; treatment should be undertaken immediately.
      5. Malignant or accelerated hypertension. There is a sustained or sudden rise in diastolic blood pressure levels higher than 120 mm Hg, with accompanying evidence of end-organ damage (papilledema, decreased renal function, encephalopathy, heart failure). This constitutes a **medical emergency.** Immediate hospitalization is almost always required. (This entity is handled separately in Chapter 13.)
      6. Systolic hypertension. Systolic pressure is consistently greater than 150 mm Hg; it is accompanied by normal diastolic blood pressure.
      7. Resistant hypertension. Efforts to control blood pressure adequately (less than 140/90 mm Hg) with an appropriate regimen (provided that medications are taken as prescribed) fail.
         The interrelation of types of hypertension may be viewed in the Venn diagram found in Figure 12-1.
   D. Incidence. The prevalence of hypertension has been assessed by various epidemiologic studies. It is generally accepted that 15% to 20% of the adult population in the United States is hypertensive. It is further estimated that approximately one third to one half of this population is adequately treated. It has also been reported that many of the untreated hypertensive patients are elderly and have only moderate systolic hypertension. Although these figures are widely debated, hypertension remains a significant health problem, the most common cardiovascular disease, and a condition that every physician must understand.

TABLE 12-1. DISEASES CAUSING SECONDARY HYPERTENSION

I. Renal
   A. Renal parenchymal disease
     1. Polycystic renal disease
     2. Chronic pyelonephritis
     3. Acute and chronic glomerulonephritis
   B. Renal vascular disease
     1. Renal artery stenosis
     2. Renal infarction
   C. Most other severe renal diseases (e.g., arterial nephrosclerosis, diabetic nephropathy)

II. Endocrine
   A. Glucocorticoid excess (Cushing's disease)
   B. Mineralocorticoid excess (primary aldosteronism)
   C. Congenital or hereditary adrenogenital syndromes (enzyme defects)
   D. Pheochromocytoma
   E. Acromegaly
   F. Myxedema
   G. Diabetes mellitus
   H. Oral contraceptive pills

III. Neurogenic
   A. Psychogenic
   B. Familial dysautonomia (Riley-Day syndrome)
   C. Poliomyelitis (bulbar)
   D. Polyneuritis
   E. Increased intracranial pressure (acute)
   F. Spinal cord section

IV. Miscellaneous
   A. Hypercalcemia
   B. Drug-induced, e.g., contraceptive pills, steroids, alcohol
   C. Disseminated lupus erythematosus
   D. Scleroderma
   E. Dermatomyositis
   F. Pseudoxanthoma elasticum
   G. Periarteritis nodosa
   H. Excess salt loading
   I. Coarctation of the aorta

V. Unknown etiology
   A. Primary hypertension (>90% of all cases of hypertension)
   B. Toxemia of pregnancy
   C. Acute intermittent porphyria

    E. **Pathophysiology.** The pathophysiology of hypertension can invariably be traced to disorders in the fundamental relationship

      Blood pressure = cardiac output total × peripheral resistance

      Although different investigators have emphasized the complex nature of blood pressure control, there is general agreement that the kidney plays a primary role in hypertension. Many studies point to the kidney as the ultimate effector organ in the control of blood pressure. Many other factors play a role in the genesis of hypertension, including vascular endothelial function, complex neurohormonal control mechanisms, and various genetic factors.

II. **Diagnosis**
   A. **History.** Patients with hypertension should be questioned closely about a number of personal and family issues. The extent of the diagnostic evalua-

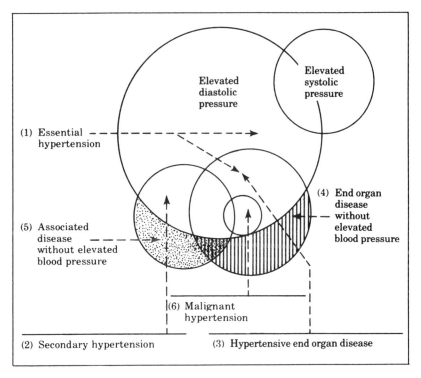

FIG. 12-1. Venn diagram illustrating the different ways that hypertensive patients may present.

tion will depend on a number of clinical parameters: (i) the patient's family history, race, and age; (ii) the severity of the hypertension; (iii) the likelihood of finding a treatable cause for the hypertension; and (iv) the cost, time, and risk of the workup. The majority of patients with hypertension present without symptoms referable to their blood pressure. Elevated levels of blood pressure in these patients generally are discovered during a workup for another disease, during a routine physical examination, or during blood pressure screening in the community or at work. Nonetheless, a careful history is important for at least two reasons: (i) to determine possible curable underlying disease and (ii) to assess possible complications and end organ damage associated with the elevated blood pressure. Significant items in the history of a hypertensive patient are listed in Table 12-2.

B. Physical examination. Most patients with mild or moderate hypertension have no physical findings referable to their disease early in the course of the illness. Abnormalities develop with time. Careful physical examination—with particular emphasis on the cardiovascular system, fundi, and central nervous system—is essential to assess possible end-organ damage and to look for typical findings of underlying curable disease. The physical findings of hypertension are listed in Tables 12-3 and 12-4.

C. Laboratory tests. Many laboratory tests are available, some of which are costly and may involve risk to the patient. A rational sequence of tests should be developed for each patient based on the likely benefit of each investigation. The nature and extent of the laboratory investigation will be suggested by findings in the history and physical examination. General guidelines are given in Table 12-5.

TABLE 12-2. ITEMS OF HISTORY IN PATIENT WITH HYPERTENSION

Category	Item	Comment
Present illness	Age of onset of hypertension	Most primary hypertension has onset between ages 20 and 50 years; if age of onset <20 or >50 years; be alert for underlying disease
	Recent flank trauma	? Renal artery partial occlusion
	History of UTI	Renal parenchymal disease
	Polydipsia, nocturia, weight change, flushing	Possible endocrine disease (including diabetes and Cushing's disease, pheochromocytoma)
	Chest pain; symptoms of cerebrovascular insufficiency; Sx of CHF; peripheral vascular disease	Vascular complications of hypertension
	Occipital headache (present on arising in A.M.), palpitations, dizziness, easy fatigability	Sx directly related to hypertension (headache less frequent than commonly assumed)
Risk factors	Cigarette smoking, diabetes mellitus, hyperlipidemia, family Hx of deaths from cardiovascular disease	Other risk factors for atherosclerotic diseases
Past medical history	Childhood disease	Particularly glomerulonephritis secondary to streptococcal infection
Family history	Relatives with hypertension	Family Hx is evidence for primary hypertension
Current medications	Oral contraceptives, steroids, monoamine oxidase inhibitors	May lead to secondary hypertension
Review of systems (constitution)	Flushing, weight loss	? Pheochromocytoma, ? thyroid disease, high-output hypertension
Head, eyes, ears, nose, throat	Headache; blurred vision	Direct Sx of hypertension, ? papilledema
Cardiovascular	Sx of vascular disease	
Renal	Sx of UTI or renal parenchymal disease	
Endocrine	Sx of thyroid disease, Cushing's disease, diabetes mellitus	
Nervous system	Sx of high sympathetic outflow	

UTI, urinary tract infection; Sx, symptoms; CHF, congestive heart failure; Hx, history.

TABLE 12-3. PHYSICAL FINDINGS THAT MAY BE ASSOCIATED WITH HYPERTENSION

System	Finding	Significance
General	Round face, truncal obesity	Cushing's disease
	Muscular development of upper extremities out of proportion to lower extremities	Coarctation of aorta
Vital signs	Blood pressure	Both arms mandatory; in young hypertensives, leg pressure mandatory to rule out coarctation; do both supine and standing blood pressure
Skin	Plethora	Cushing's disease
Head, eyes, ears, nose, throat	Ocular fundi	Funduscopic examination essential to determine duration of hypertension; Keith-Wagener-Barker classification, see Table 12-4
Cardiac/chest	Left ventricular lift; third heart sound (S3); fourth heart sound (S4)	Cardiac hypertrophy or decompensation
	Pulmonary rales	Cardiac decompensation
	Harsh systolic murmur at apex	Papillary muscle dysfunction
	Systolic murmur between scapulae	Coarctation of aorta
Peripheral vascular system	Carotid bruit or occlusion; femoral bruit	Peripheral vascular disease
Abdomen	Abdominal bruit	Renal artery stenosis (usually diastolic component, often best heard in flank)
	Palpable kidneys	Polycystic kidney disease
Neuromuscular	Focal findings; mental status changes	Previous cerebrovascular accident or lacunar infarct; hypertensive encephalopathy

D. ECG. The ECG in general provides little **diagnostic** information in hypertension. It does, however, supply useful **prognostic** data. ECG findings in hypertension may include (i) evidence of left ventricular hypertrophy and (ii) evidence of myocardial ischemia (S–T and T wave changes). Patients with such ECG findings have a worse prognosis compared with that of individuals with normal ECGs.

E. Chest x-ray examination; computed tomography (CT) and magnetic resonance imaging (MRI). Except for coarctation of the aorta (findings include aortic dilatation and rib notching), the chest x-ray film is often unremarkable. Of prognostic significance is left ventricular enlargement, suggesting decompensation and dilatation. CT and or MRI scans are often used to iden-

TABLE 12-4. KEITH-WAGENER-BARKER CLASSIFICATION OF RETINAL CHANGES ASSOCIATED WITH HYPERTENSION

Degree	Arterioles General narrowing AV ratio[a]	Focal spasm	Hemorrhages	Exudates	Papilledema
Normal	3/4	1/1	0	0	0
Grade I	1/2	1/1	0	0	0
Grade II	1/3	2/3	0	0	0
Grade III	1/4	1/3	+	+	0
Grade IV	Fine, fibrous cords	Obliteration of distal flow	+	+	+

[a]Ratio of arteriolar/venous diameters. + = present; 0 = absent.

tify renal or adrenal abnormalities in individuals with suspected secondary hypertension owing to intrinsic kidney disease, Cushing's disease, or primary hyperaldosteronism (see Section **F.** below).

F. Other radiologic studies. When renovascular hypertension is suspected, for example, because an abdominal bruit has been heard, a variety of tests may be ordered for confirmation. The gold standard test is a renal arteriogram. A number of noninvasive tests have been developed that may obviate invasive renal arteriography if they reveal normal results. Different authorities and different institutions favor one noninvasive test over another. The various noninvasive tests that have been recommended for the diagnosis of renovascular hypertension include the radioisotope renogram with or without pretreatment with an angiotensin-converting enzyme (ACE) inhibitor, digital subtraction angiography (DSA), duplex ultrasound scanning, and MRI angiography. Individual hospitals will favor one or two of these tests over the others (Table 12-5).

G. Radionuclide studies. Radionuclide studies of the heart are not done solely for the diagnosis of hypertension. If associated heart disease is suspected, for example, arteriosclerotic coronary artery disease (CAD), then studies such as a thallium exercise test are indicated. Radionuclide evaluation of the kidney, may provide useful information. The iodine 131 hippuran renogram yields data about renal vascular blood flow and is particularly helpful when the diagnosis of renovascular hypertension is being pursued.

H. Catheterization and angiography
   1. Cardiac catheterization and angiography. Except for the rare cases of hypertension in which coarctation of the aorta is suspected, cardiac catheterization and angiography have no role in the specific diagnostic workup of hypertension. Their use in the diagnosis of CAD and mitral regurgitation owing to papillary muscle dysfunction (both of which may be secondary to hypertension) is well established and discussed elsewhere in this manual.
   2. Renal catheterization and angiography. The definitive diagnosis of renal artery disease requires renal angiography. If renovascular hypertension is strongly suspected (as in patients below the age of 20 years who develop hypertension), renal angiography may be undertaken. Caution must be exercised in the interpretation of angiographic lesions, because their presence does not establish a causal link to hypertension (indeed, renal artery stenosis is a common finding at postmortem examination in normotensive patients). Therefore, differential renal vein renin determinations are often performed at the same time as renal arteriography.

TABLE 12-5. LABORATORY TESTS IN THE EVALUATION OF HYPERTENSION

I. All patients
   A. Blood: Complete blood count, electrolytes, blood urea nitrogen, creatinine, calcium, uric acid, thyroid-stimulating hormone, cholesterol (total, LDL, HDL), triglycerides, and fasting blood sugar levels
   B. Urine: routine urinalysis
   C. Other: ECG, posteroanterior and lateral chest x-ray films. Optional studies in selected patients include echocardiography and various imaging studies such as computed tomography or MRI (see below).

II. Selected patients (based on history and physical examination)
   A. Blood: Plasma cortisol, creatinine clearance, microalbuminuria, glycosolated hemoglobin, plasma renin activity/urinary sodium determination or a post-ACE inhibition plasma renin, plasma catecholamine levels, and an aldosterone suppression test as well as other tests (see below).
   B. Urine: urine culture, 24-hour urine for protein, catecholamines, normetanephrine, or urinary metanephrine-to-creatinine ratio.

III. Very particularly selected patients (based on history, physical examination, and initial laboratory results or high index of suspicion of curable underlying disease)
   A. When initial workup suggests renal artery stenosis one or more of the following may be indicated:
      1. Postcapopril plasma renin activity
      2. Radionuclide renogram with or without ACE inhibition
      3. Split renal vein renins (often performed at the same time as renal arteriography)
      4. Duplex ultrasound scanning
      5. Digital subtraction angiography, MRI angiography, or renal arteriogram
   B. When initial workup suggests primary aldosteronism one or more of the following may be indicated:
      1. Plasma aldosterone (random and with Na+ loading or postural change in levels)
      2. Plasma renin activity or the plasma aldosterone/plasma renin ratio
      3. Dexamethasone suppression test
      4. Plasma 18-hydroxycorticosterone levels
      5. Computed tomography or MRI
      6. Adrenal arteriography; adrenal venography with venous blood aldosterone levels
   C. When initial workup suggests Cushing's disease one or more of the following may be indicated:
      1. Plasma cortisol level
      2. Urinary free cortisol level
      3. Dexamethasone suppression test
      4. Plasma adrenocorticotropic hormone level

LDL, low-density lipoprotein; HDL, high-density lipoprotein; MRI, magnetic resonance imaging; ACE, angiotensin converting enzyme.

The plasma renin value should be elevated in blood samples coming from the kidney with the renal arterial stenosis.

Renal arteriography also helps distinguish atherosclerotic lesions from fibrous dysplasias (of prognostic benefit: fibrous disease is more amenable to surgery or percutaneous balloon catheter dilatation).

3. Split renal vein renins. When significant renal artery stenoses are found, split renal vein renins are helpful in assessing the functional significance of the lesion and the likelihood of successful surgical intervention. Catheters are passed retrograde into the renal veins bilaterally, and samples are withdrawn. When plasma renin from the involved kidney exceeds that of the uninvolved kidney by a ratio of greater than 1.5:1.0, surgical cure may be anticipated in more than 80% of patients. Other noninvasive tests to identify renovascular hypertension are listed in Table 12-5.

4. Adrenal arteriography and adrenal vein aldosterone sampling. When primary aldosteronism secondary to an adrenal tumor is strongly suspected (see Section **II.J.2.**), adrenal arteriography and split adrenal vein aldosterone measurements may be warranted.

5. CT, DSA, and MRI. These computerized, radiologic techniques—CT scanning, MRI, and DSA—are frequently useful in the workup of patients with secondary forms of hypertension. Adrenal hyperplasia or tumors (aldosteronoma, pheochromocytoma), spinal cord abnormalities, and certain renal structural abnormalities can be readily identified with these techniques.

Renal artery stenosis and coarctation of the aorta can be easily identified with DSA.

I. Public policy issues. Hypertension represents a public and a private health concern. Numerous studies have assessed the diagnostic accuracy of procedures relative to their cost. Screening protocols for diagnosing hypertension in large populations have been developed. Although such public health considerations may initially appear of little relevance to the individual physician, issues of cost, benefit, and equity are becoming increasingly pertinent.

J. Protocol for the diagnosis of hypertension

1. Criteria for making the diagnosis. The diagnosis of elevated blood pressure is based on the straightforward determination of cuff blood pressure, which should be part of every physical examination. Patients who have blood pressures in excess of 140/90 mm Hg on at least three separate consecutive visits have hypertension.

The challenge in the diagnosis and treatment of hypertension is determining that 10% of patients who have potentially curable forms of hypertension and establishing the best blood pressure control program for the remaining 90%. Figure 12-2 depicts a suggested decision tree for the diagnosis of hypertension.

2. Differential diagnosis. The critical issues in the differential diagnosis of hypertension lie not in distinguishing hypertension from other disease entities but in differentiating primary hypertension from curable forms of secondary hypertension and in distinguishing the different disease processes that cause hypertension from one another.

A listing of the disease processes known to cause hypertension is found in Table 12-1. The process of differential diagnosis should seek to divide hypertension into five general categories: (i) renal, (ii) endocrine, (iii) neurogenic, (iv) miscellaneous, and (v) of unknown etiology.

a. Renal causes. Renal causes fall into three general categories: (i) renal parenchymal disease, (ii) renovascular disease, and (iii) other severe renal disease. The mechanisms of hypertension underlying these diseases are complex; however, all involve activation of the renin-angiotensin-aldosterone system, either through disorders in the volume regulating function of the kidney or because of renal ischemia. The diagnosis of an underlying renal etiology will be suggested by history and the initial laboratory values for blood urea nitrogen, creatinine, urinalysis, and microscopic examination of the urine. Further examinations may include urine culture, plasma renin values after pretreatment with captopril, and radionuclide renography with or without ACE inhibition. Invasive and costly procedures that may involve some risk to the patient, such as renal arteriography and split renal vein renins, should be undertaken only for specific clinical indications.

The role of plasma renin measurement remains controversial. Some investigators have achieved good results with renin profiling by combining plasma renin measurements with 24-hour sodium measurements under controlled conditions (renin-sodium index). Good results have also been achieved with furosemide-provoked renin values. The capability of measuring renin is not universally

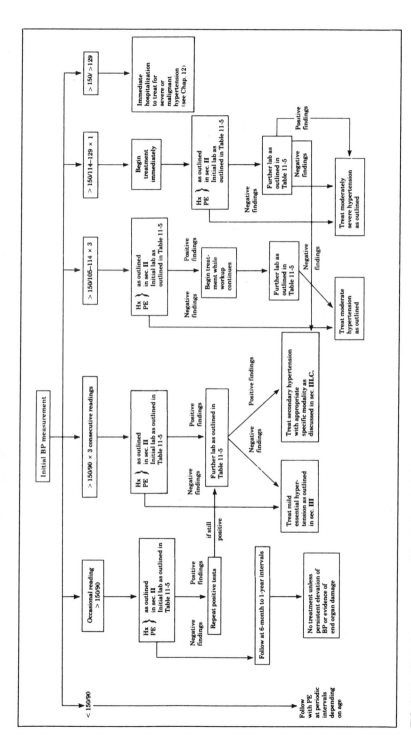

FIG. 12-2. Clinical management of the patient with hypertension.

available, but when capability and experience with the test exist, it may be valuable in the workup of renal causes of hypertension. Most patients with hypertension do **not** need plasma renin determinations.

b. Endocrine causes. Hypertension is associated with a broad spectrum of endocrine disorders (see Table 12-1). The initial workup for possible endocrine etiologies of hypertension (in addition to a careful history of endocrine symptoms and a complete physical examination) should include obtaining electrolyte values, thyroid stimulating hormone, postcibal and fasting blood sugar levels, calcium levels, and a urinalysis. More extensive examination—including 24-hour urine for potassium, metanephrine, catecholamines, and aldosterone concentrations—should be undertaken only when the initial screening tests point to a specific endocrine abnormality. Adrenal angiography, adrenal vein aldosterone measurements, and various stimulation and suppression tests should be performed only with a high index of suspicion that a remediable endocrine disorder underlies the blood pressure elevation (Table 12-5). The complete workup for endocrine abnormalities that lead to hypertension may be found in any standard textbook of medicine, cardiovascular disease, or endocrinology.

c. Neurogenic causes. The fact that a variety of specific and general neurogenic causes have been documented (Table 12-1) is not surprising, because the interplay of neural and endocrine systems on the control of blood pressure is well described. The exact mechanisms for neural etiologies of hypertension are largely unknown, although they presumably involve the sympathetic nervous system. Unfortunately, no good screening devices exist for neurogenic causes of hypertension.

d. Miscellaneous causes. Miscellaneous causes (Table 12-1) range from metabolic factors such as hypercalcemia to mechanical causes such as coarctation of the aorta. Of particular note are the diverse systemic diseases that can cause hypertension (particularly connective tissue abnormalities such as systemic lupus erythematosus, scleroderma, and polymyositis), and hypertension secondary to drug ingestion. A careful drug history should be part of every workup of hypertension. Among the drugs implicated in causing hypertension are oral contraceptives, steroids, alcohol, and monoamine oxidase inhibitors.

e. Unknown causes. The final category in the differential diagnosis of the etiologies of hypertension is also the largest. In more than 90% of patients with hypertension, no underlying cause can be found. This large category of primary hypertension represents a diagnosis of exclusion. The degree to which possible underlying etiologies will be ruled out before a patient's condition is consigned to the catchall diagnosis of primary hypertension is a function of the physician's index of suspicion.

III. Therapy. Rational therapy for primary hypertension is hindered by the fact that the disorder's etiology remains largely undefined. Thus, therapy is usually empiric and nonspecific.

The rationale for treating hypertension comes mainly from large-scale epidemiologic and interventional trials that have shown considerably more cardiovascular morbidity and mortality in patients with uncontrolled hypertension compared with individuals with controlled blood pressure. Even older patients with isolated systolic hypertension benefit from control of their blood pressure. The issue of blood pressure control is further complicated by several competing "systems" of treatment.

The present section is based on two fundamental assumptions: (i) that it is good practice to treat blood pressures greater than 140/90 mm Hg, and (ii) when possible, it is preferable to treat high blood pressure with physiologically rational treatment modalities.

A. Medical treatment

1. Drugs. Four broad classes of drugs are used, either singly or in combination, for the treatment of hypertension. They are (i) diuretics, (ii) sym-

patholytic agents, (iii) vasodilators, and (iv) selective antagonists. See Table 12-6 for specific doses, side effects, etc.

a. Diuretics. The chronic administration of diuretics to patients with hypertension lowers blood pressure **primarily by reducing peripheral resistance.** The precise mechanism by which this occurs is not known, although negative sodium balance and the altered ionic state of the arterial wall have been implicated. Maximally effective doses of diuretics may lower the blood pressure by up to 15 mm Hg by themselves and be effective single-drug therapy in mild hypertension. Diuretics are also used in combination with sympatholytic and vasodilator drugs because they prevent compensatory salt retention. Small differences in action and effectiveness may influence the choice of diuretic. Thiazides have more direct antihypertensive effect than do loop diuretics (e.g., furosemide, ethacrynic acid). Loop diuretics are most effective in the prevention of sodium retention. Spironolactone has maximal efficacy in high-aldosterone states. Diuretics often are the cornerstone for treating hypertension because they target the abnormally elevated peripheral resistance observed in hypertensive individuals. (see Section **III.C.**). Specific clinical and prescriptive information on the diuretics is found in Table 12-6. Hypokalemia can occur in hypertensive patients treated with diuretics. Cardiac arrhythmias and even sudden death may be the result of hypokalemia. Consequently, many physicians prescribe potassium supplementation together with diuretics.

b. Sympatholytic agents. The sympatholytic agents are divided according to the segment of the sympathetic nervous system they inhibit.

(1) Predominant central action. Clonidine is the prototype drug. It is thought to act by inhibiting efferent outflow from central sympathetic centers, thereby decreasing sympathetic activity to the heart, kidney, and peripheral vasculature.

(2) Predominant peripheral action. Guanethidine is the prototype. It inhibits sympathetic activity at peripheral nerve terminals by inhibiting the release of norepinephrine and depleting its supply.

(3) Central and peripheral action. Methyldopa blocks the enzymatic conversion of Dopa (3,4-dihydroxyphenylalanine) to both dopamine (the immediate precursor of norepinephrine) and 5-hydroxytryptophan (the precursor of serotonin). Methyldopa's specific antihypertensive mechanism has not been proven. It is thought to act both centrally and peripherally and may inhibit renal renin release. Reserpine (and other rauwolfia alkaloids), the other major class of drugs in this category, depletes both the heart and the blood vessels of norepinephrine. Reserpine is rarely used today for the control of hypertension.

(4) Receptor blockers

(a) Alpha-adrenergic blockers. Phentolamine and phenoxybenzamine have been used primarily in the diagnosis of pheochromocytoma and have little role in the clinical management of most individuals with hypertension. Prazosin has been used for patients with essential hypertension but is not associated with the same efficacy in reducing morbidity and mortality as many other agents, for example, beta-blockers or ACE inhibitors.

(b) Beta-adrenergic blockers. Propranolol, metoprolol, nadolol, atenolol, timolol, acebutolol, bisoprolol, carvedilol, and pindolol are the beta-blockers available for clinical use in the United States. Beta-blockers are thought to have at least two major antihypertensive actions: (i) decrease in cardiac output and (ii) a complex inhibitory effect on the renin-angiotensin-aldosterone axis. Beta-blockers have been

TABLE 12-6. DRUG THERAPY FOR HYPERTENSION

Class of drug	Drug Generic name	Drug Brand name	Available tablet size (mg)	Initial dose (mg)	Range of usual daily dose (mg)	Route of administration	Contraindications and adverse reactions	Comments
Diuretics Thiazides	Chlorothiazide Hydrochloro- thiazide	Diuril Hydrodiuril	500 25, 50	500–1000 25–50 bid	500–1000 50–100	PO PO	Hypersensitivity to drugs, hypokalemia, GI irritation, elevated blood glucose	Diabetes mellitus or gout, relative contraindication
Loop diuretics	Furosemide	Lasix	24, 40 PO 20, 100 IV	40 PO bid 10 IV	40–120 PO 10–80 IV	PO or IV	GI toxicity, elec- trolyte imbalance, hearing loss	
	Ethacrynic acid	Edecrin	25, 50	25–100 bid	50–200	PO	GI toxicity, elec- trolyte imbalance, hearing loss	
Potassium- sparing agents	Spironolactone	Aldactone	25, 50	25 qid	100–200	PO	Drowsiness, anorexia, skin eruptions, gynecomastia	
	Triamterene	Dyrenium	50, 100	100 bid	100–300	PO	Hyperkalemia, GI irritation	
Sympatholytics Predominant central action	Clonidine	Catapres	0.1, 0.2	0.1 bid	0.2–0.8	PO	Sedation, dizziness, orthostatic hypotension	
Peripheral action	Guanethidine	Ismelin	10–25	10–25 qd	10–150	PO	Dizziness, ortho- static hypoten- sion, inability to ejaculate	

	Drug	Brand	Strengths	Dose	Range	Route	Side effects	Notes
Central and peripheral action	Methyldopa	Aldomet	250, 500	250 tid	760–2000	PO	GI upset, positive Coombs' test, liver damage	
	Reserpine	(Various)	0.1, 0.25	0.25 qd	0.25–0.50	PO	CNS depression, GI irritation, depression	
Receptor blockers	Phentolamine	Regitine	50	60 qid	200	PO, IV	Tachycardia, arrhythmias	Use in control of hypertension secondary to pheochromocytoma
	Phenoxybenzamine	Dibenzyline	10	10 bid	20–120	PO	Hypotension, tachycardia, failure in ejaculation	
	Propranolol	Inderal	10, 40, 60	20 qid	80–320	PO	Fatigue, bradycardia, exacerbation of asthma, congestive heart failure	
	Metoprolol	Lopressor	50, 100	50–100 bid	50–400	PO	As for propranolol	Selective for beta$_1$-receptors at low dose
	Atenolol	Tenormin	50, 100	60–100 qd	60–100	PO	As for propranolol	Selective for beta$_1$-receptors at low dose
	Nadolol	Corgard	40, 80, 120, 160	80–320 qd	80–320	PO	As for propranolol	
	Timolol	Blocadren	10, 20	10–20 bid	10–60	PO	As for propranolol	

(continued)

TABLE 12-6. (*Continued*)

Class of drug	Drug — Generic name	Drug — Brand name	Available tablet size (mg)	Initial dose (mg)	Range of usual daily dose (mg)	Route of administration	Contraindications and adverse reactions	Comments
Calcium channel blockers	Nifedipine	Procardia	10, 20	10 tid	30–90	PO	Headache, dizziness, flushing, hypotension, leg edema	
	Diltiazem	Cardizem	30, 60, 90, 120	30 tid	90–360	PO	Bradycardia, hypotension	
	Verapamil	Calan	40, 80, 120	40 tid	120–480	PO	Hypotension, flushing, constipation, nausea, headache, dizziness	
	Pindolol	Visken	5, 10	5–10 tid	40–60	PO	As for propranolol	Partial beta-agonist at low dose
Vasodilators Predominant arterial action	Diazoxide	Hyperstat	Injection, 15 mg/ml	80–150 IV bolus	May repeat at 30 min, 4 hr, 24 hr	IV bolus	Sodium retention, hyperglycemic	
	Hydralazine	Apresoline	10, 25, 50, 100–200 mg/ml	10 qid PO	100–300 PO	PO, IV	Headache, tachycardia	

Drug	Trade name	Preparations	Parenteral dose	Initial dose	Maintenance dose	Route	Adverse effects	Comments
							SLE (dose-dependent)	
Minoxidil	Loniten	Injection, 2.5, 10	10–40 prn IV, IM	2.5 qd	10–40 PO	PO	Tachycardia, increased cardiac output	Reported particularly effective in chronic renal failure
Guancydine		Investigational		250 tid	750–1500	PO	Tachycardia, increased cardiac output, angina, gynecomastia	
Arterial and venous action								
Nitroprusside	Nipride	Injection, 50 mg	3 μg/kg/min IV infusion		0.9–8.0 μg/kg/min	IV only	GI irritation, restlessness, thiocyanate toxicity (dose-related)	
Selective antagonists								
Captopril	Capoten (converting enzyme inhibitor)	12.5, 25 mg		6.25–25.0 tid	50–150	PO	Renal, bone marrow toxicity; orthostatic hypotension with initial dose	
Enalapril	Vasotec (converting enzyme inhibitor)	2.5, 5, 10, 20 mg		5 mg	5–20	PO	Headache, rash, renal insufficiency, orthostatic hypotension	

GI, gastrointestinal; SLE, systemic lupus erythematosus.

demonstrated to be particularly effective in high-renin hypertension, and they are the cornerstone of treatment in the "renin-vasoconstrictor" theory of treating hypertension (see Section **III.C.**). The antianginal properties of beta-blockers confer added benefit when CAD complicates hypertension. Their use is contraindicated when asthma coexists with hypertension. Some of the beta-blockers have semi-selective $beta_1$ properties (cardiac), namely, metoprolol and atenolol. However, at the dosage levels usually used with these agents, they are semi-selective at best. Consequently, even these semi-selective beta-blockers should not be prescribed for patients with asthma or bronchospastic chronic lung disease. Carvedilol and labetalol combine beta- and alpha-blocking properties. Thus, they display the following pharmacological actions: decreased heart rate, decreased myocardial contractility, and peripheral arteriolar vasodilatation.

  c. Vasodilators. The vasodilators are divided according to site of action. Diazoxide, hydralazine, and minoxidil are predominantly arterial dilators while nitroprusside, ACE inhibitors, angiotensin receptor blockers (ARBs), and nitroglycerin exert effects on both arterial and venous tone. All of these vasodilators act by relaxing vascular smooth muscle and decreasing total peripheral resistance. Their clinical utility is limited by three compensatory reflexes elicited by the decrease of arteriolar pressures: (i) increased sympathetic activity, (ii) rise in plasma renin activity, and (iii) retention of sodium and water. For these reasons, they are often coadministered with beta-blockers and/or diuretics.

    (1) Calcium antagonists. Calcium antagonists have found an increasing role in the treatment of hypertension. Available calcium channel antagonists vary in terms of site and mode of action. Nifedipine and the other dihydropyridines are particularly potent peripheral vasodilators. Verapamil and diltiazem result in less peripheral vasodilatation but are nonetheless effective antihypertensives. Calcium antagonists appear to be particularly effective in elderly hypertensive patients. Some literature has suggested that blacks are less responsive than are whites to calcium antagonists. There has been considerable debate concerning the use of calcium blockers in hypertensive patients. Some authorities believe that calcium blocker therapy (particularly therapy with the dihydropyridine group of calcium blockers, i.e., nifedipine and its relatives) is associated with increased morbidity and mortality compared with other antihypertensive agents. However, most of the investigators who work in this field feel that calcium blockers are safe and highly effective in the management of hypertension.

    (2) Renin-angiotensin inhibitors. ACE inhibitors are frequently used as antihypertensives. The most commonly used ACE inhibitors for this purpose are enalapril, lisinopril, ramipril, and captopril. Other ACE inhibitors include quinapril, perindopril, benazepril, trandolapril, fosinopril, and moexipril. In patients with uncomplicated primary hypertension, ACE inhibitors appear to have an equivalent effect on blood pressure to diuretics and beta-blockers. There is some evidence that ACE inhibitors are less effective in blacks than in whites. ACE inhibitors are as effective in the elderly as in younger hypertensive patients. Initial doses of captopril for hypertension may be as small as 12.5 mg twice a day; for enalapril, as little as 5 mg per day. There may be an initial but transient fall in blood pressure, with a full

effect of any particular dosage of these medicines not seen for 7 to 10 days. The HOPE (Heart Outcomes Prevention Evaluation) trial demonstrated impressive decreases in morbidity and mortality in a group of patients with cardiovascular risk factors but no clinical evidence of atherosclerotic disease. Hypertension was one of the risk factors sought in the HOPE trial. This trial represents further evidence of the beneficial effect of ACE inhibitors in patients with potential or evident vascular disease.

(3) ARBs. These agents block the cellular receptor for angiotensin activity and are hence powerful vasodilators. They do not block the ACE as ACE inhibitors do. Therefore, they are not associated with elevated blood bradykinin levels such as those seen with ACE inhibitor therapy. The dry cough that often accompanies ACE inhibitor therapy is, at least in part, because of these elevated blood bradykinin levels. Because ARBs do not elevate bradykinin levels, the ACE inhibitor–associated cough is not observed. Commonly used ARBs are losartan, valsartan, candesartan, irbesartan, telmisartan, and eprosartan. The results of the HOPE trial have not yet been replicated with the ARBs, and so ACE inhibitors are the therapy of choice over ARBs in the category of antihypertensive vasodilators. ARBs are used when allergic or untoward reactions are seen with ACE inhibitors. Both ACE inhibitors and ARBs should be used with caution in patients with renal insufficiency because they may lead to worsening renal function and/or hyperkalemia.

2. Activity. The admission of a hypertensive patient to the hospital frequently results in a dramatic improvement in blood pressure. Hospitalization and initial bed rest are important in the acute treatment of malignant hypertension, as discussed in Chapter 13. To some extent, the decline in blood pressure during hospitalization may be attributed to reduced activity, although extricating the patient from environmental and psychological stress also undoubtedly contributes. Reduction of activity, together with the avoidance of stressful situations, was often advocated in the past for management of hypertension.

Activity restriction on a day-to-day basis has little role in the modern management of chronic hypertension, although it remains an acute modality when severe elevations of pressure are present. Moderate exercise programs should indeed be recommended, particularly for sedentary patients in whom high sympathetic outflow is thought to contribute to elevated pressure. Regular exercise leads to weight loss, improved arterial function, and a drop in blood pressure.

3. Diet. Dietary management of hypertension may be broken down into four areas.

a. Sodium restriction. Sodium has long been known to be a key determinant of extracellular fluid volume and plasma volume. Severe sodium restriction was previously a component of blood pressure control. Although low-salt diets had some efficacy, they were frequently accompanied by orthostatic hypotension and postural syncope. With the advent of oral diuretics, it is practical to prescribe mild sodium restriction of up to 5 g per day. (The normal diet contains 6 to 15 g of sodium chloride a day.) Removing the salt shaker from the table usually reduces the sodium intake to 4 to 7 g per day.

Eliminating salt from cooking generally lowers intake to 2 to 4 g per day. One level teaspoon of salt contains 6 g of sodium chloride.

b. Weight reduction. A clear link between hypertension and obesity has been established by epidemiologic studies. Obese patients are five times as likely to develop hypertension as nonobese patients are. Moreover, weight reduction is effective in reducing blood pressure. In general, a patient may expect a reduction of 1 mm Hg for each 1.8 kg lost. Overweight hypertensive subjects also suffer an increased incidence of the vascular complications of stroke and CAD. For all these reasons, weight control or reduction is an important component of comprehensive blood pressure management.

Caloric restriction should be coupled with a moderate exercise program. The combination of diet and exercise is of demonstrated benefit in weight reduction and blood pressure control.

Because weight reduction may take some time to accomplish and be difficult to maintain (approximately one person in three is able to sustain initial weight loss), pharmacologic therapy of hypertension should be instituted simultaneously with caloric restriction.

   c. Cholesterol and saturated fats. Because a reduction in dietary intake of cholesterol and saturated fats may diminish the incidence of atherosclerotic disease, a modest restriction of both generally is recommended. Fat intake should be reduced to 40 to 50 g per day, and cholesterol intake should remain below 300 mg per day in the hypertensive patient. As noted in Chapter 14 (hyperlipidemia), some patients who have failed to lose weight with a low-fat diet may respond to the low-carbohydrate diet. However, careful monitoring of serum lipids should be performed in patients on low-carbohydrate/high-protein/high-fat diets. Diets rich in fruits and vegetables, for example, the Mediterranean diet, are beneficial in patients with hypertension. The Mediterranean diet is discussed in Chapter 14.

   d. Alcohol, coffee, and cigarettes. Alcohol consumption in moderate quantities probably has no adverse effect on blood pressure. A larger intake of alcohol can increase blood pressure. Moderate coffee drinking (0 to 6 cups per day) has also been shown to have no adverse effect on either systolic or diastolic blood pressure. Cigarette smoking has been linked to so many cardiovascular complications that its cessation should be urged for patients regardless of blood pressure levels.

4. Environmental and psychological factors. A variety of environmental, behavioral, and psychological modalities have been advocated for lowering blood pressure, including psychotherapy, relaxation, biofeedback, meditation, and environmental modification.

   a. Psychotherapy. Trials of psychotherapy have reported disparate results in control of hypertension. Blood pressure reductions of 20 to 40/10 to 30 mm Hg have been achieved by therapy continued for several years, although "escape" during stressful situations is common. Supportive therapy from the patient's primary physician is appropriate and may have both a direct effect through lowering anxiety and an indirect effect through augmenting compliance.

   b. Relaxation. Relaxation methods that have been advocated for blood pressure control include hypnosis, hatha yoga, transcendental meditation, and the meditational state or relaxation response. Although some decrements in blood pressure have been described in patients using each of these techniques, the numbers of patients in the studies undertaken are small and controls are lacking. These techniques may confer the additional benefit of a sense of well-being on the practitioner. They suffer from the disadvantage that many patients will consider them too "far-out" for serious consideration.

   c. Biofeedback. Decreases in blood pressure up to 20/10 mm Hg have been recorded in small series of patients using various biofeedback techniques. Although results are modest, compliance may be less of a problem in patients electing this form of treatment in conjunction with pharmacologic therapy than in those using medication alone.

   d. Environmental modification. The concept that modifying a patient's environment will help lower blood pressure is based on the theory that stressful environmental stimuli contribute to elevated pressures. Epidemiologic evidence showing that urban populations have higher blood pressures than do rural ones tends to support this belief, as does the common clinical experience of falling blood pressure during a patient's hospitalization; however, no controlled studies of the long-term effects of environmental change on blood pressure are currently available. If the patient relates a history suggestive of extreme environmental stress, the physician should counsel the patient or advise counseling from a psychiatrist/psychologist.

B. Surgery. Surgical management of hypertension is reserved for situations in which elevated blood pressure is secondary to a correctable lesion. Because surgery exposes the patient to risks, which are compounded in the hypertensive patient (particularly if vascular disease accompanies hypertension), caution must be exercised in recommending surgery. Surgically correctable causes of hypertension are as follows:

Systolic hypertension	Diastolic hypertension
Arteriovenous fistula	Pheochromocytoma
Thyrotoxicosis	Primary aldosteronism
Aging	Cushing's syndrome
	Coarctation of the aorta
	Renovascular hypertension
	Unilateral renal parenchymal disease

Arteriovenous fistula, thyrotoxicosis, and aging are causes of systolic hypertension and are thought to have fewer sequelae than do the remaining lesions in the list, which result in primarily diastolic hypertension.

1. Pheochromocytoma. Once the diagnosis of pheochromocytoma has been established, careful preoperative pharmacologic preparation assumes utmost importance. Alpha-adrenergic blockade is essential to bring blood pressure under control and to counteract catecholamine-induced vasoconstriction. This is accomplished with 40 to 100 mg of phenoxybenzamine for several days, including the day of surgery. Beta-blockade is also beneficial. The surgeon should be prepared to explore both adrenal glands and the entire abdominal cavity for extraadrenal tumors, and should be able to perform major vascular surgery if a large vessel is involved.

2. Primary aldosteronism. The vast majority of aldosterone-producing tumors are single. The left adrenal should be explored first because it is twice as likely to contain tumor as the right. Controversy exists about the percentage of patients who can expect a cure from adrenal surgery (estimates range from 50% to 75%). If blood pressure can be corrected with spironolactone, 300 to 400 mg every day before surgery, the chance of surgical cure is greater.

3. Cushing's syndrome. In the great majority of patients with hypertension secondary to Cushing's syndrome, blood pressure can be controlled with an appropriate regimen of antihypertensives and diuretics. Surgery has been attempted in such patients (bilateral adrenalectomy followed by pituitary irradiation), although results have been mixed. For the one third of patients who have Cushing's syndrome secondary to an adrenal tumor, the treatment of choice is complete surgical excision of the tumor.

4. Coarctation of the aorta. Coarctation of the aorta is a rare congenital cause of hypertension. The treatment of choice is surgical excision of the coarctation and reconstruction of the aorta or balloon catheter dilatation of the narrowed aortic segment. These procedures result in remission of hypertension in approximately 95% of patients.

5. Renovascular hypertension. Renovascular hypertension is defined as hypertension secondary to an occlusion in the main renal artery of one kidney or in a branch of the artery large enough to stimulate a systemic vasoconstrictor response (mediated by renin). The renal arterial lesion may be either fibrous or atherosclerotic. Before recommendation of sur-

gical or balloon catheter intervention, an anatomic lesion with functional significance must be demonstrated. The recommended sequence for diagnostic tests is:

Non-invasive evaluation, for example, isotope renogram → renal ateriography → differential renal vein renin determination → surgery or angioplasty

The surgical treatment of choice is vascular reconstruction or balloon angioplasty. A variety of surgical techniques are available for this. Balloon angioplasty of the renal artery is equivalent to surgical repair in many patients (see Section **III.B.6.a.** below).

6. Unilateral renal and parenchymal disease. Some patients have hypertension and one atrophic kidney with a contralateral normal or hypertrophic kidney.

Possible underlying etiologies include posttraumatic fibrosis, radiation fibrosis, unilateral pyelonephritis, and congenital hypoplasia. Before recommendation of surgical intervention, both the presence of an atrophic kidney and its functional significance (split renal vein renins) must be demonstrated. Treatment of choice is surgical excision of the atrophic kidney.

a. Localized renal artery stenoses can be opened with a special balloon catheter that is passed across the stenotic area and then inflated, with or without placement of an intravascular metal stent, thereby dilating the stenotic segment of renal artery. This form of percutaneous renal arterial reconstruction has been shown to be effective in relieving renovascular hypertension with consequent lowering of renin production by the treated kidney.

C. Protocol for therapy of hypertension

1. General strategy. No one system of therapy for hypertension is completely rational or universally effective. The extent to which cardiac output, total peripheral resistance, intravascular volume, sympathetic nervous system stimulation, and the functional status of the renin-angiotensin-aldosterone system influence blood pressure differs from patient to patient. The goals for maximizing the effectiveness of treatment for the patient with hypertension are as follows:

a. Therapy should be individualized as much as possible for each patient.

b. Therapy should be directed to the physiologic abnormality when known.

c. Arterial pressures should be reduced to the normal range when possible.

d. Therapy should not cause side effects that threaten compliance with the prescribed regimen.

e. Continued monitoring and support are essential to help the patient deal with the emotional and physical aspects of this chronic condition.

2. Treatment protocol. The following general protocol will be effective for more than 90% of hypertensive patients.

a. Secondary hypertension should be treated with specific modalities directed at the underlying disease.

Malignant hypertension is a medical emergency. Immediate hospitalization and reduction of blood pressure are imperative (see Chapter 13).

b. For patients with chronic primary hypertension (greater than 90% of patients with hypertension), the physiologic abnormality is increased peripheral resistance.

(1) Begin therapy with a diuretic and/or a beta-blocker or ACE inhibitor (Table 12-6). Use calcium channel blockers, central or peripheral sympatholytics, and angiotensin receptor blockers as additional or substitute therapy based on the response to the initial therapy and any observed adverse reactions to initial therapy (see below).

(2) Restrict salt to 5 g sodium every day (no-added-salt diet). Encourage the patient to lose excess weight and to use a Mediterranean diet (see Chapter 14).

(3) After a thorough physical examination and ECG, prescribe a moderate exercise program.

(4) If patient is overweight, begin caloric restriction.

(5) Some patients elevate their blood pressure each time they visit the physician, a stress-related response. Such patients can often monitor their blood pressure at home with the aid of an inexpensive Doppler blood pressure device that can be purchased in most drug stores. If the patient carefully records blood pressure readings several times per week and if the values demonstrate good control, then it is usually not necessary to increase the dosage or complexity of the patient's blood pressure regimen.

c. For patients with inadequate control on the above regimen, a second drug is added.

(1) If the patient was begun on a beta-blocker, add an ACE inhibitor. If the patient was begun on an ACE inhibitor, add a beta-blocker. (see Table 12-6 for contraindications); dosage of all medications may be increased gradually.

(2) A less physiologic alternative to the addition of a beta-blocker or ACE inhibitor is the addition of methyldopa, reserpine, clonidine, or guanethidine to the initial diuretic.

d. For patients who achieve inadequate control, add a third drug (e.g., an ACE inhibitor or beta-blocker if not already used): hydralazine 25 to 50 mg three or four times a day, or a calcium channel blocker such as long-acting nifedipine 30 to 60 mg, amlodipine 5 to 10 mg, or long-acting diltiazem 120 to 180 mg (see Table 12-6 for contraindications); drug dosages may be increased gradually.

e. For patients who fail to achieve adequate control on three-drug therapy:

(1) Question the patient concerning compliance.

(a) Does the patient understand the medication schedule?

(b) Are there troubling side effects?

(2) Initiate diagnostic workup seeking underlying cause of refractory hypertension.

(3) It may be necessary to add a fourth drug if no other strategy is successful in lowering the patient's blood pressure. Drugs such as minoxidil or guanethidine may be required in addition to the patient's original program.

SELECTED READINGS

Abascal VM, Larson MG, Evans JC, et al. Calcium antagonists and mortality risk in men and women with hypertension in the Framingham Study. *Arch Intern Med* 1998;158:1882–1886.
There were no differences in mortality among patients with hypertension who received calcium antagonists compared with those who received other antihypertensive medications.
Carretero OA, Oparil S. Essential hypertension, II: treatment. *Circulation* 2001;101: 446–453.
A succinct review of therapeutic modalities in patients with hypertension.
Casale PN, Devereux RB, Milner M, et al. Value of echocardiographic measurement of left ventricular mass in predicting cardiovascular morbid events in hypertensive men. *Ann Intern Med* 1986;105:173–178.
Left ventricular hypertrophy by echo identifies patients at high risk for cardiovascular morbid events.
Glynn RJ, Chae CU, Guralnik JM, et al. Pulse pressure and mortality in older people. *Arch Intern Med* 2000;160:2765–2772.

Pulse pressure is the single best measure of blood pressure for predicting mortality in older people.

Hyman DJ, Pavlik VN. Characteristics of patients with uncontrolled hypertension in the United States. *N Engl J Med* 2001;345:479–486.

Most cases of uncontrolled hypertension in the United States consist of isolated, mild systolic hypertension in older adults.

Kaplan NM. Non-drug treatment of hypertension. *Ann Intern Med* 1985;102:359–373.

Use of dietary changes, exercise, relaxation, and mineral supplements in the management of hypertension.

Kaplan NM, Carnegie A, Raskin P, et al. Potassium supplementation in hypertensive patients with diuretic-induced hypokalemia. *N Engl J Med* 1985;312:746–749.

Short-term potassium supplementation ameliorates diuretic-induced hypokalemia and can further decrease blood pressure.

Kaplan NM. Systemic hypertension: mechanisms and diagnosis. In: Braunwald E, ed. *Heart disease,* 6th ed. Philadelphia: Saunders, 2001.

An excellent up-to-date chapter on pathophysiology and treatment of systemic hypertension.

Klungel OH, Heckbert SR, Longstreth WT, et al. Antihypertensive drug therapies and the risk of ischemic stroke. *Arch Intern Med* 2001;161:37–43.

Including a thiazide diuretic in an antihypertensive drug program reduces the risk of stroke.

Major cardiovascular events in hypertensive patients randomized to doxazosin vs chlorthalidone: the Antihypertensive and Lipid-Lowering Treatment to Prevent Heart Attack Trial (ALLHAT). ALLHAT Collaborative Research Group. *JAMA* 2000;283:1967–1975.

The alpha-blocker doxazosin was less effective in preventing cardiovascular events compared with the effectiveness of chlorthalidone.

Mosterd A, D'Agostino RB, Silbershatz H, et al. Trends in the prevalence of hypertension, antihypertensive therapy, and left ventricular hypertrophy from 1950 to 1989. *N Engl J Med* 1999;340:1221–1227.

Increasing use of antihypertensive medication correlates with the decline in cardiovascular mortality over the past 30 years.

Perry HM, Davis BR, Price TR, et al. Effect of treating isolated systolic hypertension on the risk of developing various types of stroke and subtypes of stroke: the Systolic Hypertension in the Elderly Program (SHEP). *JAMA* 2000;284:465–471.

Treating isolated systolic hypertension in the elderly reduces the incidence of all types of stroke.

Rowlands DB, Glover DR, Ireland MA, et al. Assessment of left ventricular mass and its response to antihypertensive treatment. *Lancet* 1982;467–470.

Mean arterial blood pressure correlates with left ventricular mass; ventricular hypertrophy regresses with effective antihypertensive therapy.

Sacks FM, Svetkey LP, Vollmer WM, et al. Effects on blood pressure of reduced dietary sodium and the dietary approaches to stop hypertension (DASH) diet. *N Engl J Med* 2001;344:3–10.

A diet low in salt and rich in fruits and vegetables is beneficial for patients with hypertension.

The sixth report of the Joint National Committee on prevention, detection, evaluation, and treatment of high blood pressure. *Arch Intern Med* 1997;157:2413–2445.

The standard guideline for evaluation and management of hypertension.

Whelton PK, He J, Cutler JA, et al. Effects of oral potassium on blood pressure: meta-analysis of randomized controlled clinical trials. *JAMA* 1997;277:1624–1632.

Potassium supplementation reduces blood pressure in patients with hypertension.

Yarows SA, Julius S, Pickering TG. Home blood pressure monitoring. *Arch Intern Med* 2000;160:1251–1257.

Home blood pressure monitoring is useful in the management of patients with hypertension.

13. HYPERTENSIVE CRISIS

I. **Definition.** Hypertensive crisis is a medical emergency requiring immediate action. Hypertensive crises are often categorized into *emergencies* and *urgencies* (Table 13-1). This chapter focuses on hypertensive emergencies. A hypertensive emergency is characterized by some or all of the following signs: (i) sudden or sustained blood pressure rise to diastolic greater than 120 mm Hg, (ii) papilledema (not always present), (iii) evidence of progressive decrease in renal function, (iv) presence of heart failure or dissection of the aorta, and (v) presence of neurologic dysfunction.

An alternative term for hypertensive crisis is **malignant hypertension.** In this chapter, the terms are used interchangeably.

Hypertensive crisis may present in a variety of ways demanding emergency treatment (Table 13-1). Treatment should assume higher priority than diagnostic procedures. Many of the complications of hypertensive crisis can be avoided or diminished by prompt and effective treatment. Management of hypertensive crisis is often performed in the hospital and by means of intravenous drugs. However, potent oral antihypertensive agents can be used, and under specific, carefully controlled circumstances, some patients can be managed as out-patients.

II. **Incidence.** The true incidence of hypertensive crisis is difficult to assess. In patients with previously diagnosed hypertension, it is estimated that malignant hypertension arises in 2% to 7% of patients at some time during the course of their illness. Those at highest risk are 40 to 60 years old with a 2-to 10-year history of poorly controlled blood pressure. Malignant hypertension arising in a previously normotensive patient is extremely rare, although isolated cases exist.

III. **Pathophysiology.** The most significant lesion associated with malignant hypertension is focal necrosis of arteries and arterioles known as "fibrinoid necrosis." Although this pathologic change may be found in any end organ, it is most common and significant in the kidney, retina, and brain.

Hypertensive crisis may be associated with a variety of underlying and intercurrent conditions and illnesses (Table 13-2).

IV. **Diagnosis.** The initial diagnostic workup should be minimal, with emphasis placed on blood pressure reduction. Parts of the detailed diagnostic plan presented in this section may be performed during the patient's hospitalization.

A. **History.** A brief history should be taken on admission (Table 13-3). Of particular importance is a history of hypertension and the drugs have been used for its treatment. The history should focus on neurologic, renal, and cardiac symptoms, both to assess the degree of end organ damage and to rule out other cardiac, renal, or neurologic emergencies.

B. **Physical examination.** Physical examination (Table 13-4) should focus on accurate assessment of blood pressure and evidence of end-organ damage (particularly funduscopic and neurologic examinations). It is important to attempt to distinguish complications of hypertensive crisis from other neurologic emergencies or other causes of congestive heart failure and pulmonary edema. Evidence of significant intercurrent disease (such as coronary artery disease [CAD]) should be noted. Intercurrent diseases will influence how rapidly and with which agents blood pressure can be treated.

C. **Laboratory tests.** Laboratory tests in the workup of hypertensive crisis are divided into two categories: (i) emergency (a rapidly obtainable laboratory profile should be made) and (ii) further diagnostic laboratory tests based on clinical impression and initial laboratory results (should be obtained after therapy is in progress). Valuable time should not be wasted on detailed diagnostic tests before therapy to reduce blood pressure is undertaken. The recommended laboratory tests are outlined in Table 13-5.

TABLE 13-1. HYPERTENSIVE CRISES

Emergencies
  Hypertensive encephalopathy
  Acute aortic dissection
  Pulmonary edema
  Pheochromocytoma crisis
  Monoamine oxidase inhibitor/tyramine interaction
  Intracranial hemorrhage eclampsia
  Immediately following coronary artery bypass surgery
  Clonidine withdrawal hypertensive crisis

Urgencies
  Hypertension associated with coronary artery disease
  Accelerated and malignant hypertension
  Severe hypertension in the kidney transplant patient
  Postoperative hypertension
  Uncontrolled hypertension in the patient requiring emergency surgery
  Hypertension complicating cerebral hemorrhage
  Hypertension in association with postoperative bleeding

D. ECG. It is essential to examine the ECG carefully, because evidence of myocardial ischemia may influence the choice of therapy. In patients with CAD, blood pressure reduction must proceed cautiously (see Section **V.**). Evidence of left ventricular hypertrophy is of prognostic value (left ventricular hypertrophy carries a poor prognosis in hypertensive crisis particularly if ST–T wave changes are present). Serial ECGs should be taken as therapy is initiated (particularly during the first half-hour; when rapid-acting vasodilators are used, patients should have continuous ECG monitoring). Daily ECGs should be obtained for a short period of time to assist in the diagnosis of myocardial necrosis.

E. Chest x-ray examination. A good quality posteroanterior chest x-ray film to examine cardiac chamber size and lung fields should be taken once therapy has commenced. Except for rare cases of coarctation of the aorta, the film will not yield a diagnosis in patients with hypertensive crisis.

F. Other radiologic studies. Other radiologic studies should be undertaken only for specific clinical reasons, namely, intravenous pyelogram, renal angiography, and computed tomography scanning (Table 13-5).

TABLE 13-2. CONDITIONS AND DISEASES ASSOCIATED WITH HYPERTENSIVE CRISIS

Essential hypertension
Chronic pyelonephritis
Chronic glomerulonephritis
Acute glomerulonephritis
Polyarteritis nodosa
Unilateral renal artery obstruction
Postpregnancy
Congenital small kidney
Hydronephrosis
Cushing's disease
Nephrocalcinosis
Scleroderma
Tuberculous and polynephritic kidney
Tyramine ingestion with monoamine oxidase inhibitor use
Atheromatous embolization of kidney

TABLE 13-3. IMPORTANT ITEMS OF HISTORY IN PATIENT
WITH HYPERTENSIVE CRISIS

Category	Item	Comment

Present illness	History of hypertension
	Age
	Weight loss
	Neurologic symptoms
	   Visual impairment
	   Headache
	   Dizziness
	   Mental status change
	   Anxiety
	Renal symptoms
	   Gross hematuria
	   Decreased urinary output
	Cardiac symptoms
	   Symptoms of congestive
	     heart failure and pul-
	     monary edema
	   Chest pain
		Most common history
		Most common 40–60 years old
		
		Looking for end organ
		  damage, must distinguish
		  between hypertensive
		  encephalopathy and other
		  neurologic events or anxiety
		
		Looking for end organ damage
		  (renal)
		
		Looking for end organ damage,
		  must distinguish from other
		  causes of pulmonary edema;
		  must worry about myocardial
		  infarction or dissection of
		  thoracic aorta; history of
		  coronary artery disease
		  important because it limits
		  therapeutic options

Past medical history	History of glomerulonephritis History of pyelonephritis	
Ob/gyn history	Problems with pregnancy	Hypertensive crisis with severe toxemia or eclampsia
Current medications	? Monoamine oxidase inhibitors ? Hypertensive medications	Issue of compliance important

G. Catheterization and angiography. Cardiac catheterization and angiography have no role in the diagnostic workup of hypertensive crisis with two exceptions.

First, catheterization and aortography are important in the rare instance in which one suspects that coarctation of the aorta underlies hypertensive crisis. Aortography may be undertaken later after therapy has reduced blood pressure. Second, when dissection of the aorta is suspected as a complication of hypertensive crisis, emergency aortography is important. Renal catheterization and angiography may be undertaken with a high clinical suspicion that renal artery embolization underlies hypertensive crisis. These procedures, however, usually have no role in the initial diagnostic workup.

H. Protocol for the diagnosis of hypertensive crisis
  1. Criteria for the diagnosis. At least two of the following must be present: (i) sudden or sustained blood pressure rise to greater than 120 mm Hg diastolic, (ii) papilledema, (iii) evidence of progressive decrease in renal function, (iv) evidence of neurologic dysfunction, and (v) evidence of pulmonary edema.
  2. Differential diagnosis. Two critical issues arise in the differential diagnosis of hypertensive crisis: (i) distinguishing between hypertensive crisis and other entities for which the treatment would be markedly different

TABLE 13-4. PHYSICAL FINDINGS THAT MAY BE ASSOCIATED WITH HYPERTENSIVE CRISIS

System	Finding	Significance/comment
General	Anxiety, restlessness	Hypertensive encephalopathy vs. anxiety
Vital signs	Blood pressure >180/120 mm Hg (must be taken on both arms and legs)	May have very high blood pressure readings without true hypertensive crisis (e.g., no end organ damage: papilledema)
Head, eyes, ears, nose, throat	Hemorrhages and exudates in fundus; papilledema	Papilledema is not always present
Cardiac/chest	Rales Third heart sound (S3) Fourth heart sound (S4)	Evidence of left ventricular decompensation
Peripheral vascular system	Arterial bruits Diminished pulses	Evidence of intercurrent carotid artery disease or atherosclerotic peripheral vascular disease Beware of too rapid lowering of blood pressure
Neurologic	Focal findings	Major distinction is hypertensive encephalopathy vs. neurologic emergency of another etiology

TABLE 13-5. RECOMMENDED LABORATORY TESTS IN WORKUP OF HYPERTENSIVE CRISIS

A. Emergency (obtain immediately on all patients)
   1. Blood: CBC, BUN, creatinine, electrolyte, and glucose levels
   2. Urine: urinalysis and urine culture
   3. 12-lead ECG
   4. Chest x-ray film (must be posteroanterior, may wait until after therapy is begun)

B. Further diagnostic workup (based on initial lab results and clinical suspicion; obtain *after* therapy underway)
   1. If renal pathology suspected
      IVP or CT scan of the abdomen with contrast
      Renal angiography (very particularly selected patients)
      Renal biopsy (very particularly selected patients)
   2. To rule out surgically correctable neurologic disease
      CT scan of the head with contrast
      Spinal tap
   3. If pheochromocytoma suspected
      24-hour urine for catecholamines, metanephrine, or vanillylmandelic acid
   4. Rule out myocardial infarction protocol in selected patients

CBC, complete blood cell count; BUN, blood urea nitrogen; IVP, intravenous pyelogram; CT, computed tomography.

and (ii) recognizing intercurrent diseases and conditions that would modify the course of treatment. These two categories are outlined in Table 13-6 and discussed here.

3. Entities that must be distinguished from hypertensive crisis
   a. Severe hypertension. It has been clearly established that one may have blood pressure elevations as high as 180/120 mm Hg or more without the end-organ damage associated with hypertensive crisis. Although such elevations also require urgent medical attention, they should be distinguished from hypertensive crisis, in which delay of even a few hours may be disastrous. Both severe hypertension and hypertensive crisis are most frequently the result of uncontrolled essential hypertension. Both may demand immediate hospitalization, possibly in a coronary care unit or intensive care unit. As noted earlier, selected, stable patients may be managed with meticulous and frequent out-patient visits. The rapidity with which the blood pressure must be lowered, and hence, the choice of therapeutic agents differs. In hypertensive crisis, an attempt is made to achieve significant blood pressure reductions within minutes to hours, whereas in severe hypertension, bed rest plus immediate two- or three-drug therapy administered orally will usually bring blood pressure under control within 24 to 48 hours.
   b. Surgically correctable neurologic emergencies. Neurologic emergencies can occur both as a result of hypertensive crisis and independently of it.
      All patients with neurologic changes that are possibly secondary to hypertensive crisis must receive a careful neurologic examination and appropriate laboratory studies to rule out potentially correctable neurologic disease of other origin. Neurologic disorders that must be ruled out include (i) infiltrating and rapidly growing cerebral and glial tumors, (ii) pseudotumor cerebri, (iii) significant intracerebral bleeding, (iv) seizure disorders secondary to cortical scars in patients with hypertension, (v) edematous cerebral infarcts, and (vi) high brainstem lesions causing elevated blood pressure. In each of these conditions, headache, convulsions, or focal neurologic signs may be present. The key distinction between these conditions and neurologic dysfunction based on severe hypertension is that, in the latter, reduction in blood pressure results in symptomatic improvement. Spinal tap may be warranted in some settings. Cerebrospinal fluid findings in hypertensive crisis include elevated pressure and elevated protein; gross blood is rare. Computed tomography scanning is usually

TABLE 13-6. DIFFERENTIAL DIAGNOSIS OF HYPERTENSIVE CRISIS

Entities to be distinguished from hypertensive crisis
  Severe hypertension without major end-organ damage or dysfunction
  Surgically correctable neurologic emergency
  Anxiety with labile hypertension
  Pulmonary edema with left ventricular failure secondary to primary cardiac disease
Intercurrent diseases for which special precautions must be observed in the treatment of
  hypertensive crisis
  Toxemia of pregnancy
  Pheochromocytoma
  Stroke
  Dissecting aortic aneurysm
  Renal insufficiency
  Coronary artery disease

helpful in ruling out mass lesions or acute central nervous system bleeding.
c. Anxiety with labile hypertension. Occasionally, it is necessary to distinguish between hypertensive encephalopathy and anxiety accompanying labile hypertension. The distinction is significant because anxiety will respond to sedatives, tranquilizers, or both, whereas hypertensive encephalopathy requires immediate blood pressure control. In general, the patient with anxiety expresses multiple complaints, often including dizziness. Physical examination of this patient shows normal retinal vasculature, normal cardiac findings, and no focal neurologic findings. Treatment should be directed toward relief of anxiety. As the patient's psychological distress recedes, blood pressure returns to lower levels, at times, even normalizing.
d. Pulmonary edema with left ventricular failure. Patients with pulmonary edema secondary to cardiac disease occasionally present with marked elevation of blood pressure. In this situation, blood pressure will respond to the standard therapy as outlined in Chapter 5.
4. Intercurrent diseases for which special precautions must be observed in the treatment of hypertensive crisis
a. Toxemia of pregnancy. The diagnosis of toxemia will be apparent from the clinical setting. This diagnosis has important treatment implications, discussed in Section **V.A.5.**
b. Pheochromocytoma. The presence of a pheochromocytoma is suggested by elevated catecholamines, metanephrine, or vanillylmandelic acid in a 24-hour urine. Treatment is discussed in Section **V.A.5.b.**
c. Stroke. The diagnosis of stroke is important because it will influence the rate of blood pressure reduction (slower if a stroke is thought to have occurred or to be in process). Diagnosis is made by history, either from patient or family, or by complete neurologic examination. Computed tomography scan and spinal tap are often helpful.
d. Dissecting aortic aneurysm. Diagnosis is largely by history, with sudden onset of severe thoracic, back, or abdominal pain. Chest x-ray films usually show a widened mediastinum. Emergency transesophageal echocardiography and/or aortography is essential to confirm the diagnosis. Treatment is discussed in Section **V.A.5.d.**
e. Renal insufficiency. Patients presenting with severely elevated blood pressure and blood urea nitrogen greater than 60 have a poor long-term prognosis. Some investigators believe that these patients have irreversible renal insufficiency with progressive renal dysfunction despite blood pressure reduction and dialysis. Others point out that renal function may return after long periods of dialysis (up to 6 months). The return of renal function is a rare phenomenon. There is no evidence that rapid reduction of blood pressure contributes to long-term deterioration of renal function.
f. CAD. The increased afterload that accompanies marked elevation of blood pressure increases myocardial oxygen demand and can exacerbate the symptoms of CAD. Chest pain generally diminishes when blood pressure is brought under control. The diagnosis is made by history and ECG.
   Agents such as hydralazine and diazoxide should be avoided because of the added cardiac work load owing to sympathetic reflex stimulation with resultant increased heart rate (see Section **V.A.5.f.**).
V. Therapy. Once the diagnosis of hypertensive crisis has been established and initial laboratory work rapidly completed (within 30 minutes), the first priority is to reduce the blood pressure as rapidly and safely as possible. A good general target is reduction of diastolic blood pressure to 100 to 110 mm Hg. A wide variety of drugs with different properties, times of onset, and durations of action are

available for use in hypertensive crisis. Furthermore, the intercurrent conditions outlined in the previous section may dictate different approaches.

A. Medical treatment
   1. Drugs. The clinical properties, dosage schedules, and side effects of the drugs discussed here are listed in Table 13-7. There are basically two types of drugs available: (i) rapid-acting agents (nitroprusside, nitroglycerin, diazoxide), which act quickly but require close monitoring, and (ii) slower acting drugs (hydralazine, methyldopa), which are more gradual but smoother in onset of action, thus requiring less monitoring.

   The drugs most commonly used are all administered parenterally. An important goal of therapy is to switch to long-term oral antihypertensive therapy as soon as the clinical situation allows. Selected patients may be managed with oral agents alone (Table 13-7).

      a. Hydralazine. Hydralazine can be employed either intramuscularly or intravenously. It works by directly dilating peripheral resistance vessels (arterioles). The onset of action of hydralazine is approximately 15 minutes. Its chief disadvantages are that (i) it is not predictably effective in blood pressure reduction, and (ii) it provokes reflex cardiac sympathetic stimulation (this reflex arc can be blunted by administering intravenous beta-blockade [metoprolol, atenolol, propranolol] or pretreating with reserpine or methyldopa).

      b. Diazoxide. Acting through the same mechanism as hydralazine, diazoxide is more powerful and more predictably effective. It may be less effective in severely uremic patients. It must be administered intravenously and rapidly (10 to 20 seconds) and if not effective may be readministered in 30 minutes. The reflex tachycardia it provokes may be blunted by intravenous beta-blockade. Because it causes sodium retention, diazoxide should always be coadministered with a diuretic (intravenous furosemide 10 to 40 mg).

      c. Nitroprusside. Nitroprusside is a potent and predictably effective drug for hypertensive emergency. It works primarily through arteriolar dilatation but has some venous effects as well. It acts immediately and requires constant blood pressure monitoring (arterial line). Thiocyanate toxicity may be a problem in long-term use.

      d. Nifedipine. Oral nifedipine is a potent arteriolar vasodilator that can rapidly control marked hypertension. The drug is a calcium channel blocker. Some patients experience an excessive drop in blood pressure that may be dangerous. Therefore, nifedipine is **not advised** for the therapy of patients with hypertensive crisis.

      e. Labetalol. Although several beta-blockers can be given parenterally (e.g., propranolol, esmolol, metoprolol and atenolol), labetalol is one of the most commonly employed beta-blockers in the intensive care unit for hypertensive emergencies. Labetalol is a racemic mixture of a selective alpha$_1$ agonist and a nonselective beta-blocker. It promptly reduces both peripheral vascular resistance and cardiac contractility. Because the beta-blocker component of labetalol prevents significant changes in cardiac output or reflex tachycardia, it is particularly valuable when CAD and hypertensive crisis coexist.

   2. Activity. During the acute phase of a hypertensive crisis, the patient should be confined to strict bed rest. For many of the parenteral therapies just outlined, 30-degree elevation of the head of the bed is beneficial. Activity may be increased once blood pressure is controlled.

   3. Diet. In the acute phase of hypertensive crisis, patients are given nothing by mouth. Once pressure is controlled, only moderate salt restriction, used as part of long-term antihypertensive therapy, is necessary. In patients with renal failure complicating hypertensive crisis, protein restriction may also be necessary.

TABLE 13-7. DRUGS USED TO TREAT HYPERTENSIVE CRISIS

Drug		Time and course of action		Dosage			Mechanism of action	Effect on cardiac output	Adverse reactions	Comment
Generic name	Trade name	Onset	Maximum duration	Intra-muscular (mg)	Intravenous (mg)	Interval (hr)				
Hydralazine	Apresoline	10–20 min	20–40 min 3–8 hr	10–40	10–40	3–6	Direct dilatation of arterioles	Increased	Tachycardia, palpitations, flushing; contraindicated in angina or aortic dissection	Causes reflex tachycardia
Diazoxide	Hyperstat	1–2 min	2–3 min 4–12 hr		80–150	3–10	Direct dilatation of arterioles	Increased	Sedation and somnolence, sodium retention, hyperglycemia, tachycardia, palpitations, chest pains	Must be given rapidly in bolus (10–20 sec)

				IV infusion rate					
Nitroprusside	Nitropress	0.5–1 min	1–2 min 3–5 min	0.3–10 µg/kg/min	4–12	Direct dilation of arterioles and veins	Decreased	Nausea, vomiting, apprehension	Requires arterial line
Methyldopa	Aldomet	2–3 hr	3–5 hr 6–12 hr	500–1,000	4–8	Decreased sympathetic vasomotor stimulation	Unchanged	Sedation, drowsiness, positive Coombs' test, liver damage, drug fever, rarely thrombocytopenia	Slow onset; response highly variable
Labetalol	Normodyne	5–10 min	5–10 min	20–80 mg over 10 min		Decreased resistance, decreased contractility	Unchanged	Orthostatic hypertension, nausea, vomiting, flushing, dizziness, headache	Relative contraindicators include asthma and significant congestive heart failure

CNS, central nervous system; GI, gastrointestinal.

    4. Environmental support. Patients with a hypertensive crisis are acutely ill and often extremely anxious. A quiet supportive atmosphere is beneficial.

    5. Specific diseases with accelerated or malignant hypertensive potential. A number of disease states can be complicated by severe or accelerated hypertension. These entities may require special diagnostic or therapeutic intervention.

      a. Toxemia of pregnancy. Two drugs are as a rule contraindicated: (i) reserpine, tends to increase the likelihood of seizures; and (ii) trimethaphan, causes fetal ileus and stops labor.

      b. Pheochromocytoma. Phentolamine (Table 13-7) is the treatment of choice for paroxysmal hypertension in previously diagnosed pheochromocytoma. Oral phenoxybenzamine (10 to 40 mg per day) should also be begun immediately. Oral and/or intravenous beta-blockade is a useful adjunct to blunt tachycardia and prevent angina in patients with CAD.

      c. Stroke. Blood pressure should be diminished more gradually if the possibility of an intercurrent stroke exists. The risk of "completing" an occlusive stroke may be decreased by using drugs that increase cardiac output such as hydralazine or diazoxide.

      d. Dissecting aortic aneurysm. Agents that either leave cardiac output unchanged or reduce it (beta-blockade, methyldopa, reserpine, trimethaphan) are recommended for lowering blood pressure when aortic dissection is suspected. Agents that increase cardiac output and hence pulse pressure (hydralazine, diazoxide, nitroprusside) are contraindicated unless the patient is first treated with intravenous beta-blockade, for example, metoprolol, atenolol, propranolol, or esmolol.

      e. Renal insufficiency. Treatment for renal insufficiency complicating hypertensive crisis may include dialysis and may rarely include nephrectomy and transplantation. The drug of choice in the acute setting is diazoxide (which increases cardiac output and renal perfusion). Calcium channel blockers are also indicated in this setting. ACE inhibitors are contraindicated.

      f. CAD. Hydralazine and diazoxide are contraindicated because of their effect on heart rate (reflex tachycardia). The drugs of choice are beta-blockers, alone or in combination with nitroprusside or ACE inhibitors.

B. Surgery. Surgery has little role in the acute management of hypertensive crisis. With two conditions, however, surgical intervention is necessary: (i) pheochromocytoma and (ii) dissection of the aorta.

    1. Pheochromocytoma (see Chapter 11 for details). Surgery should be undertaken under pharmacologic coverage of both alpha- and beta-adrenergic blockade.

    2. Dissecting aortic aneurysm. Some controversy exists over the relative merits of surgical versus medical therapy for acute dissection of the thoracic aorta (see Chapter 26). Evidence seems to support surgical treatment for ascending aortic dissections or any dissection complicated by acute bleeding. Stable descending aortic dissections can often be treated medically but eventually may require surgery.

C. Protocol for acute treatment of hypertensive crisis. The following sequence is recommended:

    1. Brief history (special attention paid to cardiovascular and neurologic systems, renal function, and medications)

    2. Physical examination (look for end-organ damage—central nervous system, cardiac, renal)

    3. 12-Lead ECG

    4. Intravenous line started (central venous pressure obtained if possible)

    5. Arterial line needed if trimethaphan or nitroprusside is to be given

    6. Baseline blood and urine (complete blood cell count, blood urea nitrogen, creatinine, electrolytes, glucose levels, urinalysis, urine culture)

7. Parenteral (occasionally oral) therapy begun based on clinical situation (Table 13-7)
8. Chest x-ray study (posteroanterior)
9. Admission to hospital usually indicated. ECG monitoring necessary.
10. Reassessment and alteration of therapy on the basis of initial clinical response and laboratory studies
11. Further laboratory investigation considered to elucidate the cause of the hypertensive crisis or the resultant end-organ damage

SELECTED READINGS

Heyka RJ. Evaluation and management of hypertension in the ICU. In: Rippe JM, Irwin RS, Fink MP, et al., eds. *Intensive care medicine.* Boston: Little, Brown and Company, 1995.
A thorough and up-to-date summary of treatment options for hypertensive crisis.
Kincaid-Smith, P. Malignant hypertension: mechanisms and management. *Pharmacol Ther* 1980;9:245–269.
Updates Dr. Kincaid-Smith's classic article of 1958.
Kincaid-Smith P, McMichael J, Murphy E. The clinical course and pathology of hypertension with papilledema (malignant hypertension). *Q J Med* 1958;27:117.
The classic article on malignant hypertension; describes clinical characteristics and natural history in detail; out of date in terms of therapy.
The sixth report of the Joint National Committee on prevention, detection, evaluation, and treatment of high blood pressure. *Arch Intern Med* 1997;157:2413–2446.
Consensus recommendations on all aspects of hypertension by the Joint National Committee supported by the National Institutes of Health, Bethesda, Maryland.
Varon J, Marik PE. The diagnosis and management of hypertensive crises. *Chest* 2000;118:214–227.

14. HYPERLIPIDEMIA

I. Introduction. Compelling scientific evidence now demonstrates that reduction of risk factors in patients with coronary artery disease (CAD) and peripheral vascular disease improves long-term survival and quality of life, decreases the need for interventional procedures such as coronary bypass surgery and angioplasty, and reduces the incidence of subsequent myocardial infarction (MI). One of the most critical risk factors requiring control is hyperlipidemia.

Much of the data supporting the recommendations that follow have been obtained in patients with CAD and peripheral vascular disease. However, several studies exist supporting the concept that the recommendations made for patients with CAD can be generalized for all patients with atherosclerotic disease, regardless of the vascular territory affected, and for individuals at high risk for developing atherosclerotic vascular disease. Modest regression (10% to 15%) of atherosclerotic vascular disease can be achieved with control of hyperlipidemia. Nevertheless, this modest regression of atherosclerotic vascular disease is associated with significant decreases in cardiovascular morbidity and mortality.

Tight control of serum glucose in patients with diabetes mellitus also reduces vascular complications and aids in controlling the dyslipidemia that frequently accompanies diabetes. Lipid lowering therapy has three goals: (i) decrease total cholesterol and low-density lipoprotein (LDL)–associated cholesterol levels in the blood; (ii) decrease blood triglyceride levels; and (iii) raise high-density lipoprotein (HDL)–associated cholesterol blood levels. Oxidized LDL cholesterol plays a major role in the genesis of atherosclerosis in both men and women, although women develop clinical atherosclerotic disease an average of 10 to 15 years later than do men. LDL cholesterol is often referred to as "bad cholesterol," whereas HDL cholesterol is called "good cholesterol" in the lay media.

II. Diagnosis. Serum lipid levels should be measured in all adults 20 years of age and older at least once every 5 years. Such measurements should quantitate both LDL and HDL cholesterol as well as total cholesterol and triglyceride levels. In individuals **free** of clinical atherosclerotic disease, cholesterol levels less than 200 mg/dl are ideal; cholesterol levels between 200 to 239 mg/dl are considered modestly elevated, and values of or more than 240 mg/dl are classified as definitely elevated. HDL cholesterol values below 40 mg/dl are said to be "low." Levels of LDL cholesterol equal to or greater than 160 mg/dl are considered markedly elevated; LDL cholesterol levels of 130 to 159 mg/dl are modestly elevated; LDL cholesterol levels between 100 to 129 mg/dl are borderline elevated; and LDL levels less than 100 mg/dl are desirable.

In patients with **known CAD or peripheral atherosclerotic disease,** many clinicians seek to lower LDL and total cholesterol levels well below the "desirable" level. For example, some physicians (ourselves included) seek total cholesterol levels in the range of 150 to 170 mg/dl and LDL cholesterol levels in the range of 60 to 80 mg/dl. Triglyceride values are also determined and used to guide therapy (see Section **III.C.**). Ideal triglyceride levels are below 150 mg/dl.

III. Therapy. Diet, regular exercise, and various drugs are used **to treat hyperlipidema** (Section **III.C.**)

A. Diets used to treat hyperlipidemia. Two levels of diet are used to treat hyperlipidemia, step I and step II. The step I diet is less rigorous than the step II diet. The step I diet contains 30% or fewer of its calories as fat, with 8% to 10% of total calories as saturated fat. In addition, daily cholesterol is less than 300 mg. In the step II diet, saturated fat is reduced to less than 7% of daily calories, and cholesterol is reduced to less than 200 mg. Detailed dietary information is available from nutritionists or in the third report of the Expert Panel on Detection, Evaluation, and Treatment of High Blood Cholesterol in Adults (see Selected Readings). Some obese patients have great difficulty losing weight on the above-mentioned diets. These obese individuals are often at high risk for developing atherosclerotic vascular disease. They demonstrate abdominal obesity, insulin resistance, and dyslipidemia. Some of these patients will have dramatic weight loss with improved insulin sensitivity and serum lipid patterns when placed on the so-called low-carbohydrate, protein-sparing diet. Many versions of this diet are touted in the lay media. Some forms of this diet are very rich in saturated fat and cholesterol. However, one version of the low-carbohydrate diet is not excessively rich in saturated fat. It resembles somewhat the diet eaten in the Mediterranean region and has been called the "Mediterranean diet" for this reason. The essential features of this diet are as follows:

1. Increase the amount of fish and lean poultry in the diet, especially oily fish (salmon, mackerel, sardines, tuna, and swordfish).
2. Decrease the quantity of mammalian animal products (whole-fat milk, high-fat cheese, and red meat) in the diet.
3. Use olive oil as the principal fat in the diet.
4. Decrease the quantity of simple carbohydrates (refined flour products, white rice, and pasta) in the diet.
5. Avoid *trans* fatty acids in products such as margarine and commercial baked goods.
6. Maintain a diet that emphasizes vegetables, fruits, whole grains, and seafood.

   It is essential in all therapy of hyperlipidemia that patients exercise regularly. Exercise moderately every day, for example, 40 to 60 minutes of exercise such as brisk walking, jogging, cycling, rowing, or swimming.

B. Drugs used to treat hyperlipidemia
   1. Bile acid sequestrants. The major effect of bile acid sequestrants is to lower LDL cholesterol. The sequestrants are anion exchange resins that bind bile acids in the intestinal lumen. They thereby interrupt the enterohepatic circulation of bile acids and promote conversion of cholesterol to bile acids in the liver. Reducing liver cholesterol content stimulates the formation of LDL receptors, which reduces serum cholesterol levels. The two most commonly used bile acid sequestrants are cholestyramine and colestipol. Their use is associated with significant gastrointestinal side effects (e.g., constipation, bloating, nausea, and flatulence). The usual dose of cholestyramine is 4 to 16 g per day; the usual dose of colestipol is 5 to 20 g per day.
   2. Nicotinic acid. This agent lowers all serum lipid and lipoprotein values when given in large doses. Nicotinic acid reduces the production of very low density lipoproteins (VLDLs) in the liver, which in turn lowers serum LDL cholesterol levels. Nicotinic acid also raises serum HDL cholesterol levels. Nicotinic acid comes in two forms, crystalline (short-acting) and sustained-release capsules.

      The usual dose is 1.5 to 3 g per day for crystalline nicotinic acid and 1 to 2 g per day for the sustained-release formulation. Adverse reactions are common and include flushing, hyperglycemia, hyperuricemia, gastrointestinal complaints, and hepatic toxicity. Serum liver function tests should be monitored during therapy. Flushing is at times countered by administering one to two aspirin tablets per day.
   3. Hepatic hydroxymethyl glutaryl coenzyme A (HMG CoA) reductase inhibitors (statins). These agents are among the most effective drugs currently available for lowering serum cholesterol. They inhibit the enzyme HMG CoA reductase, a key rate-limiting component in the biochemical pathway for the synthesis of cholesterol. Inhibition of this pathway results in increased synthesis of LDL receptors, which lowers serum cholesterol. Five HMG CoA reductase inhibitors are currently available: atorvastatin, lovastatin, pravastatin, simvastatin, and fluvastatin. Side effects include dyspepsia, flatus, constipation, abdominal pain and cramps, and hepatic toxicity. Serum hepatic function tests should be monitored during ther-

apy. The usual doses are as follows: lovastatin, 10 to 80 mg per day; pravastatin, 10 to 40 mg per day; simvastatin, 5 to 40 mg per day; atorvastatin, 10 to 80 mg per day; and fluvastatin, 20 to 40 mg per day. Muscle injury and even fatal rhabdomyolysis rarely occur with these agents. Any patient reporting diffuse muscle aches and/or cramps should have serum creatine kinase measured. If it is more than mildly elevated, statin therapy should be discontinued.

4. Fibric acid derivatives. There are currently three fibric acid derivatives available in the United States: gemfibrozil, fenofibrate, and clofibrate (Atromid-S). Gemfibrozil (Lopid) is the most commonly used product. These agents increase the activity of the enzyme lipoprotein lipase, which enhances catabolism of VLDLs and intermediate density lipoproteins, and reduces serum triglycerol levels. HDL cholesterol levels are increased by fibric acid derivative therapy. Side effects include gastrointestinal complaints and increased gall stone formation. The usual dose of gemfibrozil is 600 mg twice a day; the usual dose of clofibrate is 500 mg three or four times a day.

Combining statins with either nicotinic acid or fibrates increases the risk for adverse reactions and toxicity. Therefore, patients receiving combination hypolipidemic therapy should be monitored closely.

C. Protocol for treating hyperlipidemic patients
   1. Determine the patient's lipid profile on a fasting specimen (no alcohol for 24 hours before the determination, fasting for 12 hours).
   2. Primary prevention is used in patients without evidence of atherosclerotic vascular disease. Everyone should probably adhere to at least a step I diet.

      Patients with borderline or high LDL cholesterol levels should definitely adhere to a step I diet. Exercise and weight loss should be advised. If the LDL cholesterol level is not reduced to desirable levels, a step II diet should be introduced. If the step II diet fails to lower LDL cholesterol to the desirable level, then drug therapy should be initiated as follows and pursued until LDL cholesterol levels fall into the desirable range:

      a. Treat the patient with a statin to lower LDL cholesterol below 100 mg/dl. At that point, if serum triglyceride levels are less than 200 mg/dl, patients may continue with the current regimen or statin dosage may be increased, thereby lowering serum triglyceride levels to less than 150 mg/dl.

      b. If serum triglyceride levels are between 200 to 499 mg/dl, patients should be treated with either an increased dose of statin or addition of niacin or fibrates.

      c. If serum triglyceride levels are greater than 500 mg/dl, patients should be treated with combination therapy (niacin and fibric acid derivatives are the first choice followed by the addition of statins).

      d. In all patients, if monotherapy fails to lower LDL cholesterol into the desirable range, combination therapy should be considered.

   3. In patients with clinically evident atherosclerotic vascular disease, secondary prevention should be initiated. It is similar to the protocol for primary prevention (see Section **III.C.2.**), but lower levels of LDL cholesterol are sought before the patient is declared as having a "desirable" blood LDL cholesterol level (see discussion above). Thus, in a patient with known atherosclerotic vascular disease, the physician seeks to lower LDL cholesterol levels well below 100 mg/dl, whereas primary prevention measures seek to lower serum LDL cholesterol to approximately 100 mg/dl. The same protocol as that outlined in Section **III.C.2.** is used.

   4. Regular aerobic exercise is advised for all hyperlipidemic patients. A minimum of 30 to 60 minutes three or four times per week is encouraged. Maximum benefit probably occurs at 5 to 6 hours per week.

   5. Patients should be strongly urged to achieve 120% or **less** of ideal body weight through exercise and diet.

SELECTED READINGS

Bjerre LM, LeLorier. Do statins cause cancer?: a meta-analysis of large randomized clinical trials. *Am J Med* 2001;110:716–723.
There is no evidence that statins cause cancer.

Executive summary of the third report of The National Cholesterol Education Program (NCEP) Expert Panel on detection, evaluation, and treatment of high blood cholesterol in adults (adult treatment panel III). *JAMA* 2001;285: 2486–2497.
Standard reference for guidelines concerning treatment of hyperlipidemia in adults.

Furberg CD, Adams HP Jr, Applegate WB, et al. Effect of lovastatin on early carotid atherosclerosis and cardiovascular events. *Circulation* 1994; 90:1679–1687.
Statin drugs decrease atherosclerosis in high risk settings.

Gotto AM Jr. Low high-density lipoprotein cholesterol as a risk factor in coronary heart disease: a working group report. *Circulation* 2001;103:2213–2218.
Low HDL cholesterol is an important risk factor in the development of coronary artery disease.

Gould AL, Rossouw JE, Santanello NC, et al. Cholesterol reduction yields clinical benefit: a new look at old data. *Circulation* 1995;91:2274–2282.
Further proof that elevated serum cholesterol leads to atherosclerosis and that lowering serum cholesterol decreases the risk for atherosclerosis.

Hunt D, Young P, Simes J. Benefits of pravastatin on cardiovascular events and mortality in older patients with coronary heart disease are equal to or exceed those seen in younger patients: results from the LIPID trial. *Ann Intern Med* 2001;134:931–940.
The absolute benefit of statin therapy is greater in older patients than in younger ones.

Knopp RH. Drug treatment of lipid disorders. *N Engl J Med* 1999;341:498–511.
A thorough review of the management of hyperlipidemia.

LaRosa JC, He J, Vupputuri S. Effect of statins on risk of coronary disease: a meta-analysis of randomized controlled trials. *JAMA* 1999;282:2340–2346.
Reduction of LDL cholesterol with statin drugs decreases the risk of developing coronary artery disease and all-cause mortality.

Maron DJ, Fazio S, Linton MRF. Current perspectives on statins. *Circulation* 2000;101: 207–213.
A review of the many effects of statin therapy.

Robins SJ, Collins D, Wittes JT, et al. Relation of gemfibrozil treatment and lipid levels with major coronary events: VA-HIT, a randomized controlled trial. *JAMA* 2001;285:1585–1591.
Patients with low HDL cholesterol benefit from gemfibrozil therapy.

Schwartz GG, Olsson AG, Ezekowitz MD, et al. Effects of atorvastatin on early recurrent ischemic events in acute coronary syndromes: the MIRACL study, a randomized controlled trial. *JAMA* 2001;285:1711–1718.
Atorvastatin at a dose of 80 mg per day lowers recurrent ischemic events in patients who present with an acute coronary syndrome.

Superko HR, Krauss RM. Coronary artery disease regression: convincing evidence for the benefit of aggressive lipoprotein management. *Circulation* 1994;90:1056–1069.
Further evidence that lowering cholesterol reduces atherosclerotic tendency.

15. ISCHEMIC HEART DISEASE

I. Myocardial infarction (MI). MI is one of the most common life-threatening diseases occurring in technically advanced countries. In the United States, it is the number one cause of death. MI is the result of coronary thrombosis. Mortality from MI is the highest during the first few hours after the onset of infarction. It is therefore important to make the diagnosis of MI quickly to expedite admission of the patient to the coronary care unit (CCU) and to provide possible thrombolytic therapy.

A. Diagnosis
1. History. Patients complain of chest discomfort that builds in intensity, eventually becoming severe and unrelenting. The pain frequently lasts for 30 minutes or more and is usually located in the region of the sternum, precordium, or epigastrium. Pain is usually characterized as constricting, crushing, oppressing, or compressing but may be stabbing, boring, knife-like, or burning. The discomfort often spreads to engulf both sides of the anterior chest, with predilection for the left side. Pain of MI may radiate down the inner aspect of the left arm, to the left or both shoulders, and/or to the jaw or interscapular region. As many as 25% of patients with MI may have minimal or no chest discomfort. Patients are likely to complain of associated feelings of weakness, cold perspiration, dizziness, palpitation, and a sense of impending doom. In many individuals, the discomfort of MI is confused with that of indigestion.

2. Physical examination. Patients with MI often appear restless and ashen, with anguished facies. The skin is usually cool and clammy. Respiratory distress occurs in individuals with left ventricular failure. Patients may be normotensive, hypertensive, or hypotensive. A low-grade fever (38° to 39°C) is common during the first 48 hours after infarction. Funduscopic examination may reveal hypertensive changes, atherosclerotic changes, or both. If right ventricular failure is present (secondary to left ventricular failure or right ventricular infarction), jugular venous distention should be evident.

Chest examination may be normal or may reveal rales and rhonchi secondary to left ventricular failure. Occasionally, wheezing occurs in individuals with severe left ventricular failure. Patients with MI invariably have a fourth heart sound (S4) as a result of ischemic changes in left ventricular compliance. The presence of a third heart sound (S3) denotes more severe left ventricular compliance alteration, which occurs with more extensive left ventricular damage (Table 15-1). Systolic murmurs may be the result of varying quantities of mitral valvular regurgitation stemming from ischemia, necrosis, or rupture of part or all of a papillary muscle or from left ventricular dilatation. Rupture of the ventricular septum, which occasionally accompanies transmural septal infarction, produces a loud holosystolic murmur (Table 15-1). Pericardial rubs are heard only in patients with transmural infarction (Table 15-1).

Hepatomegaly is seen in individuals with right ventricular failure. Peripheral edema occurs in patients with left or right ventricular failure or with peripheral venous disease that antedates the acute MI. Peripheral vascular disease with associated pulse and skin changes often accompanies coronary artery disease (CAD) and is therefore often present in individuals with MI. Localizing neurologic deficits can occur after cerebral embolization from a left ventricular mural thrombus.

3. ECG. Development of Q waves or loss of R waves usually follows or accompanies S–T segment elevation and is the ECG hallmark of Q wave infarction (formerly called transmural MI). Non–Q wave infarction (formerly called nontransmural MI) may be accompanied by persistent minor or marked S–T or T wave changes in the ECG. ECG abnormali-

TABLE 15-1. CARDIAC EXAMINATION IN ACUTE MYOCARDIAL INFARCTION

Finding	Description	Etiology
Small-amplitude carotid pulse	Small volume in carotid systolic pulse	Low cardiac output
Jugular venous distention	Jugular veins distended with estimated pressure >10 cm H_2O	Right ventricular failure secondary to left ventricular failure or right ventricular infarction
Abnormal apical impulse (anterior or apical infarcts only)	Diffuse or dyskinetic apical impulse	Paradoxical bulging of infarcted myocardium during systole
Soft heart sounds	Barely audible heart tones	Decreased left ventricular contractility
Paradoxical S2	S2 split widens on expiration, narrows on inspiration	Severe left ventricular dysfunction or left bundle branch block
S4	Soft, low-pitched presystolic sound	Decreased left ventricular compliance
S3	Soft, low-pitched early diastolic sound	Markedly decreased left ventricular compliance
Systolic murmur of mitral regurgitation	Holosystolic (occasionally crescendo-decrescendo) murmur, often with wide radiation	Ischemia; necrosis; rupture of papillary muscle
Systolic murmur of ventricular septal rupture	Holosystolic murmur often localized to lower left sternal border	Rupture of ventricular septum with resultant left-to-right shunt
Precordial rub	One-, two-, or three-component raspy rub	Pericarditis accompanying transmural infarction

S2, second heart sound; S3, third heart sound; S4, fourth heart sound.

ties are most specific when they are new (i.e., represent a change from patterns seen on previous ECGs). MI can occur in the absence of ECG changes. Localization of infarction by ECG is presented in Table 15-2.

In patients with S–T segment elevation, the following ECG changes are indicative of myocardial ischemia: new or presumed new S–T segment elevation at the J point in two or more contiguous leads or at least 0.2 mV in leads V_{1-3} and at least 0.1 mV in all other leads. In patients without S–T segment elevation, the following changes may be indicative of myocardial ischemia: S–T segment depression and/or T wave abnormalities. Q waves should be at least 0.3 milliseconds in duration (three fourths of a small box) on the ECG.

ECG localization of infarction is inaccurate. Thus, pathologic transmural infarction can be associated with ECG S–T and T wave changes only. The converse may also occur (pathologic nontransmural infarction associated with the presence of Q waves on the ECG). In addition, the localization of an infarct in the left ventricle (e.g., septum, inferior wall) cannot be accurately discerned by an examination of the ECG. It appears that the most that can be said about ECG localization of an infarct within the left ventricle is that it is in the anterior half of the ventricle

TABLE 15-2. ECG CRITERIA FOR LOCALIZATION OF TRANSMURAL MYOCARDIAL INFARCTION

1. Anteroseptal infarction
   Q–S pattern in V_1, V_2
   Absence of small Q waves in V_5, V_6
   S–T elevation and T wave changes may occur in other leads

2. Anterior or anteroapical infarction
   Initial R wave maintained in V_1 or V_2
   Appearance of abnormal Q wave in one or more of the following leads: V_2, V_3, V_4 or a decrease in the R waves without their disappearance in precordial leads V_2 through V_6
   No abnormal Q waves in leads V_5, V_6, aVL, I, II, and III

3. Anterolateral infarction
   Abnormal Q waves in V_5 and V_6 or in V_4, V_5, and V_6 as well as in leads aVL and I

4. Extensive anterior infarction
   A combination of the findings of nos. 1, 2, and 3 (above)
   Q waves are usually present in all precordial leads (except occasionally V_1), in lead aVL, and in lead I

5. High anterolateral or high lateral infarction
   Abnormal Q waves in leads I and aVL
   No changes in precordial leads; occasionally, V_5 and V_6 show minor changes

6. Inferior or diaphragmatic infarction
   Appearance of abnormal Q waves along with characteristics S–T and T wave changes in leads II, III, and aVF, or in leads III and aVF

7. Inferolateral infarction
   Same criteria as in no. 6 (above) plus abnormal Q waves in lead V_6 and sometimes in leads I, aVL, and V_5

8. Posterior infarction
   Appearance of an RSR pattern or a tall, slurred, wide R wave with an R:S ratio ≥ 1 in lead V_1

9. Posterolateral infarction
   Same criteria as in no. 8 (above) plus abnormal Q waves in lead V_6 and sometimes in leads I, aVL, and V_5

Source: Lipman BS, Massie E, Kleiger RE. *Clinical scalar electrocardiography.* Chicago: Year Book, 1973.

(ECG diagnoses: anteroseptal, anterolateral, anterior, lateral infarcts) or the posterior half of the ventricle (ECG diagnoses: inferior, inferior-posterior, posterior infarcts).

Right ventricular infarction may be inferred from the ECG. Individuals with right ventricular infarction usually have S–T segment elevation in one of the following leads: V_1, V_3R, or V_4R, as well as evidence of inferior or posterior MI on the ECG.

4. Chest x-ray examination. Pulmonary vascular redistribution and interstitial and alveolar pulmonary edema occur in patients with increased left ventricular filling pressures (Table 15-3). Cardiomegaly implies left ventricular dilatation, a finding usually seen only in individuals with left ventricular dysfunction antedating their acute MI. Discrepancies occur between chest x-ray findings and the level of left ventricular filling pressure. Such discrepancies are the result of lag time required for interstitial pulmonary edema fluid to accumulate or be resorbed secondary to directional changes in left ventricular filling pressure and increased pulmonary capillary permeability in acute MI.

TABLE 15-3. RELATIONSHIP BETWEEN CHEST X-RAY FINDINGS AND LEFT VENTRICULAR FILLING PRESSURES

Left ventricular filling pressure	Chest x-ray findings
<13 mm Hg	Normal
13–18 mm Hg	Pulmonary vascular redistribution
19–25 mm Hg	Interstitial pulmonary edema, Kerley B lines
>25 mm Hg	Alveolar pulmonary edema

    5. Laboratory tests
       a. Chemistry. Characteristic elevations in serum levels of a number of myocardial cell biomarkers occur after MI.
         (1) Creatine phosphokinase (CK). Serum CK-MB levels rise within 6 to 8 hours of onset of infarction, peaking at 24 hours and falling back to normal within 3 to 4 days after MI. Serum total CK levels are too nonspecific for routine diagnostic use in patients with suspected MI.
         (2) Glutamic-oxaloacetic transaminase (GOT); Lactic dehydrogenase (LDH), including LDH subfraction 1. GOT and LDH levels are too nonspecific for routine diagnostic use in patients with suspected MI.
         (3) Troponin, myoglobin, and other biomarkers of myocardial necrosis. Injured myocardial cells release numerous intracellular components into the circulation. Myoglobin is released rapidly into the circulation, often appearing within 1 to 2 hours after the onset of myocardial necrosis. Troponin appears in the blood at 4 to 6 hours (occasionally as late as 12 hours) after the onset of necrosis and remains in the blood for 7 to 10 days. Experimental biomarkers include various components of the myosin molecule. Troponin is the preferred biomarker and currently serves as the basis for the new definition of MI (see below). Assays exist for two forms of troponin, I and T.
       b. Hematology
         (1) White blood cell (WBC) count. The WBC count rises soon after the onset of infarction, receding after 2 to 3 days and returning to normal within a week after MI. The WBC count usually varies between 12,000 and 15,000 cells/l, with a rare individual reaching 20,000 cells/l.
         (2) Erythrocyte sedimentation rate (ESR). The erythrocyte sedimentation rate rises 48 to 72 hours after infarction, peaking on day 4 or 5 after MI. The erythrocyte sedimentation rate often remains elevated for 3 weeks or longer.
    6. Echocardiography and cardiac graphics
       a. Echocardiography. Echocardiographic abnormalities seen in infarction patients include regional hypokinetic, akinetic, and dyskinetic wall motion secondary to ischemia or necrosis; increased left ventricular cavity size secondary to dilatation; reduced left ventricular compliance; and small pericardial effusions secondary to post-MI pericarditis or left ventricular failure. Aneurysm formation with or without mural thrombus can be observed. Doppler echocardiography can be used to detect and quantitate mitral regurgitation and ventricular septal rupture with resultant left-to-right shunt.
    7. Radionuclide techniques
       a. Infarct scintigraphy. There are two types of infarct scintigraphy, "hot spot" and "cold spot" imaging. With the hot spot techniques, radioisotopes such as technetium 99m bound to inorganic pyrophosphate, or labeled antimyosin antibodies are injected intravenously,

localizing in the vicinity of infarcted myocardium and thereby producing an area of increased uptake (hot spot) on the scintigram. With the cold spot technique, a radioisotope such as thallium 201 is injected intravenously. This radioisotope is taken up by viable, perfused myocardial cells. The scintigram reveals an area of reduced tracer uptake (cold spot) in the region of the infarct.

b. Radionuclide ventriculography. Left ventricular ejection fraction, end-diastolic and end-systolic volume, and regional wall motion can be measured by means of radionuclide ventriculography. Such studies quantitate the severity of left ventricular dysfunction after MI. Ejection fraction obtained by means of radionuclide ventriculography correlates well with clinical estimates of the degree of left ventricular failure that occurs after MI. Left-to-right shunts through a ruptured ventricular septum can also be detected and quantitated with this method.

8. Cardiac catheterization and angiography. Patients with acute MI may undergo cardiac catheterization for angioplasty (mechanical) thrombolytic therapy. Many cardiologists routinely study postinfarction patients days to weeks after MI to determine prognosis. Elevated left ventricular filling pressures and regional wall motion abnormalities (hypokinesis and akinesis) are the rule in such individuals. Left ventricular aneurysm, mitral regurgitation, mural thrombus, or all three may be identified during such studies. Coronary angiography usually demonstrates total obstruction or high-grade stenotic lesions of coronary arteries supplying infarcted zones of myocardium. Approximately 10% to 20% of infarction patients under the age of 40 years will have normal coronary arteries despite documented MI.

Flow-directed, balloon-tipped catheters can be placed with relative ease in the pulmonary artery of patients with acute MI. Indications for hemodynamic monitoring in acute MI are as follows:

Hypotension
Sinus tachycardia with left ventricular failure
Severe left ventricular failure for which vasodilator therapy is planned
Suspected ventricular septal rupture or acute mitral regurgitation

Elevated left ventricular filling pressures and depressed cardiac output usually are seen in individuals with acute infarction. Patients with cardiogenic shock after MI have left ventricular filling pressures greater than 20 mm Hg in the face of cardiac indexes less than 1.8 liters per minute per m^2. See Chapter 9 for an in depth discussion of indications, uses, and risks of hemodynamic monitoring.

Individuals with ventricular septal rupture demonstrate a marked increase in blood oxygen content (secondary to the left-to-right shunt) in samples from the right ventricle. Patients with mitral regurgitation can be distinguished from those with ventricular septal rupture by normal right ventricular oxygen content and the presence of large regurgitant V waves seen in the pulmonary capillary wedge pressure tracing. Patients with acute MI can be classified into four hemodynamic subsets on the basis of left ventricular filling pressure and cardiac output measurements (Table 15-4).

9. Protocol for the diagnosis of MI

a. Patients suspected of having acute MI should have serum troponin and CK-MB activity measured q8h for 24 hours. Daily ECGs should be recorded for the first 3 days after admission. Radionuclide examinations (myocardial scintigraphy or ventriculography) or echo/Doppler study is performed in selected patients to evaluate residual left ventricular function and/or to identify possible complications of MI such as mitral regurgitation.

TABLE 15-4. HEMODYNAMIC CATEGORIES IN ACUTE MYOCARDIAL INFARCTION

Clinical subset	Cardiac index (L/min/m²)	Pulmonary capillary wedge pressure (mm Hg)	Approximate mortality
No pulmonary congestion or systemic hypoperfusion	2.7±0.5	12±7	2
Isolated pulmonary congestion	2.3±0.4	23±5	10
Isolated systemic hypoperfusion	1.9±0.4	12±5	22
Both pulmonary congestion and systemic hypo- perfusion	1.6±0.6	27±8	55

Source: Adapted from Forrester JS, Diamond GA, Swan HJC. Correlative classification of clinical and hemodynamic function after acute myocardial infarction. *Am J Cardiol* 1977;39:137.

   b. The diagnosis of MI is made when patients meet the criteria indi-
      cated in one of the following categories:
      The definition of MI has been revised as follows:
      Criteria for acute, evolving or recent MI
      Either one of the following criteria satisfies the diagnosis for an
      acute, evolving or recent MI:
      (1) Typical rise and gradual fall (troponin) or more rapid rise and
          fall (CK-MB) of biochemical markers of myocardial necrosis with
          at lease one of the following:
          (a) Ischemic symptoms
          (b) Development of pathologic Q waves on the ECG
          (c) ECG changes indicative of ischemia (S–T segment eleva-
              tion or depression)
          (d) Coronary artery intervention (e.g., coronary angioplasty)
      (2) Pathologic findings of an MI at autopsy
              Criteria for established MI
              Any one of the following criteria satisfies the diagnosis for es-
          tablished MI:
          (a) Development of new pathologic Q waves on serial ECGs.
              The patients may or may not remember previous symp-
              toms. Biochemical markers of myocardial necrosis may
              have normalized, depending on the length of time that has
              passed since the infarct developed.
          (b) Pathologic findings of a healed or healing MI at autopsy
   c. Differential diagnosis. Other entities that may simulate MI include
      the following:
      (1) Chest wall pain. Often atypical in character and long-lasting,
          chest wall pain is localized to a specific area of the anterior chest
          without radiation. It is occasionally made worse by a deep inspi-
          ration or arm exercise and is often associated with tenderness to
          palpation over the area of discomfort. Patients with this syn-
          drome are likely to be young, anxious, and without obvious risk
          factors for CAD. The correct diagnosis is suggested by history
          and physical examination as previously noted, together with a
          normal ECG. Exercise testing and coronary angiography may be
          required to rule out CAD in individuals whose presentation re-
          sembles that seen with ischemic heart disease.

(2) Gastrointestinal disorders. Epigastric discomfort secondary to esophagitis, esophageal spasm, gastric and duodenal peptic ulcer, various forms of gallbladder disease, and pancreatitis can mimic the pain of MI.

Gastrointestinal etiology for discomfort is suggested when symptoms are precipitated or relieved by eating. Relief of the distress by antacids, H_2-blockers, or proton pump inhibitors is suggestive but not conclusive evidence that the pain is gastrointestinal in origin. Radiation of the discomfort to abdominal regions or the lower back is also suggestive but not conclusive evidence that the pain is gastrointestinal in origin. The correct diagnosis is suggested by history (as already noted) and abdominal physical findings such as epigastric or right upper quadrant tenderness to palpation. Various combinations of gastrointestinal roentgenographic studies, endoscopy, exercise testing, and coronary angiography are often indicated in selected individuals.

(3) Cervical osteoarthritis. Pressure exerted on cervical dorsal root nerves secondary to osteoarthritic encroachment on cervical spine foramina occasionally results in upper chest discomfort that radiates to the arms, a syndrome resembling ischemic myocardial discomfort. The discomfort may last only 1 or 2 seconds, or it may persist for hours; both situations suggest that the pain is not myocardial in origin. Cervical spine films demonstrate narrowed nerve foramina, and use of a soft cervical or Thomas collar usually results in significant relief. Exercise testing or coronary angiography or both are required in an occasional patient to rule out CAD.

(4) Pericarditis. The pain of pericarditis may closely resemble that of MI with respect to character and radiation. However, pericarditic pain is usually made worse by a deep inspiration or by lying down. Characteristic diffuse S–T and T wave changes are seen on the ECG, and the discomfort almost always responds to salicylates, ibuprofen, indomethacin, or steroids (see Chapter 19).

B. Therapy
  1. Medication
    a. Thrombolytic therapy. Recent attention has centered on the dissolution of the obstructing coronary arterial thrombus that is the cause of most MIs.

      If coronary thrombolysis is performed successfully within 12 hours of the onset of symptoms of MI, the size of the eventual resulting infarct and mortality will be reduced. The agents of choice for coronary thrombolysis are either mechanical (i.e., percutaneous transluminal coronary angioplasty [PTCA]), or pharmacological (i.e., streptokinase, urokinase, tissue plasminogen activator, reteplase, tenecteplase, and APSAC, a form of streptokinase). Streptokinase and urokinase can be infused directly into the coronary artery at the time of cardiac catheterization. Alternatively, all of these agents may be administered intravenously. In most instances, rapid mechanical dissolution of the thrombus by PTCA is preferred, assuming that the procedure will be performed by an experienced team. If no catheterization laboratory is available, patients should receive intravenous thrombolytic therapy. Thereafter, the patients may be transferred to a facility where angioplasty is available. If successful reperfusion is achieved, PTCA is avoided. However, if pharmacological reperfusion has failed or is inadequate, then mechanical reperfusion with PTCA is performed. The best patients for mechanical reperfusion are those with extensive infarction, particularly if the infarct is anterior in location or inferoposterior associated with significant right ventricular infarction. Other patient subgroups that benefit particularly from mechanical reperfusion are (i) those with heart failure and/or shock complicated acute infarction or (ii) patients in whom pharmacological thrombolysis is contraindicated because of a risk of hemorrhage.

Reentrant ventricular arrhythmias such as ventricular tachycardia are seen commonly at the moment that coronary arterial reperfusion is established. Patients with unstable angina may also have fresh thrombus in a coronary artery but such individuals apparently do **not** benefit from thrombolytic therapy. After coronary thrombolysis, patients should be treated with intravenous or low molecular weight heparin and aspirin. Commonly used thrombolytic regimens include 500,000 U of streptokinase administered intravenously over 2 hours; 100 mg of tissue plasminogen activator administered using a variety of intravenous protocols; 30 mg of intravenous APSAC, administered over 5 minutes; 10 units of intravenous reteplase administered over 2 minutes, with a second dose of 10 intravenous units given 30 minutes later; and 30 to 50 mg of intravenous tenecteplase using a weight-adjusted protocol.

b. Anticoagulants. Anticoagulants are commonly used in patients with acute MI. Systemic heparinization followed by 3 to 6 months of oral warfarin therapy is indicated in patients with cardiogenic shock, severe left ventricular failure (e.g., pulmonary edema), mural thrombus, and arterial or venous thromboembolism complicating acute MI. Heparin, either unfractionated or low molecular weight, is administered to essentially all patients with acute MI unless strongly contraindicated. Low-dose or mini-dose heparin (5,000 U subcutaneously two or three times a day) is advocated routinely for **all** patients in the CCU who are not already receiving intravenous heparin to prevent deep venous thrombosis.

There is currently considerable enthusiasm for treating MI patients with agents that reduce platelet adherence or stickiness. Aspirin, dipyridamole, and clopidogrel have all been suggested as appropriate agents for long-term therapy in patients with MI. Aspirin or clopidogrel are the drugs of choice for this indication.

c. Agents to reduce infarct size. A number of different agents have been shown to reduce infarct size in experimental animals and clinical trials. Agents that may reduce infarct size include, among others, beta-blockers and nitrates.

Patients who develop unstable angina soon after Q wave MI or individuals with small or moderate-sized non–Q wave infarctions are candidates for immediate beta-blockade, nitrate therapy, or non-dihydropyridine calcium channel blockers.

d. Antiarrhythmics. Patients with acute MI who manifest very frequent ventricular ectopic beats (VPCs) or ventricular tachycardia usually receive antiarrhythmic therapy during the first day or two after MI. Intravenous followed by oral beta-blockers (e.g., metoprolol, atenolol) seems to be the best strategy for this indication because of proven efficacy and safety. Metoprolol and atenolol are administered as 5 mg intravenous boluses followed by 25 to 50 mg by mouth. The daily dosage is increased so that patients eventually receive 50 mg of atenolol every day or 50 mg of metoprolol twice a day. Intravenous lidocaine can also be employed (bolus of 50 to 200 mg followed by infusion of 1 to 4 mg per minute). If marked ventricular ectopic activity persists, procainamide may be substituted for lidocaine (intravenous boluses of 100 mg q3–5min to a total of 1 g, followed by an infusion of 1 to 4 mg per minute). Procainamide is a peripheral vasodilator, and hypotension may occur after its administration. An occasional patient still demonstrates significant ventricular ectopic activity despite lidocaine, beta-blocker, or procainamide administration. Such an individual may be treated cautiously with intravenous or oral amiodarone or oral sotalol. Intravenous antiarrhythmic drug regimens are listed in Table 15-5. Patients who fail to respond to these

TABLE 15-5. GUIDE TO INTRAVENOUS ADMINISTRATION OF ANTIARRHYTHMIC DRUGS

Drug	Dose	Therapeutic plasma level (ng/ml)	Side effects	Comment
Lidocaine	200 mg IV bolus over several minutes, followed by 2–4 mg/min constant infusion, 100-mg IV bolus for patients with pulmonary edema and 50-mg bolus for patients in shock	1.4–6.0	Focal seizures, grand mal seizures, respiratory arrest, dizziness, heart block (usually associated with preexisting abnormal His-Purkinje conduction), sinuatrial arrest	Significant reduction in dose in patients with heart failure, moderate reduction in dose in patients with hepatic disease; no oral form available; no significant myocardial depression; toxicity usually seen at high plasma levels; toxicity at low plasma levels may be caused by metabolites
Procainamide	100 mg IV slowly (25–50 mg/min) q5min (or more often in life-threatening situations), up to 1000 mg	4–8	Hypotension, prolonged atrioventricular and His-Purkinje conduction	Myocardial toxicity usually only at high plasma levels or after rapid administration
Verapamil	2.5–5.0 mg IV bolus: repeat to total dose of 10 mg	—	Headache, nausea, constipation, hypotension, heart block	Only effective for supraventricular arrhythmias; do not use verapamil and beta-blockers concomitantly; asystole may result
Propranolol	1 mg/min IV, up to 10 mg	40–85	Hypotension, bradycardia, prolonged atrioventricular conduction and heart block, myocardial depression, bronchospasm	Probably should not be considered in the presence of severe heart failure; many of the side effects reversed by large doses of isoproterenol

Drug	Dose		Adverse Reactions	Comments
Metoprolol	5 mg IV every 5 min, up to 15 mg	—	Same as for propranolol	Same as for propranolol
Atenolol	5 mg IV initial dose; 5 mg second dose 10 min after initial dose	—	Same as for propranolol	Same as for propranolol
Esmolol	500 µg/kg/min loading dose followed by an infusion dose of 60–300 µg/kg/min, depending on heart rate and blood pressure response	—	Hypotension, bradycardia, prolonged atrioventricular conduction, heart block, bronchospasm	Primarily useful for supraventricular dyarhythmias
Adenosine	6-mg IV initial dose; if no response in 1–2 min, a second and third dose of 12 mg may be administered	—	Flushing, headache, palpitations, hypotension, dyspnea, nausea, dizziness	Serum half-life is <10 sec; adverse reactions are short-lived
Atropine	0.5–1.0 mg IV as a rapid bolus	—	Sinus tachycardia, glaucomic crisis, urinary retention, psychosis	Occasionally precipitates paradoxical slowing of heart rate or ventricular tachycardia
Digoxin	0.25 mg IV q8h for 2 days and then 0.25 mg qd	1.0–2.0	Gastrointestinal toxicity, cardiac arrhythmias, atrioventricular conduction disturbances, insomnia, visual disturbances	May be given PO with the same dose and rate of administration; should not be given IM
Bretylium tosylate	5–10 mg/kg loading dose over 10 min, followed by maintenance infusion of 1–2 mg/min	—	Hypotension, nausea, vomiting, transient increase in heart rate and blood pressure	Dose should be reduced in patients with renal failure; patient response may be better when drug is used alone rather than with other antiarrhythmic drugs
Amiodarone	1200 mg/24 hr for 2–4 days	—	Hypotension, left ventricular failure	

agents may be candidates for intraaortic balloon counterpulsation (see Section **I.B.9.c.**). Selected patients may also be candidates for invasive electrophysiologic study (EPS).

Patients with chronic, severe, ventricular ectopic activity may be candidates for maintenance oral antiarrhythmic therapy. Unfortunately, cardiologists do not agree on what constitutes appropriate therapy or even on which patients to treat. It seems reasonable to treat patients in whom ECG monitoring (e.g., Holter ECG tape recordings) demonstrates frequent episodes of ventricular tachycardia. Based on the Cardiac Arrhythmia Suppression Trial (CAST), it seems clear that patients with multifocal or frequent unifocal VPCs should **not** receive chronic antiarrhythmic therapy. Patients who do (e.g., for atrial fibrillation) should be monitored by Holter monitor recordings and determinations of serum levels of antiarrhythmic medications. Antiarrhythmic drug regimens for patients with chronic ventricular ectopic activity include various agents singly and in combination (Table 15-6). EPSs frequently are performed in survivors of acute MI who manifest ventricular tachycardia.

During an EPS, electrode catheters are placed in various locations in the right heart chambers, and a series of ectopic beats are induced by a sophisticated programmable pacemaker attached to the electrode catheters. Patients who have a propensity to develop reentrant ventricular arrhythmias (ventricular tachycardia) usually develop an episode of ventricular tachycardia or ventricular fibrillation during programmed stimulation. Serial EPS may be performed during trials of many different antiarrhythmic drugs to determine which of these agents is effective in preventing ventricular tachycardia. EPS performed in this manner can be somewhat helpful in predicting those drug regimens that may prevent the development of potentially life-threatening arrhythmias. Antiarrhythmic agents may **worsen** ventricular arrhythmias, the so-called pro-arrhythmic effect. CAST demonstrated that the agents encainide and flecainide increased mortality and cardiac arrest in MI patients with frequent VPCs. Moricizine tended to do the same thing. Therefore, great caution should be exercised in using antiarrhythmic drugs in these patients. Results with beta-blockers and amiodarone have been more encouraging. Patients with severe bradycardia with associated evidence of low cardiac output should be treated with atropine (0.5 to 1.0 mg intravenous boluses q5–10min to a total dose of 2 mg). If bradycardia persists, such patients are candidates for temporary transvenous pacing (see Section **I.B.5.**).

e. Vasodilators. Patients with severe or persistent left ventricular dysfunction with or without clinical signs of failure may be treated with vasodilators (so-called afterload reduction therapy). To be a candidate for vasodilator therapy, a patient should have a systolic blood pressure in excess of 100 mm Hg. Intravenous nitroglycerin or nitroprusside is best used in individuals in whom pulmonary arterial and systemic arterial pressures are being monitored. Long-acting nitrates, such as nitroglycerin ointment and sublingual or oral isosorbide dinitrate, are instituted as maintenance therapy in patients who respond to intravenous vasodilators. Long-acting transcutaneous, sublingual, or oral nitrate preparations may be administered to patients who are not undergoing hemodynamic monitoring but who demonstrate evidence of left ventricular failure. Patients with low cardiac output frequently complain of severe fatigue; systemic blood pressure is low (systolic, 90 to 100 mm Hg), as is urine output in such individuals. Patients with low cardiac output may be treated with oral hydralazine (25 to 50 mg four times a day) in addition to long-acting nitrates.

TABLE 15-6. GUIDE TO ORAL ADMINISTRATION OF ANTIARRHYTHMIC DRUGS

Drug	Usual total daily dose	Frequency of administration	Therapeutic plasma level (μg/ml)	Half-life (hr)	Side effects	Comments
Propranolol	80–480 mg	q6h	40–85	3–4.6	Myocardial depression, prolonged atrioventricular conduction and heart block, bradycardia, bronchospasm, fatigue, depression, peripheral vascular insufficiency, hyperglycemia, hypoglycemia, alopecia, gastric distention	Active metabolites may play a role in clinical effect; dose chosen empirically; should be tapered slowly in patients with angina; caution needed in patients with cardiac function dependent on sympathetic tone
Metoprolol	50–200 mg	bid	—	3–7	Same as propranolol	—
Atenolol	50–200 mg	qd	—	6–9	Same as propranolol	—
Nadolol	40–80 mg	qd	—	20–24	Same as propranolol	—
Procainamide	2–6 g	q3–4h	4–8	3–4	Nausea, vomiting, agranulocytosis, lupuslike syndrome, myocardial depression, prolonged atrioventricular and His-Purkinje conduction	Toxic myocardial effect usually only at toxic plasma levels; half-life markedly prolonged in renal failure or alkaline urine

(continued)

TABLE 15-6. (Continued)

Drug	Usual total daily dose	Frequency of administration	Therapeutic plasma level (μg/ml)	Half-life (hr)	Side effects	Comments
Quinidine	1.0–2.4 g	q6h	2.3–5.0	7	Hypotension, nausea, vomiting, diarrhea, tinnitus, vertigo, prolonged His-Purkinje conduction, rash, fever, thrombocytopenia, hepatic dysfunction, hemolytic anemia, ventricular arrhythmias	Minor gastrointestinal side effects controlled with symptomatic therapy; clinically significant decrease in plasma binding in hypoproteinemia and hepatic disease; myocardial toxicity usually only at toxic plasma levels; accumulation of metabolites in renal disease
Disopyramide	400–800 mg	q6h	2–5	7	Myocardial depression, hypotension, prolonged atrioventricular conduction and heart block, glaucoma, urinary retention, dry mouth, constipation, blurred vision, nausea, anorexia	Reduced dosage in hepatic or renal insufficiency, or both; hypotension can occur in patients with myocarditis or cardiomyopathy, or both; 300-mg loading dose advised in patients with life-threatening arrhythmias
Amiodarone	200–600 mg	qd	1.0–2.5 μg/ml (steady state)	30–100 days	Tremor, dizziness, pulmonary fibrosis, anorexia, nausea, vomit-	Extremely long half-life, requires 7–10 days of loading with PO

					...ing, alopecia, peripheral neuropathy, insomnia, depression, bradycardia, atrioventricular block	amiodarone; marked enhancement of anticoagulant action of warfarin
Tocainide	600–1800 mg	tid	5–15 µg/ml	14	Light-headedness, tremor, nausea, twitching, diplopia, anorexia, abdominal pain, constipation, rash, fever	Response to tocainide can be predicted by the response of the ventricular arrhythmia to IV lidocaine
Mexiletene	600–900 mg	tid	0.75–2.0 µg/ml	8–12	Same as for tocainide	Similar structure to tocainide
Moricizine	600–900 mg	tid	—	3.4 (0.8–4.2)	Proarrhythmia, heart block, dizziness, nausea, headache	Not shown to prevent sudden death in post-infarction patients with ventricular ectopy
Propafenone	300–900 mg	tid	0.5–3.0	2–24	Central nervous system events, elevated liver function tests, agranulocytosis, anemia, alopecia	Has beta-blocking qualities: can cause bronchospasm
Flecainide	50–200 mg	bid	0.2–1.0	12–27	Proarrhythmia, dizziness, visual disturbances	—
Sotalol	80–160 mg	bid	q12h	15–17 hr	Fatigue, torsades de pointes	Sotalol is a combination beta-blocker and type III antiarrhythmic drug
Diltiazem	120–240 mg	tid or qd with long-acting forms	0.05–0.3	2–11	Same as for verapamil	—

Angiotensin converting-enzyme (ACE) inhibitors (captopril, 6.25 to 50 mg three times a day; enalapril, 2.5 to 10 mg twice a day; lisinopril, 10 to 40 mg; ramipril, 2.5 to 20 mg; as well as others) are particularly effective in managing left ventricular failure and have been shown to increase long-term survival in patients with reduced left ventricular function (ejection fraction greater than 40%) after MI. These latter agents decrease the tendency of the infarct zone and the entire left ventricle to dilate after MI. Hence, they attenuate left ventricular remodeling. ACE inhibitor therapy is best initiated during the first week after the onset of MI. ACE inhibitors have been shown to reduce postinfarction short-term and long-term mortality and morbidity even in patients without reduced left ventricular ejection fraction. Many cardiologists treat infarct patients with a combination of beta-blockers and ACE inhibitors, reducing systolic blood pressure as much as the patient can tolerate: Commonly, systolic blood pressure is reduced to 100 to 110 mm Hg unless the patient exhibits symptoms of orthostatic hypotension.

f. Analgesics. Morphine, hydromorphone (Dilaudid), and meperidine (Demerol) are opiate analgesics that can be used to relieve the discomfort of MI. Ischemic myocardial discomfort results in activation of the sympathetic nervous system with attendant potentially deleterious increases in heart rate and blood pressure. It is therefore important to relieve the patient completely of any ischemic pain. Nitrous oxide inhalation (30 to 60% with 70 to 40% oxygen) is also efficacious in easing ischemic myocardial discomfort.

g. Sedation. Anxiety, like ischemic discomfort, activates the sympathetic nervous system with potentially deleterious effects on the infarcted heart.

Patients with acute MI should be sedated for several days (longer if deemed necessary). A short-acting benzodiazepine (alprazolam, 0.125 to 0.5 mg two or three times a day) is the tranquilizer of choice. A sleeping medication such as flurazepam is often helpful as well, during the first few days or weeks after infarction.

h. Stool softeners and laxatives. Because the Valsalva maneuver decreases coronary blood flow, straining at stool should be avoided in postinfarction patients. Consequently, sufficient bulk in the diet (see Section I.B.3.) and stool softeners such as dioctyl sodium sulfosuccinate should be part of all postinfarction regimens. An occasional individual will require a laxative to prevent straining at stool.

i. Diuretics. Patients who develop evidence of left ventricular failure after MI may be candidates for diuretic therapy. Evidence of left ventricular failure includes one or more of the following: tachypnea, tachycardia, rales, S3, pulmonary vascular congestion or edema by x-ray film, and arterial hypoxia. Patients who are comfortable and stable despite minimal or moderate evidence of left ventricular failure should be treated initially with modest doses of intravenous furosemide (10 to 20 mg). Patients who fail to respond to this dose or who have more severe degrees of left ventricular failure (e.g., pulmonary edema) may be treated with larger doses of furosemide with or without concomitant administration of vasodilators.

j. Digitalis. The use of digitalis glycosides in patients with acute MI is controversial. Studies of experimental MI in animals have shown increases in infarction size when digitalis is administered to animals without heart failure. Animals with experimental MI and heart failure seem to benefit from digitalis administration. Clinical studies (e.g., the DIG trial) concerning possible beneficial or detrimental effects of digitalis administration after MI have shown that digoxin therapy decreases hospitalization for heart failure in these patients. Mortality is unaffected. Recommendations for the use of digitalis preparations in acute MI are as follows: (i) patients without evidence of left ventricular failure do not receive digitalis except for control of ventricular response with atrial fibrillation, and (ii) patients with severe left ventricular failure, particularly if it is associated with left ventricular dilatation, may be treated with a digitalis glycoside such as digoxin. Objective evidence of severe left ventricular dysfunction or dilatation or both may be obtained by means of chest x-ray film, echocardiogram, radionuclide ventriculogram, hemodynamic monitoring, or left ventricular angiography. However, vasodilators and diuretics are the preferred first-line therapy. Digitalis is administered to individuals who continue to demonstrate signs and/or symptoms of heart failure despite therapy with vasodilators and diuretics.

k. Volume therapy. Patients with hypotension or sinus tachycardia whose left ventricular filling pressures are less than 18 mm Hg should receive volume therapy to raise the filling pressure to 18 to 20 mm Hg. Colloid infusions such as plasma and dextran are preferred because they remain in the vascular space longer than crystalloid solutions.

l. Oxygen. In an effort to correct arterial hypoxia, which commonly occurs in patients with MI, most CCUs routinely administer supplemental inspiratory oxygen. Although such therapy has not been shown conclusively to be of benefit, it seems reasonable to treat MI patients with modest amounts (2 to 4 liters per minute) of supplemental inspiratory oxygen.

2. Activity. Current ambulation schedules for postinfarction patients are considerably more liberal than earlier programs. Patients with uncomplicated MI (absent or short-lived arrhythmias, left ventricular failure, pericarditis, etc.) may begin ambulation by day 2 or 3 after infarction. They can be discharged from the hospital in 4 to 7 days; however, the physician should ascertain that such "early discharge" patients have made adequate psychological adjustments to their infarctions before discharge. Patients with complicated MI remain in the hospital for 1 week or longer. Hospitalization schedules of 4 to 7 days and of 10 to 14 days are recorded in Table 15-7. Sexual activity between familiar partners does

TABLE 15-7. ACTIVITY SCHEDULE AFTER MYOCARDIAL INFARCTION: 4- TO 7-DAY SCHEDULE

4- to 7-day schedule	
Days 1–2	Bed rest in the CCU; may use chair in the CCU 1 day after admission as tolerated
Days 3–6	Low-level ambulation initially, with increasing levels of activity subsequently in the intermediate cardiac unit; may use chair most of the day; patients may use the bathroom as soon as they can sit up comfortably. Patients may shower and wash hair on days 3–7, depending on comfort and stability when standing.
10- to 12-day schedule	
Days 1–3	Bed rest in the CCU/intermediate cardiac unit with bedside commode; chair use as tolerated from day 2 onward.
Days 3–7	Patient may go to bathroom aided by nurse or aide; may begin to walk, not more than 1 hr/day
Days 8–12	Patient may walk to bathroom and elsewhere as needed; may shower

CCU, coronary care unit.
Source: Adapted from Alpert JS, Francis GS. *Manual of coronary care,* 6th ed. Boston: Little, Brown and Company, 2000.

not require marked increases in left ventricular work. Hence, moderate sexual activity may be resumed a few days after patients are discharged from the hospital.

3. Diet. Most CCUs reduce dietary intake of calories, cholesterol, and saturated fat. It is reasonable to offer patients a diet rich in potassium and bulk to combat hypokalemia and constipation, both common problems in MI patients.

Every encouragement should be given for patients to discontinue smoking. Alcohol in moderate quantities has not been shown to be detrimental to patients following MI.

4. Environmental and psychological support. Three psychological mechanisms occur commonly in post-MI patients: anxiety, denial, and depression. Psychological upset in MI patients can result in increased heart rate, blood pressure, and incidence of cardiac arrhythmias. Therefore, a psychologically supportive environment is essential for post-MI patients. As already noted, tranquilizing medication is also of benefit in this respect.

5. Pacemakers. Third-degree heart block is a greatly feared complication of acute MI. Unfortunately, placement of temporary transvenous pacing catheters in patients with acute MI in anticipation of complete heart block has not been shown to affect mortality. Moreover, complete heart block does not necessarily result in hemodynamic embarrassment if the ventricular escape rhythm is sufficiently rapid (e.g., 45 to 55 beats per minute). This is often the case after inferior infarction when the only indication for temporary pacing is bradycardia (secondary to sinus bradycardia or any form of heart block) sufficient to cause clinical deterioration such as worsening left ventricular failure or decreasing urinary output.

The development of third-degree heart block after anterior or anteroseptal MI is associated with very slow ventricular escape rhythms (25 to 40 beats per minute). Because anterior infarcts tend to be larger than inferior infarcts, and because ventricular escape rhythms in third-degree heart block are slower with anterior than with inferior MI, it is not surprising that severe hemodynamic decompensation frequently accompanies complete heart block after anterior infarction. Therefore, prophylactic, temporary pacing wires are often placed in patients with anterior infarction and threatened third-degree heart block. Table 15-8 lists indications for the use of prophylactic pacing catheters in anterior infarction. Thrombolytic therapy is associated with a decreased incidence of heart block.

The development of the external pacemaker has simplified the protocol for patients who are at risk for developing symptomatic, high degree atrioventricular block. The electrode pads are placed prophylactically on the chest of such patients awaiting the development of third-degree atrioventricular block before the external pacer is activated. Thereafter,

TABLE 15-8. INDICATIONS FOR PLACEMENT OF PROPHYLACTIC PACING CATHETERS FOLLOWING ANTERIOR OR ANTEROSEPTAL MYOCARDIAL INFARCTION

Secure indications
  Mobitz type II block
  Third-degree heart block
  New left bundle branch block
  New right bundle branch block, especially if accompanied by
    1. Left anterior hemiblock (marked left axis deviation)
    2. Left posterior hemiblock (marked right axis deviation)

Controversial indication
  Mobitz type I block

under the protection of external pacing, a transvenous pacing wire can be placed. This system offers the advantage of not placing a pacing electrode wires in patients who subsequently prove not to need them.

6. Cardioversion. Electric reversion is reserved for arrhythmias that are so serious as to require immediate termination or for arrhythmias that fail to respond to the administration of antiarrhythmic medication. Ventricular fibrillation and ventricular tachycardia without obtainable blood pressure both demand immediate electrical reversion. The full output of the defibrillator is required to revert ventricular fibrillation, but 100 W per second or less may be sufficient to interrupt ventricular tachycardia. Patients who maintain an adequate blood pressure despite ventricular tachycardia should receive intravenous lidocaine or procainamide (both, should either drug alone fail to terminate the arrhythmia). If ventricular tachycardia persists despite medical therapy, cardioversion should be performed under diazepam, midazolam, or other short-acting barbiturate anesthesia.

Atrial flutter, fibrillation, or tachycardia is usually treated with intravenous beta-blockers, verapamil, diltiazem, or digitalization in patients who are not hemodynamically compromised. If these fail to revert the arrhythmia to sinus rhythm, procainamide (500 mg intravenous bolus over 25 minutes followed by an infusion of 1 to 2 mg per minute) may be tried for 24 hours. Alternatively, one may administer oral propafenone or sotalol or intravenous amiodarone. Oral dofetilide has also been shown to promote return to sinus rhythm, perhaps more effectively than any other antiarrhythmic agent. However, dofetilide use is associated with the development of torsades de pointes (multifocal ventricular tachycardia).

Patients who are still not in sinus rhythm are candidates for electrical cardioversion under diazepam or short-acting barbiturate anesthesia. Patients who have been in atrial fibrillation for 48 hours or more without anticoagulation should receive warfarin anticoagulation for 3 to 4 weeks before electrical cardioversion is attempted. Warfarin therapy should continue for approximately 2 weeks after successful cardioversion. Sinus tachycardia is not an arrhythmia that requires electrical reversion or antiarrhythmic drugs. It is a sign of increased sympathetic nervous stimulation of the heart. When sinus tachycardia occurs after infarction, the following should be sought: pain, agitation, hypovolemia, and left ventricular failure.

7. Postinfarction rehabilitation. The objective of postinfarction rehabilitation is the restoration of the individual's physiological, social, and vocational status. As noted earlier, psychological problems are common after MI. Open discussions among the patient, family, physician, and cardiac nurse are often helpful in alleviating psychological distress. Many localities have organized cardiac rehabilitation programs that emphasize conditioning and risk factor reduction. Table 15-9 presents a general outline for cardiac rehabilitation.

8. Associated medical disorders. Hypertension, diabetes mellitus, hyperlipidemia, gout, and chronic obstructive pulmonary disease commonly accompany ischemic heart disease and MI. These conditions should be sought and appropriate diagnostic and therapeutic measures instituted.

9. Treatment of specific complications following acute MI
   a. Left ventricular failure. Elevated left ventricular filling pressures are almost universally present in patients with acute MI. These elevated filling pressures can cause pulmonary vascular congestion with resultant transudation of fluid into the pulmonary interstitial space. The higher the left ventricular filling pressure and the longer it remains elevated, the greater the amount of pulmonary interstitial fluid.

   In some individuals, signs and symptoms of left ventricular failure are mild, requiring no therapy. In other patients, severe left ventricular failure develops, necessitating vigorous treatment. Figure 15-1 is a flow chart for the treatment of left ventricular failure in patients

TABLE 15-9. POST–MYOCARDIAL INFARCTION REHABILITATION SCHEDULE

1. Rehabilitation begins once the patient has been discharged from the coronary care unit. Patient education should be offered throughout the period of convalescence.
2. Before discharge, the patient should be carefully instructed concerning medicines and activities. Moderate activity, including walking, is allowed at this time (but no isometric exercises such as lifting). The patient is given sublingual nitroglycerin tablets and is instructed in their use.
3. At discharge or 1–3 weeks thereafter, the patient undergoes a submaximal treadmill test (maximal heart rate = 120 beats/min). If this is performed without angina, S–T segment change, or arrhythmias, the patient is allowed to walk progressively longer distances each day and to resume sexual activity.
   If angina, S–T segment change, or arrhythmia occur, further pharmacologic intervention is probably indicated (e.g., nitrates, beta-blockers, calcium channel blockers, or diuretics, depending on patient status); cardiac catheterization should be strongly considered.
   Patients with markedly abnormal treadmill responses should not increase their activity level until improvement has occurred, as documented by a subsequent treadmill test or Holter monitor tape. Such patients usually undergo cardiac catheterization as well as coronary angioplasty or coronary bypass surgery.
4. Approximately 3–6 weeks after discharge, the patient walks for 30–60 minutes/day comfortably and may return to work.
5. Approximately 6–8 weeks after discharge, the patient may undergo another treadmill exercise test performed to 70% predicted maximal heart rate (about 150 beats/min). If this treadmill test is performed without incident, the patient can participate in a medically supervised exercise program if desired (e.g., jogging, bicycling, weight lifting).

Source: Adapted from Alpert JS. Francis GS. *Manual of coronary care,* 6th ed. Boston: Little, Brown and Company, 2000.

with acute MI. Its use requires that the physician know the patient's heart size (physical examination, chest x-ray film, or echocardiogram) and heart rate.

b. **Cardiogenic shock.** The most severe example of left ventricular failure after MI is cardiogenic shock, in which so much myocardium has been damaged that inadequate systemic perfusion occurs secondary to low cardiac output. The definition of cardiogenic shock is as follows: (i) MI (usual Q wave) by the usual criteria, (ii) systolic blood pressure less than 90 mm Hg, and (iii) organ hypoperfusion as manifested by low urinary output (less than 20 to 30 ml per hour), cool clammy skin, or mental obtundation.

It is important to rule out other causes of hypotension such as hypovolemia, medications, arrhythmias, blood gas or electrolyte disturbances, and marked bradycardia.

Patients in cardiogenic shock should have pulmonary arterial, systemic arterial, and urinary catheters inserted to monitor therapy. Pressors such as dobutamine, dopamine, or norepinephrine should be administered in sufficient amount so that systemic arterial pressure rises above 90 mm Hg and at least 30 ml of urine is produced each hour. Patients who require such support for more than 24 to 48 hours or who had severe shock from the outset are candidates for intraaortic balloon counterpulsation. Selected cardiogenic shock patients benefit from urgent coronary artery angioplasty or coronary bypass grafting performed as soon as possible after infarction. Unfortunately, the majority of shock patients who are without mechanical defect (i.e., acute mitral regurgitation, ventricular septal defect) do not survive, despite counterpulsation and cardiac surgery or angioplasty.

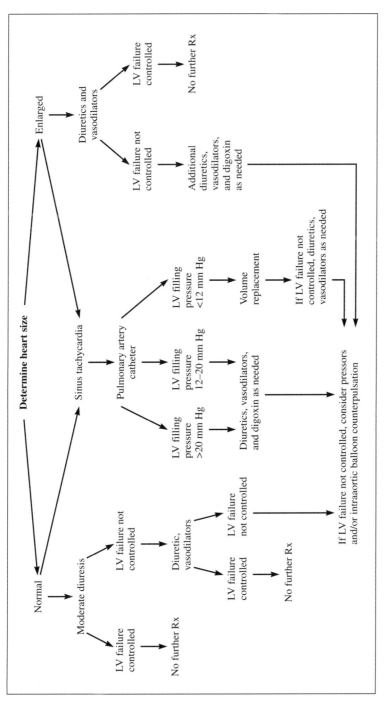

FIG. 15.1. Treatment of left ventricular failure complicating acute myocardial infarction.

c. Ventricular septal rupture and acute mitral regurgitation. Sudden clinical deterioration accompanied by a loud systolic murmur is usually the result of rupture of the ventricular septum or part of a papillary muscle. The resultant volume overload placed on an already compromised left ventricle generally produces severe left ventricular failure with or without shock.

The patient may require pressors, digitalis, diuretics, vasodilators, or intraaortic balloon counterpulsation to effect stabilization (Fig. 15-2). Patients who can be stabilized can undergo elective surgical repair of their defect at a later date at modest risk. Patients who require counterpulsation to maintain systemic perfusion must

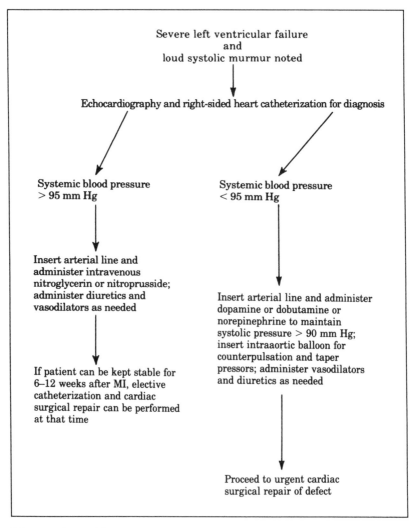

FIG. 15.2. Protocol for patients with ventricular septal rupture or acute mitral regurgitation after myocardial infarction.

be operated on as soon as possible. Mortality from such surgery is substantial.

d. Hypertension during acute MI. An occasional patient will have significant residual hypertension (blood pressure greater than 160/100 mm Hg) after pain and initial anxiety have been relieved with analgesics, tranquilizers, and reassurance. Hypertension is not infrequently noted when patients arrive in the CCU, but the "pain and anxiety" pressor response usually abates within 2 to 3 hours of admission.

Individuals who demonstrate continued hypertension after relief of pain and anxiety should be strongly considered for intravenous beta-blockade. If this fails to reduce blood pressure or is contraindicated, the physician should consider a moderate diuresis (1,000 ml) initiated with intravenous furosemide (10 to 20 mg bolus). Persistent hypertension (blood pressure greater than 160/100 mm Hg) should be treated with oral, sublingual, or transcutaneous long-acting nitrates. Most physicians employ intravenous vasodilators (nitroprusside, nitroglycerin) or beta-blockers (propranolol, metoprolol, or esmolol) in patients with hypertension and MI. Intraarterial measurement of blood pressure is often employed in patients with severe hypertension who receive intravenous nitroprusside or nitroglycerin. The physician should attempt to lower the blood pressure to approximately 130 to 140/80 to 90 mm Hg.

e. Angina after MI. Anginal episodes during the immediate (1 to 3 weeks) postinfarction period are considered unstable because they usually occur when the patient is rather inactive. Unless significant and overt left ventricular failure is present, the patient should receive oral propranolol or other beta-blockers in a rapidly increasing dosage schedule: for oral propranolol, initiate 10 mg four times a day and increase to 20 mg four times a day and 40 mg four times a day on successive days. For metoprolol, dosage begins with 25 mg twice a day and advances to 50 or 100 mg twice a day, depending on heart rate and blood pressure response. For atenolol, dosage begins with 25 mg and advances to 50 to 100 mg, depending on heart rate and blood pressure response. A rapid increase in dosage may be necessary in patients with recurrent anginal episodes. Long-acting nitrates such as isosorbide dinitrate (oral or sublingual) or nitroglycerin ointment are also usually given to patients with postinfarction angina. Patients with overt left ventricular failure often tolerate beta-blockade without further decompensation. If heart failure symptoms develop or worsen, intravenous furosemide should be used. Often, beta-blocker therapy can be continued following diuresis. On the other hand, such patients may benefit from nondihydropyridine calcium channel blocker therapy (e.g., diltiazem 30 to 90 mg three times a day, or verapamil 80 to 120 mg three times a day). Those who fail to respond to beta-blockers, calcium channel blockers, and nitrates should be considered for intraaortic balloon counterpulsation and urgent coronary bypass grafting. Most patients with postinfarction angina should undergo coronary arteriography and possibly coronary angioplasty or bypass surgery.

f. Postinfarction risk stratification. Most cardiologists perform some type of exercise or pharmacologic "stress" test (ECG or thallium exercise test or intravenous dipyridamole or adenosine) before discharge in patients with MI. These examinations seek to identify patients with residual myocardial ischemia who need further medical, surgical, or angioplasty therapy. Most patients with a positive exercise or pharmacologic stress test should undergo coronary arteriography.

g. Pericarditis. The discomfort of postinfarction pericarditis can mimic that of postinfarction angina. Usually the pain of pericarditis has some pleuritic or positional component to it. Evanescent or sustained one-, two-, or three-component rubs may be heard. Fever and even sinus tachycardia may be the result of pericarditis. Pericarditis with its attendant discomfort may occur soon after MI (1 to 5 days) or develop late in the convalescence (1 to 12 months after MI). Salicylates, ibuprofen, and indomethacin are effective in relieving the discomfort of pericarditis. An occasional patient will be refractory to this regimen, requiring moderate doses of oral prednisone.

Weaning from steroids may be difficult in such patients, with multiple recrudescences of pericarditis.

h. Arterial and venous embolism. Patients with MI may develop arterial embolism from an endocardial mural thrombus or venous thromboembolism secondary to bed rest and elevated blood sedimentation rate, or both.

Fortunately, both forms of embolism are uncommon. Episodes of arterial embolism should be treated with systemic heparinization for 1 to 2 weeks followed by oral warfarin for 2 to 6 months or longer if a left ventricular aneurysm is present. Patients with episodes of cerebral embolism should receive anticoagulants only after a computed tomography scan has demonstrated the absence of cerebral hemorrhage. Peripheral embolism should be removed by a vascular surgeon employing a Fogarty embolectomy catheter. Venous embolism, formerly common in infarction patients, is now quite unusual because of early ambulation schedules and the use of minidose heparin (5,000 U subcutaneously q8–12h of unfractionated heparin or 0.5 mg/kg once or twice a day of low-molecular-weight heparin). Patients with documented episodes of deep vein thrombophlebitis or pulmonary embolism should be treated with intravenous unfractionated heparin or subcutaneous low molecular weight heparin for 1 to 2 weeks, followed by 2 to 6 months of oral warfarin. Patients with strong contraindications to anticoagulation should have an inferior vena caval umbrella filter inserted under local anesthesia.

i. Ventricular free wall rupture. Ventricular free wall rupture is almost invariably fatal. Patients who develop this complication frequently have a normal ECG rhythm in the absence of any blood pressure.

Emergency pericardiocentesis and cardiac surgical repair salvage an occasional patient.

j. Aneurysms. Left ventricular aneurysms are circumscribed, noncontractile segments of ventricular wall composed mostly of fibrous tissue. They are usually noted months to years after infarction. Aneurysms may be associated with significant left ventricular failure or repetitive ventricular arrhythmias. When such problems cannot be controlled with appropriate medications, surgical extirpation of the aneurysm is indicated. Medical therapy in such patients often includes lifelong anticoagulation with warfarin.

II. Angina pectoris. The diagnosis of angina pectoris secondary to ischemic heart disease traditionally has been based on clinical criteria. Particular emphasis has been placed on the history. A number of objective tests have been developed to aid in the diagnosis of ischemic heart disease.

Chest discomfort has several diverse etiologies, and objective demonstration of myocardial ischemia is helpful in differentiating myocardial ischemic discomfort from other forms of chest pain. Indeed, the diagnosis of ischemic heart disease can be difficult in some individuals because (i) anginal chest discomfort can occur in patients with normal coronary arteriograms, and (ii) conversely, severe ischemic heart disease can exist in the absence of chest discomfort. Most clinicians, however, still strongly emphasize clinical information in making the diagnosis of angina pectoris.

Angina pectoris is ischemic heart discomfort that results when myocardial metabolic demand outruns myocardial blood flow. This imbalance in supply and demand of myocardial nutrition may be caused by decreased supply (e.g., atherosclerotic CAD or coronary vasospasm) or increased demand (e.g., aortic stenosis). In rare instances, angina pectoris is the result of unknown factors (e.g., angina with normal coronary arteries).

Two clinical syndromes of angina pectoris exist: stable and unstable. Stable angina pectoris implies that the discomfort predictably occurs with exertion of certain intensity and abates promptly with cessation of activity and/or administration of nitroglycerin. Unstable angina pectoris occurs with minimal activity, after meals, or at rest. Discomfort is often severe and prolonged, requiring two or more nitroglycerin tablets for relief. Individuals with unstable angina have a greater risk of developing MI or dying suddenly than do patients with stable angina. Unstable angina is associated with rupture or ulceration of an atherosclerotic plaque. Patients with unstable angina require immediate hospitalization. Survival after the onset of angina pectoris depends on several factors, including the number of coronary arteries involved by the atherosclerotic process, the state of left ventricular function, and other patient lifestyle and physical characteristics (Tables 15-10 and 15-11).

A. Diagnosis

    1. History. The symptom of angina pectoris is often not described as pain but as discomfort, distress, or a disagreeable feeling that resembles indigestion. The discomfort may be associated with belching, causing both patient and physician to ascribe the symptom to gastrointestinal disease. Anginal discomfort is most commonly located in the center of the chest, over the sternum or just to the left of it. Occasionally, anginal discomfort is described as precordial or near the apical impulse. Angina pectoris discomfort may be described in a variety of anatomic locations including any area between the epigastrium and the root of the neck with radiation down the arms, through the back, or to the neck, jaw, lower teeth, or shoulders. Radiation is more commonly to left-sided rather than to right-sided structures.

    Angina is usually described as constricting, tightening, burning, or choking. Some individuals say they have a sense of fullness or just an uncomfortable feeling. Anginal discomfort is often confused with indigestion, which it resembles in quality and location. Stable angina comes on rather abruptly during effort. Walking is the type of exertion that ordinarily precipitates an anginal episode. Walking produces angina more rapidly if it is performed after meals, in the cold, early in the day, or up a slight grade. Other kinds of exertion such as sexual intercourse, mental excitement, or agitation can also cause angina pectoris.

    Unstable anginal episodes occur with minimal or no exertion. In fact, episodes of unstable angina often develop during rest or sleep. The discomfort of unstable angina is frequently severe, prolonged, and unresponsive to a single nitroglycerin tablet. Patients with unstable angina

TABLE 15-10. FACTORS ASSOCIATED WITH WORSENING OF PROGNOSIS IN PATIENTS WITH ISCHEMIC HEART DISEASE

Increased number of coronary arteries involved by the atherosclerotic process
Impaired left ventricular function
Diabetes mellitus
Cigarette smoking
Uncontrolled hypertension
Obesity
Ventricular tachyarrhythmias
Conduction defects in the ECG
Male sex
Elevated serum cholesterol
Progressive elevation in C-reactive protein levels

TABLE 15-11. MORTALITY IN PATIENTS WITH ANGINA RELATED TO THE NUMBER OF INVOLVED VESSELS AND THE STATE OF LEFT VENTRICULAR FUNCTION

	Yearly mortality (%)
Vessel involvement	
Single-vessel disease	0–3
Double-vessel disease	2–6
Triple-vessel disease	3–10
Left ventricular function	
Normal left ventricular function	5
Localized area of abnormal left ventricular wall motion	6
Presence of left ventricular aneurysm	9
Diffusely hypokinetic left ventricle	14

have intracoronary thrombus narrowing the lumen of the artery. Thrombus overlies a ruptured or ulcerated atherosclerotic plaque. It is likely that episodic coronary spasm is also involved, at least in part, in the pathophysiologic sequence of unstable angina. Although unstable angina does not always lead to MI, the latter is more likely to occur in patients with unstable compared with stable angina pectoris. This fact has led some authorities to use the term *crescendo* or *preinfarction angina* rather than *unstable angina*. Patients with normal coronary arteriograms sometimes describe chest discomfort resembling that described by individuals with CAD. Chest discomfort in patients with normal coronary arteriograms is more likely to occur at rest and with emotion or agitation. These patients often describe their discomfort as sharp or heavy and lasting more than 10 minutes. Pain location and radiation are not different from that noted in persons with angina pectoris secondary to CAD.

Prinzmetal's angina is an unusual variant form of angina that generally occurs at night or when the patient is quiet. It seldom occurs with exertion. ECGs taken during episodes of Prinzmetal's angina demonstrate S–T segment elevation. Prinzmetal's angina is a severe form of unstable angina. It can be associated with potentially lethal arrhythmias or conduction defects.

Patients with **silent ischemia** (i.e., individuals with ECG or radionuclide scan evidence of myocardial ischemia in the absence of symptoms) represent a special problem. Should they be treated in a manner similar to that employed for patients with symptomatic myocardial ischemia, or is their natural history different requiring another approach? In individuals with known atherosclerotic heart disease, silent ischemic episodes occur more frequently than symptomatic episodes (angina pectoris). The implications of silent ischemia are not entirely understood. However, most authorities favor treating such episodes in the same way that symptomatic angina pectoris is managed.

2. Physical examination. Between attacks of angina, physical findings may be relatively normal except for the presence of atherosclerotic changes in the fundus and a fourth heart sound. During ischemic episodes, findings similar to those in patients with acute MI may be noted (Table 15-1). In both instances, the abnormal physical findings are caused by failure of the involved left ventricular myocardium to contract and relax normally as the result of ischemia.

3. ECG. Between attacks of angina pectoris, the ECG may be normal or may show evidence of prior MI; during episodes of angina, reversible horizontal or downsloping depression of the S–T segment may occur or the ECG may be unaffected. Careful comparison of the tracing obtained during pain with prior tracings may reveal subtle S–T segment alter-

ations. Such changes usually resolve within a few minutes or hours after anginal discomfort disappears.

During silent ischemic episodes, ST–T changes in the ECG tracing occur without accompanying angina pectoris. In an effort to improve the clinician's ability to diagnose ischemic heart disease, exercise ECG tests have been developed: the maximal bicycle and treadmill test. In these tests, patients are exercised to the point of pain, fatigue, a predetermined heart rate, or a certain level of exercise. ECGs are recorded before, during, and after exercise. The development of 0.5 to 1.0 mm or more of horizontal or downsloping S–T segment depression is considered a positive test. Between 60% and 80% of patients with significant CAD demonstrate a positive response to maximal bicycle or treadmill exercise. A maximal test is one in which the patient's peak heart rate reaches 85% or 90% of its predicted maximum.

Most cardiologists perform a low-level or limited exercise test in patients who have sustained an MI. The test is performed at the conclusion of the patient's hospital admission. Patients with ST–T changes, poor exercise tolerance, or angina pectoris usually undergo coronary arteriography.

Some patients with exertional chest discomfort have false-positive exercise tests in that their coronary arteriograms are normal despite S–T segment depression during and after exercise. Women tend to have a higher incidence of false-positive exercise tests than men, although this may, in part, be owing to the higher incidence of CAD in younger men. The percentage of false-positive (specificity) and false-negative (sensitivity) tests obtained depends on the stringency of the criteria used to define a positive test and the incidence of atherosclerotic CAD in the subset of patients being tested. The protocol for the maximal exercise test is recorded in Table 15-12.

4. Chest x-ray examination. No acute changes have been noted in chest roentgenograms taken during anginal episodes. Heart size and evidence of pulmonary vascular congestion depend on prior left ventricular functional status.

    Cardiac fluoroscopy in patients with angina pectoris may demonstrate calcification of the coronary arteries.

5. Serologic tests. Serum levels of troponin and cardiac enzymes are normal in individuals with angina pectoris, because the ischemic disturbance

---

TABLE 15-12. MULTISTAGE SUBMAXIMAL OR MAXIMAL EXERCISE TEST

1. Patients exercise on a treadmill or bicycle ergometer.
2. Patients exercise until a predetermined heart rate is reached or until exhaustion or clinical condition warrants terminating the test prematurely.
3. The submaximal test is usually performed until the patient achieves a heart rate of 110 or 120 beats/min. The maximal exercise test continues until the patient's heart rate reaches 85% or 90% of predicted maximum heart rate for age and sex.
4. The speed and grade of the treadmill or the resistance of the bicycle ergometer is increased every 3 min until the target heart rate is achieved or until exhaustion or clinical condition warrants termination of the test.
5. A baseline resting ECG is recorded before the test. ECG and blood pressure monitoring are performed during the exercise period. ECGs are recorded at 0, 1, 2, 5, and 10 min after exercise.
6. A diagnosis of functional myocardial ischemia is based on 1.0 mm of horizontal or downsloping S–T segment depression.

For further information, consult Fletcher GF, Froelicher VF, Hartley LH, et al. Exercise standards: a statement for health professionals from the American Heart Association. *Circulation* 1990;82: 2286–2322.

to myocardial cell function is reversible. Likewise, sedimentation rate and WBC count are unaffected by episodes of angina pectoris. However, levels of C-reactive protein, a measure of inflammation, are elevated in patients with atherosclerotic heart disease. The atherosclerotic process involves inflammation in the arterial wall and elevated C-reactive protein levels apparently reflect the extent of the inflammatory atherosclerotic process.

6. Echocardiography. Echocardiographic visualization of the left ventricle during an ischemic episode reveals decreased or absent contractile activity in the ischemic zone. After resolution of ischemia, wall motion returns to normal. Previously infarcted regions of the left ventricle demonstrate persistently abnormal contractile function. The opening velocity of the anterior mitral valve leaflet may be decreased during angina pectoris secondary to decreased left ventricular compliance. Doppler echocardiography may also demonstrate abnormal left ventricular diastolic compliance.

After MI or in patients suspected of having atherosclerotic heart disease, myocardial ischemia may be identified by observing newly developed regions of hypokinesis or akinesis during dipyridamole or dobutamine infusion. The dobutamine echocardiographic test for myocardial ischemia is highly accurate, with sensitivity approaching 90%. Some reversibly hypokinetic or akinetic regions of the left ventricle can show improved wall motion after coronary bypass grafting or angioplasty. The implication is that the reduced wall motion noted in the echo image was the result of ischemia rather than fibrosis. This phenomenon is the result of myocardial stunning or hibernation—brief or long periods of myocardial hypokinesis or akinesis secondary to transient ischemic injury. That these myocardial zones represent living but nonfunctioning myocardium is of great interest to the clinician because these zones of reduced myocardial function can be "rejuvenated" by restoring myocardial blood flow with angioplasty or bypass surgery.

7. Radionuclide studies. As noted earlier, some patients have anginal chest pain despite normal coronary arteries, and others have significant ischemic episodes without chest discomfort. The electrocardiographic exercise test attempts to identify those patients with chest discomfort who actually have CAD.

Unfortunately, specificity and sensitivity are both approximately 70% to 80% for maximal exercise tests, even in the best hands. The search for an objective test with higher sensitivity and specificity for CAD resulted in the development of the radionuclide thallium (or other radionuclide tracer such as that using sestamibi) exercise test. In this examination, a maximal exercise test is performed as described in Table 15-12; however, just before the end of exercise, a bolus of a radioactive tracer is injected intravenously, and a postexercise scintigram of the heart is recorded. Thallium and other tracers used in such tests are taken up by myocardial cells in a uniform manner if myocardial blood flow delivers the tracer to the cells. In patients with ischemia during exercise, the radionuclide tracer does not reach the ischemic myocardial zones, and the resultant scintigram demonstrates a defect corresponding to the ischemic areas. Radionuclide exercise tests are more sensitive and specific than are ECG exercise tests, but the radionuclide tests are also more expensive and involve ionizing radiation.

Instead of exercise, one may administer oral or intravenous dipyridamole or intravenous adenosine followed by radionuclide scanning. Dipyridamole or adenosine produces maximum coronary vasodilation, thereby exposing regions of myocardial hypoperfusion resulting from atherosclerotic coronary arterial stenoses. As already noted, radiolabeled technetium sestamibi or other compounds can be substituted for thallium.

Another radionuclide examination useful in the diagnosis of CAD is the exercise radionuclide ventriculogram. This test uses red blood cells or serum albumin labeled with radioactive technetium. Diastolic and systolic ventriculographic images of the left ventricle are obtained before and during exercise. Ejection fraction and regional wall motion are calculated during rest and exercise. Patients with ischemia during exercise demonstrate abnormally reduced exercise ejection fraction and regional wall motion.

8. Catheterization and angiography. If hemodynamic measurements are made during an episode of angina pectoris, several alterations are recorded.

Systemic arterial and left ventricular filling pressures increase. The left ventricular diastolic pressure-volume relationship shifts in the direction of reduced compliance (increased stiffness). Cardiac index often falls slightly. Coronary sinus lactate and pyruvate levels increase, and the heart produces lactate and pyruvate rather than consuming these metabolites as it normally does. The production of lactate and pyruvate demonstrates that myocardial metabolism has shifted from the usual aerobic pathways to anaerobic metabolic routes.

Left ventriculography in patients with ischemic heart disease demonstrates myocardial zones with reduced or absent contractile motion. Wall motion in these zones may be improved after an extrasystolic beat or nitroglycerin administration. Such reversibly hypokinetic or akinetic regions of the left ventricle often show improved wall motion after coronary bypass grafting or angioplasty. The implication is that the reduced wall motion noted on the ventriculogram was the result of ischemia rather than fibrosis. This phenomenon is the result of myocardial stunning or hibernation—brief or long periods of myocardial hypokinesis or akinesis secondary to transient ischemic injury. As noted earlier, high-grade coronary arterial stenotic lesions (diameter reduced 50% or more) occur in the proximal coronary arterial tree of most patients with angina pectoris. Some individuals with angina pectoris and positive maximal electrocardiographic exercise tests are found to have normal coronary arteriograms.

Patients with Prinzmetal's angina fall into two categories: those with minimal or no coronary arterial stenoses and those with severe proximal coronary arterial narrowing. Anginal episodes in the first group are the result of coronary arterial spasm, which can be provoked in the catheterization laboratory by the administration of intravenous ergonovine.

9. Protocol for the diagnosis of ischemic heart disease
   a. The diagnosis of angina pectoris secondary to ischemic heart disease is made in the following individuals:
      (1) Patients over age 50 years with a history of classic angina pectoris and at least one major risk factor (smoking, hypertension, hypercholesterolemia, positive family history, diabetes mellitus), whose chest discomfort abates with nitrate, beta-blocker, or calcium channel blocker therapy.
      (2) Patients of any age with a history of classic angina pectoris and at least one major risk factor who have a positive electrocardiographic exercise test, and whose chest discomfort abates with nitrate, beta-blocker, or calcium channel blocker therapy.
      (3) Patients with atypical chest pain, a positive exercise test, and a coronary arteriogram demonstrating significant narrowing (greater than 50% luminal diameter) of at least one major coronary artery. Note that it may be possible to substitute a positive radionuclide or echocardiographic stress test result for the arteriographic criterion.
      (4) Patients with unstable angina (severe, prolonged anginal episodes that occur with minimal exertion or at rest) should not

exercise. In such individuals, the diagnosis of unstable angina pectoris is made on the basis of history, ECG S–T segment depression during pain, and decrease in chest discomfort after the administration of nitrate, beta-blocker, or calcium channel blocker. Many of these patients will require a coronary arteriogram to confirm the presence of clinically important coronary arterial stenoses.

(5) The diagnosis of unstable angina is also made in patients with an appropriate history (see Section **II.A.9.a.(4)**), at least partial amelioration of chest discomfort from nitrate, beta-blocker, or calcium channel blocker therapy, and a coronary arteriogram demonstrating significant (see Section **II.A.9.a.(3)**) CAD.

Note. Not all coronary arterial narrowings result in myocardial ischemia. The combination of chest pain and coronary arterial narrowing is not sufficient for the diagnosis of angina pectoris (stable or unstable) secondary to ischemic heart disease. Myocardial ischemia secondary to coronary arterial narrowings should be suggested either by exercise ECG S–T segment depression, by an equivalent radionuclide or echocardiographic test response, or by response of the chest pain to nitrates, betablockers, or calcium channel blockers. A standardized definition of unstable angina is as follows: recurring angina pectoris at rest or with minimal effort lasting 20 to 30 minutes or more. At least two episodes should occur within a 1-week period. The discomfort is more severe than that of stable exertional angina, and frequently two or more nitroglycerin tablets are required to obtain relief. At least one episode of angina should be associated with characteristic ST–T changes on ECG without elevation in serum troponin or CK-MB.

b. Differential diagnosis. Other entities that may simulate angina pectoris are the same conditions discussed in the section on the differential diagnosis of MI (see Section **I.A.9.c.**): chest wall pain, gastrointestinal disorders, cervical osteoarthritis, and pericarditis.

B. Therapy
1. Medical treatment
a. Nitrates. Short-and long-acting nitrates should be employed for patients with angina pectoris. Patients should be instructed in the proper use of nitroglycerin (Table 15-13). Those with more than occasional anginal episodes should be placed on a long-acting nitrate preparation. There are sublingual, oral, and transcutaneous preparations with prolonged duration of action. Because some patients may develop nitrate tolerance with loss of efficacy, patients who receive long-acting nitrate preparations should have a daily "nitratefree" interval of 8 to 10 hours built into their therapeutic regimen. Physicians should be familiar with one or two preparations, such as sublingual or oral isosorbide dinitrate (10 to 30 mg q8–12h; duration of action, 2 to 4 hours) or nitroglycerin ointment (duration of action approximately 4 hours). A common side effect is headache. This usually can be suppressed with aspirin or acetaminophen and gradually disappears with continued use of the drugs.

Patients with Prinzmetal's angina who have minimal or no CAD are often much improved with high-dose nitrate or calcium channel blocker therapy, for example, slow release nifedipine, diltiazem, or verapamil (Section **II.B.1.c.**).

b. Beta-blockers. Many investigations support the concept that betablockade prolongs life in patients with CAD who have sustained an MI. Experienced physicians treat all their patients with ischemic heart disease with beta-blockers. Beta-blocker therapy should especially be administered to patients with ischemic heart disease whose

TABLE 15-13. GUIDELINES FOR THE PROPER USE OF NITROGLYCERIN

1. Nitroglycerin tablets are placed under the tongue and allowed to dissolve. This process takes 20–30 sec.
2. Nitroglycerin can also be chewed with good effect; however, it should not be swallowed because it is absorbed directly into the bloodstream from the oral mucosa.
3. The action of nitroglycerin is prompt, and relief of chest discomfort generally is obtained within 1–2 min.
4. Nitroglycerin provokes a minor tingling or stinging sensation in the mouth, which indicates that the pill has not lost its potency.
5. Patients often experience a fullness, a warm sensation, or a throbbing in the head after taking nitroglycerin.
6. Nitroglycerin should be used immediately and without hesitation at the first hint of chest discomfort.
7. Nitroglycerin is not habit forming. Patients can take nitroglycerin many times a day.
8. Patients should carry nitroglycerin at all times.
9. To retain maximum potency of nitroglycerin tablets, keep the tablets in the original glass bottle with the metal top securely screwed on.
10. When taking nitroglycerin, patients should sit up or stand.
11. If a single nitroglycerin tablet does not relieve chest discomfort within 2–3 min, the patient should take a second one. If discomfort is constant or if the relief is transient and then recurs, a third pill is taken. If, however, the discomfort is not completely controlled or continues to recur, the patient should be driven to the nearest hospital emergency ward for further attention.
12. When chest discomfort is promptly relieved by nitroglycerin, it is unnecessary to interrupt activity. A moderate decrease in the pace of activity is advisable, however.
13. Nitroglycerin is most helpful when taken at the onset of discomfort rather than after discomfort has been present for several minutes.
14. If the patient knows that a certain activity, exertion, or excitement will bring on an anginal episode, angina can be prevented by taking a nitroglycerin tablet before the discomfort emerges.

Source: Adapted from Alpert JS. *The heart attack handbook,* 3rd ed. Yonkers, NY: Consumer Reports Books, 1993.

angina pectoris is regularly provoked by exertion. The drug should be initiated at low doses and gradually increased until angina is completely abolished or resting heart rate is in the range of 50 to 60 beats per minute. Side effects include bronchospasm, fatigue, gastrointestinal upset, and symptoms of left ventricular failure.

Patients frequently develop marked sinus bradycardia (heart rate as low as 40 to 50 beats per minute) during beta-blocker therapy. This is not of major concern as long as symptoms of heart failure or orthostatic hypotension are absent. A summary of the various beta-blockers available in the United States can be found in Tables 15-5 and 15-6.

   c. Calcium channel blockers. Calcium channel blockers are potent vasodilators.

In addition, they can preserve cellular integrity during episodes of severe myocardial ischemia. Calcium channel blockers have been shown to be of benefit in abolishing episodes of stable or unstable angina pectoris. Moreover, calcium channel blockers have proved exceedingly effective in preventing coronary arterial spasm, which is an important factor in the development of episodes of unstable or Prinzmetal's angina. A number of different calcium channel blockers are available in the United States, including nifedipine (10 to 40 mg four times a day), diltiazem (30 to 120 mg four times a day), and verapamil (80 to 120 mg three times a day). All calcium channel blockers are now available in extended release, once-a-day formulations. These long-acting preparations are preferred over their short-acting counterparts. Verapamil has significant negative inotropic activity. Both verapamil and diltiazem have potent electrophysiologic properties: They slow conduction through the atrioventricular node. This property can be used to abolish supraventricular arrhythmias such as atrial tachycardia or to slow ventricular response in atrial fibrillation and atrial flutter. Conversely, heart block or asystole may develop in patients with atrioventricular nodal or sinus nodal disease. Other calcium channel blocker side effects include headache, ankle swelling, and gastrointestinal upset. Calcium channel blockers are often effective in combination with long-acting nitrate preparations. They may also be combined with beta-blockers; however, nifedipine and diltiazem seem best in this regard, because excessive bradycardia and even asystole have been reported when beta-blockers and verapamil have been combined.

d. Sedation. Anxiety or other emotional agitation precipitates anginal episodes in certain patients. Such individuals may benefit from the regular use of a minor tranquilizer such as diazepam or alprazolam.

e. Tobacco and alcohol. Smoking should be strongly discouraged in patients with ischemic heart disease. Moderate intake of alcoholic beverages has not been shown to be of any harm.

f. Antiarrhythmic agents. Ventricular ectopic activity is common in patients with ischemic heart disease; however, ventricular ectopic activity in patients with angina pectoris does not have the same significance as when the ectopic beats occur in patients with acute MI. There is considerable disagreement among cardiologists as to both indications and drug regimens employed in patients with ischemic heart disease and ventricular ectopic activity. Certain guidelines may be offered: (i) patients with unstable angina should be treated as if they had suffered an acute MI; (ii) patients with stable ischemic heart disease should be further evaluated if they have ventricular tachycardia or if they have symptoms as a result of ventricular ectopic activity; and (iii) frequent multifocal or unifocal VPCs are usually not treated unless patients are symptomatic or manifest unstable angina. EPS may be appropriate to help decide which patients should receive chronic antiarrhythmic therapy.

g. Treatment of other medical conditions. Hypertension, diabetes mellitus, and hyperlipidemia should be appropriately treated with diet and medication.

h. Activity. Patients with angina pectoris should remain as active as they were before symptoms of ischemic heart disease developed, if possible. There is increasing evidence that regular exercise and improved fitness are beneficial in the long-term management of patients with ischemic heart disease.

Aerobic exercises such as walking, jogging, bicycling, and swimming are preferred. Isometric exercises such as heavy weight lifting are contraindicated in individuals with angina pectoris, since they result in sudden increases in heart rate and blood pressure. However, moderate levels of weight lifting are now thought to be beneficial. Prophylactic use of nitroglycerin (Table 15-13) is often helpful in preventing anginal episodes during exercise.

i. Diet. Obese patients with angina pectoris should attempt to reduce their body weight to normal levels for their sex and height. Patients with ischemic heart disease should adhere to a low-cholesterol, low—saturated fat diet, which emphasizes decreased intake of animal fats and increased intake of plant fats. A moderate sodium restriction (no added salt) is advised for patients with clinically overt left ventricular failure. Patients who have repeatedly failed to lose weight despite multiple attempts may benefit from a protein-sparing, low-carbohydrate diet.

j. Smoking. It is essential that patients with angina pectoris discontinue smoking.

2. Surgery/coronary angioplasty. Certain categories of patients should be considered strong candidates for coronary angioplasty or bypass surgery. These individuals should have cardiac catheterization and coronary arteriography performed in preparation for cardiac surgery or angioplasty. Categories of patients to be considered include (i) patients with unstable angina, (ii) individuals with stable angina pectoris whose symptoms are so severe that they interfere with the patient's normal lifestyle, (iii) patients with markedly positive (greater than 2 mm S–T segment depression) exercise tests at low levels of exercise, (iv) patients whose blood pressure falls with exercise; (v) patients found to have significant (50% or more luminal narrowing) left main coronary artery stenosis, (vi) patients with Prinzmetal's angina and severe CAD; (vii) patients with triple-vessel CAD and reduced left ventricular function, and (viii) patients with double vessel disease, including proximal left anterior CAD and reduced left ventricular function.

Intraaortic balloon counterpulsation is rarely necessary in the treatment of angina pectoris. An occasional patient will continue to manifest unstable angina despite adequate sedation, beta-blockade, nitrates, and calcium channel blockers. Such a patient, along with unstable individuals with left main coronary artery stenosis, benefits from intraaortic balloon counterpulsation in the immediate preoperative and postoperative period.

SELECTED READINGS

Alpert JS, Francis GS. *Manual of coronary care,* 6th ed. Philadelphia: Lippincott Williams & Wilkins, 2000.
Concise, multifaceted approach to the patient with acute MI, with references.
Armstrong PW, Collen D. Fibrinolysis for acute myocardial infarction: current status and new horizons for pharmacological reperfusion, part I. *Circulation* 2001;103: 2862–2866.
Armstrong PW, Collen D. Fibrinolysis for acute myocardial infarction: current status and new horizons for pharmacological reperfusion, part II. *Circulation* 2001;103: 2987–2992.
An extensive and authoritative two-part review of pharmacological thrombolysis for acute MI.
Crawford MH. The role of triple therapy in patients with chronic stable angina pectoris. *Circulation,* 1987;75(Suppl V):V122–V127.
A critical review of triple therapy for patients with stable angina pectoris.
Cruickshank JM. Beta blockers continue to surprise us. *Eur Heart J* 2000;21:354–364.
A thorough review of beta-blocker therapy for a variety of cardiovascular conditions, including ischemic heart disease.
Forrester JS, Diamond G, Chatterjee K, et al. Medical therapy of acute myocardial infarction by application of hemodynamic subsets. *N Eng. J Med* 1976;295:1356–1362.
Hemodynamic classification of patients with acute MI in planning therapy.
Gibbons RJ, Chatterjee K, Daley J, et al. ACC/AHA/ACP-ASIM guidelines for the management of patients with chronic stable angina: a report of the American College of Cardiology/American Heart Association Task Force on Practice Guidelines (Committee on Management of Patients With Chronic Stable Angina). *J Am Coll Cardiol* 1999;33: 2093–2197.
Extensive discussion of diagnosis and management of patients with angina pectoris.
Goldman LE, Eisenberg MJ. Identification and management of patients with failed thrombolysis after acute myocardial infarction. *Ann Intern Med* 2000;132:556–565.

A thoughtful review of the data and the options for clinicians in patients with failed thrombolytic therapy following acute MI.

Grines CL, Cox DA, Stone GW, et al. Coronary angioplasty with or without stent implantation for acute myocardial infarction. *N Engl J Med* 1999;341:1949–1956.

Coronary stenting produces better long-term results than does balloon angioplasty alone in patients with acute MI.

Guth BD, Tajimi T, Seitelberger R, et al. Experimental exercise-induced ischemia: drug therapy can eliminate regional dysfunction and oxygen supply demand imbalance. *J Am Coll Cardiol* 1986;7:1036–1046.

Antianginal therapy eliminates exercise-induced ischemic myocardial dysfunction in experimental animals.

Joshipura KJ, Hu FB, Manson JE, et al. The effect of fruit and vegetable intake on risk for coronary heart disease. *Ann Intern Med* 134:1106–1114.

Consumption of fruits and vegetables appears to have a protective effect against coronary heart disease.

Kawanishi DT, Reid CL, Morrison EC, et al. Response of angina and ischemia to long-term treatment in patients with chronic stable angina: a double-blind randomized individualized dosing trial of nifedipine, propranolol and their combination. *J Am Coll Cardiol* 1992;19:409.

Benefits of combination therapy in patients with stable angina.

Kim CB, Braunwald E. Potential benefits of late reperfusion of infarcted myocardium: the open artery hypothesis. *Circulation* 1993;88:2426–2436.

Why reperfusion strategy in acute MI is so important.

Krauss RM, Eckel RH, Howard B, et al. AHA Dietary Guidelines: revision 2000: a statement for healthcare professionals from the Nutrition Committee of the American Heart Association. *Circulation* 2000;102:2284–2299.

Updated recommendations for antiatherosclerotic diets from the American Heart Association.

Kris-Etherton P, Eckel RH, Howard BV, et al. AHA Science Advisory: Lyon Diet Heart Study: benefits of a Mediterranean-style, national cholesterol education program/American Heart Association step I dietary pattern on cardiovascular disease. *Circulation* 2001;103:1823–1825.

Mark DB, Lam LC, Lee KL, et al. Effects of coronary angioplasty, coronary bypass surgery, and medical therapy on employment in patients with coronary artery disease: a prospective comparison study. *Ann Intern Med* 1994;120:111–117.

No real difference in return to employment for different management strategies in patients with ischemic heart disease.

Nademanee K, Intarachot V, Josephson MA, et al. Prognostic significance of silent myocardial ischemia in patients with unstable angina. *J Am Coll Cardiol* 1987;10:1–9.

Episodes of silent myocardial ischemia assessed by Holter monitoring predict poor short-term outcome in patients with unstable angina.

O'Keefe JH, Wetzel M, Moe RR, et al. Should an angiotensin-converting enzyme inhibitor be standard therapy for patients with atherosclerotic disease? *J Am Coll Cardiol* 2001;37:1–8.

A review of the many benefits of long-term therapy with ACE inhibitors in patients with atherosclerotic cardiovascular disease.

Picard MH, Wilkins GT, Ray P, et al. Long-term effects of acute thrombolytic therapy on ventricular size and function. *Am Heart J* 1993;126:1–10.

Thrombolytic therapy prevents ventricular dilatation and preserves left ventricular function in patients with acute MI.

Pryor DB, Shaw L, McCants CB, et al. Value of the history and physical in identifying patients at increased risk for coronary artery disease. *Ann Intern Med* 1993;118:81–90.

History and physical examination predict outcome in patients with CAD.

Ridker PM, O'Donnell C, Marder VJ, et al. Large-scale trials of thrombolytic therapy for acute myocardial infarction: GISSI-2, ISIS-3, and GUSTO-1. *Ann Intern Med* 1993;119:530–532.

Update on most recent multicenter trials of thrombolytic therapy.

Ross J. Assessment of ischemic regional myocardial dysfunction and its reversibility. *Circulation* 1986;74:1186–1190.
Review of experimental and clinical data that examines regional myocardial function during ischemia.

Strauss WE, Parisi AF. Combined use of calcium-channel and beta adrenergic blockers for the treatment of chronic stable angina: rationale, efficacy, and adverse effects. *Ann Intern Med* 1988;109:570–581.
Careful review of pluses and minuses involved in using combination therapy for angina pectoris.

Tuzcu EM, Kapadia SR, Rutar E, et al. High prevalence of coronary atherosclerosis in asymptomatic teenagers and young adults: evidence from intravascular ultrasound. *Circulation* 2001;103:2705–2710.
Coronary atherosclerosis begins at a young age: Lesions are present in one in six teenagers in the United States.

Weiner DA, Ryan TJ, McCabe CH, et al. Significance of silent myocardial ischemia during exercise testing in patients with coronary artery disease. *Am J Cardiol* 1987;59:725–729.
Silent myocardial ischemia is associated with a negative prognosis compared with a normal exercise test result.

Yusuf S, Sleight P, Pogue J, et al. Effects of an angiotensin-converting-enzyme inhibitor, ramipril, on cardiovascular events in high-risk patients: the Heart Outcomes Prevention Evaluation Study Investigators. *N Engl J Med* 2000;342:145–153.
An ACE inhibitor, ramipril, markedly reduced cardiovascular events in patients at high risk for atherosclerotic cardiovascular disease during long-term follow-up.

Yusuf S, Zhao F, Mehta SR, et al. Effects of clopidogrel in addition to aspirin in patients with acute coronary syndromes without ST-segment elevation: the Clopidogrel in Unstable Angina to Prevent Recurrent Events Trial Investigators. *N Engl J Med* 2001;345:494–502.
The antiplatelet agent, clopidogrel, has long-term beneficial effects in patients who are admitted to the hospital with an acute coronary syndrome.

Zijlstra F, Hoorntje JCA, de Boer MJ, et al. Long-term benefit of primary angioplasty as compared with thrombolytic therapy for acute myocardial infarction. *N Engl J Med* 1999;341:1413–1419.
Primary coronary angioplasty gives better results than pharmacological thrombolysis in patients with acute MI.

16. VALVULAR HEART DISEASE

I. Introduction. A number of factors play a part in pathologic valvular changes. Valvular disease may be caused by genetic factors, infectious agents, trauma, chemicals, and a variety of other agents. Specific factors affect one valve more often than another. Thus, rheumatic valvular disease affects the mitral valve most frequently, with the aortic valve next in frequency, and the tricuspid valve least frequent in involvement. The pulmonic valve seems to be minimally affected by the rheumatic process. Valvular damage can result in either stenosis or insufficiency of the valve, depending on factors such as physical stresses on the valve, immunological competence, and the presence of comorbid conditions.

II. Mitral stenosis. Rheumatic fever is the major cause of mitral stenosis. Acute rheumatic fever usually occurs during childhood or adolescence. A long latency period then ensues, with patients first becoming symptomatic in middle adult life.

The natural history of mitral stenosis has been altered significantly by modern antimicrobial and cardiac surgical therapy.

A. Diagnosis

1. History. Approximately 50% of patients with mitral stenosis report an episode of acute rheumatic fever in childhood. Many patients relate that they had rheumatic fever as a child, but often the diagnosis was made solely on the basis of a murmur heard during childhood. The classic features of rheumatic fever (carditis, arthritis, rash, subcutaneous nodules, and chorea) were not present. Approximately 50% to 60% of children who have acute rheumatic fever will develop valvular heart disease as adults. Women are affected three times as often as men.

   In the United States, patients with mitral stenosis usually remain asymptomatic until early middle life (30 to 40 years), although mild symptoms may be present during pregnancies that occur in the early 20s. The first symptom to appear is dyspnea on exertion, at times accompanied by hemoptysis. When the effective mitral valve area reaches 1 cm^2, dyspnea lessens, hemoptysis disappears, and fatigue becomes a major symptom. Later, in the course of the disease, when the mitral orifice falls below 1 cm^2, dyspnea returns, frequently accompanied by complaints of ankle swelling (Table 16-1).

   The New York Heart Association (NYHA) symptomatic classification is not the same as the Dexter classification noted in Table 16-1. Patients with NYHA class III symptoms (severely limited) may be in Dexter class II, although they are often in Dexter class III. Complications in patients with mitral stenosis include atrial fibrillation with or without rapid ventricular response, pulmonary edema, arterial or venous embolism, and right ventricular failure.

2. Physical examination. The blood pressure is usually low normal in patients with mitral stenosis. The pulse may be irregularly irregular secondary to atrial fibrillation. A malar flush may be present, so that female patients with mitral stenosis often do not need to use rouge. The carotid pulse upstroke and amplitude are unremarkable. The left ventricular impulse is small or absent; a parasternal right ventricular impulse may be palpable.

   On auscultation, the first heart sound (S1) is loud, an easily audible opening snap occurs shortly after the second heart sound (S2), and a low-pitched rumbling murmur is audible during diastole. The murmur is most easily heard if one listens at the apex with the bell of the stethoscope while the patient lies in the left lateral decubitus position. Most patients in sinus rhythm (and a few in atrial fibrillation) will have presystolic accentuation of the diastolic rumble. Patients with more severe degrees of mitral stenosis have a holodiastolic murmur and a short interval between S2 and the opening snap. An occasional patient with

TABLE 16-1. LEWIS DEXTER'S FOUR STAGES OF MITRAL STENOSIS

Stages	I	II	III	IV
Size of mitral orifice (cm²)	>1.2	1.0–1.2	0.8–1.0	<0.8
Symptoms				
Dyspnea	±	+++	+	+++
Fatigue	+	0	+++	+
Ankle edema	0	±	±	++
Signs				
Accentuated M1	+++	+++	+++	+++
Diastolic rumble	+++	+++	+++	+++
Right ventricular failure (↑ jugular venous pressure, hepatomegaly, peripheral edema)	0	±	+	++
ECG				
Right ventricular hypertrophy	0	±	+	+
Chest x-ray film				
Left atrial size	++	++	++	++
Pulmonary arterial size	Normal	Normal or ↑	↑↑	↑↑↑
Right ventricular size	Normal	Normal or ↑	↑↑	↑↑↑

0, not present; ±, occasionally present; +, often present; ++, almost always present; +++, always present; ↑, slightly increased; ↑↑, moderately increased; ↑↑↑, severely increased; M1, mitral component of first heart sound.

severe pulmonary hypertension secondary to long-standing mitral stenosis has an early diastolic blowing murmur of pulmonary insufficiency, the Graham Steell murmur. The pulmonic component of S2 is usually accentuated in patients with pulmonary hypertension. The murmur of tricuspid regurgitation is often heard in patients with severe pulmonary hypertension and right ventricular failure. Patients with right ventricular failure manifest jugular venous distention, hepatomegaly, and peripheral edema. Physical findings in patients with mitral stenosis are summarized in Table 16-2.

3. ECG. The P wave is often broad, notched, or both in patients with mitral stenosis, so-called P-mitrale. Individuals with pulmonary hypertension and right ventricular hypertrophy (RVH) frequently demonstrate right axis deviation and R > S in lead V_1. ECG findings in patients with mitral stenosis often include:

Atrial fibrillation
Broad, notched P waves (P-mitrale)
Right axis deviation
R > S in V_1 or V_2 (RVH)

4. Chest x-ray examination. Left atrial enlargement and pulmonary vascular redistribution secondary to pulmonary venous hypertension are the most common findings on the routine chest x-ray film of patients with mitral stenosis. Late in the course of the illness, right ventricular enlargement, mitral valvular calcification, enlargement of the pulmonary artery, and signs of extensive interstitial pulmonary edema are frequently present. The radiographic findings in patients with mitral stenosis are summarized in Table 16-3.

5. Echocardiography and cardiac graphics. A specific, abnormal pattern of motion of the anterior and posterior leaflets of the mitral valve is almost invariably present in patients with mitral stenosis. The leaflets of the

TABLE 16-2. PHYSICAL FINDINGS IN PATIENTS WITH MITRAL STENOSIS[a]

Irregularly irregular pulse (atrial fibrillation)
Malar flush
Pulmonary congestion (rales, pleural effusion)
Parasternal right ventricular impulse
Accentuated first heart sound
Increased P2 in patients with pulmonary hypertension
Early diastolic opening snap
Diastolic rumbling murmur
Presystolic accentuation of diastolic murmur in patients in normal sinus rhythm

Findings in patients with right ventricular failure
    Jugular venous distention
    Right ventricular impulse
    Hepatomegaly
    Hepatojugular reflux
    Peripheral edema
    Early diastolic blowing murmur of pulmonic regurgitation (Graham Steell)
    Holosystolic murmur of tricuspid regurgitation

[a]Not all findings are present in every patient with mitral stenosis.

valve are thickened and often redundant, moving in the same direction rather than away from each other during diastole. Marked leaflet calcification may be present. Left ventricular cavity size and wall motion are usually normal. Right ventricular cavity size is often increased.

Left atrial dilatation is almost always present. Doppler echocardiography enables the physician to quantitate noninvasively the mitral valve area. Such noninvasive data correlate well with valve area measurements obtained during cardiac catheterization.

6. Radionuclide studies. Left ventricular function may be accurately measured by radionuclide ventriculography. The presence of mitral stenosis cannot at present be inferred from any radionuclide examination.
7. Catheterization and angiography. A gradient across the mitral valve is the hemodynamic hallmark of mitral stenosis. Such a gradient usually is inferred from the marked difference between pulmonary capillary wedge pressure (PCWP) and left ventricular diastolic pressure, with the former significantly higher than the latter throughout diastole. Pulmonary hypertension frequently is present in patients with mitral stenosis.

TABLE 16-3. RADIOGRAPHIC FINDINGS IN PATIENTS WITH MITRAL STENOSIS

Left atrial enlargement
    Straightening or convexity of the left heart border
    Posterior displacement of the left atrium on barium swallow
    "Double density"
    Elevation of the left main stem bronchus

Pulmonary venous hypertension
    Pulmonary vascular redistribution
    Interstitial edema
    Pleural effusion

Pulmonary arterial enlargement
Right ventricular enlargement
Mitral valvular calcification

Pulmonary arterial pressure may approach systemic arterial pressure levels late in the course of the disease. Right ventricular failure is also common in individuals with more severe degrees of pulmonary hypertension. The effective orifice size of the stenotic mitral valve can be calculated if one knows the heart rate, cardiac output, and mitral valvular gradient. Patients with mitral valve areas less than 1 cm^2 are said to have severe mitral stenosis. Individuals with valve areas between 1.1 and 1.5 cm^2 have moderate mitral stenosis, and those with valve areas greater than 1.5 cm^2 have only mild mitral stenosis. The normal mitral valve area is 4 cm^2.

Mitral valve immobility and calcification are usually apparent on the left ventriculogram. An occasional patient with mitral stenosis has reduced left ventricular function, a finding as yet not adequately explained. Varying degrees of mitral regurgitation may coexist with mitral stenosis. Functional tricuspid regurgitation may be present in patients with severe pulmonary hypertension and right ventricular failure. Balloon mitral valvuloplasty may be performed at the time of catheterization.

8. Protocol for the diagnosis of mitral stenosis. The diagnosis of mitral stenosis usually can be made without difficulty on the basis of appropriate history, physical examination, and noninvasive examinations (ECG, chest x-ray film, and echocardiogram). Information obtained from noninvasive tests often enables the physician to quantitate the severity of mitral stenosis with considerable accuracy. Some patients may even be referred for mitral valvular surgery without catheterization when the diagnosis is firmly made by means of noninvasive examination. The following is a tentative flowchart for the diagnosis of mitral stenosis. (The dashed arrow indicates that this step is optional.)

History and physical examination
↓
ECG, chest x-ray film
↓
Echocardiogram and Doppler study
↓
Catheterization **in selected patients**

Severity of mitral stenosis is estimated on the basis of the following findings:

Severe mitral stenosis	**Mild to moderate mitral stenosis**
Severe symptoms	Mild symptoms
S2–OS interval narrow	S2–OS interval wide
Holodiastolic murmur	Early or late diastolic murmur only
Atrial fibrillation, RVH on ECG	Normal sinus rhythm, no ventricular hypertrophy by ECG
Left atrial enlargement, valve calcification, and pulmonary	Modest left atrial enlargement, no valve calcification, and minimal pulmonary congestion by x-ray film
Markedly thickened valve with severely restricted motion by echocardiography; Doppler estimate of valve area < 1.2 cm^2	Modest valvular abnormality by echocardiography; Doppler estimate of valve area ≥ 1.2 cm^2

a. The diagnosis of mitral stenosis is ensured in individuals who meet the following criteria: (i) a history of effort intolerance or undue fatigue is coupled with the finding of an opening snap and a diastolic rumbling murmur on physical examination, and (ii) chest x-ray and ECG demonstrate left atrial enlargement or atrial fibrillation, and echocardiography reveals thickened mitral valve leaflets with reduced mobility. Catheterization is not required to make the diagnosis of mitral stenosis but may be indicated to aid in planning mitral valvular surgery.

b. Differential diagnosis

(1) Mitral regurgitation. Patients with considerable quantities of mitral regurgitation may have a diastolic rumbling murmur secondary to the large amount of blood traversing the mitral valve during diastole. Such individuals can be distinguished from patients with mitral stenosis through the presence of prominent holosystolic murmurs of mitral regurgitation and evidence of left ventricular enlargement or hypertrophy on physical examination, ECG, chest x-ray study, and echocardiogram with Doppler study.

(2) Hyperthyroidism. Patients with hyperthyroidism may, on occasion, have such a high cardiac output that a diastolic flow rumble is heard secondary to the large quantity of blood traversing the mitral and tricuspid valves during diastole. The clinical presentation of these individuals with their hyperactive cardiovascular, central, and peripheral nervous systems differs considerably from that of patients with mitral stenosis. The echocardiogram invariably demonstrates a hyperactive left ventricle and a normal mitral valve in patients with hyperthyroidism.

(3) Cor triatriatum. Cor triatriatum is an unusual congenital malformation resembling mitral stenosis in its pathophysiology and clinical presentation. A membrane subdivides the left atrium and is an obstacle to the free passage of blood from the pulmonary veins to the left ventricle.

Patients with cor triatriatum have systolic and diastolic murmurs that do not resemble those heard in individuals with mitral stenosis. In addition, patients with cor triatriatum never develop atrial fibrillation. Their echocardiograms reveal a normal mitral valve and left atrial membrane. If performed, catheterization demonstrates hemodynamics similar to that seen in patients with mitral stenosis.

(4) Congenital stenosis of pulmonary veins. A rare entity that can reproduce (as with cor triatriatum) the pathophysiology and clinical picture of mitral stenosis is congenital stenosis of pulmonary veins. The murmur is atypical for mitral stenosis, and the echocardiogram demonstrates a normal mitral valve. Catheterization reveals physiology similar to that of mitral stenosis.

(5) Left atrial myxoma. Left atrial myxoma is a benign tumor that frequently obstructs the mitral orifice, producing symptoms and signs resembling those of mitral stenosis. The murmur changes in intensity and timing when the patient changes position, a finding not present in individuals with mitral stenosis. The echocardiogram is distinctive in patients with left atrial myxoma, demonstrating the tumor in the left atrium behind the mitral valve. Left atrial myxoma will not be confused with mitral stenosis if an echocardiogram is obtained.

(6) Atrial septal defect (ASD). High flow across the tricuspid valve occurs in patients with ASD and a large left-to-right shunt. This large transvalvular flow can produce an early diastolic filling sound followed by a flow rumble, findings that may lead the clinician to diagnose mitral stenosis. The chest x-ray film of patients with ASD demonstrates hypervascularity secondary to increased pulmonary flow, and the echocardiogram reveals a normal mitral valve and a dilated right ventricle. A radionuclide angiocardiogram or Doppler study shows a left-to-right shunt.

B. Therapy
   1. Medical treatment
      a. Pharmacologic agents
         (1) Antibiotics. Patients with a history of prior rheumatic fever should receive prophylactic antibiotic therapy to prevent recurrences of rheumatic activity. Some authorities advise lifelong prophylaxis; others discontinue routine antibiotic therapy at 40 years of age. Table 16-4 lists the current antibiotic recommendations for rheumatic fever prophylaxis.

            Prophylactic antibiotics also are administered to patients with established valvular disease who undergo dental or surgical procedures. Although not proved efficacious in rigorous double-blind trials, such regimens, in the view of most authorities, decrease the incidence of bacterial endocarditis in these patients. Tables 16-5 to 16-7 list the current recommendations for antibiotic prophylaxis against endocarditis in patients with valvular heart disease.

         (2) Digitalis. Patients with mitral stenosis who are in sinus rhythm do not benefit from digitalis therapy. Patients in atrial fibrillation should receive a sufficient daily dose of digoxin as well as one or more of the following: verapamil, diltiazem, and/or beta-blockers, so that the resting ventricular response is in the range of 60 to 80 beats per minute. It is often helpful to exercise such individuals to observe the ventricular response. Many persons whose heart rate is well controlled at rest have inappropriate increases in rate with only modest degrees of exercise. An increased digitalis dosage or the addition of small doses of any of the agents just listed (calcium channel blockers/beta-blockers) to the regimen of such individuals usually results in adequate control of the exercise heart rate.

         (3) Diuretics. Patients with pulmonary congestion or peripheral edema often benefit from judicious administration of diuretics. Cardiac output may be decreased by diuresis secondary to reduced ventricular filling. Thus, patients with mitral stenosis who undergo diuresis may exchange the symptom of dyspnea for the symptom of fatigue.

         (4) Anticoagulation. Patients with mitral stenosis who are in sinus rhythm do not require anticoagulation. Individuals who have an episode of arterial or venous embolism or who develop sustained or transient episodes of atrial fibrillation or atrial flutter should receive long-term anticoagulant therapy with warfarin.

         (5) Antiarrhythmic drugs. Individuals with mitral stenosis who develop atrial fibrillation should have at least one attempt at restoration of sinus rhythm. Medical cardioversion with intravenous procainamide or amiodarone; oral propafenone, sotalol, dofetilide, or amiodarone; or electrical cardioversion are often

---

TABLE 16-4. ANTIBIOTIC PROPHYLAXIS AGAINST RHEUMATIC FEVER

I. Patients who have had an episode of acute rheumatic fever or Sydenham's chorea should receive continuous antibiotic prophylaxis until at least age 40 and possibly for life.

II. Recommended treatment regimens
  A. IM injection of 1.2 million U of benzathine penicillin G every 4 weeks, *or*
  B. Penicillin G, 200,000 or 250,000 U PO bid, *or*
  C. Sulfadiazine, 1 g/day, PO, *or*
  D. Erythromycin, 250 mg PO bid

TABLE 16-5. PROPHYLACTIC REGIMENS FOR DENTAL, ORAL, RESPIRATORY TRACT, OR ESOPHAGEAL PROCEDURES

Situation	Agent	Regimen
Standard general prophylaxis	Amoxicillin	Adults: 2 g; children: 50 mg/kg PO 1 hr before procedure
Unable to take oral medications	Ampicillin	Adults: 2 g IM or IV; children: 50 mg/kg IM or IV within 30 min before procedure
Allergic to penicillin	Clindamycin *or* Cephalexin[a] *or* cefadroxil[a] *or* Azithromycin or clarithromycin	Adults: 600 mg; children: 20 mg/kg PO 1 hr before procedure Adults: 2 g; children: 50 mg/kg PO 1 hr before procedure Adults: 500 mg; children: 15 mg/kg PO 1 hr before procedure
Allergic to penicillin and unable to take oral medications	Clindamycin *or* Cefazolin[a]	Adults: 600 mg; children: 20 mg/kg IV within 30 min before procedure. Adults: 1 g; children: 25 mg/kg IM or IV within 30 min before procedure

[a] Cephalosporins should not be used in individuals with immediate-type hypersensitivity reaction (urticaria, angioedema, or anaphylaxis) to penicillins.

successful in restoring sinus rhythm. Patients who are converted electrically should continue to receive sustained action oral procainamide (500 to 750 mg four times a day), oral disopyramide (100 to 200 mg four times a day), propafenone (150 to 300 mg three times a day), sotalol (80 to 160 mg two times a day) or amiodarone (200 mg per day). If the patient remains in sinus rhythm for only a brief time (days to weeks), antiarrhythmic drug therapy should be discontinued and the patient allowed to remain in atrial fibrillation. Ventricular response is controlled with daily digitalis, diltiazem, verapamil, or beta-blocker administration. Patients who have been in atrial fibrillation for 2 or more days should receive warfarin anticoagulation for 3 to 4 weeks before and 2 to 4 weeks after cardioversion.

   b. **Activity.** Patients with mitral stenosis gradually restrict their activity as the degree of valvular stenosis worsens with time. It is important to question them closely about their current level of activity compared with that of an earlier time. An objective measure of exercise limitation may be obtained by means of a treadmill or bicycle exercise tolerance test. Marked limitation is an indication for surgical therapy.

   c. **Diet.** Modest sodium restriction (no-added-salt diet) is indicated for patients with symptoms of pulmonary congestion (dyspnea on exertion, orthopnea, paroxysmal nocturnal dyspnea).

   d. **Cardioversion.** As noted in Section **II.B.1.a.(5),** patients with new-onset atrial fibrillation deserve at least one attempt at conversion to sinus rhythm. If the patient remains in sinus rhythm for only a brief time, further attempts to restore and maintain sinus rhythm will almost certainly be in vain.

  2. **Surgery or catheter balloon valvuloplasty.** Indications for valvuloplasty or valve replacement in patients with mitral stenosis include (i) relief of marked symptoms of pulmonary congestion, (ii) relief from atrial arrhythmias refractory to medical therapy, and (iii) cardiac surgery indicated for another reason, mitral stenosis being of only moderate severity.

TABLE 16-6. PROPHYLACTIC REGIMENS FOR GENITOURINARY/
GASTROINTESTINAL (EXCLUDING ESOPHAGEAL) PROCEDURES

Situation	Agents[a]	Regimen[b]
High-risk patients	Ampicillin plus gentamicin	Adults: ampicillin 2 g IM or IV plus gentamicin 1.5 mg/kg (not to exceed 120 mg) within 30 min of starting procedure; 6 hr later, ampicillin 1 g IM/IV or amoxicillin 1 g PO Children: ampicillin 50 mg/kg IM or IV (not to exceed 2 g) plus gentamicin 1.5 mg/kg within 30 min of starting the procedure; 6 hr later, ampicillin 25 mg/kg IM/IV or amoxicillin 25 mg/kg PO
High-risk patients allergic to ampicillin/ amoxicillin	Vancomycin plus gentamicin	Adults: vancomycin 1 g IV over 1–2 hr plus gentamicin 1.5 mg/kg IV/IM (not to exceed 120 mg); complete injection/infusion within 30 min of starting procedure Children: vancomycin 20 mg/kg IV over 1–2 hr plus gentamicin 1.5 mg/kg IV/IM; complete injection/infusion within 30 min of starting procedure
Moderate-risk patients	Amoxicillin or ampicillin	Adults: amoxicillin 2 g PO 1 hr before procedure, or ampicillin 2 g IM/IV within 30 min of starting procedure Children: amoxicillin 50 mg/kg PO 1 hr before procedure, or ampicillin 50 mg/kg IM/IV within 30 min of starting procedure
Moderate-risk patients allergic to ampicillin/ amoxicillin	Vancomycin	Adults: vancomycin 1 g IV over 1–2 hr; complete infusion within 30 min of starting procedure Children: vancomycin 20 mg/kg IV over 1–2 hr; complete infusion within 30 min of starting procedure

[a]Total children's dose should not exceed adult dose.
[b]No second dose of vancomycin or gentamicin is recommended.

For example, an individual with severe coronary artery disease (CAD), in whom coronary bypass grafting was to be undertaken, would be a candidate for a mitral valvuloplasty even if the mitral stenosis was only moderately severe.

a. Mitral valvuloplasty. During surgical or balloon valvuloplasty at the time of cardiac catheterization, adhesions that cause the mitral orifice to be narrowed are lysed mechanically (by the balloon catheter, by hand, or by a dilator).

This procedure can be performed only in patients with minimal or no mitral valvular calcification and, at most, mild mitral regurgitation. After 7 to 10 years, the valve usually restenoses, and mitral valve replacement is usually indicated. Mitral valvuloplasty may be repeated a second and occasionally a third time by balloon catheter. However, if the valve is heavily calcified or fibrotic, the likelihood of success with repeat balloon valvuloplasty is markedly diminished.

TABLE 16-7. OTHER PROCEDURES AND ENDOCARDITIS PROPHYLAXIS

Endocarditis prophylaxis recommended
   Respiratory tract
      Tonsillectomy and/or adenoidectomy
      Surgical operations that involve respiratory mucosa
      Bronchoscopy with a rigid bronchoscope
   Gastrointestinal tract[a]
      Sclerotherapy for esophageal varices
      Esophageal stricture dilation
      Endoscopic retrograde cholangiography with biliary obstruction
      Biliary tract surgery
      Surgical operations that involve intestinal mucosa
   Genitourinary tract
      Prostatic surgery
      Cystoscopy
      Urethral dilation

Endocarditis prophylaxis not recommended
   Respiratory tract
      Endotracheal intubation
      Bronchoscopy with a flexible bronchoscope, with or without biopsy[b]
      Tympanostomy tube insertion
   Gastrointestinal tract[b]
      Transesophageal echocardiography
      Endoscopy with or without gastrointestinal biopsy
   Genitourinary tract
      Vaginal hysterectomy[b]
      Vaginal delivery[b]
      Cesarean section
      In uninfected tissue
         Urethral catheterization
         Uterine dilatation and curettage
         Therapeutic abortion
         Sterilization procedures
         Insertion or removal of intrauterine devices
  Other
      Cardiac catheterization, including balloon angioplasty
      Implanted cardiac pacemakers, implanted defibrillators, and coronary stents
      Incision or biopsy of surgically scrubbed skin
      Circumcision

[a] Prophylaxis is recommended for high-risk patients; it is optional for medium-risk patients.
[b] Prophylaxis is optional for high-risk patients.

   b. Mitral valve replacement. During the replacement procedure, the stenotic and often severely calcified and distorted mitral valve is excised, and a prosthetic valve is sewn in its place. Individuals who receive a xenograft (usually porcine) or a homograft (cadaver) valve do not usually require long-term anticoagulation after surgery. A markedly enlarged left atrium and/or the presence of atrial fibrillation, however, may require that patients with xenograft or homograft valves receive long-term anticoagulation with warfarin. Patients with plastic and metal prosthetic valves **must take warfarin for the rest of their lives. Mitral valve replacement can be performed in individuals with good left ventricular function, with mortality under 5%.**

III. Mitral regurgitation. Once thought to be a rare complication of rheumatic heart disease, mitral regurgitation or insufficiency is now known to be one of the most common valvular lesions. It can be the result of many different pathologic processes:

Rheumatic heart disease
CAD
Bacterial endocarditis
Myxomatous degeneration of the mitral valve resulting in mitral valve prolapse or ruptured chordae tendineae
Mitral annular calcification
Left ventricular dilatation
Idiopathic hypertrophic subaortic stenosis
Abnormal mitral valve structure associated with various forms of congenital heart disease (e. g., primum ASD, corrected transposition)
Miscellaneous, rare: tumors, granulomas, amyloid, hemochromatosis, Hurler's syndrome, syphilis, ankylosing spondylitis, chest trauma

A. Diagnosis
   1. History. Patients with chronic mitral regurgitation may remain asymptomatic for decades. The left ventricle compensates for the volume overload imposed by the valvular incompetence by dilatation and hypertrophy. Eventually, however, left ventricular failure develops, and patients note exercise intolerance, orthopnea, paroxysmal nocturnal dyspnea, and fatigue. Late in the course of the illness, right ventricular failure develops as a result of left ventricular failure with secondary pulmonary hypertension.
   Atrial fibrillation is common late in the natural history of mitral regurgitation. This arrhythmia results from marked left atrial dilatation and left ventricular failure. Complications of mitral regurgitation include arterial or venous embolism, bacterial endocarditis, and left and right ventricular failure.
   Acute mitral regurgitation can occur as a result of bacterial endocarditis, ruptured chordae tendineae, or ischemic necrosis of part or all of the papillary muscle. Left ventricular and left atrial dilatation and compensation are often inadequate when severe mitral regurgitation develops suddenly; there may be a fulminant course with refractory left ventricular failure requiring urgent surgical replacement of the mitral valve. Acute and chronic mitral regurgitation are very different clinical entities.
   The presentation of the patient with mitral regurgitation depends on the etiology of the valvular lesion. Patients with rheumatic mitral regurgitation often develop effort intolerance gradually over many years; patients with ruptured chordae tendineae secondary to myxomatous degeneration of the mitral valve may present with the sudden onset of pulmonary edema. Mitral annular calcification usually occurs in elderly individuals, although young patients with Marfan's syndrome may experience this pathologic change. Mitral valve prolapse, or Barlow's syndrome, rarely produces large quantities of mitral regurgitation. Patients are asymptomatic, or they complain of atypical chest pain, palpitations, or both. They may demonstrate a wide spectrum of atrial or ventricular arrhythmias. Sudden death occurs in a rare individual with mitral valve prolapse.
   2. Physical examination. A holosystolic blowing murmur, heard best at the apex with radiation to the axilla, is the most common physical finding in patients with mitral regurgitation. The murmur may radiate over the entire thorax, however, and its characteristics and timing are of greater use than radiation in identifying its source. Significant quantities of mitral regurgitation are accompanied by evidence of left ventricular dilatation and hypertrophy (displaced, active left ventricular impulse). A prominent third heart sound (S3) in patients with mitral regurgitation does not necessarily imply left ventricular decompensation, as in individuals with CAD or cardiomyopathy. The S3 in mitral regurgitation is frequently the result of a large amount of blood entering the left ventri-

cle during early diastole from a dilated left atrium. Physical findings in patients with mitral regurgitation are summarized in Table 16-8.

3. ECG. Patients with significant quantities of chronic mitral regurgitant blood flow usually show left ventricular hypertrophy (LVH) on the ECG. A biventricular hypertrophy pattern may be seen late in the course of the illness when significant pulmonary hypertension exists, resulting in concomitant RVH. ECG findings in patients with mitral regurgitation can include the following:

Atrial fibrillation
Left axis deviation
Left atrial enlargement (deep negative terminal deflection of P wave in lead V_1)
LVH
Biventricular hypertrophy late in the course of the illness when pulmonary hypertension exists

Patients with acute mitral regurgitation often fail to demonstrate LVH by ECG.

4. Chest x-ray examination. Left ventricular enlargement secondary to dilatation and hypertrophy are often noted on the chest roentgenogram of patients with chronic mitral regurgitation. Left atrial enlargement, often of severe degree, is also commonly seen. Signs of pulmonary congestion are present in patients with left ventricular decompensation. Severe pulmonary congestion with normal heart size may be seen in patients with acute mitral regurgitation. Left ventricular function and the severity of mitral regurgitation can be quantitated by means of magnetic resonance imaging.

Possible roentgenographic findings in patients with mitral regurgitation are the following:

Left ventricular enlargement
Left atrial enlargement (may be massive)
Pulmonary congestion (vascular redistribution, interstitial edema, pleural effusion)
Mitral valvular or annular calcification in selected cases
Enlargement of pulmonary artery and right ventricle late in course of illness when pulmonary hypertension is well established

5. Echocardiography. The echocardiogram demonstrates a dilated, hyperactive left ventricle in most patients with mitral regurgitation. Of course, the echocardiographic findings depend on the underlying etiology of mitral regurgitation. Thus, patients with mitral valve prolapse may have

TABLE 16-8. PHYSICAL FINDINGS IN PATIENTS WITH MITRAL REGURGITATION[a]

Irregularly irregular pulse (atrial fibrillation)
Pulmonary congestion (rales, pleural effusion)
Soft or normal first heart sound
Increased P2 in patients with pulmonary hypertension third heart sound, fourth heart sound
Midsystolic click(s) with late systolic murmur in patients with mitral valve prolapse

Findings in patients with right ventricular failure
    Jugular venous distention
    Right ventricular impulse
    Hepatomegaly
    Hepatojugular reflux
    Peripheral edema

[a] Not all findings are present in every patient with mitral regurgitation.

a completely normal echo study, except for the presence of late systolic posterior motion (prolapse) of the mitral valve leaflets. Ruptured chordae tendineae often can be identified in the echocardiograms of patients with myxomatous degeneration of the mitral valve and acute mitral regurgitation. Individuals with congestive cardiomyopathy, in whom mitral regurgitation is the result of left ventricular dilatation, demonstrate dilated, poorly contractile ventricles on echocardiography. Patients with mitral regurgitation secondary to idiopathic hypertrophic subaortic stenosis (hypertrophic cardiomyopathy) demonstrate a thickened, hypocontractile septum and abnormal systolic anterior motion of the anterior mitral valve leaflet. Vegetations on the mitral valve may be identified in patients with mitral regurgitation secondary to bacterial endocarditis. Doppler echocardiography is very sensitive for demonstrating and quantitating mitral regurgitation.

6. Radionuclide studies. The status of left ventricular function can be measured by means of radionuclide ventriculography. Moreover, radionuclide ventriculography can be used to quantitate the amount of mitral regurgitation. With this useful technique, it is possible to obtain noninvasively almost all the information (except for wedge pressure) available by means of catheterization. Early deterioration in left ventricular systolic function can be detected with radionuclear ventriculography.

7. Catheterization and angiography. Patients with mitral regurgitation and well-compensated left ventricular function will have normal hemodynamic measurements. Left ventricular ejection fraction is often high-normal or even increased in such individuals. As left ventricular function decreases, ejection fraction falls and left ventricular filling pressure rises. The symptomatic patient with mitral regurgitation has normal or reduced ejection fraction, elevated PCWP, and moderate pulmonary hypertension. Right ventricular failure occurs late in the course of the illness. Patients with acute mitral regurgitation have very high left ventricular filling pressures with large V waves in the PCWP tracing. Patients with chronic mitral regurgitation have elevated PCWP with normal-sized or moderately enlarged V waves.

   Left ventricular angiography documents the presence and severity of mitral regurgitation (graded as 1 to 4 + mitral regurgitation) and the state of left ventricular contraction. Left atrial size usually is increased markedly in patients with chronic mitral regurgitation but is often normal in those with acute mitral regurgitation.

8. Protocol for the diagnosis of mitral regurgitation
   a. The sequence of tests for determining the diagnosis of mitral regurgitation and estimating its severity is as follows (dashed arrow indicates optional step):

   History and physical examination
   ↓
   ECG and chest x-ray study
   ↓
   Echocardiogram + Doppler radionuclide ventriculography
   ↓
   Catheterization **in selected patients**

   Severity of mitral regurgitation and left ventricular dysfunction are estimated from the following findings:

Severe mitral regurgitation	Mild to moderate mitral regurgitation
Severe symptoms	Mild to moderate symptoms
Prominent S3	No S3
Holosystolic murmur	Early or late systolic murmur only

Atrial fibrillation, LVH on ECG	Normal sinus rhythm, no ventricular hypertrophy or voltage criteria alone for LVH on ECG
Very large left atrium and left ventricle, signs of pulmonary congestion on chest x-ray film	Moderate or no left atrial enlargement, modest or no pulmonary congestion on x-ray film
Dilated, hypercontractile or hypocontractile left ventricle, marked left atrial enlargement; ruptured chord seen on echocardiography; Doppler study, severe regurgitation	Normal left ventricular wall motion and modest or no left ventricular or left atrial enlargement on echocardiography; Doppler study, mild regurgitation

b. The diagnosis of mitral regurgitation is based on an appropriate history and the finding of a systolic murmur consistent with mitral regurgitation. Confirmation of the mitral origin of the murmur rests on evidence from the ECG (atrial fibrillation, left atrial enlargement, LVH), chest x-ray film (left atrial and left ventricular enlargement, mitral valvular or annular calcification), and echocardiography with Doppler study (dilated, hypercontractile or hypocontractile left ventricle, abnormal mitral valve motion, such as prolapse or ruptured chord, enlarged left atrium, presence of mitral regurgitation by Doppler). Patients with acute mitral regurgitation usually present with signs and symptoms of left ventricular failure, including prominent S3 and fourth heart sounds (S4). The murmur of acute mitral regurgitation is usually easily appreciated, although it may not be as loud as that heard with some forms of chronic mitral regurgitation. Left ventricular enlargement may not be apparent. The echocardiogram reveals hyperdynamic left ventricular wall motion and normal or only slightly increased left atrial diameter. Doppler study documents the presence of mitral regurgitation.

c. Differential diagnosis

   (1) Mitral stenosis. Patients with predominant mitral stenosis often have a small quantity of mitral regurgitation that produces an easily appreciated holosystolic murmur. Evidence favoring mitral stenosis as the predominant lesion includes (i) narrow S2–OS interval; (ii) absence of left ventricular dilatation or hypertrophy on physical examination, ECG, chest x-ray film, or echocardiogram; (iii) presence of RVH on physical examination, ECG, or echocardiogram; and (iv) echocardiographic demonstration of marked thickening and reduced mobility of the mitral valve, and Doppler quantitation of the severity of mitral regurgitation (mild to moderate).

   (2) Aortic stenosis. The prominent systolic murmur of aortic stenosis may be confused with that of mitral regurgitation, particularly when the former is loudest at the apex, an occasional finding. Evidence in favor of aortic stenosis includes (i) slow carotid upstroke, (ii) decreased or absent aortic component of S2, (iii) a crescendo-decrescendo murmur, and (iv) calcification of the aortic valve by roentgenography or echocardiography. Evidence favoring mitral regurgitation includes (i) normal carotid pulse and S2, (ii) holosystolic blowing murmur, and (iii) normal aortic valve leaflets by echocardiography.

   (3) Idiopathic hypertrophic subaortic stenosis (IHSS, or hypertrophic cardiomyopathy). IHSS can result in two murmurs: an out-

flow tract murmur from the subaortic obstruction, and a mitral regurgitant murmur secondary to abnormal traction on the anterior leaflet of the valve and the papillary muscles. These murmurs overlap and frequently confuse the auscultator. Evidence favoring IHSS includes (i) **increase** in the intensity of the murmur during Valsalva maneuver or standing and (ii) **decrease** in the intensity of the murmur during squatting. The echocardiogram demonstrates specific septal thickening in patients with IHSS. The murmur of mitral regurgitation **decreases** in intensity during Valsalva maneuver and standing.

(4) Ventricular septal defect (VSD). The murmur of VSD is holosystolic, resembling that of mitral regurgitation; however, the former tends to be localized to the lower left sternal border. A history of a murmur since early childhood favors VSD. The ECG, chest x-ray picture, and echocardiogram may be identical in mitral regurgitation and VSD except for the presence of shunt vessels on the chest x-ray.

Radionuclide angiocardiography or Doppler study demonstrates a left-to-right shunt in patients with VSD. In some patients, the VSD can be visualized by echocardiography. Selected patients may require catheterization.

(5) Functional systolic murmur. A functional murmur can be confused with that of mitral regurgitation. Functional murmurs, however, are rarely holosystolic, and there is usually no S3. The chest x-ray film, ECG, and echocardiogram are completely normal in patients with functional murmurs. Functional murmurs usually decrease markedly in intensity or disappear when the patient stands.

B. Therapy
  1. Medical treatment
    a. Pharmacologic agents
      (1) Antibiotics. Prophylaxis against acute rheumatic fever should be prescribed for all individuals with a firm history of prior rheumatic fever (Table 16-4). Prophylaxis against bacterial endocarditis should be prescribed for all those with mitral regurgitation (Tables 16-5 to 16-7). Individuals with mitral valve prolapse who have only midsystolic clicks without a late systolic murmur and without valve thickening by echo probably do not require antibiotic prophylaxis against bacterial endocarditis.

      (2) Digitalis. Patients with atrial fibrillation benefit from control of the ventricular response with digitalis, atrioventricular (AV) blocking calcium channel blockers and beta-blockers. Digitalis administration is also indicated in patients with signs and symptoms of left ventricular failure. Patients with manifest left ventricular decompensation, however, should be considered for mitral valve replacement.

      (3) Diuretics. Patients whose signs and symptoms of left ventricular failure do not adequately resolve with digitalization should receive concomitant diuretic therapy. Most of them will also require daily potassium supplementation.

      (4) Vasodilators. Patients with signs and symptoms of left ventricular failure should be considered for vasodilator therapy. Some cardiologists favor vasodilator therapy even in the absence of left ventricular failure. Small doses of vasodilators—usually ACE inhibitors—are administered initially, followed by a gradual increase in the dosage until signs and symptoms of failure improve or symptomatic hypotension occurs. Systolic blood pressures of 90 to 100 mm Hg are acceptable. An alternative and less effective vasodilator regimen for patients with heart

failure involves the combination of long-acting nitrates and hydralazine (see Chapter 4). Angiotensin-converting enzyme (ACE) inhibitors (e.g., captopril, enalapril, lisinopril, ramipril) are the favored agents for this indication.

(5) Anticoagulation. Patients with atrial fibrillation and/or very large left atria should receive long-term oral (warfarin) anticoagulation. Clearly, individuals with arterial or venous embolism should be anticoagulated permanently.

(6) Antiarrhythmic drugs. As noted earlier, sinus rhythm can at times be restored or maintained in patients with atrial fibrillation by means of therapy with procainamide, disopyramide, propafenone, sotalol, or amiodarone with or without electrical cardioversion. If sinus rhythm cannot be maintained, antiarrhythmic drugs are discontinued and the ventricular response is controlled with digitalis, AV blocking calcium channel blockers, and/or beta-blockers.

b. Activity. Restriction of activity is not required for patients with mitral regurgitation. Patients gradually restrict their activity as symptoms of left ventricular decompensation develop. Restriction of activity secondary to symptoms of left ventricular failure is an indication for mitral valve replacement (see Section **III.B.2.b.**).

c. Diet. A modest degree of salt restriction (no-added-salt diet, 5-g sodium) is indicated in patients with signs and symptoms of left ventricular failure.

d. Cardioversion. Cardioversion is indicated in patients with new-onset atrial fibrillation. Maintenance of sinus rhythm with arrhythmic drugs after cardioversion is mentioned in Section **III.B.1. a.(6).**

2. Surgery. The indication for surgical intervention in patients with mitral regurgitation is the development of signs and symptoms of left ventricular decompensation. The risk of surgery in these individuals is directly proportional to the contractile state of the left ventricle. Thus, it is important to identify signs and symptoms of left ventricular decompensation at an early stage. Delay may result in irreversible changes in left ventricular structure, with resultant high risk at the time of subsequent surgery and persistent left ventricular failure despite successful mitral valvular surgery.

a. Mitral valve reconstruction. A number of operations have been devised for reconstructing the regurgitant mitral valve so that it regains its competence. One example is the Carpentier ring reconstruction. The advantage of these procedures is that the patient does not have the native mitral valve resected; hence, long-term anticoagulation is not necessary. Successful mitral valve reconstruction can be performed in individuals with pure mitral regurgitation and mitral valve architecture that is not grossly distorted. Thus, individuals with ruptured chordae tendineae or dilated mitral valve annuli are the best candidates for mitral valve reconstruction. Patients with rheumatic mitral valve disease often do not respond well to this procedure.

b. Mitral valve replacement. The most common surgical intervention in patients with mitral regurgitation and left ventricular failure is mitral valve replacement. Prosthetic (plastic and metal), xenograft (porcine), and homograft (cadaver) valves all have been successfully implanted in individuals with severe mitral regurgitation. Patients with prosthetic valves or those with atrial fibrillation and very large left atria, regardless of valve type, should be anticoagulated for life with warfarin. Mortality for this procedure is less than 5% if left ventricular function is adequate.

IV. Aortic stenosis. Aortic stenosis in patients less than 30 years of age is almost invariably the result of a congenitally abnormal valve with fused commissures.

Aortic stenosis in elderly patients (greater than 60 to 70 years) is usually due to atherosclerotic and calcific changes in a tricuspid valve. Aortic stenosis secondary to rheumatic heart disease is always accompanied by mitral stenosis or regurgitation. Bicuspid aortic valves become stenotic during middle-age or later in two thirds to three fourths of individuals in whom this congenital abnormality occurs. The percentage of bicuspid aortic valves that become stenotic increases with age. The multiple etiologies of aortic stenosis are as follows:

Atherosclerotic, calcific: older individuals
Congenital: younger individuals
Bicuspid: percentage of individuals manifesting aortic stenosis increases
  with age
Rheumatic: combined with mitral valve disease
Subvalvular: membranous and muscular forms
Supravalvular: rare, associated with infantile hypercalcemia

A. Diagnosis
  1. History. Patients with aortic stenosis remain asymptomatic until late in the course of the illness. At that time they usually develop one of three symptoms: angina, syncope, or left ventricular failure. The appearance of symptoms in a patient with aortic stenosis heralds the start of a period of increased risk of sudden death. It is therefore important for physicians to recognize aortic stenosis in symptomatic patients and to initiate appropriate diagnostic and therapeutic measures.

    Angina can occur in patients with aortic stenosis in the absence of significant CAD. In such individuals, angina and even MI are the result of myocardial ischemia secondary to excessive myocardial oxygen demand. Approximately 50% of persons with critical aortic stenosis have associated CAD. In the latter group, angina pectoris is due to increased myocardial metabolic demand coupled with decreased myocardial blood flow secondary to coronary arterial stenosis. Syncope in aortic stenosis can be caused by atrial or ventricular arrhythmias, or it can occur secondary to exercise-induced peripheral vasodilatation together with fixed reduced cardiac output. In the latter situation, hypotension with decreased cerebral perfusion and syncope results. Vertiginous episodes often occur between frank syncopal attacks. Left ventricular failure in aortic stenosis comes from LVH, fibrosis, and ischemia. Patients complain of exercise intolerance and fatigue. Paroxysmal nocturnal dyspnea, orthopnea, and even pulmonary edema may occur. The development of right ventricular failure is an ominous sign in patients with aortic stenosis. Survival following the onset of signs of right ventricular failure (peripheral edema, hepatomegaly, jugular venous distention) is likely to be a matter of weeks to months.

  2. Physical examination. A loud, rasping, crescendo-decrescendo systolic murmur loudest along the right sternal border is the hallmark of aortic stenosis. The degree of narrowing of the aortic valve orifice can be estimated from a careful examination of the carotid pulse and the left ventricular apical impulse.

    Patients with critical aortic stenosis have a slowly rising diminutive (**parvus et tardus,** "small and late") carotid pulse and an enlarged, sustained apical impulse (left ventricular lift or heave). A prominent notch (anacrotic notch) may be noted on the carotid upstroke. A shudder or thrill is often palpated in the carotid pulse. The thrill is the result of vibrations that produce the systolic murmur radiating from the heart and heard over the carotid vessels.

    Physical findings in aortic stenosis are as follows (not all findings are present in every patient with aortic stenosis):

Narrow pulse pressure
Pulsus alternans
Slow rising, diminutive carotid pulse with prominent anacrotic notch

Systolic thrill along the upper right sternal border

Enlarged, sustained left ventricular impulse

Normal S1

Early systolic ejection click

Decreased or absent aortic component of S2

Rasping, crescendo-decrescendo (ejection) systolic murmur along the
  right sternal border, radiating to the right clavicle and the carotid
  vessels

S4 common; S3 when left ventricular failure is present

Elderly patients may have carotid pulses that feel surprisingly normal, despite the presence of severe aortic stenosis.

3. ECG. Patients with critical aortic stenosis almost invariably have LVH with associated ST–T changes. An occasional patient (usually female) will have a normal ECG or a tracing that demonstrates only left axis deviation or ST–T changes. Left atrial enlargement often accompanies LVH. Patients with aortic stenosis may have a variety of conduction defects in the ECG, including complete left and right bundle branch block or intraventricular conduction delays. Conduction defects in patients with aortic stenosis are often the result of extension of the calcific process from the aortic valve into the septum with involvement of the bundle of His. Atrial fibrillation rarely occurs in patients with severe aortic stenosis. Those who develop atrial fibrillation often manifest hemodynamic deterioration secondary to the loss of the atrial kick. ECG findings in aortic stenosis are

Atrial fibrillation (unusual and often accompanied by hemodynamic
  deterioration)

Left ventricular hypertrophy

Left atrial enlargement

Conduction defects: left and right bundle branch block, intraventricular
  conduction delay

4. Chest x-ray examination. The overall heart size is often normal in patients with aortic stenosis, even when the valve is critically narrowed. Left ventricular prominence may be noted, however. The ascending aorta is dilated (poststenotic dilatation) and can be seen to the right of the sternum. Calcification of the aortic valve is frequently apparent on the plain chest film. Fluoroscopy readily demonstrates the calcified valve. In elderly patients, calcification is a requirement for the diagnosis of severe aortic stenosis. Roentgenographic findings in aortic stenosis are

Left ventricular enlargement

Prominent ascending aorta

Aortic valve calcification

5. Echocardiography. The fibrotic and calcified aortic valve usually can be visualized by echocardiography. Often the narrowed aortic valve orifice can be seen, and the severity of aortic stenosis can be estimated. Doppler study enables the physician to calculate the aortic valve gradient. Other echocardiographic findings that point toward severe aortic stenosis are LVH and dilatation and left atrial enlargement. Left ventricular function can be quantitated.

6. Radionuclide studies. Left ventricular function can be quantitated from the radionuclide ventriculogram. A false-positive technetium pyrophosphate scan (suggesting MI) can be obtained in patients with calcific aortic stenosis because of a high concentration of the tracer in the calcified valve.

7. Cardiac catheterization and angiography. As with mitral stenosis, the gradient across the stenotic aortic valve can be measured at the time of cardiac catheterization. Heart rate, cardiac output, and valvular gradient are determined and used to calculate effective aortic valve orifice size. Patients with an orifice size equal to or less than 0.7 cm^2 are said to have critical aortic stenosis, those whose valve area is between 0.8 and 1.0 cm^2

have moderately severe aortic stenosis, and individuals with aortic valve areas greater than 1 cm^2 have mild to moderate stenosis. Left ventricular filling pressures are frequently elevated in patients with severe aortic stenosis because of (i) decreased left ventricular function and (ii) markedly increased left ventricular stiffness secondary to hypertrophy.

Angiography documents the presence or absence of aortic regurgitation, the state of left ventricular contraction, and the condition of the coronary arteries. Half the patients with severe aortic stenosis have concomitant CAD. Balloon valvuloplasty can be performed at the time of cardiac catheterization.

8. Protocol for the diagnosis of aortic stenosis

a. Testing sequence and protocol for making the diagnosis. The diagnosis of aortic stenosis usually can be made on the basis of appropriate history and physical examination, combined with an ECG demonstrating LVH and a chest x-ray film revealing a prominent ascending aorta. Confirmation of the diagnosis rests on echocardiographic visualization of the stenotic aortic valve and Doppler calculation of the aortic valve gradient. A suggested protocol for the evaluation of patients with suspected aortic stenosis is the following. The dashed arrow indicates that this step is optional.

History and physical examination
↓
Chest x-ray study and ECG
↓
Echocardiography and Doppler study
↓
Cardiac catheterization: for consideration of surgery, coronary arteriography usually mandatory; other information obtained **in selected individuals**

b. Criteria for the diagnosis. Individuals with angina, syncope, or heart failure, an abnormal carotid pulse (slow upstroke, small volume, or both), a systolic ejection murmur, and evidence of left ventricular enlargement on physical examination, ECG, or chest x-ray film should be suspected of having aortic stenosis. Heavy calcification of the aortic valve on fluoroscopy or chest x-ray is strong supporting evidence. The diagnosis is confirmed by obtaining an abnormal echocardiogram revealing heavy calcification or fibrosis (or both) of the aortic valve, together with a Doppler demonstration of an aortic valve gradient. Catheterization may be required to make the diagnosis in a rare individual.

c. Differential diagnosis

(1) Aortic sclerosis. Elderly individuals frequently have some fibrosis or atherosclerosis of the aortic valve. This can give rise to a systolic ejection murmur in the absence of significant aortic valve obstruction. The benign nature of the murmur is confirmed by documenting a normal carotid pulse, absence of LVH by physical examination and ECG, and a normal or mildly reduced aortic valve orifice as disclosed by echocardiography and Doppler study.

(2) Mitral regurgitation. The systolic murmur of mitral regurgitation can be confused with that of aortic stenosis. Both conditions give rise to left ventricular enlargement and hypertrophy; however, the murmur of mitral regurgitation is likely to be holosystolic and loudest at the apex, with radiation to the axilla, whereas the murmur of aortic stenosis is ejection in type and loudest at the base with radiation to the neck. The carotid pulse is normal in mitral regurgitation, and the echocardiogram and Doppler study reveal a normal aortic valve.

(3) VSD. The holosystolic murmur of VSD is often heard only in the vicinity of the lower left sternal border. Left ventricular enlargement and hypertrophy may occur with this defect, and hence it may be confused with aortic stenosis. As with mitral regurgitation, the carotid pulse is normal, and the echocardiogram and Doppler study reveal a normal aortic valve and a left-to-right shunt.

(4) Idiopathic hypertrophic subaortic stenosis (hypertrophic cardiomyopathy). IHSS, a subvalvular form of aortic stenosis, is discussed at length in Chapter 18. It can resemble valvular aortic stenosis in its presentation, with a systolic ejection murmur at the base and evidence of LVH on physical examination and ECG. The carotid pulse is brisk in IHSS, however, and the echocardiogram reveals a distinctive pattern with a normal aortic valve, a markedly thickened septum, and abnormal motion of the anterior mitral valve leaflet. Myocardial scintigraphy with thallium reveals a disproportionately thick septum in patients with muscular subaortic stenosis.

(5) Supravalvular aortic stenosis. Supravalvular aortic stenosis is a rare variant of aortic stenosis in which the obstruction occurs as a result of a circumferential stenosis or constriction of the ascending aorta just above the aortic valve. This is a congenital condition that often accompanies infantile hypercalcemia. Mental retardation is commonly associated as well. The clinical presentation resembles that of valvular aortic stenosis, except for the absence of aortic valvular calcification on x-ray examination, the demonstration of a normal aortic valve on echocardiography, and considerable difference between blood pressures taken in both arms. Angiography is often required to demonstrate the supravalvular stenotic segment.

(6) Pulmonic stenosis. The murmur of pulmonic stenosis often resembles that of aortic stenosis, although it is usually most prominent along the left sternal border and fails to radiate to the neck. Right ventricular enlargement and hypertrophy are noted on the physical examination, ECG, and chest x-ray film; the echocardiogram demonstrates a normal aortic valve.

(7) Aortic regurgitation. The large stroke volume associated with aortic regurgitation often produces a prominent systolic ejection murmur.

The left ventricle is dilated and eccentrically hypertrophied, and the ascending aorta is prominent on the chest x-ray picture. The carotid pulse is brisk and the pulse pressure wide in aortic regurgitation. In addition, the echocardiogram demonstrates a dilated, hypercontractile left ventricle with distinctive diastolic vibrations of the anterior mitral valve leaflet. Doppler study documents and quantitates the amount of aortic regurgitation.

B. Therapy
  1. Medical treatment
    a. Left ventricular failure. Patients with aortic stenosis who require medical therapy should be considered for aortic valve replacement, because symptoms in aortic stenosis signal the onset of a phase in the natural history of the disease in which sudden death becomes increasingly common. Patients who present with signs and symptoms of left ventricular failure, however, should be digitalized. Careful administration of diuretics also may be necessary. Patients with aortic stenosis depend on adequate preload (ventricular filling) to maintain cardiac output. Overdiuresis (surprisingly easy) in patients with aortic stenosis can rapidly decrease cardiac output to the point at which azotemia and even hypotension occur. Vasodilators should be used with great caution if at all, because they may lead to a drop in car-

diac output and rapidly progressive renal insufficiency or hypotension in patients with aortic stenosis. In patients with aortic stenosis and heart failure who are not candidates for aortic valve replacement, small doses of an ACE inhibitor may be administered with careful monitoring of blood pressure and renal function.

    b. Activity. Physical exertion should be limited in individuals with moderate to severe aortic stenosis. Isometric forms of exercise are contraindicated, although routine light exertion such as walking is permitted. As noted already, many of these individuals should have definitive surgical therapy.

    c. Antibiotics. Patients with any form or degree of severity of aortic valve disease should receive prophylactic antibiotics with dental and surgical procedures (Tables 16-5 to 16-7).

    d. Cardioversion. Patients with aortic stenosis who develop atrial fibrillation may suffer marked hemodynamic deterioration owing to the loss of the atrial kick. Rapid electrical cardioversion to sinus rhythm is indicated.

  2. Surgery. Symptomatic patients with aortic stenosis should be strongly considered for definitive surgical therapy. Medical therapy is used to temporize until surgery can be scheduled. Unless **very severe** left ventricular dysfunction is present (ejection fraction less than or equal to 10%), all patients with aortic stenosis are candidates for surgical therapy.

    a. Valvuloplasty. Aortic valvuloplasty consists of incision of the aortic valve in an attempt to open congenitally fused commissures. The operation is performed only in young persons with congenital aortic stenosis whose valve is not calcified. The valve eventually restenoses, and aortic valve replacement becomes necessary. Aortic valvuloplasty may be performed at the time of cardiac catheterization by use of a balloon catheter. Benefit from aortic balloon valvuloplasty is almost invariably short-lived in older adult patients. Hence, balloon valvuloplasty of aortic stenosis is used primarily in children with congenital aortic stenosis.

    b. Aortic valve replacement. A variety of valves can be inserted into the aortic position after excision of the distorted, calcified native valve. Most patients with aortic stenosis who become symptomatic will require aortic valve replacement rather than valvuloplasty. Plastic and metal prosthetic devices or tissue valves (porcine xenograft or homograft) can be sewn into the aortic annulus. Often a small residual gradient (mild aortic stenosis) persists after successful aortic valve replacement. The surgical mortality for patients with good left ventricular function should be less than 5%.

V. Aortic regurgitation. Described for the first time in the seventeenth century, aortic regurgitation has always held great interest for physicians. Numerous eponyms are attached to the various physical findings associated with it. Many different factors can cause it. The most common causes of this valvular lesion are rheumatic heart disease, degenerative changes in a tricuspid or bicuspid valve, and bacterial endocarditis.

Etiologic agents that result in aortic regurgitation are listed in Table 16-9. As with mitral regurgitation, there is a considerable difference in natural history and prognosis between chronic and acute aortic regurgitation. Chronic regurgitation may be tolerated by individuals for decades without symptoms, whereas patients may develop refractory left ventricular failure and a rapid downhill course secondary to acute aortic regurgitation.

  A. Diagnosis

    1. History. Patients with aortic regurgitation are usually asymptomatic for decades because the left ventricle is able to compensate for the volume overload imposed by the valvular regurgitation. Late in the course of the disease (usually the fourth decade or later), symptoms of left ventricular failure (dyspnea on exertion, orthopnea, paroxysmal nocturnal dyspnea) often occur. Syncope is rare, and angina pectoris in the absence of

TABLE 16-9. ETIOLOGY OF AORTIC REGURGITATION

I. Inflammatory
   A. Rheumatic heart disease
   B. Ankylosing spondylitis
   C. Rheumatoid arthritis
   D. Systemic lupus erythematosus
   E. Syphilis

II. Structural
   A. Atherosclerosis
   B. Bicuspid or unicuspid valve
   C. Dissection
   D. Endocarditis
   E. Ventricular septal defect
   F. Sinus of Valsalva aneurysm
   G. Trauma
   H. Myxomatous degeneration

III. Genetic
   A. Marfan's syndrome
   B. Mucopolysaccharidoses

IV. Stress
   A. Hypertension
   B. Renal failure

CAD is also unusual. The development of right ventricular failure is an ominous sign.

Some individuals remain asymptomatic despite dilated, poorly functioning left ventricles.

2. Physical examination. The high-pitched early diastolic murmur of aortic regurgitation is often missed by inexperienced auscultators. It is best to listen for this murmur with the diaphragm of the stethoscope, with the patient sitting upright, leaning forward, and deeply expiring. The murmur is loudest along the left sternal border in aortic regurgitation secondary to rheumatic heart disease and loudest along the right sternal border when regurgitation is secondary to factors that result in a dilated aortic root (e.g., syphilis or Marfan's syndrome). A prominent aortic systolic ejection murmur is often heard secondary to the increased volume of blood flowing through the aortic valve during each systole. A low, rumbling, middiastolic or presystolic apical murmur resembling that of mitral stenosis is likely to be heard in pure aortic regurgitation. This murmur is termed the **Austin Flint murmur.** Its cause is disputed. It is probably the result of either (i) functional mitral stenosis secondary to closure of the anterior mitral valve leaflet by the regurgitant jet or (ii) filtered vibrations of the aortic regurgitant murmur heard at the apex. S1 is often soft, and the aortic component of the S2 is often increased. Peripheral pulses are usually bounding, and many physical signs have been described over the past 150 years that relate to the hyperdynamic peripheral circulation. These signs and the eponyms attached to them are listed in Table 16-10. Other physical findings in aortic regurgitation are as follows (see Table 16-10 for peripheral signs):

Thrill or shudder felt in the carotid pulse
Bisferiens carotid pulse
Hyperdynamic left ventricular impulse
Soft S1
Loud S2

TABLE 16-10. SIGNS SECONDARY TO HYPERDYNAMIC PERIPHERAL CIRCULATION IN AORTIC REGURGITATION

Eponym	Sign
Wide pulse pressure	
Corrigan's pulse	Pulse brisk when it initially strikes the finger only to suddenly fade away; also called a waterhammer pulse
Quincke's pulse	Capillary pulsation seen in the skin with each systole
Hill's sign	Popliteal arterial pressure ≥60 mm Hg than brachial arterial pressure
Pistol-shot pulse (femoral)	Loud systolic sound heard over femoral artery with each cardiac cycle
Traube's sign	Double sound heard over femoral artery with each cardiac cycle
Duroziez's sign	Systolic and diastolic bruit heard if femoral artery is slightly compressed with stethoscope
de Musset's sign	Head bobbing with each systole
Müller's sign	Uvular pulsation with each systole
Rosenbach's sign	Liver pulsation with each systole
Gerhardt's sign	Pulsation in an enlarged spleen with each systole
Landolfi's sign	Changes in pupillary size with each systole

Blowing, high-pitched diastolic murmur heard along either sternal border
Austin Flint murmur
S3, S4

3. ECG. ECG changes in aortic regurgitation are usually limited to LVH. Initially the ECG reveals only increased left ventricular voltage. Late in the course of the illness associated ST–T changes may be present.
4. Chest x-ray examination. Aortic regurgitation produces a prominent ascending aorta, left ventricular enlargement, and, late in the course of the illness, signs of left ventricular failure in the chest roentgenogram. Aortic valve calcification may be present. Roentgenographic findings in aortic regurgitation are as follows:

Dilated ascending aorta
Enlarged left ventricle (may be massively enlarged)
Calcification of the aortic valve
Signs of left ventricular failure (pulmonary vascular redistribution, interstitial edema)

5. Echocardiography. The echocardiogram in aortic regurgitation demonstrates a dilated, hyperdynamic left ventricle. Aortic root and left atrial enlargement are also often present. The anterior mitral valve leaflet echo contains a characteristic marginal band of high-frequency vibrations. Similar vibrations can be seen in some patients in the left ventricular septal echo. Patients with acute aortic regurgitation demonstrate early closure of the mitral valve secondary to rapidly rising left ventricular diastolic pressure. Doppler echocardiography is very sensitive for demonstrating and quantitating the volume of aortic regurgitant flow. Many cardiologists perform serial echocardiography to monitor changes in left ventricular function.
6. Radionuclide studies. Left ventricular function can be quantitated both at rest and during exercise by radionuclide ventriculography in patients with aortic regurgitation. It has been suggested that failure of the ejection fraction to increase with exercise in these patients is an early sign of left ventricular decompensation. The exact role of serial rest and ex-

ercise radionuclide ventriculograms in monitoring patients with aortic regurgitation has not yet been defined. Using differential stroke volume ratios of the right and left ventricles, radionuclide ventriculography can estimate semiquantitatively the severity of aortic regurgitation.

7. Catheterization and angiography. Hemodynamic changes in patients with aortic regurgitation include a marked increase in left ventricular end-diastolic pressure and low aortic diastolic pressure. The left ventricular systolic pressure may be normal or elevated. A small systolic gradient (5 to 19 mm Hg) may exist across the aortic valve, even though no significant aortic stenosis is present. The gradient is the result of markedly increased systolic flow across an aortic valve that is distorted and stiff.

Angiography is used to quantitate the amount of aortic regurgitation and the state of left ventricular function. The quantity of aortic regurgitation is expressed semiquantitatively as 1 to 4+. Aortic root angiography may also demonstrate the etiology of the aortic regurgitation (e.g., dissection, sinus of Valsalva aneurysm, or luetic aortic aneurysm). Some individuals have mixed aortic valve disease with moderate aortic stenosis and moderate aortic regurgitation. It is not possible to have both severe aortic stenosis and severe aortic regurgitation.

8. Protocol for the diagnosis of aortic regurgitation
    a. Testing sequence for the diagnosis. The diagnosis of aortic regurgitation is based on appropriate history, physical examination, chest x-ray film, and ECG with confirmation by echocardiography and occasionally catheterization. An appropriate diagnostic sequence is as follows (dashed arrow indicates optional step):

    History suggesting one of the etiologies of aortic regurgitation
    ↓
    Murmur and peripheral findings of aortic regurgitation
    ↓
    ECG and chest x-ray film
    ↓
    Echocardiogram + Doppler radionuclide ventriculography
    ↓
    Cardiac catheterization **in selected individuals**

    b. Criteria for the diagnosis
        (1) A significant degree of aortic regurgitation can exist in individuals with or without symptoms of left ventricular failure. Patients have one of the conditions that causes aortic regurgitation (Table 16-9), with a high-pitched diastolic blowing murmur heard at the base and a hyperdynamic left ventricle and peripheral circulation. The ECG usually demonstrates increased left ventricular voltage; the chest x-ray picture reveals a prominent ascending aorta and left ventricle; the echocardiogram demonstrates a hyperdynamic left ventricle and characteristic high-frequency vibrations of the anterior mitral valve leaflet; and Doppler study documents and quantitates aortic regurgitation.
        (2) Individuals with mild aortic regurgitation may have only a short, early diastolic aortic regurgitant murmur and the characteristic anterior mitral valve leaflet vibrations on echocardiography. Left ventricular enlargement and hyperactivity are usually absent in these patients, as are peripheral circulatory signs of aortic regurgitation. Mild aortic regurgitation is demonstrated by Doppler study.
        (3) Individuals with acute aortic regurgitation usually present with signs and symptoms of left ventricular failure, including a prominent S3. The murmur of aortic regurgitation may be difficult to appreciate, and left ventricular enlargement is often absent. Left ventricular and peripheral circulatory hyperactiv-

ity is less marked than with chronic forms of aortic regurgitation. The echocardiogram reveals a hyperdynamic left ventricle and, frequently, early closure of the mitral valve. Doppler study demonstrates aortic regurgitation.

   c. Differential diagnosis

     (1) Aortic stenosis. A prominent aortic systolic ejection murmur may be heard in patients with predominant or pure aortic regurgitation. This finding can be distinguished from aortic stenosis on the basis of the different peripheral circulatory findings in the two conditions: Aortic stenosis produces a slowly rising, small carotid pulse, whereas aortic regurgitation is associated with rapidly rising, bounding carotid pulsations. The echocardiogram reveals a dilated, hyperdynamic left ventricle and characteristic mitral valve vibrations in aortic regurgitation, findings not present in patients with aortic stenosis. Doppler study documents and quantitates aortic regurgitation.

     (2) Pulmonic insufficiency. Usually the result of severe pulmonary hypertension (Graham Steell murmur), pulmonic insufficiency is often secondary to mitral stenosis or Eisenmenger's syndrome secondary to a congenital defect. The murmur can resemble that of aortic regurgitation, but **right** ventricular enlargement and hypertrophy are present with pulmonic regurgitation, and **left** ventricular involvement occurs with aortic regurgitation. The peripheral circulatory findings of aortic regurgitation are likewise absent in patients with Graham Steell murmurs. Doppler study documents and quantitates aortic regurgitation. If doubt still exists, aortic angiography can settle the issue by demonstrating the presence or absence of aortic regurgitation.

     (3) Mitral stenosis. As noted earlier, the Austin Flint murmur may mimic the murmur of mitral stenosis. The disappearance of the Austin Flint murmur with inhalation of amyl nitrite and the presence of a normal mitral valve echo rule out mitral stenosis as the cause of the diastolic rumbling murmur.

     (4) Patent ductus arteriosus. The continuous murmur of patent ductus arteriosus occasionally is confused with the systolic and diastolic murmurs often present in aortic regurgitation. A wide pulse pressure frequently accompanies both conditions; however, the murmur of patent ductus is continuous (i.e., it continues through the S2 and, in fact, peaks in loudness at that point). The chest x-ray film reveals pulmonary shunt vasculature in patients with a patent ductus, and radionuclide angiocardiography, Doppler echocardiography and cardiac catheterization demonstrate a left-to-right shunt. Both the latter findings are absent in patients with aortic regurgitation.

B. Therapy

  1. Medical treatment

    a. Digitalis, diuretics, and vasodilators. Patients with aortic insufficiency who manifest left ventricular failure should be digitalized. If signs and symptoms of left ventricular failure do not respond adequately to therapy with digitalis alone, a diuretic should be added to the regimen. Most cardiologists favor early vasodilator therapy with ACE inhibitors. The combination of hydralazine and long-acting nitrates can be used in patients who cannot tolerate ACE inhibitors. Patients who develop signs and symptoms of left ventricular failure (or rarely angina or syncope) should be strongly considered for aortic valve replacement (see Section **V.B.2.**). Many cardiologists advocate the use of prophylactic ACE inhibitors or other arteriolar vasodilator in patients with asymptomatic aortic regurgitation. A number of studies have documented that left ventricular function is preserved and remodeling of the ventricle is prevented with such a strategy.

    b. Antiarrhythmic drugs. Occasionally patients with aortic insufficiency develop atrial fibrillation. This arrhythmia is not as devastating for individuals with aortic insufficiency as it is for those with aortic stenosis. Hence, cardioversion may be undertaken electively, with ventricular response controlled in the interim by digitalis, AV blocking calcium channel blockers and/or beta-blockers. High-grade ventricular arrhythmias (e.g., ventricular tachycardia) can be controlled by a variety of medications, as with other cardiac conditions (see Chapter 3). Large doses of beta-blockers should generally be avoided in patients with severe aortic insufficiency because they may precipitate left ventricular failure.

    c. Prophylactic antibiotics. Antibiotics should be administered to patients with all degrees of aortic insufficiency at the time of dental or surgical procedures (Tables 16-5 to 16-7).

    d. Activity. There is no need to limit activity in asymptomatic patients with aortic insufficiency. When left ventricular failure develops, moderate limitation of activity is prudent (see Chapter 4).

    e. Diet. There is no need to limit salt intake in asymptomatic patients with aortic insufficiency. Those who show signs or symptoms of left ventricular failure should restrict salt intake modestly (see Chapter 4).

  2. Surgery. Patients who develop signs or symptoms of left ventricular failure should be strongly considered for aortic valve replacement. Left ventricular function should be carefully determined (echocardiography, radionuclide angiography, catheterization with angiography), because a minority of such individuals will have developed irreversible left ventricular dysfunction.

    Most cardiologists advise aortic valve replacement at the earliest signs of left ventricular failure. In many patients, the earliest sign of left ventricular failure is progressive dilation of the left ventricle by echocardiography. Many cardiologists advise aortic valve replacement for patients with severe aortic regurgitation when the end-systolic diameter of the left ventricle exceeds 55 mm on an echocardiographic examination. Therefore, patients with severe aortic regurgitation are followed with serial echocardiographic studies every 6 to 12 months, depending on the degree of left ventricular dilation present.

    Patients with moderately severe aortic insufficiency who are undergoing mitral valve replacement probably should have concomitant aortic valve replacement.

VI. Tricuspid stenosis. Tricuspid stenosis is an unusual valvular lesion. It is almost invariably associated with rheumatic mitral stenosis. Rheumatic aortic valve disease also can be present, resulting in triple valve disease. Other rare causes of tricuspid stenosis include congenital fusion of valve cusps, obstruction of the tricuspid valve orifice by vegetations of bacterial endocarditis or thrombus, and carcinoid neoplasms.

    The clinical picture is dominated by signs and symptoms of right ventricular failure (jugular venous distention, hepatomegaly, peripheral edema) secondary to tricuspid stenosis, as well as by signs and symptoms of pulmonary congestion secondary to associated mitral valve disease. The jugular venous pulse shows a very prominent A wave. The ECG reveals right atrial enlargement or atrial fibrillation; the chest film discloses an enlarged right atrium projecting to the right of the sternum. The echocardiogram demonstrates a thickened tricuspid valve with reduced motion. Echocardiography and Doppler study demonstrate and quantitate the degree of tricuspid stenosis present by documenting the severity of the tricuspid valve gradient. Catheterization documents a gradient across the tricuspid valve. The approach to therapy is dominated by the associated valvular lesions, with tricuspid valvuloplasty or replacement occurring at the time of mitral valve surgery. The clinical findings in tricuspid stenosis are summarized in Table 16-11.

VII. Tricuspid regurgitation. Tricuspid regurgitation can be the result of primary valvular disease, or it may occur secondary to right ventricular dilatation and failure. Table 16-12 lists primary and secondary etiologies of tricuspid regurgi-

TABLE 16-11. CLINICAL FINDINGS IN PATIENTS WITH TRICUSPID STENOSIS

History
  Invariably associated with rheumatic mitral stenosis; symptoms usually originate from
    mitral valve disease, including dyspnea on exertion, orthopnea, and paroxysmal
    nocturnal dyspnea

Physical examination
  Pulsating neck veins with prominent, giant A waves
  Tender, enlarged, pulsating liver
  Rumbling diastolic murmur at left sternal border, increasing with inspiration
  Opening snap
  Ascites
  Peripheral edema

ECG
  Right atrial enlargement or atrial fibrillation

Chest x-ray film
  Enlarged right atrium

Echocardiogram, Doppler
  Thickened tricuspid valve with decreased motion; tricuspid valve gradient

Catheterization
  Diastolic gradient across the tricuspid valve

Treatment
  Prophylactic antibiotics with dental or surgical procedures
  Valvuloplasty or valve replacement for signs and symptoms of right ventricular failure

---

tation. Primary tricuspid regurgitation is said to be organic in origin, whereas
secondary tricuspid regurgitation is termed **functional.** Rheumatic valvular involvement is the most common cause of organic tricuspid regurgitation. Tricuspid
valvular involvement in rheumatic heart disease does not occur alone but always
accompanies mitral or aortic valvular disease. Ebstein's anomaly is an unusual
form of congenital heart disease in which a morphologically abnormal tricuspid
valve is displaced down into the right ventricle. The result is a large, poorly functioning right atrium; a small, stiff right ventricle; and tricuspid regurgitation.
  A. Diagnosis
      1. History. Patients with tricuspid regurgitation present with the clinical
         picture of severe right-sided heart failure. Fatigue, peripheral edema,

---

TABLE 16-12. ETIOLOGY OF TRICUSPID REGURGITATION

Primary or organic
  Rheumatic heart disease
  Bacterial endocarditis
  Tricuspid valve prolapse from myxomatous degeneration
  Ebstein's anomaly
  Trauma
  Right ventricular infarction involving papillary muscles
  Carcinoid tumors

Secondary or functional
  Right ventricular dilatation and failure caused by
    1. Left ventricular failure
    2. Pathologic right-sided heart conditions (e.g., pulmonic stenosis, Eisenmenger's
       syndrome, primary pulmonary hypertension)

anorexia, and abdominal swelling are the main symptoms. Dyspnea occurs only as a result of associated, pathologic left-sided heart conditions. Often dyspnea on exertion and orthopnea resolve when patients with left ventricular failure develop tricuspid regurgitation, probably because of decreased right ventricular output into the pulmonary circulation. Pain in the right upper quadrant secondary to hepatic congestion is occasionally the presenting complaint.

2. Physical examination. Tricuspid regurgitation produces signs of right ventricular failure including jugular venous distention, hepatomegaly, and peripheral edema. The morphology of the jugular venous pulse is distinctive in most forms of tricuspid regurgitation, with large V waves accompanying each systole. Patients with Ebstein's anomaly do not demonstrate cervical venous V waves because the tricuspid regurgitant bolus is delivered into a grossly dilated right atrium, so that only a minimal rise in pressure occurs. Hepatic systolic pulsation, hepatojugular reflux, ascites, anasarca, and pleural effusion can all occur in patients with severe tricuspid regurgitation. Peripheral cyanosis secondary to low cardiac output and icterus resulting from hepatic congestion and dysfunction occur in individuals with long-standing tricuspid regurgitation.

Patients with Ebstein's anomaly have a distinctive cardiac examination: A loud tricuspid component of the S1 is followed by a murmur of tricuspid regurgitation and loud S3 or S4 or both. The auscultatory findings in Ebstein's anomaly have been likened to the sounds of a steam locomotive. Physical findings in patients with tricuspid regurgitation are as follows:

Irregularly irregular pulse (atrial fibrillation)
Icterus
Jugular venous distention with prominent v waves
Pleural effusion
Right ventricular impulse along left sternal border
Holosystolic murmur at lower left sternal border, which often increases with inspiration
Hepatomegaly
Systolic hepatic pulsations
Hepatojugular reflux
Ascites
Peripheral edema and occasionally anasarca

3. ECG. The ECG often demonstrates right atrial enlargement or RVH (or both) in patients with organic tricuspid regurgitation. Atrial fibrillation is common. Patients with Ebstein's anomaly demonstrate right bundle branch block, prolonged P–R interval (when sinus rhythm is present), and frequently the Wolff-Parkinson-White syndrome.

ECG findings in patients with tricuspid regurgitation are summarized in Table 16-13.

4. Chest x-ray film. The transverse diameter of the heart is increased secondary to right atrial enlargement. In the posteroanterior view, the right heart border is displaced approximately 2 inches or more beyond the

TABLE 16-13. ECG FINDINGS IN TRICUSPID REGURGITATION

Atrial fibrillation
Right atrial enlargement
Right ventricular hypertrophy

Ebstein's anomaly
  First-degree atrioventricular block (when sinus rhythm is present)
  Right bundle branch block
  Wolff-Parkinson-White syndrome

right sternal border. Right ventricular enlargement is also frequently present. Enlarged left-sided heart chambers and pulmonary congestion are observed in patients with functional tricuspid regurgitation secondary to left-sided heart lesions. Individuals with Ebstein's anomaly have markedly enlarged right atria and small pulmonary arteries. Roentgenographic findings in patients with tricuspid regurgitation are shown in Table 16-14.

5. Echocardiography. The echocardiogram usually discloses right ventricular cavity dilatation and paradoxical septal motion in patients with tricuspid regurgitation. Other specific findings may include tricuspid valve prolapse, vegetations, or rheumatic thickening and decreased motion of the valve. Patients with Ebstein's anomaly often demonstrate simultaneously visualized mitral and tricuspid valve echoes with delayed tricuspid valve closure. Doppler echocardiography is very sensitive for demonstrating and quantitating tricuspid regurgitation.

6. Radionuclide studies. An enlarged right ventricle with abnormally depressed ejection fraction may be noted with radionuclide ventriculography.

7. Catheterization and angiography. Right atrial pressure is often increased, and the pressure tracing resembles the jugular venous tracing with a decreased X descent, an increased Y descent, and prominent V waves. Right ventriculography demonstrates dilated right atrial and ventricular cavities and marked tricuspid regurgitation. Patients with Ebstein's anomaly have right ventricular electrocardiographic complexes recorded simultaneously with a right atrial pressure curve.

8. Protocol for the diagnosis of tricuspid regurgitation
    a. Testing sequence. The following sequence for the workup of patients with tricuspid regurgitation is suggested (dashed arrow indicates optional step):

History and physical examination
↓
(characteristic murmur and neck veins)
↓
ECG and chest x-ray film
↓
(right atrial or right ventricular enlargement)
↓
Echocardiography + Doppler
↓
(right ventricular enlargement and paradoxical septal motion)
↓
Cardiac catheterization **in selected individuals**

TABLE 16-14. ROENTGENOGRAPHIC FINDINGS IN TRICUSPID REGURGITATION

Primary tricuspid regurgitation
  Right atrial enlargement
  Right ventricular enlargement
  Prominent superior vena cava and right innominate vein

Secondary tricuspid regurgitation
  Enlargement of pulmonary arteries
  Enlargement of left-sided heart chambers
  Pulmonary congestion

Ebstein's anomaly
  Marked right atrial enlargement
  Small pulmonary arteries
  Clear lung fields

b. Criteria for making the diagnosis. The diagnosis of tricuspid regurgitation is made when one of the following sets of criteria is met:

    (1) An individual with or without symptoms of right ventricular failure (fatigue, anorexia, peripheral edema) has neck veins with prominent V waves, a holosystolic murmur along the left sternal edge that often increases on inspiration, hepatomegaly, and peripheral edema. The ECG shows atrial fibrillation or right atrial enlargement and RVH; the chest x-ray film reveals an enlarged right atrium. Echocardiography reveals a large right ventricular cavity and paradoxical septal motion. Doppler study documents and quantitates the volume of tricuspid regurgitation flow.

        (a) Catheterization and angiography rarely are required to make the diagnosis of tricuspid regurgitation. Selected individuals will need these invasive diagnostic techniques to confirm the diagnosis, usually before surgery on the tricuspid valve.

        (b) The differentiation of organic from functional tricuspid regurgitation is based on the presence of associated heart disease (e.g., mitral stenosis) with pulmonary hypertension and the echocardiographic appearance of the tricuspid valve.

    (2) Ebstein's anomaly is diagnosed in individuals who are often cyanotic with normal jugular venous pulsations and characteristic cardiac auscultatory findings (loud tricuspid component of S1, murmur of tricuspid regurgitation, and loud S4). The ECG reveals right bundle branch block and frequently Wolff-Parkinson-White syndrome. The chest x-ray film demonstrates a very large right atrium. Catheterization is usually necessary to confirm the diagnosis: A combined pressure and electrode catheter is advanced to the right ventricle. Simultaneous right ventricular pressure and electrocardiographic pattern are recorded. The catheter is gradually withdrawn to the right atrium. In healthy individuals, the ECG pattern changes from a right ventricular to a right atrial pattern at the same time as the hemodynamic tracing shows a change from right ventricular to right atrial pressure. Patients with Ebstein's anomaly continue to demonstrate a right ventricular ECG pattern after the pressure tracing reveals a transition from right ventricular to right atrial pressure.

c. Differential diagnosis

    (1) Mitral regurgitation. The holosystolic murmur of mitral regurgitation often resembles that of tricuspid regurgitation. The correct diagnosis is suggested by inspiratory increase in the intensity of the murmur and large V waves in the jugular venous pulse in patients with tricuspid regurgitation. Also helpful is the presence of right ventricular dilatation and paradoxical septal motion by echocardiography with tricuspid regurgitation. Doppler study demonstrates mitral or tricuspid regurgitation. It is not uncommon for mitral and tricuspid valvular regurgitation to coexist.

    (2) Aortic stenosis. The systolic ejection murmur of aortic stenosis is, at times, confused with the murmur of tricuspid regurgitation. Only the latter, however, increases in loudness during inspiration. As noted in the preceding paragraph, examination of the jugular venous pulse and the echocardiogram should distinguish these two lesions.

    (3) Idiopathic hypertrophic subaortic stenosis (hypertrophic cardiomyopathy). The combined aortic outflow and mitral regurgitant murmurs of subaortic stenosis may be confused with the murmur of tricuspid regurgitation. As already noted, changes in the

intensity of the murmur with respiration, the jugular venous pulse morphology, and echocardiographic findings help distinguish these two lesions.

(4) VSD. The murmur of VSD is holosystolic and loudest along the lower left sternal edge. It therefore resembles the murmur of tricuspid regurgitation. Attention to variation in the murmur's intensity during respiration, the form of the jugular venous pulse, and the echocardiogram should help distinguish these two lesions.

B. Therapy
  1. Medical treatment
    a. Antibiotics. Prophylactic antibiotics are administered to patients with tricuspid regurgitation who undergo dental or surgical procedures (Tables 16-5 to 16-7).
    b. Diuretics, digitalis, and vasodilators. Right ventricular failure secondary to tricuspid regurgitation is treated primarily with diuretics and ACE inhibitors. Decreased activity and modest salt restriction also are indicated. Digitalization plays a minor role in the treatment of right ventricular failure. Digitalis glycosides are important, however, for heart rate control in patients with atrial fibrillation. Vasodilator therapy has not been shown to benefit patients with primary or organic tricuspid regurgitation; however, vasodilator therapy can decrease left ventricular filling pressure, with a resultant fall in pulmonary arterial pressure. Thus, right ventricular work is decreased, and secondary or functional tricuspid regurgitation may improve.
    c. Anticoagulants. Patients with right ventricular failure who are put to bed are at high risk for the development of venous thrombosis and pulmonary embolism. Low-dose heparin therapy (subcutaneous unfractionated or low-molecular-weight heparin) is indicated until such patients are ambulatory. If signs of right ventricular failure persist despite therapy, or if the patient is not fully ambulatory, long-term oral anticoagulation with warfarin should be considered.
  2. Surgery
    a. Tricuspid valvuloplasty. Tricuspid valve annuloplasty can be performed successfully in patients with dilated annuli secondary to right ventricular dilatation and failure. A number of different procedures have been devised. Organic tricuspid valve disease usually requires valve replacement if severe regurgitation is present.
    b. Tricuspid valve replacement. Insertion of a prosthetic or tissue valve into the tricuspid position is necessary in individuals with severe organic (and often functional) tricuspid regurgitation. Tricuspid valve replacement frequently accompanies mitral or aortic valve replacement for rheumatic valvular disease.

      Ebstein's anomaly is often difficult to treat surgically because of the small, stiff right ventricle. Tricuspid valve replacement may result in severe right ventricular failure because of the right ventricle's inadequate size and function. Selected individuals can undergo tricuspid valve replacement.

VIII. Pulmonic stenosis. Pulmonic stenosis is discussed in Chapter 17.
 IX. Pulmonic regurgitation. Pulmonic regurgitation is an unusual valvular lesion. It is usually functional in nature, secondary to marked pulmonary hypertension. A rare individual develops endocarditis of the pulmonic valve or is born with a congenitally regurgitant valve. Pulmonic regurgitation with normal or near normal pulmonary arterial pressure is seen in patients who undergo successful surgical correction of pulmonic stenosis (pulmonary valvulotomy) or tetralogy of Fallot (reconstruction of right ventricular outflow tract).

  Pulmonic regurgitation is extremely well tolerated, and it is rare to see right ventricular failure solely on the basis of this lesion. Right ventricular dilatation and hypertrophy do occur, however, secondary to incompetence of the pulmonic valve. Fatigue and symptoms of right ventricular failure are occasionally reported in patients with pulmonic regurgitation, particularly if the regurgitant volume is large. Pulmonic regurgitation can produce a blowing or harsh diastolic murmur heard at the upper left sternal border. When pulmonic regurgitation is functional (secondary to severe pulmonary hypertension), it is called a Graham Steell murmur. The murmur of pulmonic regurgitation often increases with inspiration. The Graham Steell murmur of functional pulmonic regurgitation is high pitched, resembling the murmur of aortic regurgitation, whereas the murmur of organic pulmonic regurgitation is low pitched and often harsh. A systolic flow murmur often accompanies the diastolic murmur of pulmonic regurgitation. The ECG can be normal, or RVH may be present. The chest x-ray film may reveal right ventricular and pulmonary arterial enlargement. Doppler echocardiography usually documents and quantitates the presence and severity of pulmonic regurgitation. Pulmonary angiography is rarely required but can demonstrate diastolic reflux of contrast medium into the right ventricle. Treatment for pulmonic regurgitation is usually limited to administration of prophylactic antibiotics with dental or surgical procedures. Heart failure rarely occurs as a result of pulmonic regurgitation, but when right ventricular failure does develop, pulmonic valve replacement is indicated. The clinical features of patients with pulmonic regurgitation are summarized in Table 16-15.

X. Prosthetic valves. A variety of prosthetic valves are available to replace stenotic or regurgitant native valves. Each model and type of valve has distinct advan-

TABLE 16-15. CLINICAL FEATURES OF PULMONIC REGURGITATION

History
  Asymptomatic, or mild symptoms of right ventricular failure (fatigue, anorexia, peripheral edema)

Physical examination
  Right ventricular impulse palpable along left sternal border
  Systolic ejection click
  Wide but physiologically split second heart sound
  Systolic ejection murmur
  High-pitched, blowing diastolic murmur along upper left sternal border (Graham Steell)
  Low-pitched, harsh diastolic murmur along upper left sternal border (organic)

ECG
  Normal
  or
  Right ventricular hypertrophy

Chest x-ray film
  Normal
  or
  Right ventricular enlargement
  Pulmonary arterial enlargement

Echocardiography/Doppler
  Normal right ventricular size
  or
  Dilated right ventricle
  Presence of pulmonic regurgitation (Doppler)

Angiography
  Pulmonary angiography reveals pulmonic regurgitation

Treatment
  Prophylactic antibiotics with dental and surgical procedures
  Rarely, pulmonic valve replacement

tages and disadvantages. No prosthetic valve functions as well as, or is as free of problems as, a normal native valve.

A. **Tissue valves.** A variety of biologic valves have been implanted in patients for more than 20 years with considerable success. Tissue valves have the distinct advantage of not requiring long-term systemic anticoagulation with warfarin. A disadvantage inherent in tissue valves is that they are not as durable as mechanical (plastic and metal) valves and tend to degenerate after 10 to 12 years of use. Stenotic tissue valves can occasionally be reopened during cardiac catheterization by a balloon catheter.

1. **Porcine xenograft.** The porcine xenograft valve is made from a glutaraldehyde pig aortic valve attached to a sewing ring. It has had widespread use and is favored as the valve of first choice by many cardiac surgeons. Smaller porcine xenografts have relatively decreased valve areas. Thus, patients with small-valve annuli usually receive mechanical prostheses. The valve can be used as a semilunar or AV valve depending on how it is inserted.

   a. **Examples.** Edwards xenograft, Hancock xenograft.

2. **Homografts.** Fresh or preserved aortic valve transplants from human cadavers have been used extensively in patients who require valve replacement. Anticoagulation is not required but degenerative changes do occur in these valves with time. It is often difficult to obtain human valves.

3. **Bovine pericardial xenografts.** The bovine pericardial xenograft valve is made from preserved bovine pericardium attached to a sewing ring. It appears to resemble porcine xenografts with respect to advantages and disadvantages. It is apparently not as durable as the porcine heterograft.

   a. **Example:** Ionescu-Shiley xenograft.

B. **Mechanical valves**

1. **Ball valves.** The first prosthetic valves implanted in patients were ball valves. Ball valves consist of a composite plastic ball contained in a metal cage. The ball moves up and down with cardiac systole and diastole, thereby opening and closing the valve orifice. Some models have a cloth covering over all metal parts in an attempt to decrease the formation of blood clots on the metal parts of the valve. Systemic anticoagulation with warfarin is required for all patients with ball valves. Individuals who require surgical or extensive dental procedures and who have a mechanical valve implanted generally have their warfarin discontinued several days to a week before the surgical procedure. Daily doses of subcutaneous unfractionated or low-molecular-weight heparin are administered in place of warfarin until it is safe to resume oral anticoagulant therapy after surgery. For most forms of dental work, it is not necessary to discontinue warfarin therapy since the risk of bleeding is modest.

   a. **Examples:** Starr-Edwards, Smeloff-Cutler, DeBakey-Surgitool.

2. **Disk valves.** Disk valves are mechanical prostheses that contain a plastic or graphite disk in a metal cage. The disk moves up and down within the cage, thereby opening and closing the valve orifice. Anticoagulation is required with this valve.

   a. **Examples:** Björk-Shiley, Cooley-Cutler, Lillehei-Kaster, Wada-Cutter, Kay-Suzuki, Starr-Edwards, Beall-Surgitool, Kay-Shiley.

3. **Mechanical leaflet.** The St. Jude valve is a mechanical valve with two composite graphite leaflets that swing open and shut, thereby opening and closing the valve orifice. This valve has excellent hemodynamic characteristics. Anticoagulation is required.

C. **Complications.** Serious, life-threatening complications may result from prosthetic valve implantation.

1. **Prosthetic valve regurgitation and dehiscence.** Prosthetic valves are sewn into the heart with a cloth-covered sewing ring. Sutures can tear loose, or tissue may retract from the sewing ring, thereby resulting in moderate to severe degrees of valvular regurgitation. Valve replacement is often required. Xenograft valves are prone to degenerative changes that usually lead to regurgitation and occasionally to stenosis.

2. Prosthetic valve endocarditis. Prosthetic valves are highly prone to bacterial or fungal infection. Antibiotic prophylaxis with dental work or surgical procedures therefore should be meticulously adhered to in patients with prosthetic valves. Prosthetic valve endocarditis that develops within a month of valve implantation carries a worse prognosis than endocarditis that develops many weeks or months after valve placement. Mortality is high (50% to 70%), and valve replacement usually is required.

3. Thromboembolism. A blood clot may form on the sewing ring, struts, ball, or disk of a prosthetic valve. Depending on the location of the valve, pulmonary or arterial embolism can result. All mechanical valves require anticoagulation for life. Patients with xenografts or homografts are often anticoagulated transiently (1 to 3 months); however, anticoagulant therapy can lead to hemorrhage. Patients who remain in atrial fibrillation, regardless of valve type, should receive warfarin anticoagulation for life.

4. Prosthetic valve mismatch. Occasionally, an implanted prosthetic valve has too small an orifice for a particular patient. Signs and symptoms of valvular stenosis are observed in such individuals.

5. Valve thrombosis. Prosthetic valves may develop such a large amount of thrombus on the valve structure itself that the valve orifice becomes acutely obstructed. Marked ventricular failure is usually the result of this complication.

6. Hemolysis. Red blood cells may become hemolyzed by contact with mechanical valves. Small leaks around prosthetic valve sewing rings can result in a powerful regurgitant jet that also leads to red blood cell lysis. Such patients are anemic and icteric and have high serum lactic dehydrogenase values.

7. Prosthetic valve structural failure. Rarely, part of the structure of a mechanical valve may break. This can lead to orifice obstruction or massive valvular regurgitation with marked signs and symptoms of heart failure.

SELECTED READINGS

Barlow JB. Idiopathic (degenerative) and rheumatic mitral valve prolapse: historical aspects and an overview. *J Heart Valve Dis* 1992;1:163–174.
An excellent review of the mitral valve prolapse syndrome.
Ben Farhat M, Ayari M, Maatouk F, et al. Percutaneous balloon versus surgical closed and open mitral commissurotomy: seven-year follow-up results of a randomized trial. *Circulation* 1998;97:245–250.
Percutaneous balloon commissurotomy for mitral stenosis gave better long-term results than those of surgical commissurotomy.
Bonow RO, Lakatos E, Maron BJ, et al. Serial long-term assessment of the natural history of asymptomatic patients with chronic aortic regurgitation and normal left ventricular systolic function. *Circulation* 1991;84:1625–1635.
Noninvasive serial evaluation of left ventricular function predicts long-term outlook for patients with chronic aortic regurgitation.
Cappell MS, Lebwohl O. Cessation of recurrent bleeding from gastrointestinal angiodysplasias after aortic valve replacement. *Ann Intern Med* 1986;105:54–57.
Gastrointestinal bleeding from angiodysplastic vessels ceases after successful aortic valve replacement for aortic stenosis.
Dalen JE, Alpert JS. *Valvular heart disease,* 3rd ed. Philadelphia: Lippincott Williams & Wilkins, 1999.
Multiauthored reviews of pathophysiology and clinical aspects of patients with different forms of valvular heart disease.
Donofrio MT, Engle MA, O'Loughlin JE, et al. Congenital aortic regurgitation: natural history and management. *J Am Coll Cardiol* 1992;20:366–372.
Careful clinical follow-up is important in these patients to detect progression of aortic regurgitation.

Dubin AA, March HW, Cook K, et al. Longitudinal hemodynamic and clinical study of mitral stenosis. *Circulation* 1971;44:381–389.

Steadily progressive disability in some patients with mitral stenosis, distinctly more gradual course in others.

Dujardin KS, Enriquez-Sarano M, Schaff HV, et al. Mortality and morbidity of aortic regurgitation in clinical practice: a long-term follow-up study. *Circulation* 1999;99: 1851–1857.

Severe aortic regurgitation is associated with significant morbidity and mortality.

Faggiano P, Ghizzoni G, Sorgato A, et al. Rate of progression of valvular aortic stenosis in adults. *Am J Cardiol* 1992;70:229–233.

Mild to moderate aortic stenosis may progress to severe aortic stenosis over a number of months.

Freed LA, Levy D, Levine RA, et al. Prevalence and clinical outcome of mitral valve prolapse. *N Engl J Med* 1999;341:1–7.

In a community-based sample of the population, the prevalence of mitral valve prolapse was lower than previously reported. There were few adverse events in this population.

Gilon D, Buonanno FS, Joffe MM, et al. Lack of evidence of an association between mitral valve prolapse and stroke in young patients. *N Engl J Med* 1999;341:8–13.

No association was demonstrated between mitral valve prolapse and ischemic stroke in young patients.

Gordon SPF, Douglas PS, Come PC, et al. Two-dimensional and Doppler echocardiographic determinants of the natural history of mitral valve narrowing in patients with rheumatic mitral stenosis: implications for follow-up. *J Am Coll Cardiol* 1992;19:968–973.

Various echocardiographic variables predict the long-term course of patients with mitral stenosis.

Grigioni F, Enriquez-Sarano M, Zehr KJ, et al. Ischemic mitral regurgitation: long-term outcome and prognostic implications with quantitative Doppler assessment. *Circulation* 2001;103:1759–1764.

Ischemic mitral regurgitation is associated with excess mortality independent of left ventricular function or baseline characteristics of the patients.

Iung B, Garbarz E, Michaud P, et al. Late results of percutaneous mitral commissurotomy in a series of 1024 patients: analysis of late clinical deterioration: frequency, anatomic findings, and predictive factors. *Circulation* 1999;99:3272–3278.

Percutaneous mitral commissurotomy can be successfully performed in many patients with mitral stenosis with excellent long-term results.

Jick H, Vasilakis C, Weinrauch LA, et al. A population-based study of appetite-suppressant drugs and the risk of cardiac valve regurgitation. *N Engl J Med* 1998; 339:719–724.

The use of fenfluramine or dexfenfluramine is associated with cardiac valve disorders, particularly aortic regurgitation.

Landzberg JS, Pflugfelder PW, Cassidy MM, et al. Etiology of the Austin Flint murmur. *J Am Coll Cardiol* 1992;20:408–413.

The Austin Flint murmur is caused by the regurgitant jet abutting the left ventricular myocardium.

Levine HJ, Gaasch WH. Vasoactive drugs in chronic regurgitant lesions of the mitral and aortic valves. *J Am Coll Cardiol* 1996;28:1083–1091.

A thoughtful review on the effect of vasodilator drugs on the pathophysiology of mitral regurgitation.

Ling LH, Enriquez-Sarano M, Seward JB, et al. Early surgery in patients with mitral regurgitation due to flail leaflets: a long-term outcome study. *Circulation* 1997;96: 1819–1825.

Early surgery is preferred over medical therapy in patients with flail mitral leaflets.

Ling LH, Enriquez-Sarano M, Seward JB, et al. Clinical outcome of mitral regurgitation due to flail leaflet. *N Engl J Med* 1996;335:1417–1423.

Surgery is the preferred treatment modality for patients with flail mitral valve leaflet; medical therapy is associated with a considerably higher mortality.

Lombard JT, Selzer A. Valvular aortic stenosis: a clinical and hemodynamic profile of patients. *Ann Intern Med* 1987;106:292–298.

A careful hemodynamic and clinical review of 397 patients with valvular aortic stenosis.
Morganroth J, Perloff JK, Zeldis SM, et al. Acute severe aortic regurgitation: pathophysiology, clinical recognition and management. *Ann Intern Med* 1977;87:223–232.
A review of clinical features of patients with acute aortic regurgitation.
Multicenter experience with balloon mitral commissurotomy: NHLBI Balloon Valvuloplasty Registry Report on immediate and 30-day follow-up results: the National Heart, Lung, and Blood Institute Balloon Valvuloplasty Registry Participants. *Circulation* 1992;85:448–461.
Balloon valvuloplasty is an effective therapy for patients with mitral stenosis.
Nitta M, Nakamura T, Hultgren HN, et al. Progression of aortic stenosis in adult men: detection by noninvasive methods. *Chest* 1987;92:40–43.
Marked progression of valvular aortic stenosis can occur in only 3 years.
Orsinelli DA, Aurigemma GP, Battista S, et al. Left ventricular hypertrophy and mortality after aortic valve replacement for aortic stenosis. *J Am Coll Cardiol* 1993;22:1679–1683.
Excessive LVH in patients with aortic stenosis is associated with increased surgical mortality.
Palta S, Pai AM, Gill KS, et al. New insights into the progression of aortic stenosis: implications for secondary prevention. *Circulation* 2000;101:2497–2502.
Progression of aortic stenosis is associated with hypercholesterolemia, cigarette smoking, elevated serum creatinine, and increased serum calcium levels.
Patel JJ, Shama D, Mitha AS et al. Balloon valvuloplasty versus closed commissurotomy for pliable mitral stenosis: a prospective hemodynamic study. *J Am Coll Cardiol* 1991;18:1318–1322.
Balloon valvuloplasty creates a larger mitral valve area than does surgical commissurotomy in patients with mitral stenosis.
Perloff JK, Roberts WC. The mitral apparatus: functional anatomy of mitral regurgitation. *Circulation* 1972;46:227–239.
Extensive review of clinical and pathologic features of mitral regurgitation.
Roberts WC. Morphologic features of the normal and abnormal mitral valve. *Am J Cardiol* 1983;51:1005–1028.
An extensive review of the pathologic features of mitral valve disease.
Roberts WC, Cohen LS. Left ventricular papillary muscles: description of the normal and a survey of conditions causing them to be abnormal. *Circulation* 1972;46:138–154.
Extensive pathologic and pathophysiologic review of papillary muscle dysfunction.
Rosenhek R, Binder T, Porenta G, et al. Predictors of outcome in severe, asymptomatic aortic stenosis. *N Engl J Med* 2000;343:611–617.
Surgery can be delayed in patients with severe aortic stenosis as long as patients remain asymptomatic. Patients with moderate to severe calcification and a rapid increase in aortic jet velocity have a poor prognosis.
Salazar E, Levine HD. Rheumatic tricuspid regurgitation: the clinical spectrum. *Am J Med* 1962;33:111.
Extensive clinical review of functional and organic tricuspid regurgitation associated with rheumatic valvular disease.
Tischler MD, Rowan M, LeWinter MM. Effect of enalapril therapy on left ventricular mass and volumes in asymptomatic chronic, severe mitral regurgitation secondary to mitral valve prolapse. *Am J Cardiol* 1998;82:242–245.
Six months of enalapril therapy reduced left ventricular volumes and mass in patients with severe mitral regurgitation.
Weissman NJ, Tighe JF, Gottdiener JS, et al. An assessment of heart valve abnormalities in obese patients taking dexfenfluramine, sustained-release defenfluramine, or placebo. *N Engl J Med* 1998;339:725–735.
There was a small increase in the prevalence of aortic and mitral regurgitation observed in patients who had received these appetite suppressant medications.

17. CONGENITAL HEART DISEASE IN THE ADULT

I. **Introduction.** Undiagnosed congenital heart disease in adults is rather rare. Adult patients with congenital heart disease manage to escape detection in childhood either because of inadequate medical attention, the subtle nature of the defect, or the close resemblance of cardiac manifestations of the lesion to so-called innocent or benign murmurs. The percentage distribution of various congenital heart lesions is different in adults and in children (Table 17-1). More than 90% of adults who present with congenital heart disease have one of five easily differentiated lesions: atrial septal defect (ASD), ventricular septal defect (VSD), pulmonic stenosis (PS), patent ductus arteriosus (PDA), and coarctation of the aorta (COARC). These five lesions usually can be distinguished from one another on the basis of strikingly different findings by physical examination, ECG, chest x-ray film, and echocardiography.

II. **ASD.** ASD is the most common form of congenital heart disease in adults. The diagnosis may be difficult to make because the associated physical findings can be subtle.

   A. Diagnosis

      1. **History.** Most patients with ASD are asymptomatic. In fact, many of them survive beyond middle age with minimal or no symptoms; however, patients with ASD are likely to shun vigorous physical activity, frequently with the excuse that they never enjoyed recreational or occupational activities that require considerable exertion.

        The development of left or right ventricular failure (or both) results in a significant increase of symptoms. Left ventricular failure in adult patients with ASD is often secondary to associated conditions such as coronary artery disease or hypertension. Left ventricular failure produces systemic rather than pulmonary venous congestion in patients with ASD because of the communication between the left and right atria.

        Most patients are asymptomatic until the third or fourth decade. At that time, dyspnea on exertion and fatigue are commonly noted. Orthopnea can also occur, apparently secondary to decreased pulmonary compliance. Pulmonary hypertension results from pulmonary vascular disease, a feared complication of all forms of congenital heart disease with left-to-right shunts. Eventually, right ventricular failure develops in patients with pulmonary hypertension. Significant pulmonary hypertension rarely occurs before 20 years of age but may happen at earlier ages in individuals who reside at higher altitudes. Initially, patients with ASD have a left-to-right intracardiac shunt in which a portion of the pulmonary venous return passes across the atrial defect to join the systemic venous blood returning to the right side of the heart. As pulmonary hypertension develops, the magnitude of the left-to-right shunt decreases. Ultimately, when severe pulmonary hypertension exists, the direction of the intracardiac shunt is reversed: Systemic venous blood passes across the atrial defect to mix with pulmonary venous return on the left side of the circulation, rendering the patient cyanotic. Patients with right-to-left shunts complain of dyspnea, fatigue, effort cyanosis, and hemoptysis. Chest discomfort resembling angina pectoris may also occur.

        Supraventricular arrhythmias are not uncommon in patients with ASD. Indeed, such rhythm disturbances may persist even after successful closure of the ASD.

      2. **Physical examination.** The hallmark of patients with ASD is the so-called fixed split second heart sound (S2). Slight respiratory variation does occur between the aortic and pulmonic components of the S2, but clearly audible splitting persists throughout the respiratory cycle. A pulmonic ejection murmur secondary to increased right ventricular cardiac output is also easily auscultated. Physical findings in patients with ASD are summarized in Table 17-2.

TABLE 17-1. APPROXIMATE PERCENTAGE OF FORMS OF CONGENITAL HEART DISEASE IN CHILDREN AND ADULTS

Disease	Children (%)	Adults (%)
Atrial septic defect	5–10	45
Ventricular septic defect	20–30	25
Pulmonic stenosis	7–10	15
Patent ductus arteriosus	8–15	5
Coarctation of the aorta	3–8	3
Tetralogy of Fallot	6–10	2
Other	25–35	5

Skeletal malformations involving the upper extremity and particularly the thumb or radius coexist with ASD in patients with the autosomal dominant Holt-Oram syndrome.

3. ECG. As noted earlier, patients with ASD are prone to atrial arrhythmias. Atrial fibrillation is the most common arrhythmia, followed by atrial flutter and atrial tachycardia. The P–R interval is often prolonged in elderly patients with ASD. Incomplete right bundle branch block (RBBB; RSR in leads V_1 or V_2 or both) is the most frequent QRS alteration in patients with ASD. Older individuals may demonstrate complete RBBB. Patients with marked pulmonary hypertension usually have ECG evidence of right ventricular hypertrophy (RVH; increasing amplitude of R with decreasing amplitude of S in lead V_1, resulting in one of the following patterns: rsR, rR, qR, or monophasic R wave with slurred upstroke).

Individuals with secundum ASD have a normal frontal plane QRS axis. Ostium primum ASD can be recognized by means of the marked left axis deviation in the limb leads. ECG findings in patients with ASD are summarized in Table 17-3.

4. Chest x-ray examination. Patients with ASD and left-to-right shunting demonstrate markedly increased pulmonary vasculature on the posteroanterior chest film. The main pulmonary artery and right ventricle are also prominent. When pulmonary hypertension supervenes, the main pulmonary arteries enlarge further, but more peripheral pulmonary vessels regress. The chest x-ray findings in ASD are listed in Table 17-3.

5. Echocardiography. Confirmation of the diagnosis of ASD can be obtained by echocardiography and Doppler study. The most common finding in

TABLE 17-2. PHYSICAL FINDINGS IN PATIENTS WITH ATRIAL SEPTIC DEFECT[a]

Gracile habitus
Prominence or bulging of the left precordium
Equality in size of jugular venous A and V waves
Carotid pulse may have reduced volume
Parasternal right ventricular impulse
Fixed split second heart sound
Systolic pulmonic ejection murmur
Diastolic tricuspid opening snap (large shunts)
Diastolic tricuspid rumbling murmur (large shunts)

Patients with pulmonary hypertension and right-to-left shunts
   Cyanosis and digital clubbing
   Right ventricular heave
   Markedly increased P2

[a] Not all findings are present in every patient with atrial septic defect.

TABLE 17-3. ECG AND CHEST X-RAY FINDINGS IN PATIENTS WITH ATRIAL SEPTIC DEFECT[a]

ECG findings
  Atrial arrhythmias
  P–R interval prolongation
  Incomplete right bundle branch block
  Complete right bundle branch block
  Marked left axis deviation with ostium primum atrial septic defect

Chest roentgenographic findings
  Prominent pulmonary vasculature (shunt vessels)
  Enlarged main pulmonary arteries
  Small aortic knob
  Enlarged right ventricle

Patients with marked pulmonary hypertension
  Right ventricular hypertrophy (rsR, rR, qR, monophasic R with slurred upstroke in lead V_1)
  Markedly enlarged main pulmonary arteries
  Reduced peripheral pulmonary vessels
  Right ventricular enlargement

[a] Not all findings are present in every patient with atrial septic defect.

ASD is an increased right ventricular cavity dimension. Other findings include abnormal septal motion and, in many individuals, mitral valve prolapse. The ASD itself can often be visualized and the left-to-right shunt quantitated.

6. Radionuclide studies. Accurate quantitation of the left-to-right shunt of ASD can be obtained by radionuclide angiocardiography. Right-to-left shunts can also be detected by this technique.

7. Cardiac catheterization and angiography. Right-sided heart catheterization demonstrates increased oxygen saturation in blood samples from the right atrium, compared with superior and inferior vena caval samples (oxygen step-up). By obtaining blood samples for determination of oxygen content from the superior and inferior venae cavae, the right atrium and ventricle, and the pulmonary and systemic arteries (diagnostic run), one can estimate the quantity of left-to-right or right-to-left blood shunting. Left ventriculography reveals a small left ventricle with a normal contraction pattern. Mitral valve prolapse also may be noted.

8. Protocol for the diagnosis of ASD
   a. Testing sequence for patients suspected of having ASD. The physical examination or routine chest x-ray film usually suggests the diagnosis of ASD. A protocol for the workup of patients with suspected congenital heart disease is as follows:

   History
   ↓
   Physical examination
   ↓
   ECG and chest x-ray film
   ↓
   Echocardiography and Doppler study
   ↓
   Radionuclide angiography **in selected patients**
   ↓
   Cardiac catheterization optional, depending on consistency of other clinical and noninvasive laboratory data, **in selected patients**

b. Criteria for making the diagnosis
 (1) Asymptomatic or minimally symptomatic individuals may have fixed split S2, systolic pulmonic ejection murmur, incomplete RBBB on ECG, increased pulmonary vasculature (shunt vessels) on chest roentgenography, and demonstration of an enlarged right ventricular cavity on the echocardiogram, with a left-to-right shunt on radionuclide angiocardiography or Doppler.

  Patients in whom all clinical and noninvasive laboratory findings are totally consistent with ASD may undergo repair of the ASD without catheterization confirmation. Individuals with inconsistencies in the clinical or noninvasive laboratory findings should undergo cardiac catheterization.

 (2) Individuals in whom a right-sided heart catheter passes from right atrium to left atrium but who lack the usual clinical or noninvasive laboratory findings of ASD should have a diagnostic run performed in the catheterization laboratory. Almost all such individuals will be found to possess a hemodynamically insignificant ASD (patent foramen ovale).

c. Differential diagnosis. Other entities may mimic ASD.
 (1) Idiopathic dilatation of the pulmonary artery. Patients with this condition have systolic pulmonic ejection murmurs and enlarged main pulmonary arteries on chest x-ray. The jugular venous pulse is normal, however, and no right ventricular impulse is palpable. Splitting of S2 is physiologic, and the ECG is normal. No shunt vessels appear on the chest x-ray picture, and echocardiography reveals a normal-sized right ventricle and normal septal motion. There is no left-to-right shunt on radionuclide angiocardiography, Doppler, or right-sided heart catheterization.

 (2) Innocent or functional murmurs. Functional murmurs are the result of turbulent blood flow somewhere in the cardiovascular system. They are rarely louder than grade III to VI in intensity and generally decrease with the Valsalva maneuver or assumption of the upright position. The S2 splits physiologically. Chest x-ray film, ECG, and echocardiogram are normal. Most such murmurs arise from turbulence in the aortic root. Other physiologic murmurs include cervical bruits, venous hums, and mammary souffles secondary to turbulent flow at branch points in the innominate or carotid arteries, in the jugular venous system, and in arterial and venous vessels of the engorged breast, respectively.

 (3) Thoracic bony abnormalities. Individuals with loss of the normal thoracic kyphosis (straight back syndrome) and those with pectus excavatum may have abnormal parasternal impulses, wide but physiologic splitting of S2, and systolic murmurs. Incomplete RBBB may even be present on the ECG. These findings may suggest the diagnosis of ASD.

  The bony thoracic abnormality, however, is evident on physical examination and chest x-ray film. Moreover, shunt vessels are not present on chest roentgenography, and echocardiography is usually unremarkable. No left-to-right shunt is detected by radionuclide angiography or catheterization, should these examinations be necessary because of confusing clinical and noninvasive laboratory data.

 (4) Bicuspid aortic valve. Patients with bicuspid aortic valves have early systolic ejection clicks and systolic ejection murmurs that may on occasion simulate the findings of ASD or PS. The S2 splits physiologically, however, and the chest x-ray picture and ECG are usually normal. Echocardiography reveals a normal right ventricle and septum and frequently an asymmetric aortic valve. Doppler, radionuclide angiography, and cardiac catheterization, if required, demonstrate the absence of any intracardiac shunt.

(5) PS. Individuals with PS frequently have left parasternal impulses, early systolic ejection sounds, wide but physiologically split second heart sounds, systolic ejection murmurs, RVH on ECG, and an enlarged pulmonary arterial trunk on chest x-ray film. Echocardiography may demonstrate an enlarged right ventricular cavity and even abnormal septal motion.

Consequently, it may be difficult to differentiate this condition from ASD. Helpful differences include (i) prominent atrial wave in the jugular venous pulse, (ii) physiologic splitting of S2, (iii) absence of shunt vessels on the chest x-ray film, and (iv) absence of intracardiac shunt on radionuclide angiography or Doppler, or, if required, cardiac catheterization in patients with PS.

(6) Mitral valve disease. In an occasional patient, mitral stenosis or mitral regurgitation can be confused with ASD because of the presence of a murmur, a parasternal impulse, RVH on ECG, and prominent pulmonary vasculature and right ventricle on chest roentgenography. Echocardiography almost invariably provides the correct diagnosis by revealing mitral valve abnormalities and left atrial enlargement. Doppler, isotope angiocardiography, and cardiac catheterization, if required, document the absence of any intracardiac shunt.

d. Unusual variants of ASD

(1) Lutembacher's syndrome. ASD associated with mitral stenosis is known as Lutembacher's syndrome. There is a higher than expected incidence of mitral stenosis in patients with ASD. The reason for this association is unknown. Clinically, patients with this syndrome are almost universally symptomatic, resembling individuals with either pure mitral stenosis or uncomplicated ASD. The physical examination suggests both lesions with the following findings: parasternal right ventricular impulse, increased first heart sound (S1), fixed split S2, and a mitral valve opening snap.

The diagnosis is made by echocardiographic and hemodynamic evidence of mitral stenosis accompanied by a left-to-right shunt at the atrial level.

(2) Patent foramen ovale. A patent foramen ovale represents a small ASD. It is usually discovered fortuitously when a right-sided heart catheter crosses the atrial septum and enters the left atrium. A diagnostic run and indicator dilution curves may demonstrate a small left-to-right shunt. The only clinical significance of a patent foramen ovale is as a route for paradoxical embolism. The presence of a patent foramen ovale can be inferred noninvasively by means of a so-called bubble study, in which the transit of tiny microbubbles through the right heart chambers is monitored by echocardiography. This study can be performed with and without a Valsalva maneuver, which transiently increases the small right-to-left shunt. If bubbles are seen crossing the interatrial septum, this strongly suggests the presence of a patent foramen ovale.

(3) Partial anomalous venous return. In partial anomalous venous return, one or more of the pulmonary veins drains into the systemic venous circulation (superior vena cava, inferior vena cava, right atrium, coronary sinus, subclavian vein, innominate vein, or portal vein), rather than into the left atrium. This entity may coexist with an ASD, or the atrial septum may be intact. Partial anomalous venous drainage with ASD resembles the latter with respect to natural history, physical examination, ECG, and chest x-ray study. The anomalous vein is occasionally evident on the

posteroanterior chest roentgenogram. Patients with anomalous venous drainage and intact septum resemble individuals with ASD except for absence of fixed splitting of S2. Identification of this syndrome usually requires cardiac catheterization, although the diagnosis is at times evident when the anomalous vein is clearly visualized by chest roentgenography.

B. Therapy

1. Medical treatment. Patients who develop right or left ventricular failure without severe pulmonary hypertension should be treated with digitalis, diuretics, or both and should be considered for elective closure of their ASD. Arrhythmias are managed conventionally (see Chapter 3).

   Patients with severe pulmonary hypertension and reversed (right-to-left) shunting are said to suffer from **Eisenmenger's syndrome.** They are usually quite cyanotic, with clubbed digits. They have marked exercise intolerance. Surgical intervention is generally impossible, resulting in increased pulmonary vascular resistance with consequent right ventricular failure and low systemic cardiac output. Medical treatment consists of diuretics and, on occasion, digitalis therapy for symptomatic left or right ventricular failure. Phlebotomy and concomitant oral iron therapy (e.g., $FeSO_4$, 300 mg four times a day after meals) are occasionally used in individuals with hematocrits above 60% to 70% who have symptoms, namely, transient ischemic attacks, related to the increased hematocrit. Antibiotic prophylaxis against subacute bacterial endocarditis is important with any dental and surgical procedure. Hyperuricemia may occur, with resultant gouty episodes. Gouty attacks are managed conventionally.

2. Surgery/interventional cardiology. Most patients with hemodynamically significant ASDs (left-to-right shunt equal to systemic cardiac output) should have elective closure of the defect, even in the absence of symptoms or signs of left or right ventricular failure. Closure of an uncomplicated ASD carries a very small risk that is less than the probability of developing severe pulmonary hypertension and reversed (right-to-left) shunting of blood. Unfortunately, it is not possible to predict which patients with uncorrected ASD will go on to develop pulmonary hypertension in middle life. It is also possible to close small- to moderate-sized ASDs by placing an occluder across the defect during an interventional catheterization. Larger defects still require surgical intervention.

III. VSD. The most common congenital defect in children, VSD is surpassed in frequency by ASD in adult patients. The incidence of VSD is decreased in adults as a result of (i) spontaneous or surgical closure of defects during childhood or adolescence and (ii) mortality from this lesion before adulthood. In addition to pulmonary hypertension and Eisenmenger's syndrome, patients with VSD may manifest aortic insufficiency, bacterial endocarditis, right ventricular outflow obstruction, and heart failure.

A. Diagnosis

1. History. Adults with VSD may be asymptomatic, or they may complain of fatigue and effort intolerance. Aortic insufficiency (secondary to prolapse of the right aortic leaflet) increases the likelihood that patients will develop symptoms of left ventricular failure. Aortic insufficiency and bacterial endocarditis in patients with VSD result in a marked increase in mortality.

   Surgical closure of a VSD does not abolish the risk of endocarditis, but endocarditis is essentially nonexistent in patients who spontaneously close a VSD.

   Pulmonary hypertension in patients with VSD usually develops in childhood. Eventually, reversal of the shunt occurs, producing peripheral cyanosis and clubbing. The development of right ventricular failure in this setting is an ominous sign. Closure of a VSD after some degree of fixed pulmonary vascular change has occurred can result in progressive obliterative pulmonary vascular disease, with increasing levels of pulmonary hypertension. Right ventricular outflow tract (infundibular) obstruction may accompany VSD in the syndrome known as tetralogy of Fallot (infundibular PS, VSD, overriding aorta, and concentric hypertrophy of the right ventricle). Many patients have severe subpulmonic stenosis and right-to-left shunting with peripheral cyanosis. Most of these individuals are recognized during childhood.

2. Physical examination. Patients with large VSDs may be frail and of small stature. The carotid pulse is of diminished volume in individuals with large shunts or heart failure. The carotid upstroke is usually brisk. The jugular venous pulse is often surprisingly normal in patients with VSD. A systolic thrill is palpable parasternally in the third or fourth left intercostal space of most patients with VSD. Those with sizable left-to-right shunts have a vigorous apical impulse. As pulmonary hypertension develops, the left ventricular impulse becomes less evident, while a parasternal right ventricular impulse becomes more apparent. Physical findings in patients with VSD are summarized in Table 17-4.

3. ECG. The ECG in VSD reflects the magnitude of the shunt and the presence of associated complications. Patients with small defects may have normal ECGs. Increasing quantities of left-to-right shunt flow or the presence of aortic insufficiency results in the pattern of left ventricular hypertrophy (LVH). Marked pulmonary hypertension or infundibular PS (tetralogy of Fallot) produces the RVH pattern in the ECG. Normal QRS axis is the rule in most patients with VSD. Marked left axis deviation suggests that one is dealing with an endocardial cushion defect. ECG findings in VSD are summarized in Table 17-5.

4. Chest x-ray examination. Small defects generally are associated with a normal chest x-ray film. With moderate to large left-to-right shunts or aortic insufficiency, left ventricular prominence can be detected. Dilatation of the main pulmonary arteries and left atrium also is commonly noted in individuals with large left-to-right shunts. Patients with marked pulmonary hypertension demonstrate right ventricular enlargement and large central pulmonary arteries with oligemia of peripheral pulmonary zones. Patients with tetralogy of Fallot have right ventricular enlargement, small or normal-sized pulmonary arteries, and oligemic lung fields. Roentgenographic findings in VSD are summarized in Table 17-5.

TABLE 17-4. PHYSICAL FINDINGS IN PATIENTS WITH VENTRICULAR SEPTIC DEFECT[a]

Asthenic habitus (large shunts)
Carotid pulse may have reduced volume
Hyperdynamic left ventricular impulse (large shunts)
Systolic thrill in third, fourth intercostal space, left sternal border
Wide, physiologic splitting of second heart sound
Uniform, holosystolic murmur
Early diastolic murmur of aortic insufficiency in approximately 10% of ventricular septic defect patients
Short, rumbling middiastolic murmur (large shunt)
Third heart sound (large shunt or left ventricular failure)

Patients with pulmonary hypertension and right-to-left shunts
   Cyanosis and digital clubbing
   Right ventricular heave
   Markedly increased P2
   Minimal or no systolic murmur or the early diastolic murmur of pulmonary insufficiency (Graham Steell murmur)

[a] Not all findings are present in every patient with ventricular septic defect.

TABLE 17-5. ECG AND CHEST X-RAY FINDINGS IN PATIENTS WITH VENTRICULAR SEPTIC DEFECT

ECG findings
   Atrial arrhythmias (uncommon)
   Left ventricular hypertrophy
   Marked left axis deviation (endocardial cushion defect)
Chest roentgenographic findings
   Left ventricular prominence
   Prominent pulmonary vasculature (shunt vessels)
   Enlarged main pulmonary arteries
   Left atrial enlargement
   Small aortic knob
Patients with marked pulmonary hypertension or infundibular stenosis
   Right ventricular hypertrophy by ECG
   Right ventricular enlargement by chest x-ray

---

5. Echocardiography. Noninvasive evaluation by echocardiography confirms the presence of a hyperactive (volume overloaded) left ventricle. Enlarged left atrium and right ventricle are also usually noted. The VSD itself can often be visualized by two-dimensional echocardiography, and the volume of the shunt can also be estimated by Doppler echocardiography.
6. Radionuclide studies. Accurate quantitation of left-to-right and right-to-left shunting of blood through a VSD can be obtained by radionuclide angiography. Left and right ventricular function (ejection fraction) can be determined by radionuclide ventriculography.
7. Cardiac catheterization and angiography. Right heart catheterization demonstrates increased oxygen saturation in blood samples from the right ventricle and pulmonary artery compared with the right atrium. The quantity of blood shunting left-to-right can be measured. The VSD can be seen, and its location in the ventricular septum can be documented by left ventriculography in the left anterior oblique position.
8. Protocol for the diagnosis of VSD
   a. Testing sequence for patients suspected of having VSD. The history, physical examination, or routine chest x-ray film usually suggests the presence of a VSD. The sequence for diagnostic evaluation of ASD suggested earlier can also be used for patients with a suspected VSD.
   b. Criteria for making the diagnosis. Asymptomatic or symptomatic individuals may have a holosystolic murmur, physiologically split S2, LVH on ECG; left ventricular prominence and increased pulmonary vasculature (shunt vessels) on chest x-ray film; hyperdynamic left ventricle on the echocardiogram; and left-to-right shunt on Doppler, radionuclide angiocardiography, or right heart catheterization. Cardiac catheterization is indicated before surgical closure of a VSD. Complicating factors such as aortic insufficiency and right ventricular outflow tract obstruction should be specifically sought at catheterization.
   c. Differential diagnosis. Other entities may mimic VSD.
      (1) Mitral regurgitation. The pathophysiology of mitral regurgitation is not very different from that of VSD. The holosystolic murmur of pure mitral regurgitation together with the presence of a hyperactive (volume overloaded) left ventricle produces a clinical picture resembling that of VSD; however, the murmur of mitral regurgitation is best heard at the cardiac apex with radiation to the axilla, whereas the murmur of VSD is localized to the lower left sternal border. Patients with mitral regurgitation lack the systolic thrill often palpated along the lower left sternal

border in individuals with VSD. Shunt vessels are not seen on the chest x-ray of patients with mitral regurgitation, and Doppler, radionuclide angiography, or right heart catheterization (if required) documents the absence of a left-to-right shunt in patients with mitral regurgitation.

(2) Valvular or subvalvular aortic stenosis. These conditions produce systolic murmurs that are often ejection in type but are occasionally confused with the murmur of VSD. The murmurs of valvular or subvalvular aortic stenosis are usually heard best at the upper right sternal border with radiation to the right clavicle and to the carotid arteries. The carotid pulse demonstrates specific abnormalities (see Chapters 16 and 18), and shunt vessels are absent in the chest x-ray picture. Specific echocardiographic findings point to the aortic valve or left ventricular outflow tract as the site of origin of the systolic murmur.

(3) Tricuspid insufficiency. The holosystolic murmur along the left sternal border produced by tricuspid insufficiency may mimic that seen with VSD. Severe tricuspid insufficiency usually results as a late complication of mitral valve disease or severe chronic left ventricular failure with pulmonary venous hypertension. The murmur of tricuspid insufficiency usually demonstrates marked respiratory variation, increasing on inspiration concomitant with increasing venous return to the heart. The jugular venous pulse has large V waves in tricuspid insufficiency, and the chest x-ray reveals right ventricular enlargement and absence of shunt vessels. Radionuclide angiocardiography documents the absence of a left-to-right shunt in patients with tricuspid insufficiency. Doppler study reveals the presence of tricuspid regurgitation.

(4) PS. PS is more likely to be confused with aortic stenosis than with VSD because it produces a systolic ejection murmur at the base of the heart. PS can usually be easily distinguished from VSD because it produces right ventricular as opposed to left ventricular overload. Thus, patients with PS have a palpable parasternal right ventricular impulse, right ventricular enlargement and absent shunt vessels on the chest roentgenogram, and absence of a left-to-right shunt on Doppler or radionuclide angiocardiography.

B. Therapy
   1. Medical treatment. Patients who develop left or right ventricular failure without severe pulmonary hypertension should be treated with digitalis or diuretics or both. Vasodilator (afterload reduction) therapy with hydralazine and long-acting nitrates or angiotensin-converting-enzyme inhibitors is also helpful in patients with VSD. If left ventricular function is adequate, and if a significant left-to-right shunt (pulmonary blood flow at least twice systemic blood flow) exists through the VSD, the patient should be offered elective closure of the defect. Bacterial endocarditis is a dreaded complication of VSD. It should be treated with intravenous antibiotics (see Chapter 20), and patients also should be considered for elective closure of their VSD.
   2. Surgery. Patients with VSD and pulmonary to systemic blood flow ratios of 2:1 or greater should have elective closure of the defect. Associated lesions such as aortic insufficiency and right ventricular outflow tract obstruction should be sought at preoperative cardiac catheterization. Right ventricular outflow obstruction is corrected at the time of VSD closure. Whether concomitant aortic valve replacement for aortic insufficiency is performed when the VSD is closed depends on the severity of the valvular lesion and the patient's age. Because aortic insufficiency is often well tolerated for decades, it is probably best to avoid aortic valve replacement if possible, particularly in younger individuals.

IV. PS. Acquired valvular PS is essentially nonexistent. Patients with this entity have almost invariably had the lesion since birth. Those with severe PS usually are discovered and treated by a pulmonary valvuloplasty during childhood; however, a number of them escape detection and reach adulthood with surprisingly few symptoms.

A. Diagnosis

1. History. Adult patients with mild or moderate PS are without symptoms. The lesion usually is discovered because a systolic murmur is noted on a routine physical examination. Even patients with severe PS may be asymptomatic.

Symptomatic patients with PS complain of effort dyspnea and undue fatigue, both symptoms being the result of inadequate rise in cardiac output during exercise. Orthopnea does not occur because pulmonary venous pressure is normal in patients with PS. Eventually, right ventricular failure develops in individuals with severe PS, and its appearance is an ominous sign. Syncope or lightheadedness is occasionally experienced by patients with PS, but sudden death (as in aortic stenosis) does not occur. Chest pain resembling angina may occur in severe PS, and right ventricular infarction has been noted in the hypertrophied right ventricles of patients with severe PS. Endocarditis is rare in PS, but it may develop even after successful pulmonary valvuloplasty.

2. Physical examination. Patients with PS have systolic ejection murmurs that are often confused with those arising from aortic stenosis. Early systolic ejection sounds are very common in PS. Differentiation of PS from aortic stenosis can be readily accomplished if the physician determines which ventricle is hypertrophied. Patients with moderate to severe PS have easily palpable right ventricular parasternal impulses and normal or small apical left ventricular impulses. Cyanosis occasionally occurs in patients with severe PS secondary to low cardiac output or a right-to-left shunt through an ASD or patent foramen ovale. Physical findings in PS are summarized in Table 17-6.

3. ECG. Patients with mild PS usually have normal ECGs. Right atrial hypertrophy and RVH patterns are seen in patients with more severe degrees of PS. The severity of PS correlates reasonably well with the $R:S$ ratio in lead V_1, with increasingly severe PS resulting in greater R wave preponderance. Individuals with severe PS demonstrate tall monophasic R waves in lead V_1. ECG findings in patients with PS are listed in Table 17-7.

4. Chest x-ray examination. The peripheral pulmonary vasculature is normal or reduced in patients with PS in contradistinction to individuals

TABLE 17-6. PHYSICAL FINDINGS IN PATIENTS WITH PULMONARY STENOSIS[a]

Habitus of Noonan's syndrome (small stature, shield chest, web neck)
Cyanosis in patients with severe pulmonary stenosis and atrial septal defect or patent foramen ovale
Carotid pulse normal or reduced in volume
Jugular venous pulse with marked A waves
Systolic thrill in third, fourth left parasternal intercostal space
Right ventricular parasternal impulse
Ejection sound
Systolic ejection murmur
Wide, physiologic splitting of second heart sound with reduced P2
Right, ventricular fourth heart sound with severe pulmonary stenosis
Marked enlargement of main pulmonary artery segment
Reduced pulmonary vasculature

[a] Not all findings are present in every patient with pulmonary stenosis.

TABLE 17-7. ECG AND CHEST X-RAY FINDINGS IN PATIENTS WITH PULMONARY STENOSIS[a]

ECG findings
   Right axis deviation
   Right atrial enlargement
   Right ventricular hypertrophy

Chest roentgenographic findings
   Normal peripheral pulmonary vasculature (no shunt vessels)
   Enlarged main pulmonary arteries (left > right)
   Enlarged right ventricle

[a] Not all findings are present in every patient with pulmonary stenosis.

with left-to right shunts. The main pulmonary arteries are usually large secondary to poststenotic dilatation. The left main pulmonary artery may be particularly increased in size. Right ventricular enlargement occurs in patients with moderate to severe degrees of PS. Calcification of the pulmonic valve is rare in PS. Chest roentgenographic findings in patients with PS are summarized in Table 17-7.

5. Laboratory studies. Pulmonary function studies are often abnormal in adults with PS. Lung volumes, airway conductance, and pulmonary diffusing capacity may be reduced, probably as a result of inadequate lung development in early childhood.

6. Echocardiography. A dilated hypertrophic right ventricle and a stenotic and thickened pulmonic valve are usually visualized by echocardiography in patients with moderate to severe PS. The pulmonic valve gradient can be quantitated by a Doppler study.

7. Radioisotope studies. Radioangiocardiography may be useful in patients with PS by demonstrating that no left-to-right shunt exists.

8. Cardiac catheterization and angiography. The hemodynamic hallmark of PS is a systolic gradient across the pulmonic valve. The size of the stenotic pulmonary valve orifice can be determined at cardiac catheterization by simultaneously measuring pulmonic valve systolic gradient and cardiac output. No left-to-right shunt is detected in patients with PS, although a right-to-left shunt (usually of small size) may exist in patients with ASD or patent foramen ovale. The stenotic, domed pulmonic valve may be visualized by right ventriculography or pulmonary angiography.

9. Protocol for the diagnosis of PS
   a. Testing sequence for patients suspected of having PS. The diagnosis of PS usually can be made on the basis of physical examination combined with supportive ECG, roentgenographic, and echocardiographic data. The protocol for the evaluation of patients with suspected PS is similar to that for patients with ASD.
   b. Criteria for making the diagnosis. Asymptomatic or symptomatic individuals may have systolic ejection murmurs along the left sternal border, often associated with an early systolic ejection click. Right ventricular dilatation and hypertrophy are noted by physical examination (left parasternal impulse), ECG, chest x-ray film, and echocardiography. Doppler study demonstrates a gradient across the pulmonic valve.
   c. Differential diagnosis. Other entities may mimic PS.
      (1) ASD. Patients with ASD may be difficult to distinguish from individuals with PS. Differentiating features include fixed split S2 on physical examination, pulmonary shunt vessels on roentgenography, and documentation of a left-to-right shunt in individuals with ASD.
      (2) Idiopathic dilatation of the pulmonary artery. Patients with idiopathic dilatation of the pulmonary artery have no evidence

of right ventricular overload, in contrast to individuals with PS. Thus, they lack a palpable left parasternal impulse and RVH or enlargement on ECG, chest x-ray film, and echocardiogram. There is no gradient on Doppler across the pulmonic valve.

(3) Aortic stenosis. Patients with aortic stenosis have systolic ejection murmurs similar to those heard in patients with PS; however, the murmur of aortic stenosis is usually loudest along the upper right sternal border (compared with the upper left sternal border for PS murmurs), with radiation to the neck. Abnormal carotid artery upstroke and evidence of compensatory LVH on physical examination, ECG, chest x-ray film, and echocardiogram differentiate patients with aortic stenosis from those with PS, who manifest RVH.

(4) Bicuspid aortic valve. Patients with bicuspid aortic valves often have systolic ejection murmurs and early systolic ejection sounds resembling those heard in patients with PS. Indeed, the differentiation between mild PS and bicuspid aortic valve may be a difficult one. The difficulty, however, may not be important because expectant medical management and infectious endocarditis prophylaxis are indicated for patients with either diagnosis. Modest abnormality of the aortic or pulmonic valve by echocardiography may enable the clinician to distinguish these two entities.

(5) Mitral regurgitation. Patients with mitral regurgitation exhibit holosystolic murmurs, usually loudest at the apex and radiating to the axilla.

Besides the difference in quality and radiation of murmurs of mitral regurgitation and those of PS, evidence of compensatory LVH or dilatation is noted in patients with mitral regurgitation compared with RVH in individuals with PS. Doppler studies demonstrate mitral regurgitation.

(6) VSD. Patients with VSD have holosystolic murmurs localized to the lower left sternal border. These murmurs are quite different in character from the systolic ejection murmur heard loudest at the upper left sternal border in patients with PS. In addition, patients with VSD usually demonstrate evidence of LVH and dilatation, compared with RVH in individuals with PS.

(7) Innocent or physiologic murmurs. Early systolic flow murmurs are usually the result of turbulent blood flow just above the aortic valve. They are systolic and ejection in character, thus mimicking the murmurs of aortic stenosis and PS. They can be differentiated from the latter in several ways. Physiologic murmurs generally occupy only the initial one third to one half of systole, and ejection sounds are absent. Moreover, physiologic murmurs frequently disappear when patients sit up or stand. No evidence of ventricular hypertrophy or enlargement by physical examination, ECG, chest x-ray study, or echocardiogram is noted in patients with physiologic murmurs. The pulmonic and aortic valves appear normal by echocardiography.

B. Therapy

1. Medical and interventional cardiology therapy. Essentially all patients with mild to moderate PS can be managed medically. Heart failure rarely, if ever, develops, and most of these individuals need only prophylactic antibiotic therapy with surgical and dental procedures. Catheterization usually is not required to confirm the diagnosis. Asymptomatic patients with severe PS represent a problem in that their management is controversial. Some authorities advise expectant medical therapy in these individuals, awaiting the onset of symptoms before advising pulmonary valvuloplasty. Other authorities recommend pulmonic valve balloon valvuloplasty in all such patients. Catheterization may be helpful in patients with severe PS because it defines the degree of right ventricular compensation. Those

with severe PS who develop signs or symptoms of right ventricular failure should definitely be offered pulmonic valve balloon valvuloplasty.

Excellent relief of the pulmonary valve gradient, as well as symptoms, is usually obtained. Antibiotic prophylaxis against subacute bacterial endocarditis probably should be continued with dental or surgical procedures even after successful pulmonary valvuloplasty.

V. PDA. Very common in premature infants, PDA is rather rare in adults. It is more frequently seen in individuals born and residing at higher elevations.

A. Diagnosis

1. History. As with patients with VSD that results in large left-to-right shunts, patients with PDA may be asymptomatic or they may complain of effort intolerance. Besides left and right ventricular failure, patients with PDA are prone to develop bacterial endocarditis (endarteritis) and pulmonary vascular disease with Eisenmenger's syndrome. The larger the left-to-right shunt, the more likely that a given patient will develop heart failure. Bacterial endarteritis usually develops on the intimal "jet lesion," located in the pulmonary artery opposite the orifice of the PDA.

   Pulmonary vascular disease with reversed shunting (right-to-left shunt) may be present soon after birth or may develop gradually with time. Patients with Eisenmenger's syndrome are likely to complain of exertional dyspnea, fatigue, or both; however, symptoms may be surprisingly mild despite marked peripheral cyanosis and digital clubbing.

2. Physical examination. Patients with PDA and a left-to-right shunt usually have an easily audible continuous murmur peaking around the time of S2 and localizing to the first or second intercostal space along the left sternal edge.

   Patients with large left-to-right shunts have carotid pulses that are brisk and at times bounding, resembling those seen in patients with aortic insufficiency. Similarly, the pulse pressure is wide. Palpation along the upper left sternal border may reveal systolic pulsation of the pulmonary artery in patients with large left-to-right shunts, who ordinarily demonstrate signs of left ventricular volume overload (laterally displaced, hyperactive left ventricular impulse).

   Patients with PDA and marked pulmonary hypertension may have only a systolic murmur. Discrete systolic (turbulent flow in a dilated pulmonary artery) and diastolic (pulmonic insufficiency secondary to severe pulmonary hypertension) murmurs may be present. Cyanosis and digital clubbing develop in individuals with reversed shunts. Clubbing of the toes without involvement of the fingers is sometimes seen in patients with PDA (differential cyanosis). It occurs when all or most of the right-to-left shunt passes into the descending aorta through the PDA. Patients with severe pulmonary vascular disease and pulmonary hypertension usually have evidence of RVH (left parasternal impulse). Physical findings in patients with PDA are summarized in Table 17-8.

3. ECG. Sinus rhythm is usually present, although individuals with large left-to-right shunts may develop atrial fibrillation. Patients with normal pulmonary vascular resistance and significant left-to-right shunting have LVH on ECG. RVH patterns evolve on the ECGs of patients who develop severe pulmonary vascular disease with resultant pulmonary hypertension. ECG findings in PDA are summarized in Table 17-9.

4. Chest x-ray examination. Patients with small left-to-right shunts through a PDA may have normal chest roentgenograms. Prominent x-ray findings in patients with PDA include increased pulmonary vasculature (shunt vessels), enlarged main pulmonary arteries and ascending aorta, and left ventricular dilatation. On occasion, calcification in the ductus can be identified lying between the aortic knob and the main pulmonary artery. Patients with severe pulmonary hypertension develop further enlargement of the main pulmonary arteries together with reduced peripheral pulmonary vasculature. In addition, right ventricular enlargement de-

TABLE 17-8. PHYSICAL FINDINGS IN PATIENTS WITH PATENT DUCTUS ARTERIOSUS[a]

Wide pulse pressure
Brisk or even bounding carotid pulse
Paradoxical splitting of second heart sound
Continuous murmur in the first or second intercostal space along the left sternal border
Laterally displaced and/or hyperactive left ventricular impulse

Patients with marked pulmonary hypertension and right-to-left shunts
 Cyanosis and digital clubbing (clubbing may be localized to the toes)
 Systolic murmur only or discrete systolic and diastolic murmurs
 Right ventricular heave
 Increased P2

[a] Not all findings are present in every patient with patent ductus arteriosus.

velops in patients with severe pulmonary hypertension. Chest roentgeno-graphic findings in patients with PDA are summarized in Table 17-9.

5. Echocardiography. Echocardiography demonstrates a hyperdynamic left ventricle and a dilated aortic root and left atrium in patients with large left-to-right shunts. The ratio of left atrial to aortic root diameter correlates with shunt magnitude in infants. Whether this relationship also holds true in adults with PDA is not known. Doppler study documents and quantitates the associated left-to-right shunt.

6. Radionuclide studies. The magnitude of left-to-right and right-to-left shunts can be determined by radionuclide angiocardiography in patients with PDA.

7. Catheterization and angiography. In patients with PDA and left-to-right shunts, right-sided heart catheterization demonstrates an increase in oxygen saturation in the pulmonary artery compared with the right ventricle. The magnitude of left-to-right or right-to-left shunts can be determined. The PDA itself may be visualized during aortography.

TABLE 17-9. ECG AND CHEST X-RAY FINDINGS IN PATIENTS WITH PATENT DUCTUS ARTERIOSUS[a]

ECG findings
 Sinus rhythm usually present
 Atrial fibrillation can occur with large left-to-right shunts
 First-degree atrioventricular block
 Left ventricular hypertrophy

Chest x-ray findings
 Increased pulmonary vascularity (shunt vessels)
 Enlarged main pulmonary arteries
 Enlarged ascending aorta
 Left ventricular enlargement
 Left atrial enlargement
 Calcification of the ductus

Patients with marked pulmonary hypertension
 Right atrial enlargement by ECG
 Right ventricular hypertrophy by ECG
 Markedly enlarged main pulmonary arteries
 Reduced peripheral pulmonary vessels
 Right ventricular enlargement

[a] Not all findings are present in every patient with patent ductus arteriosus.

8. Protocol for the diagnosis of PDA
   a. Testing sequence for making the diagnosis. The diagnosis of PDA is suggested by the presence of a continuous murmur along the upper left sternal border in symptomatic or asymptomatic individuals. An appropriate testing sequence for patients with PDA is similar to that shown for patients with ASD.
   b. Criteria for making the diagnosis. The diagnosis of PDA is established when an individual satisfies the following criteria: Symptomatic or asymptomatic individuals have a continuous murmur along the upper left sternal border with evidence of left ventricular enlargement or hyperactivity on physical examination (laterally displaced, active left ventricular impulse, brisk carotid upstroke), ECG (LVH pattern), or chest x-ray film (left ventricular prominence) and with a left-to-right shunt demonstrable by Doppler or radionuclide angiography. It is prudent to perform catheterization and angiographic visualization of a PDA before surgical or catheterization closure of the ductus is attempted; however, this may not be necessary if the ductus or calcification in the ductus is visible on the chest x-ray film.
   c. Differential diagnosis. Other entities may mimic PDA.
      (1) Coronary artery arteriovenous fistula. A fistula between a coronary artery and one of the cardiac chambers or the coronary venous system can produce a continuous murmur resembling that heard in patients with PDA. The location of the murmur is atypical for PDA, however, being loudest along the right sternal edge or at the lower left sternal border. Continuous murmurs from coronary arteriovenous fistulae are usually considerably louder in either systole or diastole because of phasic flow characteristics. The continuous murmur of a PDA is equally loud in systole and diastole. Left-to-right shunts with coronary arteriovenous fistulae are generally smaller than those with PDA. For this reason a hyperactive left ventricle or LVH is seldom found in patients with coronary fistulae.
      (2) Aorticopulmonary window. Resembling PDA in many ways, because the pathophysiology of the two conditions is almost identical, aorticopulmonary window is a round or oval communication between the aorta and the main pulmonary artery. A large left-to-right shunt occurs through the defect, and severe pulmonary vascular disease is common. Few individuals survive to adulthood. Patients with this rare entity have systolic rather than continuous murmurs because severe pulmonary hypertension reduces diastolic left-to-right shunt flow. This is the major differentiating feature of aorticopulmonary window and PDA.
      (3) Aortic stenosis and insufficiency. On occasion, the systolic murmur of aortic stenosis and the diastolic murmur of aortic insufficiency can appear almost continuous—that is, extending through S2. Thus, mixed aortic valve disease may present with a seemingly continuous murmur and evidence of left ventricular enlargement and hyperactivity. The two conditions can be distinguished by noting that the systolic murmur **ends** with S2 and that a brief pause occurs before the second, diastolic murmur commences. In addition, patients with aortic valve disease have calcification in the aortic valve discernible by fluoroscopy or echocardiography. Doppler studies demonstrate an aortic valve gradient and aortic regurgitation in patients with aortic valve disease.
      (4) Ruptured sinus of Valsalva aneurysm. This entity can produce a syndrome the pathophysiology of which resembles that of PDA. When a sinus of Valsalva aneurysm ruptures into the right atrium or right ventricle, a continuous murmur results. The mur-

mur often radiates widely over the precordium, being loudest along one of the sternal edges; it is loudest in either systole or diastole, and it does not peak at the time of S2, as does the murmur of PDA. Furthermore, patients with ruptured sinus of Valsalva aneurysm usually report sudden rather than gradual onset of symptoms. Often patients experience discomfort at the time of aneurysmal rupture.

B. Therapy
  1. Medical treatment. Prophylactic antibiotics should be administered to all patients with PDA who undergo dental or surgical procedures. Left ventricular failure is treated with digitalis, diuretics, and, if necessary, vasodilator therapy. Most authorities agree, however, that long-term medical therapy should be used only for individuals in whom surgery is strongly contraindicated because of a concomitant debilitating illness. Supraventricular arrhythmias are managed conventionally. The management of **Eisenmenger's syndrome** complicating a PDA is similar to that for severe pulmonary vascular disease complicating other intracardiac communications (see Section **II.B.1.**).
  2. Surgery/interventional cardiology. Essentially all patients with a PDA and persistent left-to-right shunt should have ligation and interruption of the ductus. Surgical interruption of the ductus markedly reduces the risk of bacterial endarteritis, and because the operation can be performed without cardiopulmonary bypass, the risk is very low. In older patients, the ductus may be aneurysmal or brittle, making repair more difficult. In current practice, many patients can have their PDA closed with a plug during an interventional catheterization. This spares the patient from having to undergo a thoracotomy.

VI. COARC. COARC represents one of the surgically correctable causes of hypertension (see Chapter 12). The lesion commonly is associated with other forms of congenital heart disease such as PDA, VSD, and bicuspid aortic valve. The renin-angiotensin system appears to play an important role in the genesis of hypertension in individuals with COARC.

A. Diagnosis
  1. History. Most patients with COARC are asymptomatic. The lesion usually is discovered during a routine search for treatable forms of hypertension in individuals with elevated blood pressure. Some patients complain of intermittent claudication or easy fatigability of the lower extremities—the result of decreased perfusion distal to the COARC itself. Other complaints include headache or symptoms of left ventricular failure. Most adult patients become symptomatic between the age of 20 and 30 years. There is a high mortality for individuals with uncorrected COARC who reach middle age. Complications of COARC include accelerated or so-called malignant hypertension, saccular or dissecting aortic aneurysms, bacterial endarteritis, and accelerated coronary atherosclerosis. Berry aneurysms of the circle of Willis are also more common in patients with COARC than in the rest of the population. Nearly all patients with COARC also have bicuspid aortic valves.
  2. Physical examination. Adults with COARC frequently demonstrate marked development of the upper half of the body as contrasted with the lower half.
    Bounding carotid pulses occur, similar to those noted in patients with aortic regurgitation; however, coexisting aortic regurgitation secondary to a bicuspid aortic valve is often present in patients with COARC. Notable differences in systolic blood pressure are recorded between the arm and the leg. Normally, leg systolic blood pressure is 10 to 20 mm Hg higher than that of arm pressure. In patients with COARC, arm systolic blood pressure is much higher than leg pressure. Simultaneous palpation of the brachial and femoral arteries demonstrates that the femoral pulse is delayed and of smaller amplitude. The left ventricular

impulse is often normal in patients with mild COARC. In those with severe COARC, the thrusting sustained impulse of pressure overloaded LVH usually is palpated. Auscultatory findings in COARC include an early systolic ejection click associated with systolic, diastolic, or continuous murmurs. These murmurs are usually best heard over the back in the vicinity of the fourth or fifth thoracic vertebra either in the middle or just to the left of the spine. Continuous murmurs generated by turbulent flow in dilated intercostal collateral vessels can be heard at various locations over the entire chest, but they are usually best heard posteriorly. Third (S3) and fourth (S4) heart sounds are often encountered as well.

3. ECG. Patients with significant COARC often demonstrate LVH on the ECG. Conduction defects such as incomplete or complete right bundle branch block or left bundle branch block also occur in these patients. Conduction defects may obscure left hypertrophy patterns. ECG findings in individuals with COARC are noted in Table 17-10.

4. Chest x-ray examination. The chest x-ray picture may be pathognomonic for COARC. Notching of the inferior rib margins from dilated collateral vessels is specific for COARC. In addition, many patients with this lesion have a dilated left subclavian artery, which produces a convexity above that of the aortic knob. These two convexities along the upper left sternal border form a silhouette of a number *3*. Left ventricular enlargement with or without pulmonary congestion secondary to left ventricular failure may also be seen in the chest roentgenogram. Radiographic findings of COARC are summarized in Table 17-10.

5. Echocardiography, computed tomography, and magnetic resonance imaging. Echocardiography demonstrates increased left ventricular wall thickness and dilatation of the aortic root. Left ventricular and left atrial dilatation may be present. A bicuspid aortic valve may be observed. The coarctation itself is usually difficult to visualize with transthoracic echocardiography in adults. However, the COARC can often be visualized by transesophageal echocardiography. Alternatively, the COARC can be visualized by computed tomography or magnetic resonance imaging with contrast.

6. Radionuclide studies. No left-to-right shunt is found by radionuclide angiocardiography in patients with uncomplicated COARC. Left ventricular function can be measured by means of radionuclide ventriculography.

7. Catheterization and angiography. No evidence of left-to-right shunt is found in patients with uncomplicated COARC. Left ventricular filling pressures may be elevated in patients with marked LVH or failure. Aortography in the left anterior oblique projection visualizes the COARC and numerous dilated, tortuous collateral vessels. A bicuspid aortic valve can usually be identified by aortography.

TABLE 17-10. ECG AND CHEST X-RAY FINDINGS IN PATIENTS WITH COARCTATION OF THE AORTA[a]

ECG findings
  Left ventricular hypertrophy
  Incomplete right bundle branch block
  Complete right bundle branch block
  Complete left bundle branch block

Roentgenographic findings
  Left ventricular enlargement
  Rib notching
  Dilated left subclavian artery and aortic knob forming a silhouette of the numeral 3

[a] Not all findings are present in every patient with coarction of the aorta.

8. Protocol for the diagnosis of COARC
   a. Testing sequence for making the diagnosis. The diagnosis usually is entertained when a patient with hypertension is found to have a marked difference between arm and leg systolic blood pressure. The diagnostic sequence outlined earlier for ASD can also be followed in patients with COARC. In addition, the COARC itself can be visualized by computed tomography or magnetic resonance imaging.
   b. Criteria for making the diagnosis. The diagnosis of COARC is made when a hypertensive individual has higher systolic pressures in the arm than in the leg, a systolic or continuous murmur heard over the midthoracic spine, and rib notching noted on the chest x-ray film. Aortography should be performed before surgical correction of this lesion. Appropriate surgical intervention requires knowledge of the severity and length of the constricting aortic segment.
   c. Differential diagnosis. Other entities must be distinguished from COARC.
      (1) Aortic valve disease. Many patients with COARC have an associated bicuspid aortic valve with stenosis or regurgitation or both. The resulting physical findings are a blend of those seen from each lesion with widely heard systolic and diastolic murmurs. Differentiation of the two lesions rests on the difference between arm and leg pressures, the presence of a loud paraspinal murmur, rib notching, and the "3 sign" on the chest film in patients with COARC, as well as on echocardiographic or radiologic evidence of aortic valve disease in patients with aortic stenosis or regurgitation.
      (2) PDA. The continuous murmur of PDA is heard only in a small, localized area along the upper left sternal border, whereas the continuous murmur of COARC is localized to the midthoracic paraspinal region.
         Patients with COARC have no radiographic or radionuclide evidence of a left-to-right shunt, whereas those with PDA have normal leg pulses and blood pressure. Rib notching on the chest film is seen only in individuals with COARC.
      (3) Pulmonary arteriovenous fistula. Continuous murmurs heard over the posterior thorax may be secondary to pulmonary arteriovenous fistulae. These are usually evident on the chest x-ray film, which also fails to reveal the rib notching or "3 sign" associated with COARC. Lower-extremity pulses and blood pressure are normal in patients with pulmonary arteriovenous fistulae.
      (4) Branch stenosis of a pulmonary artery. Continuous murmurs heard over the posterior chest can be generated by turbulent flow distal to a peripheral branch stenosis of one or more pulmonary arteries. Some of the stenoses can be seen on the posteroanterior chest film. Roentgenographic findings of COARC are absent, and lower-extremity pulses and blood pressure are normal. Elevated main pulmonary arterial pressure secondary to multiple branch stenoses produces compensatory RVH and right ventricular dilatation, which may be appreciated by physical examination or ECG.

B. Therapy
   1. Medical treatment. Left ventricular failure is treated with conventional measures including rest, digitalis, diuretics, vasodilators, and decreased salt intake. Bacterial endarteritis is managed with long-term intravenous antibiotics. Antihypertensive medication also is administered, but not as primary therapy. Surgical correction of the COARC is indicated in all patients except those with other severe debilitating illnesses.
      a. Antihypertensive medication is frequently required even after successful repair of COARC.

b. Prophylactic antibiotics should be administered to individuals with unrepaired COARC and to patients with repaired COARC who have bicuspid aortic valves.

2. Surgery/interventional cardiology. All patients who can tolerate the procedure should have elective repair of the COARC. Percutaneous balloon dilatation of COARC can be performed and avoids major surgery. Despite successful correction of a COARC, there is an increased late mortality in these patients secondary to MI and cerebrovascular hemorrhage.

VII. Cyanotic congenital heart disease. Most individuals with severe cyanosis resulting in clubbing of the fingers or toes have Eisenmenger's syndrome with severe pulmonary vascular disease and a right-to-left shunt. Murmurs may be soft or absent, and the clinical picture is often dominated by the findings of right ventricular dilatation with or without failure. It may be difficult to identify the defect through which the right-to-left shunt is occurring. Echocardiography with intravenous injection of fluid containing microbubbles (contrast echocardiography) or cardiac catheterization with angiography (or both) may be required to identify the location of the defect. Management of Eisenmenger's syndrome is discussed in Section **II.B.1.**

SELECTED READINGS

Chen CR, Cheng TO, Huang T, et al. Percutaneous balloon valvuloplasty for pulmonic stenosis in adolescents and adults. *N Engl J Med* 1996;335:21–25.
Excellent results are obtained by balloon valvulotomy in adult patients with PS.

Corone P, Doyon F, Gaudeau S, et al. Natural history of ventricular septal defect: a study involving 790 cases. *Circulation* 1977;55:908–915.
A 25-year study of a large population of children and adults with VSD.

Dalen JE, Haynes FW, Dexter L. Life expectancy with atrial septal defect. *JAMA* 1967;200:442–446.
Discussion of severe pulmonary hypertension in middle-aged patients with ASD.

De Lezo JS, Pan M, Romero M, et al. Immediate and follow-up findings after stent treatment for severe coarctation of aorta. *Am J Cardiol* 1999;83:400–406.
This interventional catheter technique gives excellent early results in the management of COARC; however, restenosis within the stent can occur.

Engle MA, Perloff JK. *Congenital heart disease after surgery: benefits, residua, sequelae.* New York: Yorke, 1983.
Extensive review of long-term results of cardiac surgery for congenital heart disease. Chapters review specific lesions and specific operative repairs.

Fahmy A, Schiavone W. Unusual clinical presentations of secundum atrial septal defect. *Chest* 1993;104:1075–1078.
Examples of unusual ASD clinical presentations.

Fawzy ME, Sivanandam V, Pieters F, et al. Long-term effects of balloon angioplasty on systemic hypertension in adolescent and adult patients with coarctation of the aorta. *Eur Heart J* 1999;20:827–832.
Normalization of blood pressure occurred in 74% of patients after balloon angioplasty for COARC.

Gray DT, Fyler DC, Walker AM, et al. Clinical outcomes and costs of transcatheter as compared with surgical closure of patent ductus arteriosus. *N Engl J Med* 1993;329:1517–1523.
Surgery was better than catheter closure of PDAs with respect to clinical results and cost.

Groundstroem KWE, Iivainen TE, Talvensaari T, et al. Late postoperative follow-up of ostium secundum defect. *Eur Heart J* 1999;20:904–909.
Patients with secundum ASD should be operated on when they are young.

Hu DC, Seward JB, Puga FL, et al. Total correction of tetralogy of Fallot at age 40 years and older: long-term follow-up. *J Am Coll Cardiol* 1985;5:40–44.
Excellent results can be obtained with surgical repair of adult patients with tetralogy of Fallot.

James FW, Kaplan S. Systolic hypertension during submaximal exercise after correction of coarctation of the aorta. *Circulation* 1974;50(Suppl II):II27–II34.

Residual hypertension at rest and during exercise after surgical repair of coarctation.

Johnson LW, Grossman W, Dalen JE, et al. Pulmonic stenosis in the adult: long-term follow-up results. *N Engl J Med* 1972; 287:1159–1163.
PS in the adult consistent with long-term, asymptomatic survival.

Maron BJ, Humphries JO, Rowe RD, et al. Prognosis of surgically corrected coarctation of the aorta: a 20-year postoperative appraisal. *Circulation* 1973;47:119–126.
Cardiovascular complications and hypertension despite successful correction of coarctation.

Masura J, Burch M, Deanfield JE, et al. Five-year follow-up after balloon pulmonary valvuloplasty. *J Am Coll Cardiol* 1993;21:132–136.
Balloon valvuloplasty is an effective therapy for PS.

Moller JH, Patton C, Varco RL, et al. Late results (30 to 35 years) after operative closure of isolated ventricular septal defect from 1954–1960. *Am J Cardiol* 1991;68: 1491–1497.
VSDs should be closed at young ages; long-term results are excellent.

Murphy JG, Gersh BJ, McGoon MD, et al. Long-term outcome after surgical repair of isolated atrial septal defect. *N Engl J Med* 1990;323:1645–1650.
Patients operated on before 25 years of age do very well; those operated on later need close follow-up.

Neumayer U, Stone S. Somerville J. Small ventricular septal defects in adults. *Eur Heart J* 1998;19:1573–1582.
The course of small VSDs is not necessarily benign in adults.

Perloff JK. *The clinical recognition of congenital heart disease,* 4th ed. Philadelphia: Saunders, 1994.
A comprehensive but clear review of the major clinical features of various congenital heart diseases.

Perloff JK, Warnes CA. Challenges posed by adults with repaired congenital heart disease. *Circulation* 2001;103: 2637–2643.
A review of the various aspects of the care of adult patients with repaired congenital heart disease.

Presbitero P, Demarie D, Villani M, et al. Long-term results (15–30 years) of surgical repair of aortic coarctation. *Br Heart J* 1987;57:462–467.
Early repair of aortic coarctation improves long-term survival.

Rao PS. Balloon pulmonary valvuloplasty: a review. *Clin Cardiol* 1989;12:55–74.
Excellent results with pulmonary valvuloplasty for PS.

Rao PS, Berger F, Rey C, et al. Results of transvenous occlusion of secundum atrial septal defects with the fourth generation buttoned device: comparison with first, second, third generation devices. *J Am Coll Cardiol* 2000;36:583–592.
Excellent results were obtained with this interventional catheter technique for closure of ASD.

Rao PS, Kim SH, Choi JY, et al. Follow-up results of transvenous occlusion of patent ductus arteriosus with the buttoned device. *J Am Coll Cardiol* 1999;33:820–826.
Excellent results were obtained with this interventional catheter technique for closure of PDA.

Shaddy RE, Boucek MM, Sturtevant JE, et al. Comparison of angioplasty and surgery for unoperated coarctation of the aorta. *Circulation* 1993;87:793–799.
Balloon dilatation can reduce the gradient across a coarctation; however, careful follow-up is necessary because of late complications such as aneurysm formation.

Thilen U, Berlind S, Varnauskas E. Atrial septal defect in adults: thirty eight year follow-up of a surgically and a conservatively managed group. *Scand Cardiovasc J* 2000;34:79–83.
Surgically treated patients with ASD do better than medically managed patients.

Webb GD, Williams RG. 32nd Bethesda Conference: care of the adult with congenital heart disease. *J Am Coll Cardiol* 2001;37:1161–1198.
A comprehensive review of various aspects of congenital heart disease in the adult.

18. CARDIOMYOPATHY, MYOCARDITIS, AND RHEUMATIC FEVER

I. **Introduction.** Cardiomyopathies, or myocardiopathies, are a group of diseases of the heart muscle itself. Less information is available about cardiac muscle disorders than about other forms of cardiac disease such as valvular, congenital, or coronary heart disease. Some forms of cardiomyopathy have a clear-cut cause, whereas many other types of myocardial disease occur without explanation. Because of the scarcity of knowledge concerning heart muscle disorders, a number of different classification schemes have been suggested, based on etiology (where known) or the pathologic and hemodynamic abnormality present. We favor the classification summarized in Table 18-1. It is based on both hemodynamic and pathologic differences between the respective types of heart muscle disease. In some forms of cardiomyopathy, the etiology of the disease is known. These types of cardiomyopathy are said to be secondary, as contrasted with primary forms of heart muscle disease, for which the cause is unknown (Table 18-2).

II. **Hypertrophic cardiomyopathy.** Patients with hypertrophic cardiomyopathy develop marked hypertrophy of the left ventricle. In some individuals, the hypertrophy tends to be localized to the left ventricular septum with encroachment on the left ventricular outflow tract. In other patients, hypertrophy is more uniform and outflow obstruction is absent.

Pathologic studies have demonstrated abnormal cellular architecture in the myocardium of patients with hypertrophic cardiomyopathy. Instead of having myocardial fibers arranged in parallel bundles as in normal myocardium, patients with hypertrophic cardiomyopathy have myocardial cells arranged in whorls and in random orientation. It has been suggested that the abnormal cellular architecture of patients with hypertrophic cardiomyopathy accounts for the marked myocardial hypertrophy noted in this condition. More than 30 different gene mutations have been identified in patients with hypertrophic cardiomyopathy. Most of the mutations involve abnormal synthesis of myosin. It seems plausible that abnormalities in myosin structure would lead to abnormal myocardial cellular architecture.

A. **Diagnosis**
1. **History.** There are a number of variants of hypertrophic cardiomyopathy:
    a. Patients with asymmetric septal hypertrophy (ASH) or asymmetric hypertrophy of other zones of the left ventricle have localized hypertrophy in one or multiple areas of the left ventricle. The commonest form of asymmetric hypertrophy involves the septum (ASH). The left ventricular septum is thicker than the free wall in these patients. Occasionally, other zones of the left ventricle, for example, the apex, are involved in the asymmetric hypertrophic process. In some individuals with ASH, the hypertrophied septum and anterior leaflet of the mitral valve encroach on the left ventricular outflow tract, causing significant obstruction to left ventricular ejection (idiopathic hypertrophic subaortic stenosis [IHSS]). Some individuals with ASH have no resting gradient across the left ventricular outflow tract. Beta-adrenergic stimulation of the myocardium with isoproterenol results in the development of a gradient. Late in the natural history of IHSS, the left ventricular outflow tract gradient disappears, and increasingly severe left ventricular failure develops. A suggested classification of hypertrophic cardiomyopathy is given in Fig. 18-1.

    Patients with ASH frequently demonstrate autosomal dominant inheritance, with some family members manifesting outflow obstruction (IHSS) and others not. As noted earlier, the genetic basis of hypertrophic cardiomyopathy has been explored, and a number of genetic abnormalities have been identified.

    b. Symmetric yet marked left ventricular hypertrophy (LVH) is less common than the asymmetric form of hypertrophic cardiomyopathy.

TABLE 18-1. CLASSIFICATION OF CARDIOMYOPATHY

Hypertrophic: stiffened, thick ventricular muscle with good contractile function; often involves the heart in an asymmetric manner (e.g., idiopathic hypertrophic subaortic stenosis, asymmetric septal hypertrophy)
Congestive: dilated, poorly contracting ventricle (e.g., viral or alcoholic cardiomyopathy)
Restrictive: stiffened ventricular muscle secondary to deposition of material between or within myocardial fibers (e.g., amyloidosis)
Obliterative: obliteration of ventricular cavity; quite rare (e.g., Löffler's eosinophilic endocarditis)

Patients with hypertrophic cardiomyopathy may complain of dyspnea on exertion, orthopnea, or angina. However, in many instances, patients with hypertrophic cardiomyopathy are asymptomatic. Symptoms are the result of elevated left ventricular filling pressures and thickened, stiff left ventricular myocardium, as well as mitral regurgitation, which is often part of this syndrome. Patients with IHSS can have malignant ventricular arrhythmias and die suddenly, although this occurs infrequently. Heart failure is often progressive once it begins and may lead to death, particularly in patients who develop atrial fibrillation. Systemic embolism is a problem with both the asymmetric and the symmetric forms of the disease. Patients with IHSS often have mitral regurgitation. Bacterial endocarditis can develop on either the mitral or the aortic valve in these patients.

2. Physical examination. The carotid pulse is usually brisk in patients with hypertrophic cardiomyopathy. In some individuals with IHSS, a bisferiens pulse is noted. A systolic murmur is often heard in patients with ASH with or without outflow tract obstruction. The murmur is ejection in quality and radiation, resembling that of aortic stenosis. Mitral regurgitation is likely to be present, however, and this murmur can be superimposed on the systolic ejection murmur, thereby confusing the examiner. Maneuvers are often helpful in distinguishing the murmurs of IHSS, mitral regurgitation, and aortic stenosis (Table 18-3).

TABLE 18-2. ETIOLOGY OF CARDIOMYOPATHIES

Primary: sporadic or inherited pattern of occurrence; etiology unknown
  Idiopathic hypertrophic subaortic stenosis
  Most cases of congestive cardiomyopathy
  Most cases of obliterative cardiomyopathy

Secondary: sporadic occurrence; muscle disease the result of another disease state or toxin

Hemochromatosis	
Amyloidosis	
Sarcoidosis	Restrictive
Glycogen storage diseases	
Neoplasm	

Postpartum disorders	
Variety of toxins including alcohol, cobalt, daunorubicin	
Connective tissue diseases (e.g., systemic lupus erythematosus)	Congestive
Infectious disease (e.g., viral, parasitic, rickettsia, tuberculosis)	
Neuromuscular disease (e.g., muscular dystrophy, Friedreich's ataxia)	
Thiamine deficiency (beriberi)	

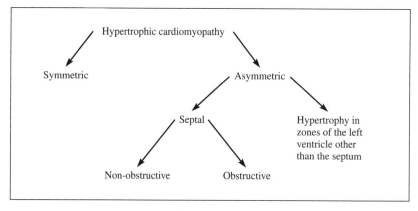

FIG. 18-1. Classification of hypertrophic cardiomyopathy.

Prominent fourth heart sounds (S4) are almost invariably heard in patients with IHSS. Physical findings in patients with hypertrophic cardiomyopathy are as follows:

Irregularly irregular pulse (atrial fibrillation; late in the course of the illness)
Brisk carotid pulse, bisferiens in quality in some patients with IHSS
Increased left ventricular apical impulse (occasionally bisferiens in quality)
Systolic ejection murmur that changes in intensity with maneuvers (Table 18-3)
Murmur of mitral regurgitation
Prominent S4
Third heart sound (S3), occasionally

3. ECG. ECG findings in patients with hypertrophic cardiomyopathy include left ventricular hypertrophy, left atrial enlargement, and various conduction disturbances such as left bundle branch block.

The Wolff-Parkinson-White syndrome is associated with IHSS. Occasionally, deep Q waves or Q–S patterns that simulate myocardial infarction (MI) occur in anterior or inferior leads. Table 18-4 lists the various

TABLE 18-3. RESPONSE OF MURMURS OF IHSS, AORTIC STENOSIS, AND MITRAL REGURGITATION TO VARIOUS MANEUVERS

Response	IHSS	Mitral regurgitation, aortic stenosis
Decrease left ventricular cavity size: Valsalva maneuver, standing, inhalation of amyl nitrite, intravenous infusion of phentolamine	↑	↓
Increase left ventricular cavity size: squatting, infusion of phenylephrine, passive elevation of patient's legs	↓	No change or ↑
Increase left ventricular contractility: infusion of isoproterenol	↑	No change or slight ↑

IHSS, idiopathic hypertrophic subaortic stenosis; ↑, increase; ↓, decrease.

TABLE 18-4. ECG AND ROENTGENOGRAPHIC FINDINGS IN IDIOPATHIC HYPETROPHIC SUBAORTIC STENOSIS

ECG findings
   Left axis deviation
   Left ventricular hypertrophy
   Left atrial enlargement
   Conduction disturbances
   Wolff-Parkinson-White syndrome
   Pseudo inferior infarction (Q waves in II, III, and AVF)
   Pseudo anterior infarction (Q–S waves in precordial leads)
   Atrial and ventricular arrhythmias

Chest x-ray findings
   Left ventricular enlargement
   Prominent ascending aorta secondary to poststenotic dilatation of the aorta
   Pulmonary congestion (late in course of disease)

ECG findings in patients with IHSS. Holter monitoring or exercise testing may reveal malignant ventricular arrhythmias.

4. Chest x-ray examination. The most common roentgenographic finding in patients with hypertrophic cardiomyopathy is left ventricular enlargement.

   Widening of the ascending aorta secondary to poststenotic dilatation is not infrequent in patients with IHSS, although it is more likely to be seen in patients with valvular aortic stenosis. The shadow of the widened ascending aorta can be observed to the right of the sternal border in the posteroanterior chest film. Calcification of the aortic valve is usually not found in patients with IHSS. Roentgenographic findings in patients with IHSS are listed in Table 18-4.

5. Echocardiography. The echocardiogram demonstrates a number of findings specific for IHSS. Disproportionate septal thickening, abnormal anterior systolic motion of the mitral valve, and midsystolic partial closure of the aortic valve leaflets can all be observed in the echocardiograms of patients with IHSS. The left ventricular outflow tract gradient can be measured by Doppler study. Disproportionate septal thickening alone—ASH—can be recorded in patients with abnormal septal hypertrophy without left ventricular outflow obstruction. Patients with IHSS (outflow obstruction present) usually manifest all the echocardiographic features mentioned previously. Patients with symmetric LVH demonstrate uniform thickening of the septum and posterior wall of the left ventricle. Patients with asymmetric hypertrophy in other zones of the left ventricle, for example, the apex, can also be identified by an echocardiographic examination.

6. Radionuclide studies. Left ventricular function can be quantitated by radionuclide ventriculography. Myocardial scintigraphy after the intravenous injection of radioactive thallium demonstrates disproportionate septal thickening in patients with ASH, and uniform left ventricular wall thickening in patients with symmetric hypertrophic cardiomyopathy. Minor perfusion abnormalities may be observed in the hypertrophied zones.

7. Catheterization and angiography. A pressure gradient occurs at rest or with provocation within the body of the left ventricle of patients with IHSS. Left ventricular filling pressures are often elevated.

   Angiography demonstrates a hypercontractile left ventricle that empties almost completely at end systole. A characteristic banana-shaped left ventricular cavity often is seen by ventriculography in patients with all forms of hypertrophic cardiomyopathy.

8. Biopsy. Samples of septal myocardium can be obtained by a cardiac bioptome. They come from the right ventricular side of the septum. Samples of septal myocardium from patients with ASH often demonstrate whorls of myocardial cells instead of the normal linear cellular array.

9. Protocol for the diagnosis of hypertrophic cardiomyopathy

a. Testing sequence for making the diagnosis. The diagnosis of hypertrophic cardiomyopathy usually is suggested when a murmur that behaves appropriately with various maneuvers is noted. The diagnosis is confirmed by echocardiography.

Symmetric hypertrophic cardiomyopathy usually presents as unexplained exertional dyspnea or LVH by ECG or chest x-ray film. An appropriate diagnostic protocol for patients with suspected hypertrophic cardiomyopathy is as follows:

History and physical examination (systolic murmur that changes appropriately with maneuvers)
↓
ECG (left ventricular hypertrophy)
↓
Chest x-ray film (left ventricular enlargement)
↓
Echocardiography or thallium myocardial scintigraphy to confirm the diagnosis; catheterization and angiography necessary only if surgery is contemplated

b. Criteria for making the diagnosis

(1) Hypertrophic cardiomyopathy without obstruction. Patients are symptomatic or asymptomatic, often with systolic murmurs that behave appropriately with maneuvers; symmetric or disproportionate septal thickening is noted by echocardiography or thallium myocardial scintigraphy. The ECG and chest x-ray may reveal LVH. Catheterization demonstrates no resting or provocable gradient across the left ventricular outflow tract. Patients with symmetric LVH are designated as having symmetric hypertrophic cardiomyopathy. Patients with disproportionate septal hypertrophy are said to have hypertrophic cardiomyopathy with ASH.

(2) Hypertrophic cardiomyopathy with obstruction (IHSS). Patients are symptomatic or asymptomatic, with systolic murmurs that behave appropriately with maneuvers. Disproportionate septal thickening and abnormal aortic and mitral valve movements are seen by echocardiography. Disproportionate septal thickening also can be observed by thallium myocardial scintigraphy. The ECG and chest x-ray film usually demonstrate LVH. Catheterization and Doppler echocardiography document the presence of a resting or provocable gradient across the left ventricular outflow tract.

c. Differential diagnosis

(1) Hypertensive heart disease. Hypertensive heart disease with marked LVH can simulate the findings of hypertrophic cardiomyopathy particularly in elderly individuals. The major difference between these two entities is the absence of hypertension or a history of hypertension in patients with hypertrophic cardiomyopathy.

(2) Aortic stenosis. Aortic stenosis frequently is confused with ASH or IHSS because systolic ejection murmurs are present in both conditions. These two entities are distinguished by the different behavior of the murmurs in the two conditions with various maneuvers (Table 18-3). A slow carotid pulse upstroke

is noted in aortic stenosis, and brisk carotid pulses occur in hypertrophic cardiomyopathy or IHSS. Moreover, patients with aortic stenosis frequently have calcified aortic valves by fluoroscopy. Disproportionate septal thickening and normal aortic valve leaflet thickness are observed in the echocardiograms of patients with ASH.

(3) Mitral regurgitation. Mitral regurgitation can be confused with hypertrophic cardiomyopathy by the similarity of the systolic murmurs in the two conditions. These entities are distinguished by the different response of the respective murmurs to various maneuvers (Table 18-3). Disproportionate septal thickening is seen, by echocardiography, only in patients with ASH. Many patients with hypertrophic cardiomyopathy have coexisting mitral regurgitation.

(4) Ventricular septal defect. Ventricular septal defect also produces a systolic murmur, which may resemble that of hypertrophic cardiomyopathy. As with mitral regurgitation, the two conditions can be differentiated by differing responses of the respective murmurs to maneuvers and by differences in the echocardiogram and Doppler study.

B. Therapy

1. Medical treatment

a. Antibiotics. Bacterial endocarditis can occur on the aortic or mitral valves of patients with hypertrophic cardiomyopathy. Consequently, prophylactic antibiotics should be administered before dental and surgical procedures are undertaken.

b. Digitalis and diuretics. Digitalis and diuretics are contraindicated in patients with IHSS because they may provoke or increase the gradient across the left ventricular outflow tract by increasing myocardial contractility and decreasing left ventricular cavity size. Late in the natural history of IHSS, left ventricular failure and atrial fibrillation may occur. In this setting, digitalis and diuretic therapy may be appropriate.

c. Vasodilators. Because vasodilators can increase or provoke the left ventricular outflow tract gradient, they too are contraindicated in IHSS. Occasionally, late in the natural history of IHSS, they can be used with or without digitalis and diuretics for the treatment of severe left ventricular failure.

d. Anticoagulation. When atrial fibrillation occurs in patients with hypertrophic cardiomyopathy, the risk of arterial embolism is great. Consequently, oral anticoagulation with warfarin should be prescribed for such individuals. All patients with hypertrophic cardiomyopathy who have had an episode of arterial embolism should be anticoagulated for life.

e. Beta-blockade and calcium channel blockade. Patients with IHSS and symptoms of angina, fatigue, or syncope may benefit from the administration beta-blockers. In the past, propranolol (usually given 40 mg four times a day or more) was noted to produce symptomatic improvement. Other beta-blockers such as atenolol or metoprolol have also been used in patients with hypertrophic cardiomyopathy. Slowing the heart rate by means of beta-blockade improves diastolic filling of the left ventricle. Administration of beta-blockade can ameliorate the signs of left ventricular outflow tract obstruction (decreasing loudness of murmur, normalization of carotid pulse morphology). Sudden death still may occur in patients with IHSS, despite adequate treatment with beta-blockade. Late in the natural history of IHSS, the gradient often disappears and severe left ventricular failure develops. At this point, beta-blockade may worsen heart failure.

Verapamil is an excellent alternative to propranolol. This negatively inotropic calcium channel blocker has been shown to abolish the gradient associated with IHSS and to ameliorate symptoms in patients with angina or dyspnea secondary to hypertrophic cardiomyopathy. Verapamil is administered in a dosage of 80 to 160 mg four times a day to patients with this condition. Beta-blockade and verapamil should be administered concomitantly with great care because severe bradycardia with hypotension may result. Patients with hypertrophic cardiomyopathy, and particularly those with malignant ventricular arrhythmias, benefit from amiodarone therapy. Disopyramide has also been used on occasion because of its negative inotropic action in symptomatic patients with hypertrophic cardiomyopathy.

2. Surgery. Patients who remain symptomatic (angina, syncope, left ventricular failure) despite adequate medical therapy should undergo cardiac catheterization. If a significant left ventricular outflow tract gradient is present and if left ventricular function is good, such patients are candidates for left ventricular septal myotomy, alcohol ablation, or mitral valve replacement. Septal myotomy/myectomy involves incising and resecting some of the asymmetrically hypertrophied septum. Excellent long-term results have been obtained with this operation with respect to symptomatic relief; however, sudden death still may occur in patients with an excellent surgical result.

Alcohol septal ablation is performed in the cardiac catheterization laboratory. After balloon occlusion of the first septal branch of the left anterior descending coronary artery, the septal artery is filled with an alcohol solution that produces myocardial necrosis in the proximal septum. Excellent relief of obstructive outflow tract gradients have been obtained with this technique. Some cardiologists advocate atrioventricular sequential pacing for symptomatic patients. However, this latter procedure has not been conclusively demonstrated to ameliorate obstructive left ventricular outflow tract gradients.

III. Congestive cardiomyopathy. Congestive cardiomyopathy has many etiologies (Table 18-2). Left ventricular contractile function deteriorates, with resultant ventricular dilatation. Autopsy specimens from patients who died of congestive cardiomyopathy demonstrate dilated ventricles and flabby, pale ventricular muscle with modest hypertrophy.

A. Diagnosis.
1. History. Patients with congestive cardiomyopathy may give a history of a systemic allergic reaction, infection, exposure to a known cardiac toxin, or recent pregnancy. More often, no causative agent is identified. Patients complain of symptoms related to pulmonary venous hypertension (dyspnea on exertion, orthopnea, paroxysmal nocturnal dyspnea), systemic venous hypertension (anorexia, peripheral edema), or low cardiac output (fatigue). Other complications include arterial and venous embolism and arrhythmias, which may result in stroke, lightheadedness, frank syncope, or sudden death. Angina is usually not present.

2. Physical examination. Patients with congestive cardiomyopathy demonstrate findings of left ventricular failure (pulmonary congestion, S3, S4) and right ventricular failure (jugular venous distention, hepatomegaly, peripheral edema). Murmurs of tricuspid or mitral regurgitation are frequently present.

These are the result of dilatation of the valve annulus secondary to ventricular dilatation. Physical findings in patients with congestive cardiomyopathy are the following (not all findings are present in all patients):

Sinus tachycardia
Atrial fibrillation with irregularly irregular pulse
Pulsus alternans
Cool, clammy skin
Peripheral cyanosis
Jugular venous distention

Carotid pulse with normal upstroke, small volume
Pulmonary congestion (rales, pleural effusion)
Diffuse, often sustained, left ventricular apical impulse
Soft heart sounds
S3, S4
Murmurs of tricuspid and mitral regurgitation
Hepatomegaly
Ascites
Peripheral edema

3. ECG. ECG findings in patients with congestive cardiomyopathy include low-voltage QRS complexes, conduction defects, and atrial or ventricular (or both) arrhythmias. Holter monitoring or exercise testing also may disclose malignant ventricular arrhythmias such as ventricular tachycardia. The ECG findings in congestive cardiomyopathy are summarized in Table 18-5.

4. Chest x-ray examination. Left ventricular and often left atrial enlargement will be apparent on the chest x-ray films of patients with congestive cardiomyopathy. Occasionally, right ventricular enlargement is also seen. Massive cardiomegaly may be observed on the chest film, and it is sometimes difficult to distinguish congestive cardiomyopathy from large pericardial effusion by chest film alone. Signs of pulmonary venous hypertension are also frequently discernible in the chest roentgenograms of patients with congestive cardiomyopathy. Roentgenographic findings in patients with congestive cardiomyopathy are summarized in Table 18-5.

5. Echocardiography. Echocardiography demonstrates a dilated, poorly contractile left ventricle; left atrial dilatation; and mitral valve motion consistent with reduced cardiac output. Doppler study often reveals mitral or tricuspid regurgitation (or both).

6. Radionuclide studies. Radionuclide ventriculography demonstrates a dilated left ventricle with decreased ejection fraction. Right ventricular ejection fraction also may be abnormally depressed.

7. Catheterization and angiography. Hemodynamic studies reveal low cardiac output and stroke volume and elevated left ventricular filling pressures (pulmonary capillary wedge and pulmonary arterial diastolic pressures). Reactive pulmonary hypertension may be present secondary to markedly elevated pulmonary venous pressure. Ventriculography reveals a dilated left ventricle with low ejection fraction and diffusely reduced contractile function. Modest quantities of functional mitral or tricuspid regurgitation may be present secondary to ventricular dilatation.

TABLE 18-5. ECG AND ROENTGENOGRAPHIC FINDINGS IN CONGESTIVE CARDIOMYOPATHY

ECG findings
  Atrial fibrillation
  Ventricular arrhythmias
  Low-voltage
  QRS complexes
  Nonspecific T wave changes (flattening, inversion)
  Conduction defects (e.g., left bundle branch block)
  Left ventricular hypertrophy
  Poor R wave progression in precordial leads mimicking anterior myocardial infarction

Chest x-ray findings
  Left ventricular enlargement
  Left atrial enlargement
  Right ventricular enlargement (less common)
  Signs of pulmonary congestion (pulmonary vascular redistribution, interstitial edema)

8. Biopsy. Cardiac biopsy often reveals fibrosis or a variety of myocardial cellular abnormalities, depending on the etiology of the congestive cardiomyopathy.

9. Protocol for the diagnosis of congestive cardiomyopathy

   a. Testing sequence for making the diagnosis. Patients with a history and physical examination suggestive of congestive cardiomyopathy should have a chest x-ray study, an ECG, and an echocardiogram. Determination of left ventricular ejection fraction by radionuclide ventriculography may be helpful in confirming the diagnosis. Cardiac catheterization, angiography, and biopsy usually are not required to make the diagnosis of congestive cardiomyopathy.

   b. Criteria for making the diagnosis. The diagnosis should be suspected in symptomatic or asymptomatic individuals with S3 or S4, nonspecific ECG abnormalities, and left ventricular enlargement (often marked) on chest x-ray examination. Confirmation of the diagnosis rests on documentation of left ventricular dilatation and diffuse hypocontractility on echocardiography or radionuclide ventriculography.

   Catheterization, angiography, and biopsy are usually not required but may be performed in younger individuals. Patients should not have a history of MI or angina pectoris.

   c. Differential diagnosis

      (1) Pericardial effusion. Massive pericardial effusion may simulate congestive cardiomyopathy in that patients with effusions often complain of dyspnea and fatigue and demonstrate tachycardia, jugular venous distension, a loud early diastolic sound similar to a S3, and peripheral edema. The ECG can reveal low-voltage and nonspecific T wave changes, and the chest film may show marked cardiomegaly in both conditions. The two conditions are differentiated by the pericardial discomfort and rubs in patients with effusion and by echocardiography that clearly demonstrates the presence of pericardial fluid.

      (2) Mitral regurgitation. Marked left ventricular dilatation and dysfunction can occur with both congestive cardiomyopathy and mitral regurgitation. Indeed, late in the natural history of the two conditions, it may be impossible to tell them apart; patients in both groups reveal moderately severe mitral regurgitation and marked left ventricular dilatation and dysfunction. When a holosystolic murmur of mitral regurgitation is discovered in a patient with left ventricular enlargement on physical examination, chest x-ray film, or ECG, echocardiography with Doppler study or radionuclide ventriculography can help to distinguish severe mitral regurgitation with preserved left ventricular function from congestive cardiomyopathy with diffuse left ventricular hypokinesis and mild to moderate functional mitral regurgitation. Cardiac catheterization and angiography may be required to differentiate these two entities.

      (3) Other forms of myocardial disease are excluded on the basis of history or noninvasive evaluation of the left ventricle. Thus, acute myocarditis is excluded because of the protracted course of patients with congestive cardiomyopathy. Echocardiography differentiates congestive from hypertrophic cardiomyopathy. Myocardial biopsy or associated clinical and laboratory data may be required to differentiate congestive and restrictive cardiomyopathy and myocarditis.

B. Therapy

   1. Medical treatment

      a. Treatment of heart failure. Digitalis, diuretics, beta-blockers, and vasodilators (especially angiotensin-converting enzyme inhibitors) are used to treat symptomatic heart failure in patients with congestive cardiomyopathy. Decreased activity and even prolonged periods of bedrest have been suggested. These measures are often helpful in the initial treatment of heart failure, but few patients will tolerate prolonged periods of forced inactivity. Modest dietary salt restriction (no-added-salt diet), 5-g sodium diet, is indicated in patients with manifest left ventricular failure. Beta-blocker therapy should be initiated with very small doses of the chosen preparation. It may be necessary to increase the dosage of diuretics because of a tendency to retain fluids when beta-blocker therapy is initiated (see Chapter 4 on heart failure for more information on beta-blocker therapy in heart failure).

b. Anticoagulation. Patients with documented arterial or venous embolism need anticoagulation. Intravenous heparin for 7 to 10 days is followed by lifelong oral anticoagulation with warfarin. Some patients require the addition of a platelet anticoagulant (aspirin, dipyridamole, clopidogrel) to warfarin to prevent recurrent embolic episodes. Patients with signs of right ventricular failure should receive prophylactic anticoagulation with warfarin to prevent venous thrombosis and subsequent pulmonary embolism.

c. Antiarrhythmics. Patients with malignant ventricular arrhythmias (e.g., ventricular tachycardia) probably should receive antiarrhythmic agents. Often, antiarrhythmic therapy is selected after careful electrophysiologic study or after multiple Holter monitoring sessions using different antiarrhythmic regimens. Amiodarone is probably the best drug in this setting, but the results of randomized clinical trials of amiodarone therapy have been contradictory in patients with congestive cardiomyopathy and malignant ventricular arrhythmias.

2. Surgery. Mitral valvuloplasty or replacement can be performed and good results obtained in the rare patient with congestive cardiomyopathy in whom left ventricular dysfunction is only moderate and mitral regurgitation is moderately severe or worse.

Cardiac transplantation can be offered to younger individuals with end-stage congestive cardiomyopathy who are otherwise healthy. This procedure is costly and carries a high risk of complications, both medical and psychological. However, functional results are often excellent. Five-year survival after heart transplantation is approximately 80%.

IV. Restrictive cardiomyopathy. The pathophysiology of restrictive cardiomyopathy resembles that of constrictive pericarditis, with restriction of ventricular filling during diastole secondary to increased myocardial stiffness (decreased compliance). Clinically, the picture of predominant right ventricular failure often overshadows the milder signs and symptoms of left ventricular decompensation. A number of disease entities can result in restrictive cardiomyopathy (Table 18-2).

A. Diagnosis

1. History. Patients with restrictive cardiomyopathy usually complain of fatigue, anorexia, and peripheral edema (as do patients with right ventricular failure). Exercise tolerance is poor, and symptoms of left ventricular decompensation are not uncommon (dyspnea on exertion, orthopnea, and paroxysmal nocturnal dyspnea). Arterial embolism is a frequent complication, as are atrial and ventricular arrhythmias. Angina-like chest discomfort also is reported on occasion.

2. Physical examination. Signs of right ventricular failure are often more common than those of left ventricular decompensation: jugular venous distention, hepatomegaly, and peripheral edema. S3, S4, and murmurs of tricuspid or mitral regurgitation are often heard. Pulsus alternans is noted late in the course of the disease and implies severe ventricular decompensation. Physical findings in restrictive cardiomyopathy are as follows:

Sinus tachycardia
Atrial and ventricular arrhythmias
Pulsus alternans

Jugular venous distention
Pulmonary congestion (rales, pleural effusion)
Diffuse right or left (or both) ventricular impulse
Soft heart sounds
Murmurs of tricuspid or mitral (or both) regurgitation, S3, S4
Hepatomegaly
Hepatojugular reflex
Ascites
Peripheral edema

3. ECG. Atrial and ventricular arrhythmias are common, atrial fibrillation being the most frequently noted arrhythmia. Low-voltage QRS complexes and nonspecific T wave inversion and flattening can be present in the ECG.

Q–S complexes in the right precordial leads, or poor R wave progression, suggestive of anterior MI, will sometimes be observed. Conduction defects such as left bundle branch block and conduction disturbances ranging from first- to third-degree heart block are not uncommon. ECG findings in restrictive cardiomyopathy are listed in Table 18-6.

4. Chest x-ray examination. Patients with restrictive cardiomyopathy often demonstrate left ventricular enlargement, left atrial enlargement, and signs of pulmonary venous hypertension on the chest roentgenogram (Table 18-6).

5. Blood tests. A number of serologic abnormalities are found in patients with restrictive cardiomyopathy, depending on the underlying etiology of the cardiac disease. Thus, patients with sarcoidosis may have hypercalcemia, whereas individuals with hemochromatosis show high serum iron levels. A number of serologic tests have been devised for the diagnosis of amyloidosis (e.g., Congo red test), but these are often replaced by biopsy demonstration of amyloid deposits (see Section **IV.A.9.**).

6. Echocardiography. The echocardiogram often reveals left ventricular dilatation and decreased contractile function. Left atrial enlargement also may be observed. Doppler studies demonstrate abnormal ventricular filling. Bright myocardial echoes may be observed in patients with myocardial amyloidosis.

7. Radionuclide studies. Radionuclide ventriculography may document reduced left and sometimes right ventricular contractile function, as well as abnormal ventricular filling. Thallium myocardial scintigraphy may reveal multiple areas of decreased radionuclide uptake scattered throughout the myocardium in patients with sarcoidosis or metastatic tumor causing restrictive cardiomyopathy.

TABLE 18-6. ECG AND ROENTGENOGRAPHIC FINDINGS IN RESTRICTIVE CARDIOMYOPATHY

ECG findings
  Sinus tachycardia
  Atrial and ventricular arrhythmias (especially atrial fibrillation)
  Low-voltage QRS complexes
  Nonspecific ST–T changes
  Q–S pattern in right precordial leads (pseudoinfarction pattern)
  Conduction defects (e.g., left bundle branch block)
  Conduction disturbances (first-, second-, or third-degree heart block)

Chest x-ray findings
  Left ventricular enlargement
  Left atrial enlargement
  Pulmonary congestion (pulmonary vascular redistribution, interstitial edema)

8. Catheterization and angiography. Right atrial and right ventricular pressures are often markedly elevated. The right atrial pressure curve has an *M* shape. The right ventricular pressure curve has a characteristic early dip and plateau during diastole, producing a pattern that resembles a square root sign (??MS 632??).

The right atrial, right ventricular end-diastolic, pulmonary arterial diastolic, pulmonary capillary wedge, and left ventricular end-diastolic pressures are often approximately equal. However, this pattern is more often found in patients with constrictive pericarditis. Patients with restrictive cardiomyopathy usually have left ventricular filling pressures (pulmonary arterial diastolic, pulmonary capillary wedge, and left ventricular diastolic) that are considerably higher than right ventricular filling pressures (central venous, right atrial, right ventricular diastolic). Arterial pulse pressure is often diminished. Hemodynamic differentiation of restrictive cardiomyopathy from constrictive pericarditis is summarized in Table 18-7. When performed, ventriculography generally reveals diminished left ventricular contractile function (reduced ejection fraction).

9. Biopsy. Right ventricular septal biopsy can be a diagnostic aid in patients with restrictive cardiomyopathy. Amyloidosis, sarcoidosis, hemochromatosis, and metastatic tumor can be identified in this manner; however, biopsy of gum, rectal mucosa, bone marrow, skin, or liver yields similar diagnostic information and may be more readily available in most hospitals.

10. Magnetic resonance imaging (MRI). MRI studies are occasionally helpful in distinguishing restrictive cardiomyopathy from constrictive pericarditis.

11. Protocol for the diagnosis of restrictive cardiomyopathy
    a. Testing sequence for making the diagnosis. A history and physical examination suggesting right ventricular failure of unknown etiol-

TABLE 18-7. HEMODYNAMIC DIFFERENTIATION OF CONSTRICTIVE PERICARDITIS AND RESTRICTIVE CARDIOMYOPATHY

Parameter	Constrictive pericarditis	Restrictive cardiomyopathy
Right atrial pressure	Almost always >15 mm Hg	Usually <15 mm Hg if PCWP is normal
Right ventricular pressure	Square root sign always present End-diastolic pressure $\geq\frac{1}{3}$ of systolic pressure	Square root sign may disappear with therapy
Pulmonary artery pressure	Systolic pressure usually <40 mm Hg	Systolic pressure usually >40 mm Hg
Left atrial pressure	Approximately equal to right atrial pressure	10–20 mm Hg higher than right atrial pressure
Cardiac output	Often normal	Often depressed
Resting pulmonary arterial blood oxygen saturation	Often normal	Often decreased
Respiratory variation in pressure tracings	Often absent	Often present

PCWP, pulmonary capillary wedge pressure.

ogy should raise the suspicion of restrictive cardiomyopathy. Chest roentgenography, ECG, and echocardiography usually suffice to confirm the diagnosis. An occasional patient requires MRI, cardiac catheterization, or cardiac biopsy.

Diagnosis of the underlying etiology (e.g., hemochromatosis) is often made by associated laboratory or biopsy data.

b. Criteria for making the diagnosis. The diagnosis of restrictive cardiomyopathy is made in individuals with signs and symptoms of cardiac decompensation; often signs and symptoms of right ventricular failure are more prominent than those of left ventricular failure. The ECG frequently reveals conduction defects, various forms of heart block, and low-voltage QRS complexes, and the chest film demonstrates left ventricular enlargement. Echocardiography shows reduced left ventricular contractile and diastolic function. Ancillary laboratory and biopsy data confirm a diagnosis associated with restrictive cardiomyopathy (e.g., hemochromatosis, sarcoidosis, amyloidosis, carcinomatosis). An occasional patient who comes to catheterization demonstrates a hemodynamic pattern similar to that seen in constrictive pericarditis with some small differences (Table 18-7).

c. Differential diagnosis. Symptoms and signs of systemic venous hypertension are seen in patients with constrictive pericarditis and restrictive cardiomyopathy. The two entities are distinguished on the basis of thickening and calcification of the pericardium on roentgenography, echocardiography, or MRI and by means of hemodynamic differences already cited (Table 18-7).

B. Therapy
1. Medical treatment
a. Therapy for restrictive myopathy is often unsatisfactory. Individual disease entities may require treatment aimed at the specific condition (e.g., repeated phlebotomy for some forms of hemochromatosis, steroids for sarcoidosis, and radiation or antimetabolites for neoplasms or amyloidosis).
b. Symptomatic pulmonary or systemic venous hypertension may improve with decreased dietary sodium intake or long-acting nitrates. Digitalis is of no benefit if ventricular contractile function is adequate.
c. Anticoagulation is indicated in severe cases of restrictive cardiomyopathy to prevent venous and arterial thromboembolism.
d. Patients with sarcoid heart disease or cardiac tumors may develop third-degree heart block, requiring permanent pacing.
2. Surgery. Cardiac transplantation is indicated in patients with severe restrictive cardiomyopathy with refractory symptoms of heart failure.
V. Myocarditis and rheumatic fever. The myocardial diseases discussed earlier in this chapter are all chronic conditions with clinical courses that evolve over a period of years. Acute forms of myocardial disease have a natural history that unfolds over a period of days, weeks, or months. Acute myocarditis may progress to a chronic cardiomyopathy, or it may resolve with minimal or no sequelae. A variety of etiologic agents can produce acute myocarditis (Table 18-8).
A. Diagnosis
1. History. Patients with acute myocarditis frequently complain of symptoms related to the underlying condition, of which myocarditis is but a part. Symptoms that often accompany myocarditis include fever, chills, weakness, palpitation, and precordial pain (secondary to a commonly associated pericarditis). Dyspnea on exertion, orthopnea, and easy fatigability are reported by individuals in whom myocarditis causes left or right ventricular (or both) decompensation.

Patients with acute **rheumatic fever** may complain of fever, arthritis, abdominal pain, epistaxis, nonspecific symptoms (fatigability, nervous irritability, "growing pains" in joints and adjacent muscles), or

TABLE 18-8. ETIOLOGY OF ACUTE MYOCARDITIS

Infectious
  Viral
  Diphtheria
  Suppurative myocarditis secondary to bacteremia with a variety of organisms
  Chagas' disease (*Trypanosoma cruzi*)
  Trichinosis
  Rheumatic fever (group A beta-hemolytic streptococcus)

Toxic
  Serum sickness
  Uremia
  Radiation
  Phenothiazines and other drugs
  Industrial exposure to toxic chemicals

Cobalt

---

cardiac symptoms (dyspnea, edema, or precordial pain secondary to pericarditis). Rheumatic fever is very uncommon in adults. It usually occurs in children 5 to 15 years of age.

2. Physical examination. Patients with myocarditis usually seek medical attention because of heart failure or arrhythmias. Signs of left or right ventricular failure, or both, may be present. The heart sounds are frequently soft or muffled. The pulse may be irregularly irregular (atrial fibrillation), or frequent extrasystoles (atrial or ventricular premature beats) may be noted.

   Findings related to the underlying cause of the myocarditis may be present (e.g., the suppurative pharyngeal membrane of diphtheria, coryza and mucosal injection in viral syndromes or arthritis, and skin rash in serum sickness). Fever and tachycardia are commonly found with all types of myocarditis.

   Besides the systemic signs of fever, tachycardia, and sweating, **rheumatic fever** is associated with five major physical findings: arthritis, carditis, chorea, subcutaneous nodules, and erythema marginatum (Table 18-9). A murmur of mitral regurgitation may be present. Other findings may include cyanosis, tendinitis, myositis, pleural rubs, and abdominal tenderness.

3. ECG. The ECG of patients with myocarditis may be normal. Intraventricular conduction defects, bundle branch blocks, or heart block may be noted. Patients with extensive and severe myocardial involvement frequently demonstrate low-voltage QRS complexes and Q waves simulating those of MI. ECG findings in patients with myocarditis are summarized in Table 18-10.

   ECG abnormalities associated with **rheumatic fever** include impaired AV conduction (first-, second-, and, rarely, third-degree heart block), S–T and T wave changes, low-voltage QRS complexes, prolongation of the Q–T interval, and atrial or ventricular (or both) arrhythmias (Table 18-10).

4. Chest x-ray examination. Cardiomegaly frequently is revealed in the chest x-ray film of patients with myocarditis. In some individuals, cardiomegaly is secondary to ventricular dilatation; in others, increased heart size is the result of pericardial effusion. Signs of left ventricular decompensation (pulmonary vascular redistribution, interstitial edema, and pleural effusion) are often seen in the chest roentgenogram. Roentgenographic findings in patients with rheumatic fever are similar to those seen with other forms of myocarditis.

TABLE 18-9. PHYSICAL FINDINGS IN RHEUMATIC FEVER

Major manifestations
  Arthritis: usually involves two or more large joints; migratory. Tenderness, erythema, heat, swelling, and limitation of motion should be present.
  Carditis: cardiomegaly; signs of left ventricular failure (rales, pleural effusion, third heart sound); pericarditis (pericarditic pain, rub, or both); murmurs of mitral stenosis, mitral regurgitation, or aortic regurgitation
  Sydenham's chorea: constant, uncoordinated, purposeless muscular activity; facial grimacing, rolling of eyes, tossing of head, and wrinkling of forehead. Holding the patient's outstretched hands for several minutes reveals exaggerated muscular twitchings.
  Subcutaneous nodules: freely movable, subcutaneous nodules 2–20 mm in diameter, tending to occur over bony prominences, tendons, and periosteum. Nodules are painless and not associated with erythema of overlying skin.
  Erythema marginatum: erythematous lesions usually occurring in the trunk, but occasionally seen on the extremities. They begin as reddish or violaceous macules or papules (1–5 mm in diameter) and develop rapidly, while one observes them, into large circles or segments of circles that join or intersect, forming scalloped, serpentine, or crescentic patterns. At the margin, the lesions are pale pink or dull red, sharply circumscribed, and slightly elevated.

Minor manifestations
  Malnutrition or wasted appearance (rare)
  Pallor
  Frequent pharyngitis
  Epistaxis
  Abdominal pain or tenderness or both
  Fever
  Laboratory findings (elevated sedimentation rate, leukocytosis, elevated antistreptolysin O titer)

5. Laboratory tests. Leukocytosis and an elevated erythrocyte sedimentation rate are often present at some point in the course of myocarditis; however, patients may first come to medical attention at a time when the white count and the sedimentation rate have returned to normal. Serum troponin and the MB fraction of creatine phosphokinase are likely to be elevated during episodes of acute myocardial inflammation.

Complement fixation tests can document the presence of infectious agents such as *Trichinella, Trypanosoma cruzi,* and various viral species. Specific laboratory findings often are present in patients with myocarditis secondary to serum sickness, uremia, cobalt intoxication, and phenothiazine toxicity. A number of different laboratory findings have been described in patients with **rheumatic fever,** including culture of

TABLE 18-10. ECG findings in myocarditis and rheumatic fever

Atrial and ventricular arrhythmias
Intraventricular conduction delay
Bundle branch block
Impaired atrioventricular conduction (first-, second-, and third-degree heart block)
Low-voltage QRS complexes
Significant Q waves (pseudoinfarction)
ST–T changes
Prolonged Q–T interval

group A beta-hemolytic streptococci from throat or skin lesions and elevated titers of antistreptolysin O (ASLO), antistreptokinase, or antihyaluronidase antibodies. Nonspecific findings include leukocytosis, elevated sedimentation rate, and increased C-reactive protein level. Laboratory findings in rheumatic fever are listed in Table 18-11.

6. Echocardiography. Pericardial effusion or decreased left ventricular contractile function may be noted in the echocardiogram of patients with myocarditis or rheumatic fever. Mitral valvular abnormalities or mitral regurgitation (or both) also may be found in patients with rheumatic fever. An echocardiographic study that demonstrates one or more of these findings is very helpful in confirming the diagnosis of acute rheumatic fever.

7. Radionuclide studies. Abnormally low left ventricular ejection fraction can be documented in many patients with myocarditis or rheumatic fever by means of radionuclide ventriculography.

8. Catheterization and angiography. Elevated ventricular filling pressures, decreased cardiac output, and abnormally reduced ejection fraction generally are noted in patients with myocarditis who undergo cardiac catheterization and angiography. Catheterization usually is not necessary to make the diagnosis of myocarditis. Indeed, catheterization findings are ordinarily nonspecific (i.e., cardiac decompensation is noted without evidence of coronary arterial, valvular, or congenital heart disease).

9. Biopsy. Biopsy of right ventricular endocardium is often performed in patients with myocarditis. Inflammatory cellular infiltration of the myocardium has been documented. This contrasts with biopsy findings in other forms of myocardial disease (hypertrophic, congestive, restrictive), in which cellular infiltration of the myocardium is sparse or absent.

10. Protocol for the diagnosis of myocarditis and rheumatic fever
    a. Testing sequence for making the diagnosis of myocarditis. A history of recent onset of symptoms of ventricular failure or arrhythmias in the absence of coronary arterial, valvular, or congenital heart disease should suggest the diagnosis of myocarditis. Specific infectious and toxic agents should be sought by history, physical examination, and laboratory testing. Confirmation of myocardial involvement and the degree of ventricular decompensation are obtained by ECG, chest x-ray film, and echocardiography.

    Cardiac catheterization and myocardial biopsy may be required to make the diagnosis of myocarditis. The following is a diagnostic pro-

TABLE 18-11. LABORATORY FINDINGS IN RHEUMATIC FEVER

Nonspecific findings
  Leukocytosis (usually 10,000–16,000/L)
  Anemia
  Elevated serum C-reactive protein level
  Elevated erythrocyte sedimentation rate
  Elevated serum levels of myocardial biomarkers (troponin, creatine kinase MB)
  Reversed albumin-globulin ratio

Streptococcus-related findings: elevated and especially rising serum titers of
  Antistreptolysin O
  Antistreptokinase
  Antihyaluronidase
  Antideoxyribonuclease B
  Antidiphosphopyridine nucleotidase

tocol for patients suspected of having myocarditis (dashed arrow indicates optional step):

History and physical examination
↓
ECG and chest x-ray film
↓
Laboratory tests (white blood cell count, erythrocyte sedimentation rate, complement fixation tests, etc.)
↓
Echocardiography
↓
Cardiac catheterization and myocardial biopsy (may be required)

b. Testing sequence for making the diagnosis of rheumatic fever. Because the diagnosis of rheumatic fever is based on clinical data, the protocol for making the diagnosis is straightforward: A careful history and physical examination and selected laboratory tests (e.g., throat culture, ASLO titer, erythrocyte sedimentation rate, white blood cell count) are required.

c. Criteria for making the diagnosis of myocarditis. The diagnosis of myocarditis is made in individuals with recent-onset ventricular decompensation or arrhythmias without evidence of coronary, valvular, or congenital heart disease. Documentation of myocardial involvement is obtained from the ECG (Table 18-10), the chest x-ray film (signs of left ventricular decompensation), and the echocardiogram (pericardial effusion, decreased left ventricular contractile function). The etiology of the myocarditis may be obvious (e.g., recent radical radiotherapy to the mediastinum) or occult (e.g., exposure to industrial toxins). Laboratory testing should be used to seek the specific causative agent. Cardiac catheterization or myocardial biopsy may be necessary to confirm the diagnosis. Confirmation often is obtained in retrospect when resolution of heart failure and arrhythmias occur. Catheterization and biopsy may be indicated in individuals with progressive heart failure.

d. Criteria for making the diagnosis of rheumatic fever. According to Jones, rheumatic fever is diagnosed in any individual with two major manifestations (Table 18-9). The diagnosis is probable in individuals with one major and two minor manifestations, except when the major manifestation is arthritis.

e. Differential diagnosis of myocarditis. Other forms of myocardial disease must be excluded to make the diagnosis of myocarditis. In general, other forms of myocardial disease have a history of chronic symptoms, whereas the course is acute with myocarditis. Echocardiography distinguishes hypertrophic cardiomyopathy. Catheterization and myocardial biopsy may be required to differentiate myocarditis from other forms of myocardial disease.

f. Differential diagnosis of rheumatic fever
   (1) Subacute bacterial endocarditis. Fever, valvular murmurs, skin lesions, and arthralgias occurring in a patient with bacterial endocarditis may simulate acute rheumatic fever. Differentiation of these two entities depends on positive blood cultures, the differing skin lesions of the two conditions, and the age of the patient: Rheumatic fever is rare in adults, but bacterial endocarditis on a chronic rheumatic valve is common.
   (2) Viral syndromes. Viral infections can cause fever, arthralgias, skin rash, and pericarditis-myocarditis, a combination of features that mimics rheumatic fever. Viral syndromes can be differentiated from rheumatic fever because, except for myocardial

involvement, clinical findings associated with rheumatic fever (arthritis, chorea, subcutaneous nodules, erythema marginatum, streptococcal infection, elevated ASLO titers) are absent.

(3) Primary arthritic disease. Rheumatoid arthritis (adult or juvenile form), systemic lupus erythematosus (SLE), and osteomyelitis may mimic rheumatic fever. Myocardial involvement is unusual in these conditions; when it occurs, myocardial injury is very rarely associated with valvular murmurs. The ECG is generally normal in rheumatoid arthritis. SLE and rheumatoid arthritis usually involve the small joints, whereas rheumatic fever affects the large ones. In addition, arthritis in rheumatic fever is migratory, which is not the situation with rheumatoid arthritis, SLE, or osteomyelitis. Specific bony changes can be observed by roentgenography in patients with osteomyelitis. Patients with SLE, develop a pathognomonic butterfly rash on the face and bridge of the nose, as well as specific blood test reactions (lupus erythematosus cell and antinuclear antibody as well as others).

(4) Assorted other conditions have been confused with rheumatic fever, including cardiac myxoma, leukemia, thalassemia, Henoch-Schönlein purpura, scurvy, hemophilia, congenital syphilis, gonococcemia, undulant fever, rat-bite fever, and granulomatous bowel disease. A careful search for the major and minor manifestations of rheumatic fever (Table 18-9) usually clarifies the diagnostic confusion. Echocardiographic examination is always useful in ruling out cardiac abnormalities.

B. Therapy

1. Myocarditis. The treatment of patients with myocarditis depends on the underlying cause of myocardial injury. Patients with exposure to toxins should receive specific antidotes if available. Individuals with infectious forms of myocarditis should receive specific chemotherapy if available. For most patients with myocarditis (e.g., viral, radiation), no specific therapy is known. They should be treated symptomatically:

   a. Heart failure is treated with decreased activity; decreased salt intake; and diuretics, beta-blockers, afterload-reducing agents, and digitalis if required.

   b. If patients develop progressive myocardial disease with increasing cardiac decompensation, a trial of oral steroids (e.g., prednisone, 60 mg every day) is indicated. Response, if it occurs, is usually seen within 1 to 2 weeks.

   c. If a myocardial biopsy has demonstrated an inflammatory cellular infiltrate in the myocardium, therapy with steroids, immunosuppressive agents, or both, may be indicated. Data supporting the use of immunosuppression are, however, highly controversial, with some studies showing benefit and others not.

2. Rheumatic fever. Therapy of rheumatic fever is based on a number of traditional elements.

   a. Bedrest. Moderate decrease in activity seems wise, particularly in patients with carditis. Strict bedrest is not necessary.

   b. Dietary salt. Patients with heart failure should have moderate dietary salt restriction (e.g., no-added-salt diet: 4- to 5-g sodium).

   c. Antibiotics. Penicillin should be given for 10 days to eradicate any residual group A beta-hemolytic streptococci. Oral penicillin V (250 mg four times a day) is acceptable. Oral erythromycin (250 mg four times a day for 10 days) may be substituted for penicillin in patients who are allergic to penicillin. Long-term antibiotic prophylaxis is administered to patients who have had an episode of rheumatic fever (Table 16-4).

   d. Salicylates. Buffered acetylsalicylic acid (aspirin) is administered to patients with rheumatic fever to relieve arthralgia, fever, and malaise. The dosage is 40 to 70 mg/lb of body weight in divided doses (q4 or 6h), up to a maximum of 10 per day. Low doses often are given initially and gradually increased. Salicylates generally are continued for 12 weeks, with tapering dosage toward the end of that time. Serum salicylate levels should be checked if toxic manifestations appear (tinnitus, deafness, vertigo, headache, nausea, vomiting, and occasionally diarrhea).

e. Corticosteroid therapy. Patients with high fever and severe rheumatic carditis with marked cardiac decompensation benefit from treatment with steroids. Such individuals should receive prednisone, 60 to 80 mg per day for 4 weeks, followed by a gradual tapering regimen over the next 6 to 8 weeks.

Patients with milder cases of rheumatic fever may also receive corticosteroid therapy, but there is no evidence that it benefits them more than salicylate therapy alone.

f. Diuretics, beta-blockers, vasodilators, and digitalis. These drugs can be administered to patients with overt heart failure.

VI. Obliterative cardiomyopathy. Obliterative cardiomyopathy is extremely rare in North America and Europe. Two conditions, endomyocardial fibrosis (a tropical disease usually limited to Africa) and the rare Löffler's fibroplastic eosinophilic endocarditis, result in gradual obliteration of the ventricular cavities. The hemodynamic pattern resembles that seen with restrictive cardiomyopathy. Complications include heart failure, atrial and ventricular arrhythmias, and arterial embolism. There is no satisfactory therapy.

SELECTED READINGS

Abelmann WH, Lorell BH. The challenge of cardiomyopathy. *J Am Coll Cardiol* 1989;13: 1219–1239.
Extensive review of pathogenesis, therapy, and prevention of the principal forms of cardiomyopathy.
Ammash NM, Seward JB, Bailey KR, et al. Clinical profile and outcome of idiopathic restrictive cardiomyopathy. *Circulation* 2000;101:2490–2496.
A clinical series of 94 patients with restrictive cardiomyopathy carefully analyzed.
Anderson JL, Gilbert EM, O'Connell JB, et al. Long-term (2-year) beneficial effects of beta-adrenergic blockade with bucindolol in patients with idiopathic dilated cardiomyopathy. *J Am Coll Cardiol* 1991;17:1373–1381.
Beta-blockade improves left ventricular function and exercise tolerance in patients with idiopathic dilated cardiomyopathy.
Arbustini E, Morbini P, Pilotto A, et al. Familial dilated cardiomyopathy: from clinical presentation to molecular genetics. *Eur Heart J* 2000;21:1825–1832.
Current perspective on familial dilated cardiomyopathy.
Billingham M. Acute myocarditis: a diagnostic dilemma. *Br Heart J* 1987;58:6–8.
It is difficult to diagnose myocarditis even with myocardial biopsy material available.
Bisno AL. Group A streptococcal infections and acute rheumatic fever. *N Eng J Med* 1991;325:783–793.
Extensive review of the pathogenesis and epidemiology of acute rheumatic fever.
Dajani AS, Bisno AL, Chung KJ, et al. Prevention of rheumatic fever: a statement for health professionals by the Committee on Rheumatic Fever, Endocarditis and Kawasaki Disease of the Council on Cardiovascular Disease in the young, the American Heart Association. *Pediatr Infect Dis J* 1989;8:263–266.
Updated recommendations for rheumatic fever prophylaxis.
Dec GW, Palacios IF, Fallon JT, et al. Active myocarditis in the spectrum of acute dilated cardiomyopathies: clinical features, histologic correlates, and clinical outcome. *N Engl J Med* 1985;312:885–890.
Many cases of unexplained dilated cardiomyopathy result from myocarditis.
Dec GW, Waldman H, Southern J, et al. Viral myocarditis mimicking acute myocardial infarction. *J Am Coll Cardiol* 1992;20:85–89.

Severe myocarditis can mimic MI in its clinical presentation and course.

Elkayam U, Tummala PP, Rao K, et al. Maternal and fetal outcomes of subsequent pregnancies in women with peripartum cardiomyopathy. *N Engl J Med* 2001;344: 1567–1571.

Subsequent pregnancies in women with a history of peripartum cardiomyopathy is associated with further deterioration in left ventricular function and clinical status.

Fauchier L, Babuty D, Poret P, et al. Comparison of long-term outcome of alcoholic and idiopathic dilated cardiomyopathy. *Eur Heart J* 2000;21:306–314.

Patients with alcoholic cardiomyopathy had a prognosis similar to that of patients with dilated cardiomyopathy. In both cases, the prognosis was poor.

Feldman AM, McNamara D. Myocarditis. *N Engl J Med* 2000;343:1388–1398.

A comprehensive and authoritative review of the subject.

Gerzen P, Granath A, Holmgren B, et al. Acute myocarditis: A follow-up study. *Br Heart J* 1972;34:575–583.

Prognosis for normal cardiac function in uncomplicated infectious myocarditis.

Guidelines for the diagnosis of rheumatic fever: Jones Criteria, 1992 update. Special Writing Group of the Committee on Rheumatic Fever, Endocarditis, and Kawasaki Disease of the Council on Cardiovascular Disease in the Young of the American Heart Association. *JAMA* 1992;268:2069–2073.

An update of the diagnostic criteria for acute rheumatic fever.

Kaplan EL. Global assessment of rheumatic fever and rheumatic heart disease at the close of the century. *Circulation* 1993;88:1964–1972.

A review of the pathophysiology and global incidence of rheumatic fever.

Kasper EK, Agema WR, Hutchins GM, et al. The causes of dilated cardiomyopathy: a clinicopathologic review of 673 consecutive patients. *J Am Coll Cardiol* 1994;23: 586–590.

Most patients with dilated cardiomyopathy have the idiopathic form. Specific heart muscle diseases occur less frequently.

Katritsis D, Wilmshurst PT, Wendon JA, et al. Primary restrictive cardiomyopathy: clinical and pathologic characteristics. *J Am Coll Cardiol* 1991;18:1230–1235.

Review of the clinical features of 24 patients with restrictive cardiomyopathy.

Keren A, Popp RL. Assignment of patients into the classification of cardiomyopathies. *Circulation* 1992;86:1622–1633.

Classification of patients with cardiomyopathy based on echo/Doppler studies.

Marcus RH, Sareli P, Pocock WA, et al. The spectrum of severe rheumatic mitral valve disease in a developing country. *Ann Intern Med* 1994;120:177–183.

In developing countries, severe mitral regurgitation is as common as mitral stenosis in patients with acute rheumatic fever.

McCarthy RE, Boehmer JP, Hruban RH, et al. Long-term outcome of fulminant myocarditis as compared with acute (nonfulminant) myocarditis. *N Engl J Med* 2000; 342:690–695.

Fulminant myocarditis is a distinct clinical entity with an excellent long-term prognosis. These patients should be treated aggressively.

Maron BJ, Casey SA, Poliac LC, et al. Clinical course of hypertrophic cardiomyopathy in a regional United States cohort. *JAMA* 1999;281:650–655.

The prognosis for hypertrophic cardiomyopathy in the community is excellent.

Narula J, Chandrasekhar Y, Rahimtoola S. Diagnosis of active rheumatic carditis: the echoes of change. *Circulation* 1999;100:1576–1581.

Echocardiography is playing an ever increasing role in the diagnosis of acute rheumatic fever.

Pearson GD, Veille JC, Rahimtoola S, et al. Peripartum cardiomyopathy: National Heart, Lung, and Blood Institute and Office of Rare Diseases (National Institutes of Health) Workshop Recommendations and Review. *JAMA* 2000;283:1183–1188.

A consensus document on the clinical and demographic aspects of peripartum cardiomyopathy.

Seggewiss H, Gleichmann U, Faber L, et al. Percutaneous transluminal septal myocardial ablation in hypertrophic obstructive cardiomyopathy: acute results and 3-month follow-up in 25 patients. *J Am Coll Cardiol* 1998;31:252–258.

Percutaneous transluminal septal ablation is effective in abolishing the left ventricular gradient in patients with hypertrophic obstructive cardiomyopathy. Patients improved clinically after this procedure.

Sugrue DD, Rodeheffer RJ, Codd MB, et al. The clinical course of idiopathic dilated cardiomyopathy. *Ann Intern Med* 1992;117:117–123.

The clinical course of dilated cardiomyopathy may be more favorable than previously thought.

Takagi E, Yamakado T, Nakano T. Prognosis of completely asymptomatic adult patients with hypertrophic cardiomyopathy. *J Am Coll Cardiol* 1999;33:206–211.

Mortality is low for asymptomatic patients with hypertrophic cardiomyopathy.

Vasan RS, Shrivastava S, Vijayakumar M, et al. Echocardiographic evaluation of patients with acute rheumatic fever and rheumatic carditis. *Circulation* 1996;94:73–82.

Mitral valve abnormalities are very common echo findings in patients with acute rheumatic fever and carditis.

Wigle ED, Rakowski H, Kimball BP, et al. Hypertrophic cardiomyopathy: clinical spectrum and treatment. *Circulation* 1995;92:1680–1692.

A thoughtful review of the clinical aspects of hypertrophic cardiomyopathy.

19. PERICARDIAL DISEASE

I. Introduction. The patterns of pericardial disease have changed over the past 20 to 30 years, with the once common tuberculous pericarditis becoming a rare entity. Uremic pericarditis, formerly one of the most dreaded complications of renal failure, is now managed with relative ease.

Pericarditis can be acute and self-limited, subacute, or chronic. Chronic forms of pericarditis often result in cardiac constriction. A variety of agents cause pericarditis (Table 19-1). Pericarditis is likely to lead to effusion, which may be minor or large enough to interfere with ventricular filling during diastole (tamponade). Chronic forms of pericarditis often are associated with pericardial and even epicardial fibrosis, a condition that can also impede diastolic ventricular filling (restrictive filling). This chapter examines pericarditis, tamponade, and constriction in separate sections.

II. Pericarditis
   A. Diagnosis
      1. History. Much of the historical information obtained from patients with pericarditis varies according to the underlying medical condition. Thus, rheumatoid pericarditis usually accompanies severe rheumatoid arthritis, whereas radiation pericarditis follows large doses of mediastinal radiation, ordinarily administered for control of neoplasm. Systemic symptoms may occur, including fever, sweats, chills, weakness, malaise, weight loss, anxiety, and depression. The pain of pericarditis is characteristic: It is almost always precordial in position, sharp and severe, and increasing in severity, with deep inspiration or recumbency. Occasionally, pain is felt only when the patient lies on the left side and makes a maximum inspiratory effort. The pain not infrequently radiates to the neck or left arm and shoulder.

      Dyspnea usually is seen only in individuals with cardiac tamponade or constriction (see Sections **III.** and **IV.**). Palpitations are noted commonly. These are caused by atrial arrhythmias, which often accompany pericarditis.

      2. Physical examination. Patients with pericarditis may have an irregular or rapid pulse secondary to atrial arrhythmias or tamponade (see Section **III.**). A pericardial friction rub is the hallmark of the disease. This superficial scraping, scratchy, or grating sound is frequently evanescent or intermittent.

      Persistent rubs are most often heard with pericarditis secondary to neoplasm, uremia, viral infection, and tuberculosis. Evanescent rubs are common in pericarditis associated with myocardial infarction (MI). Rubs may have one, two, or three components occurring with the following stages of the cardiac cycle: (i) rapid filling in early diastole, (ii) atrial contraction in late diastole, and (iii) systole. On occasion, one- or two-component rubs are confused with systolic or to-and-fro murmurs. Sometimes a patient with pericarditis has an early diastolic sound or pericardial knock, which can be confused with a third heart sound (S3). Other systemic findings in patients with pericarditis depend on the underlying condition.

      3. ECG. The ECG is often abnormal in patients with pericarditis. ECG findings include diffusely elevated S–T segments, widespread T wave changes, and P–R segment depression. Elevated S–T segments can mimic the ECG findings of acute MI. ECG findings in pericarditis are as follows:

      Elevation of S–T segment
      Flattening and inversion of T waves
      Depression of P–R segment

      Differentiation of the ECG changes of pericarditis from the ECG changes of acute MI are listed in Table 19-2. The S–T segment elevation

TABLE 19-1. ETIOLOGY OF PERICARDIAL DISEASE

Inflammation
Collagen/vascular diseases:[a] rheumatic fever, rheumatoid arthritis, systemic lupus
  erythematosus, scleroderma
Vasculitis: polyarteritis nodosa
Allergic reaction: serum sickness, drug reactions (e.g., procainamide)
Infection[a]
Bacterial: staphylococcus, meningococcus, streptococcus, pneumococcus, gonococcus,
  tuberculosis
Viral: Coxsackie A and B, influenza A and B, varicella
Fungal: histoplasmosis
Parasitic: syphilis, echinococcus, cysticercus, *Entamoeba histolytica*
Radiation[a]
Neoplasm:[a] metastatic involvement of the pericardium
Hypersensitivity: posttraumatic, postpericardiotomy, postmyocardial infarction
Myxedema
Dissecting aneurysm
Idiopathic[a]
Uremia[a]

[a] Categories that can result in chronic constrictive pericarditis.

of early repolarization occasionally may be confused with the ECG pattern of pericarditis. However, S–T segment elevation of early repolarization usually is limited to the precordial leads, whereas that of pericarditis occurs throughout limb and precordial leads. Supraventricular arrhythmias are frequently noted in patients with pericarditis.

4. Chest x-ray examination. Patients with pericarditis with little or no effusion usually have a normal chest x-ray film. Serial chest films may reveal increasing heart size secondary to accumulation of pericardial fluid (see Section **III.**). In patients with infectious or hypersensitivity pericarditis, chest roentgenography may show pulmonary infiltrates or pleural effusions.

5. Laboratory tests. Laboratory testing may demonstrate striking abnormalities in patients with pericarditis. The nature of these abnormalities depends on the underlying condition producing pericardial irritation. Thus, infectious causes of pericarditis usually are associated with elevated

TABLE 19-2. DIFFERENTIATION OF ECG FINDINGS IN PERICARDITIS FROM ECG CHANGES IN ACUTE MYOCARDIAL INFARCTION

Pericarditis	Myocardial infarction
S–T segment elevations widespread; no S–T segment depressions present	S–T segment elevations localized to certain leads with reciprocal S–T segment depressions in other leads
S–T segment elevation with upward concavity or straight morphology	S–T segment elevation with upward convexity
Simultaneous T wave inversion in leads I, II, and III	T waves not simultaneously inverted in leads I, II, and III
Significant Q waves not seen with pericarditis	Significant Q waves frequently seen with myocardial infarction
QRS often normal	QRS often abnormal

erythrocyte sedimentation rates, white blood cell counts, and various serum globulin fractions; pericarditis secondary to allergic reactions may be associated with eosinophilia; and pericarditis induced by collagen/vascular disease may be accompanied by positive antinuclear antibody or latex fixation tests.

6. Echocardiography. Echocardiography is very sensitive in detecting small amounts of pericardial effusion. High-quality echocardiograms may even identify pericardial thickening. Often, confirmation of a diagnosis of pericarditis rests on the demonstration of a small quantity of pericardial fluid by echocardiography.

7. Radionuclide studies. Cardiac blood pool scanning after the administration of labeled erythrocytes or albumin can aid in the detection of significant quantities of pericardial effusion; however, echocardiography is more sensitive in detecting pericardial fluid.

8. Catheterization and angiography. Hemodynamic measurements are usually normal in patients with uncomplicated pericarditis. As the quantity of pericardial fluid increases, ventricular filling pressures increase (see Section III.). Angiography is less sensitive than echocardiography in detecting small amounts of pericardial fluid.

9. Biopsy. Pericardial biopsy can often be performed percutaneously or through a small subxiphoid incision. Pericardial fluid can be collected at the same time. This procedure may be important in confirming the diagnosis of bacterial (especially tuberculous) or neoplastic pericarditis.

10. Protocol for the diagnosis of pericarditis
   a. Testing sequence for the diagnosis. The history, physical examination, ECG, and echocardiogram are central in making the diagnosis of pericarditis.

   An appropriate flow chart for making the diagnosis of pericarditis follows:

   History (pleuritic, positional chest pain, and precordial rub)
   ↓
   Chest x-ray film and ECG (diffuse S–T and T wave changes)
   ↓
   Echocardiogram (pericardial fluid or thickening or both)

   b. Criteria for the diagnosis. The diagnosis of pericarditis is made in the following patients:
      (1) Individuals with substernal or precordial pleuritic or positional chest discomfort may have either (i) definite changes of pericarditis on the ECG (diffuse S–T segment elevation with or without diffuse T wave changes and P–R segment depression) or (ii) definite pericardial fluid or thickening by echocardiography.
      (2) Asymptomatic individuals in whom a pericardial rub is heard and who meet either the ECG or the echocardiographic criteria for pericarditis just noted.
      (3) Asymptomatic individuals without audible pericardial friction rub who meet both ECG and echocardiographic criteria for pericarditis just noted.
   c. Differential diagnosis
      (1) Systolic murmur. Single-component systolic rubs are occasionally mistaken for systolic murmurs. Thus, patients with pericarditis may be thought to have aortic stenosis, mitral regurgitation, or ventricular septal defect. The transient and changing nature of the rub, and associated ECG and echocardiographic evidence of pericarditis, helps to identify the correct diagnosis.
      (2) Unstable angina pectoris. Patients with post-MI pericarditis may be thought to have unstable angina because of recurrent severe substernal chest discomfort. Occasionally, the typical

pleuritic or positional nature of the pericarditic discomfort is absent, making it even more difficult to differentiate this pain from that of angina pectoris. In such circumstances, a brief trial of aspirin, indomethacin, or steroids may reveal the true diagnosis by promptly relieving the discomfort.

(3) Pulmonary infarction. The pleuritic chest pain of pericarditis may be confused with discomfort resulting from pulmonary infarction. The pain of pulmonary infarction is often posterior in location, whereas that of pericarditis is anterior. Associated findings such as abnormal arterial blood gases and pulmonary infiltrates, as well as abnormal lung scan and pulmonary arteriography, point to the diagnosis of pulmonary embolism. ECG and echocardiographic findings suggest the diagnosis of pericarditis.

(4) Pneumonia. Patients with pneumonia may have pleuritic pain simulating that of pericarditis. Differentiation of these two entities depends on a history of cough, sputum production, and fever and on the presence of an infiltrate on the chest roentgenogram of patients with pneumonia.

(5) Dissecting aneurysm. Pericarditis with an audible friction rub can occur in patients with aortic dissection secondary to leakage of blood into the pericardial space. Dissection is suspected in patients with severe, nonpleuritic precordial discomfort, abnormal mediastinal widening on the chest x-ray film, loss of one or more arterial pulses, or pulsation of one or both sternoclavicular joints.

(6) Pneumothorax. Sudden onset of chest pain associated with a crunching, to-and-fro sound over the precordium can occur in patients with pneumothorax. This loud precordial sound, the result of air in the mediastinum, may be confused with a pericardial friction rub. Pneumothorax is recognized by absence of characteristic ECG changes of pericarditis and presence of air in the pleural space and mediastinum by chest x-ray study.

(7) Because a number of different conditions can be associated with pericarditis (Table 19-1), it is important to define the etiology of pericarditis once it is identified.

B. Therapy

1. Medical treatment

a. Analgesia. Rarely, the pain of pericarditis requires opiates (meperidine or morphine) for relief. In general, aspirin, indomethacin, or ibuprofen is effective in relieving the discomfort of pericarditis. Two aspirin tablets four times a day, 50 mg of indomethacin four times a day or 400 mg of ibuprofen three or four times a day as needed and tolerated usually suffices to alleviate the discomfort within 24 to 48 hours. If discomfort persists, the dosage may be increased to three aspirin tablets four times a day or 50 mg of indomethacin four times a day. If discomfort still remains after 24 to 48 hours, patients taking aspirin or indomethacin should be given ibuprofen, and vice versa. If this regimen also fails and if the pain is disconcerting to the patient, steroid therapy should be undertaken. It may be difficult to wean patients with pericarditis from steroids once these agents have been prescribed. When steroids are withdrawn, the pain of pericarditis often recurs, so they should be tapered very gradually over weeks or months. The usual starting dose for steroids is 40 to 60 mg of prednisone (or its equivalent) daily. An occasional patient develops recurrent bouts of pain from pericarditis. Some clinicians have had excellent results with chronic oral colchicine (1 to 2 mg per day in divided doses) therapy for these patients, thereby obviating the need for prednisone.

b. Anticoagulants. Some authorities warn against using anticoagulants in patients with pericarditis because of the danger of developing hemopericardium and tamponade. Low-dose subcutaneous heparin regimens probably do not result in hemopericardium. Anticoagulation in a patient with pericarditis must be undertaken with extreme caution.

Daily or every-other-day echocardiograms are useful in monitoring such individuals.

  c. Specific therapy aimed at the underlying condition should be given (e.g., appropriate antibiotics for bacterial pericarditis).

2. Surgery. Surgical removal of the pericardium rarely is needed for relief of pain. An occasional patient with intractable discomfort despite repeated courses of steroids will require **pericardiectomy.** Patients with suppurative pericarditis usually require drainage of the pericardial space together with appropriate antibiotic therapy.

III. Pericardial effusion and tamponade. Pericarditis usually is accompanied by pericardial effusion. Often the volume of the effusion is small and does not hinder cardiac function, but larger quantities of fluid sometimes accumulate in the pericardial space, interfering with normal ventricular filling. Low cardiac output and systemic venous congestion result, a condition known as *cardiac* or *pericardial tamponade.*

  A. Diagnosis

  1. History. Patients with tamponade complain of dyspnea in addition to the symptoms (e.g., pain) that arise from the pericarditis itself. They may also complain of a dry hacking cough, hoarseness, or dysphagia. These latter symptoms are the result of compression of the trachea, bronchi, lungs, or esophagus by pericardial and, at times, pleural effusion. Patients with tamponade are usually most comfortable when sitting erect and leaning forward.

  2. Physical examination. A number of physical findings have been associated with the presence of large quantities of fluid in the pericardial space.

    a. Increased area of cardiac dullness to percussion. Normally, cardiac dullness extends laterally to the apical impulse in the fifth intercostal space. At the base of the heart, the area of dullness is much narrower, extending some 2 to 3 cm to the left of the sternal edge. Patients with large pericardial effusions have an area of increased dullness at the base of the heart in addition to generalized enlargement of the area of cardiac dullness.

    b. Dullness to percussion, bronchial breath sounds, and egophony posteriorly, below the angle of the left scapula (Pins' or Ewart's sign). These findings are the result of compression of the left lung by the heart, which is pushed posteriorly by retrosternal pericardial effusion.

    c. Decrease in intensity or absence of the apical impulse and distant or muffled heart sounds. These findings are noted in many, but not all, patients with large pericardial effusions.

    d. Sinus tachycardia, narrow pulse pressure with low systolic blood pressure, pulsus paradoxus greater than 10 mm Hg, and systemic venous congestion. These findings (Table 19-3) are almost always manifest in patients with cardiac tamponade. Beck's triad of cardiac tamponade is falling systemic arterial pressure, rising systemic venous pressure, and a small quiet heart.

    e. Jugular venous distension with a prominent X descent but without a Y descent.

  3. ECG. Besides the ECG findings associated with pericarditis (see above), a diminution in the voltage of the QRS complex may be seen in patients with pericardial effusion. Alternation in the height of every other P wave or QRS complex (electrical alternans) often is seen in patients with large pericardial effusions. Alternation in the height of the QRS complex is seen occasionally in patients with severe heart failure, but P wave alternation occurs only in individuals with pericardial effusion and tamponade.

  4. Chest x-ray examination. Serial films in the patient with pericarditis may show increasing heart size secondary to accumulation of peri-

TABLE 19-3. PHYSICAL FINDINGS IN PATIENTS WITH PERICARDIAL EFFUSION WITH OR WITHOUT TAMPONADE

Findings secondary to effusion
  Increased area of cardiac dullness
  Dullness to percussion, bronchial breathing, egophony posteriorly below angle of left scapula (Pins' or Ewart's sign)
  Decreased or absent apical impulse
  Soft or muffled heart sounds

Findings secondary to tamponade
  Tachycardia
  Low systolic blood pressure
  Narrow pulse pressure
  Pulsus paradoxus >10 mm Hg
  Systemic venous congestion: jugular venous distention, hepatomegaly, sometimes Kussmaul's sign (inspiratory swelling of the cervical veins)

cardial fluid. In general, at least 250 ml of pericardial fluid is necessary to produce an enlargement of the cardiac silhouette on the chest film. Roentgenographic findings in patients with pericardial effusion are as follows:

Symmetric cardiac enlargement
Clear lung fields
Obliteration of the normal outlines of the individual cardiac chambers and great vessels, resulting in a pear-shaped or water-bottle cardiac silhouette
Increase in the size of the cardiac silhouette in serial roentgenograms
Systemic venous engorgement with enlargement of the superior vena cava and azygos vein

Fluoroscopic examination of the right-sided heart border of patients lying on their left side after intravenous administration of a small bolus of carbon dioxide can help in the identification of significant quantities of pericardial fluid. Echocardiography has largely replaced this technique as the safest and most sensitive method of identifying pericardial effusion.

5. Echocardiography. Pericardial effusion is sensitively detected and roughly quantitated by echocardiography. A characteristic swinging motion of the heart within the pericardial effusion and compression of the right atrium and ventricle are often seen in patients with tamponade. Echocardiography can be used during pericardiocentesis to monitor the position of the needle tip. Occasionally, tumor in the pericardium mimics effusion on the echocardiogram.

Left ventricular ejection times measured from a carotid pulse tracing or an aortic valve echo tracing show marked respiratory variation (50 milliseconds). Individuals without tamponade have a maximum respiratory variation of 10 milliseconds in the left ventricular ejection time.

6. Radionuclide studies. Cardiac blood pool scanning can identify pericardial effusion. Echocardiography, however, is a more sensitive technique for recognizing the presence of pericardial fluid.

7. Catheterization and angiography. A number of hemodynamic changes can be recorded in patients with cardiac tamponade: Systemic venous pressure is elevated; right and left ventricular filling pressures are equal or nearly so; cardiac output is normal or slightly reduced, but stroke volume is diminished markedly.

The presence of pericardial effusion often can be defined at catheterization by placing a catheter against the lateral right atrial endocardium and noting the distance from the catheter tip to the lung. Patients with pericardial effusion have more than the expected 3- to 5-mm distance from the right atrial endocardium to the lateral border of the heart. Similarly, a right atrial angiogram can be obtained, and the thickness of the free wall of the right heart can be measured. An increase in this measurement of more than 3 to 5 mm suggests pericardial effusion.

8. Biopsy. Pericardial fluid can be obtained by pericardiocentesis with a needle or during an open pericardial biopsy. If the etiology of the pericarditis is clear and if signs of tamponade are not present, pericardiocentesis or pericardial biopsy is not required. When the diagnosis is obscure, however, or when tamponade is present, pericardial fluid should be removed. Pericardial fluid should be cultured for bacteria (including those of tuberculosis) and sent for cytologic analysis. Bloody pericardial effusion occurs in a variety of conditions, including tuberculosis, neoplasms, lupus erythematosus, rheumatoid arthritis, and viral infections. Purulent pericardial fluid is highly suggestive of a bacterial infection. Rheumatoid factor or lupus erythematosus cells may be found in pericardial fluid from patients with rheumatoid arthritis or systemic lupus erythematosus.

9. Protocol for the diagnosis of pericardial effusion and tamponade
   a. Protocol for making the diagnosis of pericardial effusion. A detailed history and physical examination are followed by an ECG and chest x-ray study.

   Pericardial effusion can be suspected on the basis of historical, physical, ECG, or roentgenographic findings. Confirmation of the diagnosis depends on the demonstration of pericardial effusion by echocardiography, radioisotope blood pool scanning, or angiography. Echocardiography is the easiest and most sensitive of these techniques. On occasion, small and even moderate volumes of pericardial fluid are clinically unsuspected until demonstrated by echocardiography. The protocol for making the diagnosis of **cardiac tamponade** is as follows (dashed arrow indicates optional step):

   History and physical diagnosis
   ↓
   ECG and chest x-ray film
   ↓
   Echocardiography
   ↓
   Right-sided heart or central venous catheterization
   ↓
   ? Pericardial aspiration or biopsy

   b. Criteria for making the diagnosis of pericardial effusion. The clinical diagnosis of pericardial effusion is based on the presumptive identification of pericardial fluid by echocardiography. In some individuals, a history of positional or pleuritic chest discomfort or the discovery of a friction rub leads to the echocardiographic demonstration of pericardial fluid. In other patients, pericardial effusion is discovered during an echocardiographic examination that was ordered for another reason. Patients with heart failure may develop pericardial effusion without pericardial inflammation. Thus, not all patients with pericardial effusion noted by echocardiography have pericarditis.

   c. Criteria for making the diagnosis of cardiac tamponade. Two elements must be present to make the diagnosis of cardiac tamponade: pericardial effusion and evidence of restricted ventricular filling. Pericardial effusion is diagnosed as already noted. Evidence suggesting restricted ventricular filling is usually noninvasive and should include at least three of the following: sinus tachycardia, low systolic blood pressure with narrow pulse pressure, marked pulsus paradoxus or jugular venous distention on physical examination; wide respiratory variation in left ventricular ejection times; and a swinging heart or right atrial/ventricular compression on echocardiography. Confirmation of the diagnosis requires the demonstration of elevated right atrial pressure by central venous or right-sided heart catheterization. Right-sided catheterization also documents equalization of right and left ventricular filling pressures (right atrial and pulmonary capillary wedge or pulmonary arterial diastolic pressures) in patients with cardiac tamponade.

   d. Differential diagnosis of pericardial effusion. Individuals with **cardiomyopathy** may have enlarged, globular heart outlines on the chest x-ray film that resembles those seen in patients with large pericardial effusions. Differentiation of these two conditions is by echocardiography. Cardiac blood pool scanning and the left lateral decubitus chest x-ray picture after intravenous carbon dioxide injection also can differentiate these conditions when echocardiography is not available.

   e. Differential diagnosis of pericardial effusion with tamponade. Patients with **right ventricular failure** resulting in systemic venous congestion and low cardiac output may have clinical features similar to those of patients with cardiac tamponade. For example, a patient with cor pulmonale secondary to chronic obstructive pulmonary disease or an individual with a right ventricular MI may have a low systolic blood pressure, pulsus paradoxus greater than 10 mm Hg, and systemic venous congestion. These conditions can be differentiated by chest roentgenography and echocardiography that show a normal (or even small) cardiac silhouette and absence of pericardial effusion in the patient with right ventricular failure.

B. Therapy
  1. Medical treatment
    a. Patients with **pericardial effusion,** but without evidence of tamponade, frequently do not require specific therapy directed at the pericardial effusion. Rather, therapy should be directed to the underlying condition. For example, tuberculous pericarditis with effusion, but without tamponade, is managed appropriately with antituberculous chemotherapy.

      (1) The discomfort of pericarditis is relieved with measures discussed earlier.

      (2) Some authorities feel that anticoagulants (heparin and warfarin) are contraindicated in patients with pericarditis with or without effusion because of the risk of developing hemopericardium with tamponade.

    b. When the diagnosis of **cardiac tamponade** is made in the manner outlined earlier, pericardiocentesis should be performed. It is wise to monitor intraarterial blood pressure during and after pericardiocentesis. The procedure can be performed with local anesthesia and needle aspiration.

      Some authorities favor leaving a small plastic cannula in the pericardial space for a few days to prevent reaccumulation of fluid. Except in an emergency, pericardiocentesis should be performed by an experienced physician in a catheterization laboratory, operating room, or intensive care unit. If a pericardial biopsy is indicated, simultaneous drainage of pericardial effusion can be performed.

      (1) Specific therapy is directed at the underlying cause of the pericardial effusion. For example, patients with bacterial pericarditis require specific antibiotics, patients with viral (also called benign or idiopathic) pericarditis receive nonsteroidal antiinflammatory agents or corticosteroids, and patients with uremic pericarditis are vigorously dialyzed.

       (2) Patients with neoplastic involvement of the pericardium frequently reaccumulate pericardial fluid after pericardiocentesis. Recurrent episodes of cardiac tamponade may occur. Instillation of tetracycline into the pericardial space often results in its obliteration, with control of recurrent cardiac tamponade. Antineoplastic agents can also be instilled into the pericardial space in such patients.

       (3) Because ventricular contractile function is normal in patients with cardiac tamponade, digitalis administration is of no benefit except to control the ventricular response in those individuals with atrial fibrillation.

           Diuresis is contraindicated despite the presence of edema and even ascites because the further reduction in right ventricular filling leads to a further fall in cardiac output. Hypotension with hypoperfusion may result. Patients with cardiac tamponade and hypotension should receive intravenous volume (saline, plasma, dextran) to ensure adequate right ventricular filling and cardiac output until tamponade is relieved by pericardiocentesis. In the event of severe hypotension and hypoperfusion, intravenous isoproterenol, as well as volume, should be administered.

  2. Surgery. Recurrent tamponade is an indication for surgical drainage of the pericardium. Surgical procedures that can be successful in permanently relieving tamponade include creation of a permanent pericardial window and pericardiectomy. A pericardial window can also be created by a catheter balloon technique, thereby avoiding surgery.

IV. Constrictive pericarditis. Formerly a common disease, constrictive pericarditis is seen only rarely because the advent of effective antituberculous chemotherapy. Constrictive pericarditis is usually the result of chronic pericardial inflammation and fibrosis that is often the result of a chronic infectious process (bacterial, fungal, or viral), neoplasm, or uremia (Table 19-1).

  A. Diagnosis

    1. History. Patients usually develop symptoms very gradually, with exertional dyspnea, ankle swelling, and abdominal swelling as the main complaints. Many patients note undue fatigue. The chest discomfort noted with acute pericarditis, as well as orthopnea and paroxysmal nocturnal dyspnea, does not usually occur in individuals with constrictive pericarditis.

    2. Physical examination. Tachycardia, elevated jugular venous pressure, hepatomegaly, ascites, and peripheral edema are noted commonly. The clinical presentation of the patient with constriction resembles that of the individual with tamponade except for normal pulse pressure and lack of pulsus paradoxus in constriction. Inspiratory increase in jugular venous pressure (Kussmaul's sign) is occasionally seen. Sharp X and Y descents are present in the jugular pulse.

    3. ECG. The ECG findings in constrictive pericarditis include low voltage of the QRS complexes and nonspecific T wave changes. A pattern resembling right ventricular hypertrophy is sometimes seen (Table 19-4).

    4. Chest x-ray examination. Chest roentgenography in patients with constrictive pericarditis reveals clear lung fields, normal or slightly increased heart size without specific chamber enlargement, and pericardial calcification in 50% of patients. Table 19-4 summarizes these findings.

    5. Echocardiography. The echocardiogram may demonstrate a number of findings in patients with constrictive pericarditis: (i) paradoxical septal motion; (ii) normal or increased diastolic slope of the anterior mitral valve leaflet; (iii) synchronous, parallel movement of the epicardium and parietal pericardium separated by a small echo-free space; (iv) rapid, early diastolic posterior motion of the left ventricular endocardium; (v) thickening of the pericardium; and (vi) normal right ventricular cavity dimensions.

TABLE 19-4. ECG AND ROENTGENOGRAPHIC FINDINGS IN PATIENTS WITH CONSTRICTIVE PERICARDITIS

ECG findings
  Atrial fibrillation
  Low-voltage QRS complexes
  Nonspecific T wave flattening and/or inversion
  Left atrial enlargement
  Pseudo right ventricular hypertrophy (right axis deviation and R>S in lead V_1)

Chest x-ray findings
  Clear lung fields
  Normal or slightly enlarged cardiac silhouette
  Calcification of the pericardium (approximately 50% of patients)

6. Magnetic resonance imaging (MRI). MRI may be helpful in distinguishing constrictive pericarditis from restrictive cardiomyopathy. The markedly thickened pericardium is visualized by MRI.
7. Catheterization and angiography. Hemodynamic findings include elevated right atrial pressure with a characteristic M-shaped pattern, an early diastolic dip and plateau (square root sign) in the left and right ventricular pressure tracings, and equalization of the following pressures: right atrial, right ventricular and end-diastolic, pulmonary arterial diastolic, pulmonary capillary wedge, and left ventricular end-diastolic. Cardiac output is often normal in patients with constrictive pericarditis. Hemodynamic differentiation of constrictive pericarditis from restrictive cardiomyopathy is dealt with in Table 18-7.
   Right atrial angiography may demonstrate a thickened atrial-pericardial heart border and straightening of the right atrial border.
8. Biopsy. Open biopsy of the pericardium may be undertaken through a small subxiphoid incision. Biopsy of the pericardium is important in patients suspected of having neoplastic infiltration of the pericardium. In this manner, the diagnosis can be obtained without resorting to a full thoracotomy.
9. Protocol for the diagnosis of constrictive pericarditis
   a. Testing sequence for making the diagnosis. The protocol for making the diagnosis of constrictive pericarditis is the same as that for cardiac tamponade (see above).
   b. Criteria for making the diagnosis. The diagnosis of constrictive pericarditis is made in symptomatic or asymptomatic patients with findings of elevated systemic venous pressure (jugular venous distention, hepatomegaly, ascites, peripheral edema), low-voltage QRS and nonspecific T wave changes on ECG, clear lung fields on chest x-ray film, a normal-sized right ventricle on echocardiography, equalization of all diastolic pressures (right atrial, right ventricular end-diastolic, pulmonary arterial diastolic, and pulmonary capillary wedge), and a normal cardiac output on right-sided heart catheterization.
   c. Differential diagnosis. Patients with restrictive myocardial disease (see Chapter 18) may resemble individuals with constrictive pericarditis in clinical presentation and hemodynamic findings. Echocardiography, MRI, and angiography often help to distinguish these two entities: Patients with cardiomyopathy usually demonstrate reduced left ventricular function, whereas individuals with constrictive pericarditis have a thickened pericardium and straightening of the right atrial border (Table 18-7). Occasionally, myocardial biopsy is needed to distinguish these two entities.
B. Therapy
   1. Medical treatment. Because ventricular function is not impaired in patients with constrictive pericarditis, digitalis has no role in the therapy

of this condition. Diuresis may result in deterioration by decreasing right ventricular filling further. Diuresis in the patient with constrictive pericarditis can therefore produce a dangerous fall in cardiac output. As noted in Section **III,** intravenous infusion of saline or generous oral intake of salt and fluids may be required to maintain adequate cardiac output and systemic blood pressure, despite significant ascites and peripheral edema. If hypotension with hypoperfusion occurs in a patient with constrictive pericarditis, the treatment is intravenous infusion of volume (saline, plasma, dextran) and isoproterenol.

2. Surgery. The treatment of choice for constrictive pericarditis is surgical removal of the pericardium (pericardiectomy). In some individuals, the pericardium adheres firmly to the epicardium, and pericardiectomy is an arduous procedure. In this event, some epicardium invariably is removed. The operative mortality is higher in patients with densely adherent pericardia.

Cardiac function may not return to normal after successful pericardiectomy, although the patient may experience considerable improvement. Failure of cardiac function to normalize completely after pericardiectomy is usually the result of three factors: (i) extension of the pathologic process that affected the pericardium into the underlying epicardium and myocardium, (ii) incomplete pericardiectomy, and (iii) damage to the epicardium and myocardium during removal of the pericardium.

SELECTED READINGS

Adler Y, Finkelstein Y, Guindo J, et al. Colchicine treatment for recurrent pericarditis: a decade of experience. *Circulation* 1998;97:2183–2185.
Concise summary of colchicine therapy for recurrent pericarditis.
Adler Y, Guindo J, Finkelstein Y, et al. Colchicine for large pericardial effusion. *Clin Cardiol* 1998;21:143–144.
Report of two cases of large pericardial effusion successfully treated with colchicine.
Atar S, Chiu J, Forrester JS, Siegel RJ. Blood pericardial effusion in patients with cardiac tamponade: is the cause cancerous, tuberculous, or iatrogenic in the 1990s? *Chest* 1999;116:1564–1569.
The most common cause of bloody pericardial effusion leading to cardiac tamponade is iatrogenic.
Bonnefoy E, Godon P, Kirkorian G, et al. Serum cardiac troponin I and ST-segment elevation in patients with acute pericarditis. *Eur Heart J* 2000;21:832–836.
Patients with idiopathic pericarditis often have elevated serum cardiac troponin values that probably result from epicardial injury.
Brown J, MacKinnon D, King A, et al. Elevated arterial blood pressure in cardiac tamponade. *N Engl J Med* 1992;327:463–466.
Elevated blood pressure may occur in some patients with cardiac tamponade and preexisting hypertension.
Cameron J, Oesterle SN, Baldwin JC, et al. The etiologic spectrum of constrictive pericarditis. *Am Heart J* 1987;113:354–360.
Review of clinical spectrum of 95 patients with constrictive pericarditis.
D'Cruz I. The noninvasive diagnosis of constricting pericarditis. *Am J Noninvasive Cardiol* 1990;4:65.
Two-dimensional echo/Doppler studies help to confirm the diagnosis of constrictive pericarditis.
Eisenberg MJ, Dunn MM, Kanth N, et al. Diagnostic value of chest radiography for pericardial effusion. *J Am Coll Cardiol* 1993;22:588–593.
A predominant left-sided pleural effusion and a lucent area in the vicinity of the pericardium—the pericardial fat strips—on the chest x-ray film are suggestive but not diagnostic of pericardial effusion.
Fowler NO. Cardiac tamponade: a clinical or echocardiographic diagnosis? *Circulation* 1993;87:1738–1741.

In most patients, cardiac tamponade is a clinical diagnosis; echocardiography is used to confirm the diagnosis.

Ilan Y, Oren R, Ben-Chetrit E. Etiology, treatment, and prognosis of large pericardial effusions. *Chest* 1991;100:985–987.
Excellent clinical review of 34 patients presenting with large pericardial effusions.

Ling LH, Oh JE, Breen JF, et al. Calcific constrictive pericarditis: is it still with us? *Ann Intern Med* 2000;132:444–450.
Pericardial calcification is a common finding in patients with constrictive pericarditis, in which it is an independent predictor of perioperative mortality.

Ling LH, Oh JK, Schaff HV, et al. Constrictive pericarditis in the modern era: evolving clinical spectrum and impact on outcome after pericardiectomy. *Circulation* 1999;100:1380–1386.
A review of the clinical features of constrictive pericarditis in 135 patients diagnosed and treated between 1985 and 1995.

Mehta A, Mehta M, Jain AC. Constrictive pericarditis.*Clin Cardiol* 1999;22:334–344.
A review of constrictive pericarditis in the modern era.

Meyers DG, Meyers RE, Prendergast TW. The usefulness of diagnostic tests on pericardial fluid. *Chest* 1997;111:1213–1221.
Usefulness of various laboratory tests in the differential diagnosis of pericardial effusion.

Permanyer-Miralda G, Sagrista-Sauleda J, Soler-Soler J. Primary acute pericardial disease: a prospective series of 231 consecutive patients. *Am J Cardiol* 1985;56:623–630.
A review of the clinical and diagnostic features of 231 patients with acute pericarditis.

Sagrista-Sauleda J, Barrabes JA, Permanyer-Miralda G, et al. Purulent pericarditis: review of a 20-year experience in a general hospital. *J Am Coll Cardiol* 1993;22: 1661–1665.
Extensive clinical review of 33 patients with purulent pericarditis managed between 1972 and 1991.

Sagrista-Sauleda J, Merce J, Permanyer-Miralda G, et al. Clinical clues to the causes of large pericardial effusion. *Am J Med* 2000;109: 95–101.
A study of the various causes of pericardial effusion in a large hospital practice with helpful clinical clues for identifying the etiology of the effusions.

Sagrista-Sauleda J, Permanyer-Miralda G, Soler-Soler J. Long-term follow-up of idiopathic chronic pericardial effusion. *N Engl J Med* 1999;341:2054–2059.
A careful clinical study with long-term outcomes for 461 patients with large pericardial effusions.

Shepherd FA, Morgan C, Evans WK, et al. Medical management of malignant pericardial effusion by tetracycline sclerosis. *Am J Cardiol* 1987;60:1161–1166.
Intra-pericardial infusion of tetracycline is effective in controlling malignant pericardial effusion.

Spodick DH. Pericardial friction: characteristics of pericardial rubs in 50 consecutive, prospectively studied patients. *N Engl J Med* 1968;278:1204–1207.
A study of various features of pericardial friction rubs in 50 consecutive patients with pericarditis.

Spodick DH. Differential characteristics of the electrocardiogram in early repolarization and acute pericarditis. *N Engl J Med* 1976;295:523–526.
Presentation of ECG criteria for differentiating early repolarization from pericarditis.

Spodick DH. Macrophysiology, microphysiology, and anatomy of the pericardium: a synopsis. *Am Heart J* 1992;124:1046–1051.
A review of normal and abnormal pericardial physiology.

Spodick DH. Pathophysiology of cardiac tamponade. *Chest* 1998;113:1372–1378.
A thoughtful review of the pathophysiology of cardiac tamponade.

Tsang TSM, Oh JK, Seward JB. Diagnosis and management of cardiac tamponade in the era of echocardiography. *Clin Cardiol* 1999;22:446–452.
A review of current approaches to diagnosis and therapy of pericardial tamponade.

20. INFECTIOUS ENDOCARDITIS

I. **Introduction.** The picture of subacute bacterial endocarditis (SBE) that most medical students commit to memory is very different from the current presentation of the disease. The traditional Oslerian patient with SBE and wasting, clubbing, Osler's and Janeway's skin lesions, renal failure, and splenomegaly is extremely rare, as these features usually require weeks to months to develop. Today the diagnosis of bacterial endocarditis almost always is made promptly, and appropriate therapy is administered, thus preventing those features of the disease so common three generations ago. Acute or virulent forms of bacterial endocarditis (usually secondary to *Staphylococcus aureus*) can result in death within days. Nonbacterial endocarditis (usually fungal) is not rare. For all these reasons, the term **subacute bacterial endocarditis,** or **SBE,** is anachronistic and erroneous; however, the term has become so ingrained in medical consciousness that it is still used. A more appropriate term for these infections of the heart is **infectious endocarditis (IE).**

II. **Diagnosis**

  A. **History.** Patients with IE are often minimally symptomatic or complaining of fever, chills, sweats, malaise, or anorexia. Frequently, symptoms resemble those commonly associated with a viral infection or influenza. Patients with more advanced or virulent IE may present with embolic complications such as stroke, splenic infarction, or peripheral vascular occlusion. Rarely, an individual who has not received medical attention presents with the Oslerian syndrome of SBE described earlier.

  Symptoms of left or right ventricular failure should be diligently sought, because the presence of heart failure in a patient with IE changes the prognosis and frequently alters therapy.

  1. Endocarditis can occur on any intracardiac or vascular abnormality, no matter how minor. Valvular lesions are the most common sites for endocarditis.

    Congenital lesions also serve as substrates for intracardiac infections, although patients with atrial septal defect rarely if ever acquire IE. Endocarditis can occur on presumptively normal heart valves, particularly if the infecting agent is staphylococcus aureus.

  2. Bacteremia, a necessary prerequisite to IE, has been reported to follow a number of procedures that result in the introduction of bacteria into the bloodstream. Thus, IE can occur after dental procedures including routine tooth cleaning, genitourinary manipulations including prostatic massage, normal obstetric delivery, respiratory infections, skin infections, cardiac or other surgery, and even cardiac catheterization.

  3. Complications of IE are as follows:

    Left or right ventricular failure
    Glomerulonephritis (may lead to renal failure)
    Renal infarction
    Splenic infarction
    Pulmonary infarction
    Cerebral infarction
    Meningitis
    Cerebral mycotic aneurysms result when bacteria/fungi invade the wall of an artery in the cerebral circulation; subarachnoid, intracerebral or intraventricular hemorrhage may result
    Cerebral abscess
    Encephalitis
    Mycotic aneurysms in other organs

  B. **Physical examination.** A variety of physical findings have been described in patients with endocarditis. Some are the result of the chronic infectious process (wasting, clubbing, pallor secondary to anemia), while others are caused by large or small emboli that tear loose from the vegetations of endocarditis (Osler's, Janeway's, and Roth's spots; splinter hemorrhages; stroke; splenic infarction). Regurgitant valvular murmurs are the hallmark of endocarditis. Physical findings in patients with endocarditis are one of more of the following:

Fever
Pallor (anemia)
Wasting
Clubbing
Osler's nodes (painful red nodules on tips of fingers or toes)
Janeway's lesions (painless hemorrhage nodules on palms or soles)
Splinter hemorrhages (beneath nails)
Petechiae
Roth's spots (hemorrhagic spots with central white area seen in the fundus)
Murmurs (usually valvular regurgitant murmurs)
Abdominal or flank tenderness (splenic, renal infarction)
Gangrene or pregangrene of fingers or toes
Neurologic findings: hemiplegia, convulsions, coma, toxic psychosis,
     meningeal irritation

C. ECG. ECG findings in patients with endocarditis depend on the nature and severity of cardiac involvement and preexisting heart disease. The ECG may be normal, or preexisting left or right ventricular hypertrophy may be noted. Occasionally, endocarditis develops in a patient with prior MI, in which case the ECG will show the infarct. Embolization to the coronary arteries may produce acute infarction in a patient with endocarditis. Left or right atrial enlargement may be present, usually as a result of prior cardiac disease. Atrial and ventricular arrhythmias are common. The development of conduction defects or first- or second-degree heart block in a patient with endocarditis is an ominous sign. It usually implies that a septal abscess is present and the conduction system involved. Third-degree heart block generally develops in such a patient.

D. Chest x-ray examination. The roentgenographic findings in patients with IE depend on the nature and severity of the infectious process and on preexisting cardiac disease. Serial chest films may disclose progressive dilatation of one or more cardiac chambers and signs of developing or increasing left ventricular failure (interstitial pulmonary edema, alveolar edema, pleural effusion). Signs of left ventricular failure should be sought with diligence. Patients with right-sided endocarditis usually demonstrate multiple pulmonary infiltrates secondary to septic embolism to the lungs.

E. Laboratory tests. The most important laboratory test in patients with endocarditis is the blood culture, because it confirms the diagnosis and guides appropriate therapy. A small number of patients with IE repeatedly have negative blood cultures, often as a result of prior partial treatment of the infection with antibiotics.

Four blood cultures identify more than 90% of patients with positive cultures, and six blood cultures identify almost 100% of such individuals. Cultures should be obtained over several days in patients with prior antibiotic exposure. Aerobic and anaerobic cultures should be planted. Aspiration of Osler's or Janeway's lesions occasionally enables the physician to identify the infecting organism by Gram's stain and culture. A list of organisms that can result in IE appears in Table 20-1. Hematologic findings in patients with IE include normocytic, normochromic anemia, and elevated erythrocyte sedimentation rate. The white blood cell count may be elevated, normal, or low. Phagocytic monocytes can be identified in a blood smear made from a drop of blood obtained from an earlobe puncture. Serum globulin levels often are raised. Urinalysis reveals albuminuria and hematuria. Red cell casts may be seen.

TABLE 20-1. ORGANISMS CAUSING INFECTIOUS ENDOCARDITIS

Gram-positive organisms
  Viridans streptococci
  Group D streptococcus (*S. faecalis, S. bovis, S. equinus*) (also known as enterococci)
  Staphylococcus aureus
  Staphylococcus epidermidis
  Pneumococcus

Gram-negative organisms
  Escherichia coli
  Haemophilus
  Proteus mirabilis
  Salmonella
  Serratia marcescens
  Pseudomonas aeruginosa
  Aerobacter

Fungi
  Candida
  Histoplasma
  Aspergillus
  Rhodotorula
  Blastomyces

Miscellaneous
  Rickettsia burnetti (Q fever)
  Brucella abortus
  Erysipelothrix
  Bacteroides

F. Echocardiography. Chamber dilatation or hypertrophy and valvular abnormalities may be identified echocardiographically in patients with IE. Because these abnormalities may have been present before the development of IE, their presence is not diagnostic of endocarditis. Vegetations of IE can be identified echocardiographically. Standard transthoracic echocardiography identifies valvular vegetations in the majority of patients with IE. Transesophageal echocardiography is more sensitive in identifying vegetations in these patients. Nearly all patients with IE will have vegetations identified by a transesophageal study. Therefore, echocardiography has become one of the principal means (together with blood cultures) of identifying IE. Doppler study enables the physician to quantitate the severity of the resultant valvular regurgitation.

G. Radionuclide studies. Left and right ventricular function can be quantitated in patients with IE, thereby obviating the need for ventriculography in some patients who require cardiac catheterization. Valvular vegetations have been identified by a radionuclide scintigraphic technique that uses isotope-labeled platelets, but this technique is not used routinely in the diagnosis of patients with IE.

H. Catheterization and angiography. Invasive procedures are undertaken with great care in patients with IE because of the fear of dislodging material from vegetations, with resultant embolism. The diagnosis of IE does not depend on data obtained by catheterization. There are three indications for invasive diagnostic procedures in patients with IE: (i) to monitor left ventricular filling pressures in patients treated with afterload reducing agents, (ii) to quantitate ventricular function and severity of valvular regurgitation in patients who are being considered for urgent valve replacement, and (iii) to perform coronary arteriography before surgery. The third indication is the one most commonly invoked when catheterization is performed in a patient with IE. Often, catheterization is unnecessary in patients with IE because transesophageal echocardiography identifies the affected valve, gives semiquantitative data concerning the amount of valvular regurgitation, and quantitates ventricular function. Catheterization and angiography should be performed expeditiously in such patients because of their unstable clinical status.

I. Protocol for the diagnosis of IE

   1. Testing sequence for making the diagnosis. Here is a testing sequence for making the diagnosis of IE. The dashed arrow indicates that the final step is optional.

History and physical examination
↓
Chest x-ray film and ECG
↓
Complete blood count and blood cultures
↓
Echocardiography
↓
Catheterization

   2. Criteria for making the diagnosis. The diagnosis of IE is made in the following situations:

     a. An individual has regurgitant valvular murmurs and positive blood cultures.

     b. An individual has documented, unexplained, and persistent fever (longer than 1 to 2 weeks), as well as documented organic heart disease or a prosthetic valve; vegetations are usually identified by transthoracic or transesophageal echocardiography. Blood cultures may be negative. A diagnostic search for other causes of fever should continue despite the initiation of therapy for endocarditis.

     c. An individual has repeatedly positive blood cultures but minimal or no evidence of organic heart disease (including the absence of a cardiac murmur), and no vegetations are seen during echocardiographic study.

     d. An individual has persistent fever and echocardiographic demonstration of valvular vegetations. Blood cultures may be negative, and murmurs may be absent.

     e. It has been suggested that IE may be present in individuals without fever, murmur, or positive blood cultures. How the diagnosis of IE can be made in such patients is hard to imagine because nodules on heart valves identified by echocardiographic study may be the result of calcification or other degenerative processes.

     f. Systems of clinical criteria for the diagnosis of IE have been developed by a number of different investigators (see **Suggested Readings** for several of these diagnostic systems). Like the Jones criteria for the diagnosis of acute rheumatic fever, these systems involve a scoring schema often with major and minor criteria. The diagnosis of IE is established when a prespecified number of criteria are present (see Table 20-2).

   3. Differential diagnosis

     a. Viral syndromes. Patients with organic heart disease may become quite ill as a result of a viral syndrome or influenza. Fever, chills, malaise, and anorexia suggest the diagnosis of IE. Blood cultures are negative; however, echocardiography does not demonstrate vegetations, and the patient improves spontaneously after a few days.

     b. Acute rheumatic fever. Fever and regurgitant valvular murmurs may occur in a patient with acute rheumatic fever. Differentiation of

TABLE 20-2. THE DUKE CRITERIA FOR THE DIAGNOSIS OF INFECTIVE ENDOCARDITIS

Definite endocarditis
  Pathologic criteria
    (1) microorganisms identified by culture and/or histologic examination of a vegetation or intracardiac abscess
    (2) presence of a vegetation or intracardiac abscess by histological exam with active infection present

  Clinical criteria: The presence of 2 major criteria or 1 major and 3 minor criteria or 5 minor criteria

  Major criteria
    (1) two to three positive blood cultures for infective endocarditis with the cultures obtained separately
    (2) positive echocardiogram for vegetation, abscess, or dehiscence of a prosthetic heart valve with new or increased valvular regurgitation

  Minor criteria
    (1) predisposing condition to endocarditis, e.g., mitral valve disease, or intravenous drug abuse
    (2) temperature to 38°C
    (3) peripheral vascular manifestations consistent with infective endocarditis such as arterial embolism, septic pulmonary emboli, mycotic aneurysm, intracranial hemorrhage, Osler's or Janeway lesions, petechiae, splinter hemorrhages, Roth spots, etc.
    (4) immunological phenomena such as glomerulonephritis, positive serum rheumatoid factor
    (5) atypical positive blood culture results, for example, an organism not commonly associated with endocarditis or a single positive blood culture
    (6) echocardiography consistent with but not diagnostic of a vegetation

---

rheumatic fever from IE depends on negative blood cultures, rising antistreptolysin O titers, absence of vegetations on echocardiographic study, and young age in patients with rheumatic fever.

  c. Atrial myxoma. Patients with atrial myxoma may present with fever, malaise, peripheral emboli, and a murmur. Differentiation of this endocarditis-like syndrome from true IE depends on negative blood cultures and echocardiographic visualization of the tumor in patients with atrial myxoma.

  d. Systemic lupus erythematosus. Patients with systemic lupus erythematosus may resemble individuals with IE because of the presence of fever, albuminuria, and hematuria; however, patients with systemic lupus erythematosus usually have no heart murmur or valvular vegetations, and blood cultures are negative. The antinuclear antibody test is almost always positive in such patients.

  e. Primary neurologic disorder. Some patients with IE present with signs or symptoms of cerebral infarction or embolism. In such cases, endocarditis may be overlooked as the clinician focuses on the neurologic manifestations. Fever and a cardiac murmur should alert the physician to the possible diagnosis of IE. Blood cultures and echocardiography confirm the latter diagnosis.

  f. Occult neoplasm. Patients with long-standing IE may present with cachexia, anemia, and fever, thus resembling individuals with malignant neoplasms. Blood cultures, a negative echocardiographic study, and a diligent search for tumor help to differentiate these two conditions.

III. Therapy
  A. Medical treatment
    1. Antibiotics. Patients with IE should receive prolonged courses of intravenous antibiotics to which the infecting organisms are sensitive. Bactericidal agents should be used whenever possible. Antibiotic dosage should be sufficient to achieve a serum concentration four times greater than the concentration that killed the infecting organism *in vitro.* Fever and peripheral embolic phenomena may occur during therapy; this does **not** mean that treatment is ineffective. Some form of penicillin alone or combined with an aminoglycoside, such as streptomycin or gentamicin, is the major treatment regimen for most patients with IE. Specific regimens for a variety of organisms are listed here:
        a. Viridans streptococci. Intravenous penicillin G, 10 to 20 million U, is administered in divided doses for 4 weeks, together with intravenous gentamicin, 1 mg/kg q8h, for the first 2 weeks of therapy. Intravenous vancomycin (15 mg/kg q12h) can be substituted for penicillin.
        b. Enterococcus, or group D streptococcus (*Streptococcus faecalis, S. bovis,* and *S. equinus*). Intravenous penicillin G, 20 to 30 million U, is administered in divided doses, together with intravenous gentamicin, 1 mg/kg q8h for 4 to 6 weeks. Intravenous vancomycin (15 mg/kg q12h) together with intravenous gentamicin (1 mg/kg q8h) is an acceptable alternative regimen.
        c. Staphylococcus. If the infecting organism is nonpenicillinase producing, treatment involves 20 to 30 million U of intravenous penicillin G per day in divided doses for 4 to 6 weeks. Intravenous vancomycin (15 mg/kg q12h) or cephalothin (Keflin, 12 g per day in divided doses) may be substituted for penicillin. For penicillinase-producing staphylococci, the treatment regimen is intravenous nafcillin or oxacillin, 12 g per day in divided doses, together with 1 mg/kg of intravenous gentamicin q8h for the first 5 to 7 days of therapy. Intravenous vancomycin (15 mg/kg q12h) is an acceptable alternative regimen.
        d. Gram-negative bacteria. Because Gram-negative organisms infrequently cause IE, treatment regimens have not been standardized. Intravenous ampicillin (12 g per day in divided doses) has been used successfully to treat sensitive strains of *Haemophilus, Escherichia coli, Proteus mirabilis,* and *Salmonella.* Combination therapy consisting of ticarcillin, 3 g q4h, and gentamicin (100 mg per day) or tobramycin (5 to 8 mg/kg per day in divided doses) or piperacillin (3 g q4h in divided doses) has been reported to cure some cases of *Pseudomonas* endocarditis, although valve replacement often is required for IE produced by this organism. A similar regimen has been used for patients with *Serratia* endocarditis. Third- or fourth-generation cephalosporins such as ceftriaxone or ceftazidime in combination with an extended-spectrum penicillin such as ticarcillin may be used with success in patients with Gram-negative IE.
        e. IE with negative blood cultures. Treatment of IE in which blood cultures are negative consists of administration of 20 to 30 million U of intravenous penicillin G per day in divided doses, plus intravenous gentamicin, 1 mg/kg q8h.
        f. Fungal IE. Amphotericin B alone or in combination with 5-flucytosine is the drug of choice for endocarditis secondary to *Candida, Histoplasma, Rhodotorula, Aspergillus,* or *Blastomyces.* The initial dose of amphotericin is 0.25 mg/kg body weight, with gradually increasing dosage to 0.75 mg/kg per day for approximately 6 months. Concomitant therapy with flucytosine may be used. Valve excision essentially is always required as part of the therapeutic regimen.
        g. Miscellaneous organisms. IE with *Rickettsia burnetii* is treated with tetracycline; gonococcal and pneumococcal IE are managed with 20 million U of penicillin G per day. *Bacteroides* endocarditis

is treated with metronidazole (1 g loading dose followed by 500 mg intravenously q6h for 6 weeks).
   h. Prosthetic valve endocarditis. This form of IE is particularly difficult to treat medically. Very high dose antibiotic therapy has resulted in some cures, but most patients eventually require valve replacement after a period of preparatory antibiotic therapy.
  2. Heart failure. Patients who develop heart failure as a result of IE are treated with digitalis, diuretics, and afterload-reducing agents as required. Valve replacement is often necessary. Patients with severe, acute mitral or aortic insufficiency may develop severe left ventricular failure, which requires intravenous afterload reduction therapy (e.g., nitroprusside).
  3. Anticoagulants. Anticoagulants usually are avoided in patients with IE because of the danger of hemorrhage from mycotic aneurysms. Patients with prosthetic valve endocarditis who are receiving maintenance anticoagulants before developing IE ordinarily can continue to receive these agents.
  B. Surgery
  1. Indications for cardiac surgery in patients with IE are (i) development of heart failure that does not respond well to medical management; (ii) recurrent or resistant infection despite adequate medical therapy; (iii) most cases of prosthetic valve endocarditis, particularly if early valve dehiscence is noted; and (iv) IE with organisms that usually respond poorly to medical therapy (fungi, *Pseudomonas, Serratia*).
  2. Urgent valve replacement may be required in individuals who meet any of these criteria.
  3. Because endocarditis is a life-threatening condition (in-hospital mortality of approximately 25%), it is wise to have three consultants monitoring these patients: a cardiologist, a cardiac surgeon, and an infectious disease expert.

SELECTED READINGS

Cecchi E, Parrini I, Chinaglia A, et al. New diagnostic criteria for infective endocarditis: a study of sensitivity and specificity. *Eur Heart J* 1997;18:1149–1156.
The Duke criteria was the most sensitive and specific criteria for the diagnosis of infective endocarditis.
Chen SCA, Dwyer DE, Sorrell TC. A comparison of hospital and community-acquired infective endocarditis. *Am J Cardiol* 1992;70:1449–1452.
Nosocomial endocarditis can be prevented; this entity is often more difficult to treat because of antibiotic-resistant organisms.
Churchill MA Jr, Geraci JE, Hunder GG. Musculoskeletal manifestations of bacterial endocarditis. *Ann Intern Med* 1977;87:754–759.
Musculoskeletal manifestations occur in more than 40% of patients with bacterial endocarditis.
Dajani A, Taubert KA, Wilson W, et al. Prevention of bacterial endocarditis: recommendations by the American Heart Association. *JAMA* 1997;277:1794–1801.
Latest recommendations for antibiotic prophylaxis against bacterial endocarditis in susceptible individuals.
DiSalvo G, Habib G, Pergola V, et al. Echocardiography predicts embolic events in infective endocarditis. *J Am Coll Cardiol* 2001;37:1069–1076.
The morphologic characteristics of vegetations predict arterial embolism.
Durak DT, Lukes AS, Bright DK, and the Duke Endocarditis Service: new criteria for the diagnosis of infective endocarditis. *Am J Med* 1994;96:211–219.
The Duke criteria for the diagnosis of infective endocarditis.
Hecht SR, Berger M. Right-sided endocarditis in intravenous drug users: prognostic features in 102 episodes. *Ann Intern Med* 1992;117:560–566.
A careful review of 102 episodes of IE in intravenous drug users; echocardiographic vegetation size is a useful predictor of outcome.

Heiro M, Nikoskelainen J, Engblom E, et al. Neurologic manifestations of infective endocarditis: a 17-year experience in a teaching hospital in Finland. *Arch Intern Med* 2000;160:2781–2787.
Rapid diagnosis and treatment prevents neurologic complications in patients with infective endocarditis.

Heiro M, Nikoskelainen J, Hartiala JJ, et al. Diagnosis of infective endocarditis: sensitivity of the Duke vs von Reyn criteria. *Arch Intern Med* 1998;158:18–24.
The Duke criteria are the most sensitive for the diagnosis of IE.

Jones HR, Siekert RG, Geraci J. Neurologic manifestations of bacterial endocarditis. *Ann Intern Med* 1969;71:21–28.
Bacterial endocarditis associated with a variety of neurologic syndromes.

Kjerulf A, Tvede M, Aldershvile J, Hojby N. Bacterial endocarditis at a tertiary hospital: how do we improve diagnosis and delay of treatment? *Cardiology* 1998;89:79–86.
Analysis and recommendations for strategies to speed diagnosis and treatment of patients with IE.

Mugge A, Daniel WG, Frank G, et al. Echocardiography in infective endocarditis: reassessment of prognostic implications of vegetation size determined by the transthoracic and the transesophageal approach. *J Am Coll Cardiol* 1989;14:631–638.
Transesophageal echocardiography is considerably more sensitive than transthoracic echocardiography in identifying vegetations in patients with IE.

Sanabria T, Alpert JS, Goldberg R, et al. Increasing frequency of staphylococcal infective endocarditis: experience at a University Hospital, 1981–1988. *Arch Intern Med* 1990;150:1305–1309.
Staphylococcal endocarditis is becoming more common in patients hospitalized in tertiary care centers with IE.

Verheul HA, van den Brink RBA, van Vreeland T, et al. Effects of changes in management of active infective endocarditis on outcome in a 25-year period. *Am J Cardiol* 1993;72:682–687.
Hospital mortality remains high for patients with infective endocarditis despite improved monitoring and antibiotic therapy.

Von Reyn CF, Levy BS, Arbeit RD, et al. Infective endocarditis: an analysis based on strict case definitions. *Ann Intern Med* 1981;94:505–518.
Strict clinical definitions of endocarditis are helpful in managing suspected cases of endocarditis.

21. CARDIAC TUMORS

I. Introduction. Cardiac tumors occur quite rarely, with metastatic neoplasms three times more prevalent than primary tumors. A large variety of benign and malignant tumors of the heart have been described. Table 21-1 lists some of the common primary and metastatic neoplasms of the heart.

II. Diagnosis

A. History. A number of clinical presentations are possible for patients with cardiac neoplasms. Many patients with myxomas present with dyspnea or syncope secondary to valvular obstruction. Often, left atrial myxoma mimics mitral stenosis. Myxomas can produce a picture resembling that of endocarditis or acute rheumatic fever with fever, chills, weight loss, murmurs, and systemic or pulmonary emboli. Some patients with cardiac neoplasms present with arterial embolism; others complain of palpitations secondary to arrhythmias. Chest pain, anasarca (superior vena caval syndrome), cardiac tamponade, and symptoms of left or right ventricular failure have been observed in patients with cardiac tumors. Sudden death secondary to valvular obstruction, arrhythmia, or embolism may occur.

Differentiation of myxoma from mitral valve disease can be made clinically (Table 21-2).

B. Physical examination. Patients with sessile cardiac tumors often present with arterial embolism or arrhythmias. Physical findings may therefore not involve the heart but may appear as abnormalities in the abdominal, neurologic, or peripheral vascular system. As sessile tumors enlarge, they may encroach on the outflow tract of either the right or the left ventricle, thereby mimicking the findings of pulmonic or aortic stenosis. Pedunculated tumors (particularly myxomas) are likely to involve the atria. They move with the blood flow into the tricuspid or mitral valve orifices, producing the murmurs of tricuspid or mitral stenosis. A sound resembling an opening snap may even be heard. Systemic symptoms are not uncommon in patients with myxoma, namely, fever, weight loss, pallor (secondary to anemia), and clubbing. Systemic symptoms combined with the presence of a murmur may lead to a mistaken diagnosis of endocarditis.

Physical findings in patients with cardiac tumors are summarized in Table 21-3.

C. ECG. ECG findings in patients with cardiac tumors include nonspecific ST–T changes, S–T segment elevation (pericarditis secondary to pericardial involvement), intraventricular conduction delays and bundle branch blocks, various degrees of heart block, and a wide spectrum of atrial and ventricular arrhythmias.

Patients with right ventricular outflow tract obstruction may have right ventricular hypertrophy on the ECG. ECG findings in patients with cardiac tumors are summarized in Table 21-4.

D. Chest x-ray examination. The chest roentgenogram rarely yields specific findings suggestive of cardiac tumor. Atrial myxomas occasionally contain calcium, which is visible on the plain chest film. Moreover, the calcifications can be seen prolapsing into the ventricle during diastole by fluoroscopy. Usually the chest x-ray picture is normal or resembles what is seen with the various forms of valvular heart disease that cardiac tumors mimic. Marked cardiomegaly may be noted in patients with massive pericardial effusion. Roentgenographic findings in patients with cardiac tumors are listed in Table 21-4.

E. Laboratory tests. Anemia, leukocytosis, elevated erythrocyte sedimentation rate, and hyperglobulinemia are often present in patients with myxoma. An occasional patient with right atrial myxoma may demonstrate polycythemia or thrombocytopenia.

TABLE 21-1. CARDIAC NEOPLASMS

Primary	Metastatic
Myxomas	Bronchogenic carcinoma
Rhabdomyoma	Breast carcinoma
Mesothelioma	Melanoma
Fibromas	Lymphoma
Lipomas	Leukemia
Sarcoma	Renal cell carcinoma
Leiomyoma	

TABLE 21-2. DIFFERENTIATION OF LEFT ATRIAL MYXOMA AND MITRAL VALVE DISEASE

Mitral Valve Disease	Left Atrial Myxoma
History of rheumatic fever	Absence of history of rheumatic fever
Progression of symptoms is slow	Progression of symptoms is rapid
Syncope is very rare	Syncope is common
Symptoms do not remit	Symptoms frequently remit or change
Symptoms do not vary with position	Symptoms often vary with position
Murmurs are typical	Murmurs are atypical, changeable, and often hard to hear
Severity of symptoms correlates with physical and roentgenographic findings	Severity of symptoms does not correlate with physical and roentgenographic findings

TABLE 21-3. PHYSICAL FINDINGS IN PATIENTS WITH CARDIAC TUMORS[a]

Systemic
  Fever
  Wasting
  Pallor (secondary to anemia)
  Clubbing
  Right ventricular failure (jugular venous distention, hepatomegaly, ascites, peripheral edema)
  Left ventricular failure (rales, pleural effusion)
  Abdominal tenderness and guarding (infarction of spleen, liver, kidney secondary to embolism)
  Neurologic abnormalities (infarction secondary to embolism)
  Loss of peripheral pulses (embolism)

Cardiac
  Irregular pulse (atrial and ventricular arrhythmias)
  Early diastolic sound (opening snap or "tumor plop")
  Diastolic murmurs of mitral or tricuspid stenosis
  Systolic murmurs of mitral or tricuspid regurgitation
  Pericardial friction rub

[a] Not all findings are present in all patients.

TABLE 21-4. ECG AND ROENTGENOGRAPHIC FINDINGS IN PATIENTS WITH CARDIAC TUMORS

ECG findings
    Atrial and ventricular arrhythmias
    Right atrial enlargement
    Low QRS voltage
    Intraventricular conduction delay
    Bundle branch block
    First-, second-, or third-degree heart block
    Right ventricular hypertrophy
    S–T segment elevation (pericarditis)
    Nonspecific ST–T changes

X-ray findings
    Roentgenographic findings of mitral, tricuspid, or pulmonic valve disease
      (see Chapter 16)
    Intracardiac calcifications
    Marked cardiomegaly (pericardial effusion)
    Irregular or unusual cardiac border (tumor mass itself)

    F. Echocardiography. Echocardiography is the method of choice for the identification of cardiac tumors. Right and left atrial pedunculated tumors are particularly well seen. Cross-sectional echocardiography visualizes cardiac tumors with special clarity. Pericardial effusion secondary to tumor in the pericardium is also easily identified by echocardiography.

    G. Radionuclide studies, computed tomography (CT), and magnetic resonance imaging (MRI). Gated blood pool scanning can reveal the presence and movement of pedunculated cardiac tumors. CT and MRI are also capable of imaging some cardiac tumors, but echocardiography is usually the imagining technique of choice for defining cardiac tumors.

    H. Catheterization and angiography. Left atrial myxoma is associated with pulmonary hypertension and V waves in the pulmonary capillary wedge tracing. There is a prominent notch on the upstroke of the left ventricular pressure tracing that corresponds to movement of the myxoma across the mitral valve into the left atrium. Similar findings occur in the right atrial and ventricular pressure tracings in patients with right atrial myxoma. The hemodynamic pattern of cardiac tamponade is found in patients with large pericardial effusions secondary to tumor (see Chapter 19). Extensive invasion of the myocardium by tumor can produce the hemodynamic picture of restrictive cardiomyopathy (see Chapter 18).

    Gradients across the tricuspid, pulmonic, or mitral valves are seen in individuals whose tumors produce obstruction of those valves. Angiocardiography reveals intracavitary filling defects in patients with cardiac tumors. Sessile and pedunculated tumors can be distinguished.

    I. Biopsy. Right ventricular endocardial biopsy in a patient with the hemodynamic picture of restrictive cardiomyopathy may reveal infiltration of the myocardium with tumor. Pericardial biopsy in a patient with unexplained or unusual pericardial effusion may demonstrate tumor. Histologic examination of material removed at peripheral arterial embolectomy may demonstrate tumor.

    J. Protocol for the diagnosis of cardiac tumor
        1. Testing sequence for making the diagnosis. The following protocol is suggested for the workup of a patient suspected of having cardiac tumor. The dashed arrow indicates that this step is optional.

History and physical examination
↓
ECG and chest x-ray film
↓
Echocardiography
↓
Catheterization and angiography
↓
Biopsy in selected individuals

2. Criteria for making the diagnosis
   a. The diagnosis of cardiac tumor is made in individuals with a history of left or right ventricular failure or arterial embolism in whom echocardiography, angiocardiography, or both demonstrate the presence of an intracardiac mass.
   b. The diagnosis of cardiac tumor is also made in individuals with a history of fever, weight loss, and fatigue with anemia; elevated erythrocyte sedimentation rate and serum globulin levels; and echocardiographic or angiographic demonstration of an intracardiac mass.
   c. The diagnosis of cardiac tumor also is made in individuals who present with pericardial effusion in whom echocardiography, CT scanning, or MRI of the pericardium outlines nodules of presumptive tumor or in whom biopsy of the pericardium or cytologic examination of the pericardial effusion demonstrates tumor. Patients with known metastatic tumor who develop pericardial effusion in the absence of heart failure or mediastinal radiotherapy can be assumed to have pericardial metastases.
3. Differential diagnosis
   a. Endocarditis. Fever, weight loss, anemia, and murmurs may suggest the diagnosis of endocarditis. Sterile blood cultures and echocardiographic demonstration of cardiac tumor differentiate tumor from endocarditis.
   b. Valvular heart disease. Cardiac tumors can present with signs, symptoms, ECG, and x-ray findings suggestive of tricuspid, pulmonic, or mitral valve disease. Differentiation of these conditions depends on echocardiographic or angiographic demonstration of cardiac tumor (Table 21-2).
   c. Pericarditis. Invasion of the pericardium by tumor can result in effusion with tamponade or constriction. Differentiation of tumorous pericardial involvement from other forms of pericardial disease depends on microscopic examination of a pericardial biopsy or cell block from the effusion.
   d. Restrictive cardiomyopathy. Invasion of the myocardium by tumor can produce a picture of restrictive cardiomyopathy. Differentiation of myopathy secondary to tumor from myopathy as a result of other pathologic processes (e g., amyloidosis, hemochromatosis) depends on characteristic laboratory or pathologic findings in the respective disease states. For example, amyloidosis is diagnosed by the Congo red test and a positive rectal mucosal or gingival biopsy. The diagnosis of restrictive cardiomyopathy secondary to tumor may require a right ventricular endocardial biopsy (see Chapter 18).
III. Therapy
   A. Medical treatment. The pathophysiologic changes associated with cardiac tumors are caused primarily by mechanical obstruction. Therefore, surgical excision is usually the treatment of choice. A number of tumors that involve the heart cannot be excised. Some of these neoplasms (e.g., lymphomas, leukemias, breast carcinoma) will respond to radiotherapy, chemotherapy, or both. Recurrent pericardial effusion with tamponade is often successfully

managed by intrapericardial instillation of tetracycline or antineoplastic medications (e.g., nitrogen mustard, methotrexate).

B. Surgery. Total excision of benign cardiac tumors (e.g., myxoma) is the treatment of choice and can be performed with little risk. Malignant tumors often are treated with a combination of surgical excision, radiation, and chemotherapy. Recurrent pericardial effusion with tamponade secondary to tumor involvement of the pericardium may be treated with partial or radical pericardiectomy with or without combined radiation and chemotherapy.

SELECTED READINGS

Bear PA, Moodie DS. Malignant primary cardiac tumors: the Cleveland Clinic experience, 1956–1986. *Chest* 1987;92:860–862.
Review of 11 patients with primary malignant tumors of the heart.

Freedberg RS, Kronzon I, Rumancik WM, et al. The contribution of magnetic resonance imaging to the evaluation of intracardiac tumors diagnosed by echocardiography. *Circulation* 1988;77:96–103.
Magnetic resonance imaging accurately demonstrates intracardiac tumors.

Goswami KC, Shrivastava S, Bahl VK, et al. Cardiac myxomas: clinical and echocardiographic profile. *Int J Cardiol* 1998;63:251–259.
A careful clinical review of 70 patients with cardiac myxomas.

Harvey WP. Clinical aspects of cardiac tumors. *Am J Cardiol* 1968;21:328—342.
Extensive review of clinical aspects of cardiac tumors.

Hoffman U, Globits S, Frank H. Cardiac and paracardiac masses: current opinion on diagnostic evaluation by magnetic resonance imaging. *Eur Heart J* 1998;19:553–563.
The value of MRI in the diagnosis of cardiac tumors.

Reeder GS, Khandheria BK, Seward JB, et al. Transesophageal echocardiography and cardiac masses. *Mayo Clin Proc* 1991;66:1101–1109.
Transesophageal echocardiography is a useful addition to transthoracic echo for the diagnosis and localization of cardiac mass lesions.

Sun JP, Asher CR, Yang XS, et al. Clinical and echocardiographic characteristics of papillary fibroelastomas: a retrospective and prospective study in 162 patients. *Circulation* 2001;103:2687–2693.
Cardiac papillary fibroelastomas are generally small, mobile, and capable of embolization.

Weinberg BA, Conces DJ Jr, Waller BF. Cardiac manifestations of noncardiac tumors, part I: direct effects. *Clin Cardiol* 1989;12:289–296.
Cardiac manifestations of cardiac tumors may be the result of direct mechanical effects on the endocardium, the myocardium, or the pericardium. A discussion of metastatic tumors and their effect on the heart.

Weinberg BA, Conces DJ Jr, Waller BF. Cardiac manifestations of noncardiac tumors, part II: direct effects. *Clin Cardiol* 1989;12:347–354.
Further discussion of the effects of metastatic tumors on the heart. The demonstration of such effects by echo, MRI, and CT scanning is also discussed.

22. PULMONARY EMBOLISM

I. **Introduction.** More than half a million Americans experience an episode of nonfatal pulmonary embolism each year, and approximately 200,000 of these die as a result.

Unfortunately, the diagnosis is not made nor is therapy instituted in more than two thirds of patients with pulmonary embolism. Such discouraging statistics are the result of the often confusing clinical presentation of pulmonary embolism. The diagnosis is made easily in the young, healthy surgical patient who develops dyspnea, cough, and hemoptysis 1 week after elective surgery. However, most patients with pulmonary embolism are elderly, minimally symptomatic, and suffering from preexisting cardiac or pulmonary disease (or both). Because the symptoms arising from pulmonary embolism are often the same as those that result from various cardiac and pulmonary disorders, the diagnosis is often overlooked.

II. **Diagnosis**

A. **History.** Patients with pulmonary embolism commonly present with one of four clinical syndromes: (i) unexplained dyspnea at rest, (ii) pulmonary infarction (cough, hemoptysis, pleuritic pain), (iii) cardiovascular collapse (massive embolism), or (iv) unexplained worsening in preexisting heart failure.

1. **Unexplained dyspnea at rest.** Patients note unusual and disturbing air hunger of sudden onset with minimal or no exertion. This is the commonest presentation for pulmonary embolism.

2. **Pulmonary infarction.** Patients report localized pleuritic chest discomfort, usually posterior in location. Cough, dyspnea, and hemoptysis also may be noted but are more frequently absent than present.

3. **Cardiovascular collapse.** Patients present with an obviously serious illness of sudden onset. They are often hypotensive and tachycardic and may suffer cardiac arrest. Complaints can include dyspnea, severe fatigue, a sense of impending doom, syncope, diaphoresis, and occasionally an oppressive, substernal discomfort without radiation. This latter symptom may result in the erroneous diagnosis of myocardial infarction.

4. **Unexplained worsening of preexisting heart failure.** Patients with prior heart disease and symptoms of left or right ventricular failure often describe worsening symptoms of cardiac decompensation over a relatively short time (1 to several days). Worsening symptoms may include dyspnea on exertion, orthopnea, fatigue, increasing abdominal girth, and peripheral edema.

5. **Predisposing factors.** Almost 90% of patients with pulmonary embolism relate a history of one or more factors predisposing to deep venous thrombosis and hence pulmonary embolism: (i) bedrest or prolonged inactivity such as a plane, bus, or car ride; (ii) debilitation secondary to advanced age or severe illness; (iii) heart disease, particularly if heart failure is present; (iv) recent surgical procedure (particularly high-risk procedures are lower-extremity orthopedic or gynecologic operations); (v) pregnancy, contraceptive pills, or hormone replacement therapy; (vi) leg trauma; and (vii) occult or known malignancy; (viii) hypercoagulable state.

B. **Physical examination.** Few physical findings are specific for pulmonary embolism.

The most helpful finding is a respiratory rate greater than 20 breaths per minute. The respiratory rate should be counted for a full minute, **not** for 15 seconds and multiplied by four. Physical findings that can be discovered in patients with pulmonary embolism are noted in Table 22-1. Massive embolism with resultant right ventricular failure is associated with the findings of acute cor pulmonale (Table 22-1). The diagnosis of deep venous thrombosis by physical examination can be quite difficult, because false-positive and false-negative findings are common.

339

TABLE 22-1. PHYSICAL FINDINGS IN PATIENTS WITH PULMONARY EMBOLISM[a]

Cyanosis
Diaphoresis
Tachycardia
Tachypnea
Low-grade fever (<101°F)
↑Prominent A wave in jugular venous pulse
Localized or bilateral wheezing (particularly suggestive of pulmonary embolism if new in onset)
Evidence of unilateral pleural effusion (dullness, decreased breath sounds)
↑Increased loudness of P2
Widened splitting of second heart sound
Continuous murmur over localized area of lung field (rare)
Evidence of deep venous thrombosis (calf or thigh tenderness, edema, prominent superficial veins)

Findings of acute cor pulmonale[a]
   Tachycardia
   ±Hypotension
   Jugular venous distention
   Right ventricular heave
   Right ventricular third heart sound, fourth heart sound (increases with inspiration)
   Murmur of tricuspid regurgitation
   Hepatomegaly

[a] Not all finding are present in any one patient.
↑, increased; ±, occasionally present.

C. ECG. Patients with massive pulmonary embolism almost invariably (95%) demonstrate some abnormality in the ECG. Those with submassive embolism also usually (75%) have an abnormal ECG (Table 22-2). Findings such as new S1,Q3,T3, poor R wave progression, incomplete right bundle branch block (RBBB), and right axis deviation are seen only in patients with massive embolism.

D. Chest x-ray examination, Spiral computed tomography (CT) scanning. Roentgenographic findings are unfortunately often nonspecific in patients with pulmonary embolism. Chest x-ray abnormalities in patients with pulmonary embolism include the following:

Pulmonary infiltrate
Elevated hemidiaphragm
Pleural effusion (usually unilateral)
Plump main pulmonary arteries
Atelectatic streaking
Focal oligemia
Left ventricular enlargement
Right ventricular enlargement

It is not uncommon for patients with pulmonary embolism to have a normal chest x-ray film (approximately 25% of patients with pulmonary embolism).

Spiral CT scanning with contrast administration is useful in identifying major pulmonary embolism in the central pulmonary arterial tree. Embolism in third-order (or smaller) pulmonary arteries cannot be identified. This test has approximately the same sensitivity and specificity as ventilation/perfusion lung scanning.

E. Laboratory tests. Because of the vagaries involved in the diagnosis of pulmonary embolism, a number of laboratory tests have been used to improve diagnostic acumen.

TABLE 22-2. ECG FINDINGS IN PATIENTS WITH PULMONARY EMBOLISM

P-pulmonale
Right axis deviation
Left axis deviation
Poor R wave progression in precordial leads
Incomplete right bundle branch block
Complete right bundle branch block
Right ventricular hypertrophy S1, S2, S3 pattern
Low-voltage frontal plane
Pseudoinfarction (inferior or anterior)
S–T and T wave abnormalities (depression, elevation, inversion)

Arrhythmias and conduction disturbances
   Sinus tachycardia
   Atrial premature beats
   Atrial fibrillation
   Ventricular premature beats
   First-degree atrioventricular block
   Supraventricular arrhythmias

1. Serum lactic dehydrogenase (LDH). Patients with pulmonary embolism generally demonstrate elevated serum LDH activity. Unfortunately, there are many false-positive and false-negative results, making this test of little use.
2. Triad of elevated LDH, normal glutamic-oxaloacetic transaminase, and elevated serum indirect bilirubin levels. This combination of findings sometimes occurs in patients with pulmonary embolism. The triad is not sensitive, but it is fairly specific.
3. Serum creatine phosphokinase (CK-MB or troponin). An occasional patient with pulmonary embolism will have elevated serum CK-MB and/or troponin activity. This finding usually occurs in patients with massive pulmonary embolism, resulting in right ventricular dilatation and failure. The elevated myocardial biomarkers are probably the result of small amounts of subendocardial right ventricular infarction, resulting from the marked increase in right ventricular myocardial oxygen demand.
4. Hematologic tests. White blood cell counts are moderately elevated in patients with pulmonary embolism (generally 12×10^3 to 13×10^3 µl). Hematocrit and platelet count may be mildly depressed (30% to 35% and 100×10^3 to 200×10^3 µl, respectively). Serum fibrin split product (D-dimer) levels frequently are elevated as a result of increased serum fibrinolytic activity because of the presence of intravascular clots. An elevated serum D-dimer level is a sensitive test for pulmonary embolism. Unfortunately, it is not very specific, and false-positive results abound. Elevated serum platelet factor IV levels, reflecting intravascular activation of platelets, occur in patients with pulmonary embolism.

   Elevated platelet factor IV levels are also found in individuals with acute myocardial infarction.
5. Arterial blood gases. Arterial oxygen tension (measured with the patient breathing room air) is usually less than 80 mm Hg in persons with pulmonary embolism. A few individuals (usually young patients with submassive embolism) will demonstrate arterial P_{O_2} values between 80 and 90 mm Hg, but it is very unusual for someone with pulmonary embolism to have an arterial P_{O_2} value higher than 90 mm Hg. Pulmonary embolism causes reflex hyperventilation with resultant arterial hypocarbia (decrease in P_{CO_2}) and respiratory alkalosis (increase in pH).

F. Tests of venous thrombosis. In recent years, a number of procedures have been developed to document the presence of deep venous thrombosis in the lower extremities. Plethysmography (electrical impedance or strain gauge), radioactive fibrinogen scanning, and Doppler ultrasound have all been used to this end. These noninvasive tests are reasonably sensitive and specific, but their predictive value is not as high as that of invasive venography. Their noninvasive nature, however, makes them particularly attractive. Venous echo/Doppler is the most widely used test. See Chapter 29 for a more complete description of the diagnosis and therapy of deep venous thrombosis.

G. Echocardiography. Echocardiographic findings in patients with pulmonary embolism usually are nonspecific. Right ventricular cavity dimensions may be increased, whereas left ventricular dimensions are normal or low. A thrombus in the right atrium or right ventricle may be seen. Some clinicians feel that evidence of right ventricular dilatation and/or dysfunction observed on an echocardiographic study suggests that the patient has suffered a massive episode of pulmonary embolism thereby predicting a poor prognosis. These physicians feel that patients with these patients with right ventricular dysfunction deserve very aggressive therapy for pulmonary embolism. However, other clinicians disagree with this contention and feel that only patients with clinically evident right ventricular failure and/or hypotension deserve the most aggressive forms of therapy.

H. Radionuclide studies. Multiple-view perfusion and ventilation lung scanning is the most sensitive and specific noninvasive test for pulmonary embolism. There are essentially no false-negative diagnoses when properly executed perfusion/ventilation scans are used. The false-positive rate is approximately 15%. A combination of ventilation-perfusion lung scanning and one of the noninvasive tests of venous thrombosis results in a low incidence of false-positive diagnosis for pulmonary embolism, as does the combination of ventilation/perfusion scanning and high-sensitivity D-dimer blood tests. Perfusion-ventilation lung scans demonstrate areas of the lung that ventilate but do not perfuse, the so-called ventilation-perfusion mismatch. Single mismatched defects are more commonly a false-positive result than are multiple defects. Pneumonitis usually results in an area of the lung that neither perfuses nor ventilates.

I. Catheterization and angiography. The gold standard for the diagnosis of pulmonary embolism is pulmonary angiography, just as venography is the gold standard for the diagnosis of deep venous thrombosis. Pulmonary angiography visualizes filling defects and cutoff vessels that result from blood clots in the pulmonary circulation. Pulmonary angiography can be performed even in critically ill, hypotensive individuals. A semiquantitative estimate of the percentage of obstruction of the pulmonary vascular bed can be obtained from the pulmonary angiogram. The major hemodynamic response to pulmonary embolism is pulmonary hypertension. At high levels of pulmonary arterial pressure (secondary to massive embolism), the right ventricle fails, which results in right ventricular dilatation, elevated right atrial pressure, and depressed cardiac output. Left ventricular filling pressures are usually reduced, whereas left ventricular contractile function is probably normal or nearly so. The hemodynamic derangement secondary to pulmonary embolism is directly proportional to the magnitude of embolic obstruction and the presence of preexisting cardiopulmonary disease. The presence of right ventricular failure or systemic arterial hypotension markedly worsens prognosis in patients with pulmonary embolism.

J. Suggested diagnostic protocol for pulmonary embolism. A history and physical examination suggesting pulmonary embolism should lead to a chest x-ray film and ECG. The patient then receives 5,000 to 10,000 U of intravenous heparin, followed by determination of arterial blood gases and a noninvasive test of venous function. If available, a high-sensitivity D-dimer blood test should be obtained. If these examinations are normal, the diagnosis of pulmonary embolism is very unlikely, and further testing is unnecessary; heparin therapy is discontinued. If one or more of the tests suggests pulmonary embolism, the patient should then have a multiple-view perfusion-ventilation lung scan or a spiral CT examination with contrast. If the history, physical examination, chest x-ray picture, and ECG are highly suggestive of pulmonary embolism, and if the lung scan or spiral CT are classic for pulmonary embolism (multiple areas of ventilation-perfusion mismatch), the diagnosis of pulmonary embolism is very likely, and anticoagulant therapy (see Section **III.A.1.**) should be continued. If the D-dimer blood test is negative, the diagnosis of pulmonary embolism is doubtful. Noninvasive studies of the veins of the lower extremities are also useful. If these studies are positive, this finding increases the likelihood that pulmonary embolism is present. If there is still doubt about the diagnosis, pulmonary angiography should be performed. Angiography will be required most commonly in patients with cardiac and pulmonary disease. Patients who are candidates for venous interruption or thrombolytic therapy (see Section **III.B.1.**) should have pulmonary angiography before such a medical or interventional procedure is performed.

K. Entities frequently confused with pulmonary embolism
1. Pneumonitis. Bacterial and viral pneumonitis may be difficult to distinguish from pulmonary embolism by history and physical examination alone. The white blood cell count and the febrile response are usually more marked in pneumonitis. Sputum production also suggests pneumonitis. Chest x-ray and blood gas abnormalities may be identical in pulmonary embolism and pneumonitis.

   Lung scanning or spiral CT scanning—combined with tests of peripheral venous function, sensitive D-dimer blood tests, or pulmonary angiography—is the most helpful tests for distinguishing pneumonitis from pulmonary embolism.
2. Viral pleuritis. Pleuritic discomfort and unilateral pleural effusion can be the result of viral pleuritis. This clinical picture also is seen commonly after pulmonary embolism. Blood gases and peripheral venous function are often normal in viral pleuritis, but lung scanning, spiral CT, D-dimer blood tests, and/or pulmonary angiography may be necessary to document the absence of pulmonary embolism.
3. Atelectasis. Postoperative pulmonary collapse may be confused with pulmonary embolism. Arterial blood gases are usually abnormal. Tests of peripheral venous function are helpful if normal. Otherwise, lung scanning, spiral CT scanning, and, at times, pulmonary angiography are required to rule out pulmonary embolism.
4. Sepsis or hemorrhage. Sudden onset of hypovolemia secondary to sepsis (often Gram-negative organisms) or hemorrhage sometimes resembles cardiovascular collapse secondary to pulmonary embolism. In this setting, emergency spiral CT scanning or pulmonary angiography may be necessary if the underlying bacterial infection or hemorrhage is not evident after appropriate diagnostic tests.
5. Hyperventilation syndrome. Anxiety may produce the sensation of severe dyspnea with resultant hyperventilation of sudden onset. The physical examination, chest x-ray film, and ECG are all normal. Arterial oxygen tension (PO_2) is likewise normal, but arterial PCO_2 is depressed, causing respiratory alkalosis. Peripheral venous function is almost always normal, whereas high-sensitivity D-dimer blood tests and lung scans are usually normal.
6. Bronchial asthma. Asthmatic wheezing occasionally is confused with bronchospasm secondary to pulmonary embolism. Wheezing is unusual in patients with pulmonary embolism. When it occurs, wheezing is always new in onset.

   Thus, bronchospasm in a patient with a past history of asthma does not suggest pulmonary embolism. Arterial blood gases may be quite abnormal in patients with bronchial asthma. Moreover, lung scans may demonstrate shifting perfusion defects. Pulmonary angiography or spiral CT scanning is often required in patients with bronchial asthma in whom the clinical presentation resembles that seen with pulmonary embolism.

7. Pulmonary congestion secondary to pulmonary venous hypertension. Left ventricular failure or mitral stenosis causes pulmonary venous hypertension with resultant dyspnea and hyperventilation. Physical examination, chest x-ray film, and ECG may be abnormal in a nonspecific manner, so that patients with pulmonary congestion resemble those with pulmonary embolism (hypoxia, hypocapnia, respiratory alkalosis). Lung scans may be abnormal in patients with pulmonary congestion, and spiral CT scanning or angiography may be required to rule out pulmonary embolism.

III. Therapy
   A. Medical treatment
      1. Anticoagulation. Patients in whom the diagnosis of pulmonary embolism is strongly suspected should receive 5,000 to 10,000 U of unfractionated intravenous heparin before diagnostic tests are completed. Alternatively, patients may be treated with low-molecular-weight heparin, for example, enoxaparin 1 mg/kg injected subcutaneously twice a day. If the physician is reasonably confident of the diagnosis, continuous anticoagulation therapy is initiated with heparin. Two protocols exist for intravenous unfractionated heparin administration: (i) periodic (generally q4h) bolus administration of 5,000 to 10,000 U of heparin, such that the partial thromboplastin time or the Lee-White clotting time is prolonged one and one-half to two times the control value just before the administration of the next dose of heparin and (ii) continuous infusion of heparin (1,000 to 1,500 U per hour), such that the partial thromboplastin time or the Lee-White clotting time is prolonged one and one-half to two times the control value. Continuous infusion of heparin is preferred. As noted above, low-molecular-weight heparin may be substituted for unfractionated heparin.

      Heparin therapy is given for 7 to 10 days, followed by oral warfarin therapy for 2 to 3 months in patients with reversible predisposition (bedrest, surgery, trauma, pregnancy, etc.). The international normalized ratio (INR) value for the prothrombin time is prolonged two to three times that of control. In individuals with lifelong predisposition (heart disease with cardiac decompensation), warfarin therapy may be required for the rest of the patient's life. If a reversible predisposition for venous thromboembolism is present, patients should receive warfarin therapy for approximately 6 months or more before discontinuation. Heparin and warfarin therapy generally overlap for 3 to 5 days, until the prothrombin time is increased to an INR of 2 to 3.

      Many authorities advocate the use of fibrinolytic agents (ie., urokinase, streptokinase, or tissue-type plasminogen activator) for patients with massive pulmonary embolism. There is still considerable controversy concerning which anticoagulant regimen is the best for patients with massive pulmonary embolism: heparin or fibrinolytic agents. Fibrinolytic agents produce more rapid resolution of pulmonary embolism, with earlier improvement in pulmonary hypertension than is seen with heparin; however, bleeding complications, including fatal cerebral hemorrhage, are considerably more common with fibrinolytic therapy than with heparin. Long-term results are identical with these two techniques. Therefore, fibrinolysis is usually reserved for patients with massive pulmonary embolism and hemodynamic compromise. Thrombolytic drug regimens for the treatment of pulmonary embolism are (i) urokinase, 4,400 U/kg infused over 10 minutes, followed by a continuous infusion of 4,400 U/kg per hour for 12 to 24 hours; (ii) streptokinase, 250,000 U infused over 30 minutes, followed by 100,000 U per hour for 24 to 72 hours; and (iii) tissue-type plasminogen activator, 100 mg infused over 2 to 3 hours. After fibrinolysis, the patient is treated with heparin and warfarin as detailed above.

      2. Activity. Patients should restrict their activity for 2 to 3 days after heparin therapy is started. Thereafter, patients may ambulate at will.

3. **Hypotension and right ventricular failure** require liberal administration of intravenous volume (colloid and crystalloid). It is best to place a central venous catheter to obtain measurements of central venous pressure, which should be kept in excess of 8 to 10 mm Hg (occasionally as high as 20 mm Hg). If hypotension persists beyond a brief time, intravenous isoproterenol should be administered. Patients with profound shock or those who require pressors for more than 1 to 2 hours may be candidates for surgical therapy.

B. Surgery

1. Venous interruption. Indications for venous interruption are as follows:

Contraindication to anticoagulation (e.g., gastrointestinal bleeding)
Failure of anticoagulation with recurrent embolism during therapy
Massive embolism with right ventricular failure and hypotension
Continued predisposition to pulmonary embolism

These indications for venous interruption include situations in which anticoagulation fails or is not feasible. In addition, patients with severe hemodynamic compromise secondary to pulmonary embolism are candidates for venous interruption because even a minor recurrent embolus probably would be lethal. There are three procedures for venous interruption: (i) inferior vena caval umbrella or filter, (ii) inferior vena caval ligation, and (iii) inferior vena caval clip. All three yield satisfactory results in experienced hands. In recent years, the umbrella or filter has essentially replaced the more invasive surgical approaches, namely, caval clip or ligation. It is important that patients who undergo venous interruption receive adequate intravenous volume replacement in the postoperative period.

2. Pulmonary embolectomy. Patients with refractory hypotension are candidates for pulmonary embolectomy. This is a high-risk procedure and is best done during heart-lung bypass. Patients with transient hypotension and right ventricular failure secondary to massive embolism are best treated with venous interruption and volume therapy.

SELECTED READINGS

Alpert JS, Smith R, Carlson J, et al. Mortality in patients treated for pulmonary embolism. *JAMA* 1976;236:1477–1480.
Good prognosis if diagnosis is made and appropriate therapy initiated.
Benotti JR, Ockene IS, Alpert JS, et al. Clinical profile of unresolved pulmonary embolism. *Chest* 1983;84:669–678.
Review of clinical, angiographic, and hemodynamic features of patients with unresolved pulmonary embolism.
Dalen JE, Alpert, JS. Natural history of pulmonary embolism. *Prog Cardiovasc Dis* 1975;17:259–270.
Comprehensive review of natural history of pulmonary embolism.
Dalen JE, Alpert JS, Hirsh J. Thrombolytic therapy for pulmonary embolism: is it effective? Is it safe? When is it indicated? *Arch Intern Med* 1997;157:2550–2556.
Dalen JE, Hirsh J, Guyatt GH. Sixth ACCP Consensus Conference on Antithrombotic Therapy. *Chest* 2001;119 (Suppl):1s–370s.
Goldhaber SZ, Morpurgo M. WHO/ISFC task force on pulmonary embolism: report of the WHO/International Society and Federation of Cardiology Task Force. *JAMA* 1992;268:1727–1733.
Review of current status of knowledge concerning pulmonary embolism, pointing out areas of ignorance.
Goldstein NM, Killef MH, Ward S, Gage BF. The impact of the introduction of a rapid D-dimer assay on the diagnostic evaluation of suspected pulmonary embolism. *Arch Intern Med* 2001;161:567–571.
Determination of blood D-dimer levels is useful in the diagnosis of venous thromboembolism.

Hirsh J, Hoak J. Management of deep vein thrombosis and pulmonary embolism: a statement for healthcare professionals from the Council on Thrombosis (in consultation with the Council on Cardiovascular Radiology), American Heart Association. *Circulation* 1996;93:2212–2245.

Summary of pathogenesis, diagnosis, and therapy for venous thromboembolism from a consensus conference.

Hull RD, Taskob GE, Ginsberg JS, et al. A noninvasive strategy for the treatment of patients with suspected pulmonary embolism. *Arch Intern Med* 1994;154:289–297.

Outlines a noninvasive approach to patients with suspected pulmonary embolism that avoids the need for invasive studies in most patients.

Kearon C, Gent M, Hirsh J, et al. A comparison of three months of anticoagulation with extended anticoagulation for a first episode of idiopathic venous thromboembolism. *N Engl J Med* 1999;340:901–907.

Patients with a first episode of pulmonary embolism should be treated with anticoagulation for longer than three months.

Moser KM, Daily PO, Peterson K, et al. Thromboendarterectomy for chronic, major-vessel thromboembolic pulmonary hypertension: immediate and long-term results in 42 patients. *Ann Intern Med* 1987;107:560–565.

Patients with pulmonary hypertension from chronic pulmonary embolism can benefit from late thromboendarterectomy.

Oudherk M, van Beek EJR, van Putten WLJ, et al. Cost-effectiveness analysis of various strategies in the diagnostic management of pulmonary embolism. *Ann Intern Med* 1993;153:947–954.

Examines all diagnostic strategies for pulmonary embolism in light of cost effectiveness. Pulmonary angiography remains an important technique in diagnosing pulmonary embolism.

Paraskos JA, Adelstein SJ, Smith RE, et al. Late prognosis of acute pulmonary embolism. *N Engl J Med* 1973;289:55–58.

Long-term prognosis after acute embolism depends on the presence or absence of underlying heart disease.

Paterson DI, Schwartzman K. Strategies incorporating spiral CT for the diagnosis of acute pulmonary embolism: a cost-effectiveness analysis. *Chest* 2001;119:1791–1800.

Spiral CT is a useful strategy for the diagnosis of pulmonary embolism.

Quinn DA, Thompson BT, Terrin ML, et al. A prospective investigation of pulmonary embolism in women and men. *JAMA* 1992;268:1689–1696.

Pulmonary angiography is often necessary in the diagnosis of pulmonary embolism.

Simonneau G, Sors H, Charbonnier B, et al. A comparison of low-molecular-weight heparin with unfractionated heparin for acute pulmonary embolism. *N Engl J Med* 1997;337:663–669.

Low-molecular-weight heparin is as effective as unfractionated heparin for the treatment of acute pulmonary embolism.

Sreeram N, Cheriex EC, Smeets LRM, et al. Value of the 12-lead electrocardiogram at hospital admission in the diagnosis of pulmonary embolism. *Am J Cardiol* 1994; 73:298–303.

The ECG is often abnormal in patients with pulmonary embolism.

Stein PD, Willis PW, DeMets DL. History and physical examination in acute pulmonary embolism in patients without preexisting cardiac or pulmonary disease. *Am J Cardiol* 1981;47:218–223.

Review of history and physical examination in 215 patients with documented pulmonary embolism in the absence of cardiac or pulmonary disease.

Stein PD, Gottschalk A, Henry JW, et al. Stratification of patients according to prior cardiopulmonary disease and probability assessment based on the number of mismatched segmental equivalent perfusion defects: approaches to strengthen the diagnostic value of ventilation/perfusion lung scans in acute pulmonary embolism. *Chest* 1993;104:461–471.

Analysis of diagnostic use of lung scanning in the diagnosis of pulmonary embolism.

Stein PD, Henry JW, Gottschalk A. The addition of clinical assessment to stratification according to prior cardiopulmonary disease further optimizes the interpretation of ventilation/perfusion lung scans in pulmonary embolism. *Chest* 1993;104:1472–1476.

Clinical assessment is useful when combined with lung scanning in making an accurate diagnosis of pulmonary embolism.

Stein PD, Hell RD, Saltzman HA, et al. Strategy for diagnosis of patients with suspected acute pulmonary embolism. *Chest* 1993;103:1553–1559.

Review of the diagnostic strategies most likely to result in an accurate diagnosis of pulmonary embolism.

White RH, Zhou H, Kim J, et al. A population-based study of the effectiveness of inferior vena cava filter use among patients with venous thromboembolism. *Arch Intern Med* 2000;160:2033–2041.

Insertion of a vena caval filter was not associated with a reduction in the 1-year incidence of rehospitalization for pulmonary embolism.

23. COR PULMONALE

I. Introduction. Cor pulmonale (CP) is defined as some combination of hypertrophy and dilatation of the right ventricle secondary to pulmonary hypertension that results from a process intrinsic to the lung. Because of the latter provision, mitral stenosis or congenital cardiac defects producing right ventricular hypertrophy and dilatation are not classified as CP. CP may be acute, secondary to pulmonary embolism (see Chapter 22), or chronic (present chapter). A variety of conditions can produce CP (Table 23-1).

II. Diagnosis

A. History. The historical information obtained from a patient with CP varies with the underlying etiology (Table 23-1). Thus, patients with chronic obstructive pulmonary disease (COPD) and CP complain of dyspnea and cough with sputum production, whereas patients with primary pulmonary hypertension are likely to relate a history of dyspnea and exertional syncope. Dyspnea secondary to cardiac disease such as mitral stenosis should be excluded. In general, orthopnea and paroxysmal nocturnal dyspnea are secondary to pulmonary venous hypertension, itself a result of cardiac disease. Occasionally, paroxysms of bronchospasm secondary to bronchial asthma result in orthopnea and paroxysmal nocturnal dyspnea. When right ventricular failure occurs in patients with CP, fatigue, abdominal or ankle swelling, and anorexia are common complaints.

B. Physical examination. Physical findings vary according to the underlying conditions that produced CP. Tachypnea, cyanosis, elevated jugular venous pressure, a right ventricular parasternal impulse, hepatomegaly, and peripheral edema often are noted, particularly in patients with right ventricular failure. Physical findings in CP are as follows (not all findings are present in all patients with CP):

Tachypnea
Cyanosis
Clubbing
Elevated jugular venous pressure, often with a prominent A wave
Abnormalities of the chest or lungs, depending on underlying condition causing CP
Soft or inaudible heart sounds
Right ventricular impulse palpated along left sternal border or in epigastrium
Right ventricular third (S3) or fourth (S4) heart sounds (or both)—diastolic sound louder during inspiration
Murmur of tricuspid insufficiency
Hepatomegaly
Ascites
Peripheral edema

C. ECG. The ECG usually demonstrates right ventricular hypertrophy and right atrial enlargement, although normal tracings are not uncommon in patients with CP. Atrial and ventricular arrhythmias are often found. ECG findings in CP are summarized in Table 23-2.

D. Chest x-ray examination, computed tomography (CT). Pulmonary parenchymal, pleural, or thoracic cage abnormalities may be seen in chest roentgenograms and CTs of patients with CP, in accordance with the etiology of pulmonary hypertension. In addition, pulmonary hypertension and CP result in enlargement of the main pulmonary artery and right ventricle. Pulmonary arterial branches often taper rapidly toward the periphery of the lung, giving a "pruned tree" appearance to the pulmonary vasculature. Roentgenographic findings in patients with CP are summarized in Table 23-2. Pleural effusions and interstitial pulmonary edema are not seen unless pneumonia or left ventricular failure is also present.

TABLE 23-1. ETIOLOGY FOR COR PULMONALE

Pulmonary parenchymal diseases
   Chronic obstructive pulmonary disease
   Bronchiectasis
   Cystic fibrosis
   Restrictive lung disease
   Pneumoconioses
   Sarcoidosis

Chest wall and muscles of respiration
   Kyphoscoliosis
   Amyotrophic lateral sclerosis
   Myasthenia gravis

Pickwickian syndrome and sleep apnea

Pulmonary vascular diseases
   Recurrent, chronic pulmonary embolism
   Primary pulmonary hypertension
   Sickle cell anemia
   Schistosomiasis
   Scleroderma

E. Laboratory tests. Patients with CP frequently have markedly abnormal pulmonary function tests and arterial blood gases. Depending on the underlying etiology, marked obstructive or restrictive (or mixed) pulmonary pathophysiology may be demonstrated by pulmonary function tests. Functional lung volume frequently is reduced. Arterial blood gas analysis may demonstrate notable hypoxia or even hypercapnia. Some individuals with CP have relatively normal arterial blood gases at rest but develop marked hypoxia and even hypercapnia with exercise, thus documenting the pulmonary etiology of their dyspnea. Patients with significant arterial hypoxia (arterial blood oxygen saturation greater than 90%) often develop secondary polycythemia.

TABLE 23-2. ECG AND ROENTGENOGRAPHIC FINDINGS IN PATIENTS WITH COR PULMONALE[a]

ECG findings
   Atrial and ventricular arrhythmias (especially multifocal atrial tachycardia)
   Tall, peaked P waves in inferior leads and V_1 P wave axis > +60 degrees
   Low QRS voltage
   QRS axis +90 degrees or greater
   S1, Q3, T3
   S1, S2, S3
   Poor R wave progression in precordial leads
   R > S in lead V_1
   Inversion of T and P waves in right precordial leads

X-ray findings: plain film and/or computed tomography
   Various pulmonary parenchymal, pleural, or thoracic bony abnormalities dependent on underlying etiology of cor pulmonale
   Enlargement of the main pulmonary artery
   Rapid tapering of pulmonary arterial branches toward the lung periphery
   Right ventricular enlargement
   Enlargement of superior vena cava and azygos vein

[a] Not all findings are present in all patients with cor pulmonale.

F. Echocardiography. Satisfactory transthoracic echocardiographic studies may be difficult to obtain in patients with CP, particularly if pulmonary hypertension is caused by COPD. Transesophageal echocardiographic studies are often required to delineate cardiac structures. When obtained, echocardiographic studies reveal an increased right ventricular cavity dimension and normal left-sided heart structures. The pulmonary valve echo may demonstrate loss of the normal A wave, a result of pulmonary hypertension. Doppler study often reveals tricuspid and pulmonic regurgitation and the degree of pulmonary hypertension can be quantitated.

G. Radionuclide studies. Abnormal right ventricular ejection fraction can be documented in patients with CP by radionuclide ventriculography. Thallium myocardial scintigraphy can delineate increased right ventricular wall thickness.

H. Catheterization and angiography. Right-sided pressures are usually markedly elevated in patients with CP. Pulmonary arterial systolic and mean pressures are invariably elevated, as is right ventricular systolic pressure. Pulmonary arterial diastolic pressure often is elevated, but pulmonary capillary wedge, left atrial, and left ventricular end-diastolic pressures are usually normal unless concomitant left ventricular disease is present. A number of investigators have noted abnormal left ventricular diastolic function in patients with pure CP, but the abnormalities are usually subtle and probably not of major clinical significance. Right ventricular end-diastolic and right atrial mean pressures are often normal at rest in patients with CP. Exercise or the onset of right ventricular failure results in elevated right ventricular filling pressures. Cardiac output is usually normal at rest but fails to rise appropriately with exercise.

Left ventricular ejection fraction is ordinarily normal in patients with pure CP, but right ventricular ejection fraction often is reduced. Associated coronary artery disease is not uncommon in these individuals, particularly if they have COPD secondary to many years of heavy cigarette smoking.

I. Protocol for the diagnosis of CP
1. Testing sequence for making the diagnosis. The diagnosis of CP can be made according to the following diagnostic protocol. The dashed arrow indicates an optional step.

History and physical examination
↓
Chest x-ray film/CT and ECG
↓
Pulmonary function tests and arterial blood gases
↓
Echocardiography
↓
Right and left ventricular radionuclide ventriculography or cardiac catheterization (or both)

2. Criteria for making the diagnosis. The diagnosis of CP is made in patients with severe pulmonary or thoracic cage disease (Table 23-1)—documented by chest x-ray study, CT, pulmonary function tests, and arterial blood gases—who also demonstrate right ventricular hypertrophy or dilatation by any of the following: physical examination, chest x-ray film, ECG, and echocardiogram.

Left-sided heart diseases (mitral stenosis, cardiomyopathy) must be ruled out by physical findings, chest x-ray examination, echocardiography, radionuclide ventriculography, and, if necessary, cardiac catheterization.

3. Differential diagnosis
a. Pulmonary venous hypertension. Dyspnea and right ventricular failure are frequently the result of pulmonary venous hypertension. The causes of pulmonary venous hypertension are many, commonly including mitral stenosis and various entities that lead to left ventricu-

lar failure. Dyspnea secondary to pulmonary venous hypertension (often referred to as cardiac dyspnea) usually involves orthopnea and paroxysmal nocturnal dyspnea, two symptoms usually absent in patients with pulmonary dyspnea. Mitral stenosis and the various entities that cause left ventricular failure (e.g., cardiomyopathy) can be distinguished from the numerous cases of CP by physical examination, ECG, echocardiography, and, on occasion, catheterization with measurement of pulmonary wedge pressure (normal in patients with CP).

   b. Constrictive pericarditis. Signs and symptoms resembling those of right ventricular failure are noted in patients with constrictive pericarditis. Individuals with the latter entity, however, have normal or mildly abnormal pulmonary function tests and arterial blood gases. Right ventricular enlargement or hypertrophy is almost invariably absent by physical examination, chest roentgenography, ECG, and echocardiography. Cardiac catheterization reveals the hemodynamic pattern of restriction to ventricular filling in patients with constrictive pericarditis.

III. Therapy

  A. Medical treatment

    1. Treatment of underlying disorders. General and specific measures aimed at the underlying disorder that resulted in CP include cessation of cigarette smoking or exposure to other irritants in patients with chronic parenchymal pulmonary disease; specific antibiotic therapy and pulmonary toilet for infectious processes; and various combinations of bronchodilators, expectorants, corticosteroids, and oxygen when indicated. Individuals with pickwickian syndrome may benefit from progesterone and weight loss; those with myasthenia gravis usually are treated with anticholinesterase drugs and corticosteroids. Attention should not be focused on the therapy of right ventricular failure with exclusion of therapeutic regimens aimed at amelioration of the underlying condition that produced CP.

    2. Arrhythmias. Atrial and ventricular arrhythmias are common in patients with CP. Therapy aimed at the entity that resulted in CP often produces a concomitant improvement in right ventricular failure with a decrease in arrhythmias. Bronchodilators often have both beta$_1$- and beta$_2$-agonist activity, and use of these agents may actually precipitate or worsen arrhythmias. Supraventricular arrhythmias such as atrial tachycardia, atrial fibrillation, or atrial flutter generally are best treated with diltiazem or verapamil, digitalis, and possibly other antiarrhythmic agents such as amiodarone and, if required, electrical reversion. Verapamil, diltiazem, and other calcium channel blockers with electrophysiologic properties are very often useful in the control of supraventricular arrhythmias. Beta-blockers are contraindicated in patients with CP secondary to reactive airways disease. However, if the patient does not have reactive airways disease, small doses of beta-blockers may be tried during careful clinical observation. If the patient is having paroxysms of spontaneously reverting supraventricular arrhythmia, cardioversion usually is not helpful because it merely reestablishes sinus rhythm transiently. Therapy in this situation should involve diltiazem, verapamil, digitalis, or other antiarrhythmic medication.

      Patients with arterial hypoxia should be digitalized with care because some authorities believe that hypoxic myocardium has an increased susceptibility to digitalis intoxication. Beta-blocking agents should be used with considerable caution in patients with underlying pulmonary disease. Multifocal atrial tachycardia should not be managed with digitalis or antiarrhythmic drugs. Instead, attention is focused on improving the underlying pulmonary condition.

    3. Anticoagulants. Patients with recurrent pulmonary embolism should be treated with intravenous heparin for 7 to 10 days, followed by oral

warfarin therapy for 2 to 6 months or longer. Patients with severe right ventricular failure are particularly predisposed to venous thrombosis and pulmonary embolism. Prophylactic long-term anticoagulation—often lifelong—with warfarin is often beneficial in such individuals, particularly if they are obese, are relatively inactive, and have signs and/or symptoms of heart failure.

4. Vasodilators. Patients with CP frequently have marked pulmonary hypertension that eventually leads to right ventricular failure. Some clinical investigators have used vasodilators in these patients in an effort to dilate the pulmonary vascular bed and thereby decrease pulmonary arterial pressure and diminish right ventricular work. Such therapy has met with some success in selected patients. Nifedipine, a calcium channel blocker with potent vasodilatory properties, has been the most efficacious agent with regard to lowering pulmonary arterial pressure and vascular resistance. The dosage is usually 10 to 40 mg three or four times a day. Higher doses of calcium channel blockers have been reported to be of benefit in patients with severe primary pulmonary hypertension. The major side effects include headache, ankle swelling, gastrointestinal upset, and arterial hypoxia secondary to vasodilation of pulmonary capillaries that supply poorly ventilated lung regions. Diltiazem may be used in place of nifedipine. Selected patients with primary pulmonary hypertension and scleroderma heart disease can be markedly ameliorated with continuous intravenous infusions of prostacyclin. Pulmonary hypertension and CP regress when this therapy is successful.

B. Surgery. An occasional patient with bronchiectasis or large emphysematous bullae benefits from a partial pulmonary resection. Pressure breathing devices, tracheostomy, or pharyngeal reconstruction can be of use in the management of some patients with sleep apnea. Patients with recurrent pulmonary embolism and CP may be candidates for inferior vena caval plication or interruption. Patients with chronic pulmonary embolism may benefit from pulmonary thromboendarterectomy of the chronic pulmonary arterial organized thrombus.

SELECTED READINGS

Alpert JS. Pulmonary hypertension. In: Goldman L, Bennett JC, eds. *Cecil textbook of medicine.* Philadelphia: Saunders, 2000:273–279.
Concise overview of pulmonary hypertension and its clinical concomitants.

Archer S, Rich S. Primary pulmonary hypertension: a vascular biology and translational research "work in progress." *Circulation* 2000;102:2781–2791.
A review of the vascular biology of primary pulmonary hypertension.

Badesch DB, Tapson VF, McGoon MD, et al. Continuous intravenous epoprostenol for pulmonary hypertension due to the scleroderma spectrum of disease: a randomized, controlled trial. *Ann Intern Med* 2000;132:425–434.
Continuous epoprostenol therapy improves hemodynamics and exercise capacity in scleroderma patients with pulmonary hypertension.

Braman SS, Eby E, Kuhn C, et al. Primary pulmonary hypertension in the elderly. *Arch Intern Med* 1991;15:2433–2438.
Primary pulmonary hypertension occurs surprisingly often in elderly patients.

Cohen M, Edwards WD, Fuster V. Regression in thromboembolic type of primary pulmonary hypertension during 2½ years of antithrombotic therapy. *J Am Coll Cardiol* 1986;7:172–175.
Pulmonary hypertension can be the result of recurrent episodes of pulmonary embolism; chronic anticoagulation results in regression of pulmonary hypertension in these patients.

D'Alonzo GE, Barst RJ, Ayres SM, et al. Survival in patients with primary pulmonary hypertension: results from a national prospective registry. *Ann Intern Med* 1991; 115:343–349.

Mortality in primary pulmonary hypertension is most closely associated with the degree of right ventricular dysfunction.

Hoeper MM, Schwarze M, Ehlerding S, et al. Long-term treatment of primary pulmonary hypertension with aerosolized iloprost, a prostacyclin analogue. *N Engl J Med* 2000;342:1866–1870.

Long-term treatment with aerosolized iloprost improves exercise capacity and hemodynamics in patients with primary pulmonary hypertension.

Lilienfeld DE, Rubin LJ. Mortality from primary pulmonary hypertension in the United States, 1979–1996. *Chest* 2000;117:796–800.

Mortality from primary pulmonary hypertension seems to be increasing in the United States.

Morley TF, Zappasodi SJ, Belli A, et al. Pulmonary vasodilator therapy for chronic obstructive pulmonary disease and cor pulmonale: treatment with nifedipine, nitroglycerin, and oxygen. *Chest* 1987;92:71–76.

Therapy with vasodilators does not improve survival in patients with CP who are already receiving oxygen therapy.

Murphy ML, Adamson J, Hutcheson F. Left ventricular hypertrophy in patients with chronic bronchitis and emphysema. *Ann Intern Med* 1974;81:307–313.

Left ventricular hypertrophy in patients with COPD is usually the result of associated diseases that affect the left ventricle.

Rich S, Abenhaim L, eds. Primary pulmonary hypertension (monograph). *Chest* 1994; 105:1S.

A collection of papers covering up-to-date concepts on the pathophysiology, diagnosis, and therapy of primary pulmonary hypertension.

Rich S, Brundage BH. High-dose calcium channel blocking therapy for primary pulmonary hypertension: evidence for long-term reduction to pulmonary arterial pressure and regression of right ventricular hypertrophy. *Circulation* 1987;76:135–141.

High-dose calcium channel blocker therapy is effective in reducing pulmonary hypertension and right ventricular hypertrophy in patients with primary pulmonary hypertension.

Rubin LJ. Primary pulmonary hypertension. *Chest* 1993;104:236–250.

Consensus statement concerning definitions, pathophysiology, diagnosis, and therapy of primary pulmonary hypertension.

Saito S, Miyamoto K, Nishimura M, et al. Effects of inhaled bronchodilators on pulmonary hemodynamics at rest and during exercise in patients with COPD. *Chest* 1999;115:376–382.

Bronchodilators reduce right ventricular afterload in patients with COPD.

Wax D, Garofano R, Barst RJ. Effects of long-term infusion of prostacyclin on exercise performance in patients with primary pulmonary hypertension. *Chest* 1999;116: 914–920.

Exercise capacity is markedly improved by long-term infusion of prostacyclin in patients with primary pulmonary hypertension.

24. HEART BLOCK AND SICK SINUS SYNDROME

I. **Introduction.** A number of conditions produce symptoms related to sudden or prolonged changes in heart rate with resultant fall in cardiac output. Some patients present with marked bradycardia; others have intermittent episodes of tachycardia followed by bradycardia. Degenerative changes or congenital defects in the conduction system or sinoatrial node are present in the vast majority of these patients who require permanent pacing. Traumatic, surgical, or inflammatory injury to the conduction system also can produce a situation demanding permanent pacing (Table 24-1). Most people who require permanent pacing have one of two conditions: heart block (HB) or sick sinus syndrome (SSS). Individuals with HB may have continuous or episodic periods of markedly slow heart rate because the electrical impulse initiated in the sinoatrial node fails to reach the ventricles because of conduction system malfunction. Consequently, the heart rate is regulated by a slow (20 to 40 beats per minute) junctional or ventricular pacemaker. Patients with SSS have dysfunction of the sinoatrial node, with either marked sinus bradycardia or alternating episodes of supraventricular tachycardia and bradycardia.

II. **Diagnosis**

A. **History.** Patients with HB or SSS may be asymptomatic, particularly if the resultant bradycardia is not marked. Symptomatic patients complain of episodic dizziness, giddiness, or frank syncope. Often, lightheadedness or syncopal episodes vary in length and severity because of the variable duration of episodes of bradycardia or tachycardia. Some individuals are aware of palpitations, but the majority of arrhythmic episodes are unnoticed. Individuals with HB or SSS (or both) and another form of heart disease that results in limited cardiac reserve may develop new or increased symptoms of left or right ventricular failure during episodes of bradycardia. Similarly, patients with coexisting coronary artery disease may note new or increased angina pectoris during bradycardia or tachycardia. Other symptoms that are noted occasionally include personality changes, irritability, fleeting memory losses, generalized weakness or fatigue, muscle aches, slurred speech, and insomnia.

B. **Physical examination.** Unless HB or SSS has caused new or increased heart failure, the physical examination may be unremarkable. Because the majority of patients with HB and SSS are elderly, coexisting hypertension and coronary artery disease are common. Physical findings secondary to the two latter conditions (see Chapters 12 and 15) may be noted (e.g., a prominent fourth heart sound). Patients with permanent or prolonged episodes of HB are markedly bradycardic with a wide pulse pressure. An aortic systolic flow murmur is often heard during bradycardia. It is caused by increased stroke volume secondary to an increase in left ventricular diastolic volume, which in turn is the result of bradycardia-induced prolongation of the diastolic filling period. Large A waves (cannon waves) may be seen in the jugular pulse of patients with complete HB. They are caused by atrial contraction against a closed tricuspid valve.

An occasional patient has physical findings that result from a pacemaker. Usually such findings are limited to single or multiple systolic clicks or a high-pitched, short systolic murmur; however, perforation of the ventricle by a transvenous pacing wire can result in a pericardial rub.

C. **ECG.** The scalar ECG or a Holter monitor ECG tape usually confirms the diagnosis of HB or SSS. Patients with persistent HB ordinarily have normal-appearing P waves with normal atrial rate and rhythm and some form of bundle branch block pattern of the QRS with a very slow rate. Supraventricular capture beats with normal QRS pattern can occur alongside the bizarre, widened complexes of the slower ventricular response. Episodes of HB may be sporadic and may be observed only during prolonged periods of ambulatory

TABLE 24-1. ETIOLOGY OF HEART BLOCK AND SICK SINUS SYNDROME

Heart block
  Congenital (often associated with ventricular septal defect or corrected transposition)
  Degeneration of the conduction system (Lenegre's disease, primary degeneration;
    Lev's disease, damage to conduction system from contiguous fibrosis or calcification)
  Rheumatic fever
  Myocardial infarction
  Hypoxia
  Hyperkalemia
  Drugs (digitalis, amiodarone, sotalol, procainamide, beta-blockers, diltiazem,
    verapamil, etc.)
  Calcific aortic stenosis
  Infectious endocarditis
  Trauma
  Diphtheria
  Amyloidosis
  Sarcoidosis
  Muscular dystrophy
  Friedreich's ataxia
  Syphilis
  Cardiac surgery
  Cardiac tumors

Sick sinus syndrome
  Degeneration of the sinus node
  Coronary artery disease
  Rheumatic fever
  Pericarditis
  Amyloidosis
  Collagen vascular disease
  Arteritis
  Cardiac tumors
  Cardiac surgery
  Friedreich's ataxia
  Subarachnoid hemorrhage
  Drugs (digitalis, amiodarone, sotalol, procainamide, propranolol, etc.)
  Hyperkalemia

ECG monitoring (Holter monitoring). Individuals with congenital forms of HB often have QRS complexes that appear relatively normal. These patients may demonstrate prolonged periods of first- or second-degree HB with or without occasional episodes of third-degree HB. ECG findings in patients with HB and SSS are recorded in Table 24-2. Holter monitoring for 12 or 24 hours in patients with HB demonstrates persistent or paroxysmal HB (first, second, or third degree). Holter monitoring in patients with SSS may reveal a variety of abnormalities: (i) persistent unexplained sinus bradycardia, (ii) paroxysms of supraventricular tachycardia (atrial fibrillation, flutter, or tachycardia followed by long sinus pauses), (iii) episodic sinus arrest, (iv) sinoatrial exit block, or (v) marked sinus bradycardia alternating with atrial tachycardia, atrial flutter, or atrial fibrillation (the so-called bradycardia-tachycardia, or brady-tachy, syndrome).

D. Chest x-ray examination. The chest x-ray picture of patients with HB or SSS may be unremarkable, or it may demonstrate findings that are the result of associated heart disease. For example, a patient with HB secondary to calcific aortic stenosis would have a chest roentgenogram with features consistent with aortic stenosis (see Chapter 16).

TABLE 24-2. ECG FINDINGS IN PATIENTS WITH HEART BLOCK AND SICK SINUS SYNDROME

Heart block
    Bundle branch block (complete right, complete left, left anterior or left posterior hemiblock)
    First-, second-, or third-degree atrioventricular block
    Findings associated with etiology of heart block (see Table 24-1)

Sick sinus syndrome
    Sinus bradycardia
    Wandering atrial pacemaker
    Sinoatrial exit block (absence of expected P waves)
    Sinus arrest or pauses
    Paroxysmal atrial fibrillation or other supraventricular tachycardia
    Bundle branch block (common but not part of the syndrome)

E. Echocardiography. Echocardiography in patients with HB or SSS either is normal or shows findings of associated heart disease.

F. Catheterization and angiography. Electrical events in the conduction system can be examined by intracardiac electrophysiologic study (His bundle electrocardiography). Abnormal generation of the cardiac electrical impulse in the sinus node or interruption of transmission of the impulse to the ventricles can be documented by this technique. ECG manifestations of SSS may be intermittent and, at times, difficult to elicit. For this reason, several provocative tests have been developed to test the function of the sinus node: (i) response to atropine, (ii) response to isoproterenol, (iii) response to atrial pacing, and (iv) response to premature atrial stimulation. Invasive provocative tests, however, are not always abnormal in patients with SSS.

Similarly, marked abnormalities in intracardiac conduction may be documented in individuals with first-degree atrioventricular (AV) block and bifascicular conduction system disease (right bundle branch block with left anterior or posterior hemiblock; left bundle branch block) by His bundle ECG. Despite markedly abnormal function of the conduction system, however, the majority of such persons infrequently develop high-grade (second- or third-degree) AV block. Thus, the role of His bundle ECG in diagnosis and management of patients with SSS or first-degree HB is in confirming the clinical diagnosis rather than in disclosing an unexpected entity. Other findings at catheterization depend on associated heart disease (e.g., coronary artery disease).

G. Protocol for the diagnosis of HB or SSS
    1. The diagnosis of HB and SSS usually is made by history and routine scalar ECG or Holter ECG monitoring. His bundle ECG and provocative tests may be helpful in making the diagnosis in an occasional patient. The following protocol is suggested (dashed arrow indicates optional step):

History and physical examination
      ↓
ECG, ECG monitoring (12 to 24 hours), or both
      ↓
His bundle ECG

    2. Criteria for making the diagnosis
      a. The diagnosis of HB is made in asymptomatic or symptomatic (dizzy, giddy, or syncopal) patients with first-, second-, or third-degree HB by scalar ECG or ECG monitoring. Patients with bifascicular block (right bundle branch block with left anterior or posterior hemiblock;

left bundle branch block) and abnormal His bundle ECG measurements (markedly prolonged H–V interval) who have spontaneous syncopal episodes may be assumed to have transient high-grade AV block, even if such an episode does not occur during ECG monitoring. In a rare patient with unexplained syncope, occult paroxysms of AV block may be found by repeated episodes of ECG monitoring, a home event ECG recorder, or means of an implantable ECG recorder.

   b. The diagnosis of SSS is made in asymptomatic or symptomatic (dizzy, giddy, or syncopal) patients who demonstrate at least one of the following rhythm disturbances by ECG or ECG monitoring: (i) persistent unexplained sinus bradycardia; (ii) inability of the sinus node to resume firing after cessation of paroxysmal tachycardia, atrial pacing, or electrical cardioversion; (iii) episodic sinus arrest; (iv) sinoatrial exit block; (v) marked sinus bradycardia alternating with atrial tachycardia, atrial flutter, or atrial fibrillation with rapid ventricular response (bradycardia-tachycardia syndrome); and (vi) atrial fibrillation with a slow ventricular response in the absence of digitalis, beta-blockers, diltiazem, or verapamil. His bundle ECG or provocative tests (atropine, isoproterenol, rapid atrial pacing, premature atrial stimulation) may be required to confirm the diagnosis.

3. Differential diagnosis. HB and SSS can both produce giddiness, dizziness, and frank syncope. Differentiation of the two conditions usually can be made by routine scalar ECG or Holter monitoring. Occasionally, His bundle ECG is required to distinguish these entities. HB and SSS may coexist in the same patient. The majority of differential diagnostic problems concern the identification of associated forms of heart disease or other causes of syncope or loss of consciousness (Table 24-1 and below).

   Patients with a hereditary form of heart disease characterized by a **prolonged Q–T interval** by ECG and recurrent syncopal episodes initially may be thought to have HB or SSS. ECG monitoring reveals paroxysms of ventricular tachycardia or ventricular fibrillation. The ECG Q–T interval is markedly prolonged. Congenital deafness also may occur in patients with the prolonged Q–T interval syndrome.

   a. Neurologic conditions. The most common symptoms associated with HB and SSS also are noted frequently in patients with a variety of neurologic conditions (e.g., seizure disorders, labyrinthitis, cerebrovascular disease). Thus, patients who complain of dizziness or frank syncope should always have a careful neurologic evaluation to exclude central nervous system disease as the cause of their symptoms. Such an evaluation includes a careful history and neurologic examination as well as selected laboratory tests, which may include an EEG, CT scan, MRI, and/or a lumbar puncture, among others.

III. Therapy
   A. Medical treatment
      1. Many patients with HB or SSS require no therapy because they are asymptomatic and serious bradycardia is not impending. Included in this group are (i) individuals with transient first-, second-, and even third-degree HB complicating inferior myocardial infarction; (ii) patients with asymptomatic, nonfamilial, congenital HB with narrow QRS complexes by ECG and a normal or near normal resting heart rate; (iii) asymptomatic individuals with bifascicular block with or without first-degree AV block; and (iv) asymptomatic patients with SSS.
      2. Patients with SSS may have an increased incidence of left atrial thrombosis with subsequent arterial embolism. If paroxysms of atrial fibrillation or flutter are noted, these patients should receive long-term oral warfarin anticoagulation.
      3. Some patients with SSS and marked, symptomatic bradycardia will respond to oral theophylline therapy given as 200 to 300 mg twice a day in a slow-release formulation.

B. Surgery. Patients with third-degree HB or symptomatic SSS should have a right ventricular or AV demand pacemaker placed. Patients with SSS may require concomitant antiarrhythmic medication (digitalis, procainamide, beta-blockers, verapamil, propafenone, sotalol, amiodarone, etc.) to control supraventricular tachyarrhythmias. Permanent or temporary pacing should be initiated before any of these agents (except digitalis) are administered to patients with SSS to prevent the occurrence of severe bradycardia. There is increasing data favoring the implantation of an AV sequential pacemaker in these patients unless they are chronically in atrial fibrillation.

1. Patients with bifascicular block and second-degree HB should have a permanent pacemaker implanted.

2. Patients with congenital HB and narrow QRS complexes do not require a pacemaker despite the presence of second-degree AV block, as long as they are not symptomatic and have reasonable heart rates. Frequent ECG monitoring, exercise testing, or both (every 6 months) should be performed in such individuals to search for paroxysms of complete HB. The presence of complete HB or serious ventricular escape rhythms should induce the physician to treat these patients with permanent pacing.

3. Patients with the syndrome of prolonged Q–T interval and recurrent ventricular fibrillation are treated with various combinations of implanted defibrillator, cervical sympathectomy, and/or beta-blockers.

SELECTED READINGS

Alboni P, Menozzi C, Brignole M, et al. Effects of permanent pacemaker and oral theophylline in sick sinus syndrome: the THEOPACE Study: a randomized controlled trial. *Circulation* 1997;96:260–266.
AV sequential pacing or oral theophylline therapy benefit patients with symptomatic bradycardia secondary to SSS.

Andersen HR, Nielsen JC, Thomsen PEB, et al. Atrioventricular conduction during long-term follow-up of patients with sick sinus syndrome. *Circulation* 1998;98:1315–1321.
Atrial pacing is stable over long periods of time in patients with SSS.

Brandt J, Anderson H, Fahraeus T, et al. Natural history of sinus node disease treated with atrial pacing in 213 patients: implications for selection of stimulation mode. *J Am Coll Cardiol* 1992;20:633–639.
Atrial pacing is often beneficial in patients with symptomatic bradycardia secondary to SSS.

Bryce M, Spielman SR, Greenspan AM, et al. Evolving indications for permanent pacemakers. *Ann Intern Med* 2001;134:1130–1141.
Up-to-date review of pacer therapy.

Eriksson P, Hansson PO, Eriksson H, et al. Bundle-branch block in a general male population: the study of men born 1913. *Circulation* 1998;98:2494–2500.
Bundle branch block correlates strongly with age. Bundle branch block is a marker for slowly progressive degenerative disease of the myocardium.

Gregoratos G, Cheitlin MD, Conill A, et al. ACC/AHA guidelines for implantation of cardiac pacemakers and antiarrhythmia devices: a report of the American College of Cardiology/American Heart Association Task Force on Practice Guidelines (Committee on Pacemaker Implantation). *J Am Coll Cardiol* 1998;31:1175–1209.
Most recent guidelines for the use of pacing devices including indications for pacer therapy in patients with SSS and AV block.

Hayes DL, Vlietstra RE. Pacemaker malfunction. *Ann Intern Med* 1993;119:828–835.
An extensive review of pacer malfunction: identification and management.

Hesselson AB, Parsonnet V, Bernstein AD, et al. Deleterious effects of long-term single-chamber ventricular pacing in patients with sick sinus syndrome: the hidden benefits of dual-chamber pacing. *J Am Coll Cardiol* 1992;19:1542–1549.
AV pacing is the best form of pacing for patients with SSS.

McAnulty JH, Rahimtoola SH, Murphy E, et al. Natural history of "high-risk" bundle branch block: final report of a prospective study. *N Engl J Med* 1982;307:137–143.

Patients with chronic bifascicular conduction abnormalities generally do well and do not need prophylactic pacemaker implantation.

Menozzi C, Brignole M, Alboni P, et al. The natural course of untreated sick sinus syndrome and identification of the variables predictive of unfavorable outcome. *Am J Cardiol* 1998;82:1205–1209.

Clinical cardiovascular events occur commonly in patients with SSS during long-term follow-up.

Saito D, Matsubara K, Yamanari H, et al. Effects of oral theophylline on sick sinus syndrome. *J Am Coll Cardiol* 1993;21:1199–1204.

Oral theophylline may be beneficial in patients with symptomatic bradycardia secondary to SSS.

Sigurd B, Sandoe E. Management of Stokes-Adams syndrome. *Cardiology* 1990;77: 195–208.

Careful review of Stokes-Adams attacks and their management.

Skanes AC, Krahn AD, Yee R, et al. Progression to chronic atrial fibrillation after pacing: the Canadian Trial of Physiologic Pacing. *J Am Coll Cardiol* 2001;38:167–172.

Physiologic pacing reduces the annual rate of development of chronic atrial fibrillation.

Waltuck J, Buyon JP. Autoantibody-associated congenital heart block: outcome in mothers and children. *Ann Intern Med* 1994;120:544–551.

Long-term follow-up of mothers and children affected by autoantibody congenital HB.

25. CARDIAC TRAUMA

I. **Introduction.** All regions of the heart may be damaged by penetrating or nonpenetrating chest injuries. Many cardiac injuries are overlooked transiently or permanently because of trauma to other parts of the body that demands immediate attention. Thus, many cardiac contusions undoubtedly resolve without notice in individuals with multiple traumatic injuries. Cardiac traumatic injuries can be rapidly fatal; for example, laceration or disruption of the pericardium, myocardium, and/or coronary artery or vein frequently results in hemopericardium and tamponade.

Swift recognition of the cardiac injury combined with pericardiocentesis and surgical repair of the lesion is required if the patient is to survive. Table 25-1 lists some of the many forms of traumatic cardiac injury. Myocardial rupture, contusion, and laceration account for almost 90% of deaths secondary to nonpenetrating cardiac trauma.

II. **Diagnosis**
   A. **History.** Any penetrating or nonpenetrating chest injury can involve the heart.

   The patient may not notice or be capable of reporting chest trauma. If the injury occurs in the hospital (e.g., perforation of a cardiac chamber by a cardiac catheter) in a conscious patient, the individual often complains of severe chest discomfort. Recurrent syncope may be reported in someone with tamponade or heart block after cardiac trauma. Heart failure, either immediate or delayed, may occur in individuals with valvular disruption, arteriovenous fistula, or myocardial infarction (MI) secondary to coronary arterial injury.

   A delayed form of pericarditis similar in character and natural history to post-MI pericarditis occurs in approximately 20% of patients with penetrating wounds of the heart. This syndrome can also occur in patients with nonpenetrating cardiac trauma. All patients with penetrating and nonpenetrating injury to the anterior chest should undergo evaluation for cardiac trauma.

   B. **Physical examination.** Systemic and cardiovascular findings in patients with cardiac trauma depend on the type of injury sustained. Thus, patients with acquired ventricular septal defect (VSD) may have a loud systolic murmur, a third heart sound (S3), and signs of left or right ventricular failure. Patients with aortic disruption may demonstrate pulse inequalities; patients with pericardial, myocardial, or coronary arterial lacerations often present with cardiac tamponade (see Chapter 19). Patients with pericarditis or pericardial tears or lacerations may have audible precordial rubs. Some of the physical findings in patients with cardiac traumatic injuries are as follows (not all findings are present in all forms of cardiac injury):

   Tachycardia (hypovolemia, tamponade)
   Bradycardia (conduction system injury)
   Hypotension (hypovolemia, tamponade)
   Jugular venous distention (right ventricular failure, tamponade)
   Signs of left ventricular failure: tachypnea, rales, pleural effusion, S3 (aneurysm, infarction, valvular disruption, VSD)
   Signs of right ventricular failure: jugular venous distention, hepatomegaly, peripheral edema (same conditions producing left ventricular failure)
   Signs of cardiac tamponade: tachycardia, hypotension, jugular venous distention, small quiet heart
   Systolic cardiac murmurs (mitral or tricuspid valvular injury, VSD)
   Diastolic cardiac murmurs (pulmonic or aortic valvular injury, aortic–left ventricular fistula)
   Continuous cardiac murmurs (arteriovenous fistula, fistula from aorta to atrium or right ventricle)

TABLE 25-1. CARDIAC LESIONS FROM PENETRATING AND NONPENETRATING CHEST TRAUMA

Pericardium
   Laceration or rupture with or without hemopericardium and cardiac tamponade
   Recurrent posttraumatic pericarditis
   Suppurative pericarditis

Myocardium
   Contusion, laceration, or rupture with or without delayed aneurysm formation
   Atrial or ventricular septal defect
   Fistula from aorta to atrium or ventricle
   Abscess
   Foreign body within the heart or great vessels

Valves
   Leaflet tear or disruption
   Rupture of chordae tendineae or papillary muscle

Coronary artery
   Laceration or thrombosis with or without myocardial infarction
   Arteriovenous fistula

Conduction system
   Heart block of any degree
   Conduction disturbance (e.g., bundle branch block)

Embolism
   Foreign body or thrombus

Great vessels
   Rupture or laceration with or without delayed aneurysm formation

      Rub (pericarditis, pericardial tear or laceration)
      Pulse inequalities (aortic disruption)
      Signs of splenic, renal, or cerebral infarction (foreign body or thrombotic
        embolism)

  C. ECG. Atrial and ventricular arrhythmias are common in patients with cardiac trauma. Individuals with myocardial contusions often have the same ventricular arrhythmias (ventricular premature beats, ventricular tachycardia, ventricular fibrillation) seen in patients with acute MI. First-, second-, or third-degree heart block is seen with conduction system injuries. Nonspecific ST–T changes or infarction patterns are found in patients with myocardial contusion or laceration. The S–T segment changes of pericarditis may be present, or the ECG may be normal. Tall, peaked precordial T waves often are seen in patients with hemopericardium. ECG findings in patients with cardiac traumatic injuries are the following (not all findings are present in all forms of cardiac injury):

      Atrial and ventricular arrhythmias
      Bundle branch blocks
      First-, second-, third-degree heart block
      Nonspecific ST–T changes
      Diffuse S–T segment elevation (pericarditis)
      Tall, peaked precordial T waves (hemopericardium)
      Infarction patterns

  D. Chest x-ray examination. Roentgenographic findings in patients with cardiac trauma include (i) cardiomegaly secondary to hemopericardium or pericardial effusion; (ii) signs of left ventricular failure (vascular redistribution, interstitial or alveolar edema, pleural effusion) secondary to myocardial contusion, ventricular aneurysm, valvular disruption, intracardiac fistula, or VSD; and (iii) mediastinal widening secondary to aortic disruption. Other roentgenographic findings that may be observed in patients with chest trauma include fractured ribs, pneumothorax, hemothorax, or pulmonary hemorrhage. Chest x-ray findings in patients with cardiac trauma are as follows:

Cardiomegaly (effusion or hemopericardium)
Left ventricular failure (vascular redistribution, interstitial or alveolar
    pulmonary edema, pleural effusion)
Mediastinal widening (aortic disruption)
Tracheal deviation (disruption)
Pneumothorax
Hemothorax
Pulmonary infiltrates (pulmonary hemorrhage)

E. Laboratory tests. Increased serum activities for various cardiac biomarkers are observed in patients with cardiac contusion. The time course of these enzyme elevations resembles that for MI. Because skeletal muscle trauma can result in higher serum levels of glutamic oxaloacetic transaminase, lactic dehydrogenase, and creatine phosphokinase (CK), these biomarkers are **not** useful in the diagnosis of cardiac contusion. Measurement of blood levels of cardiac specific troponin is the preferred method of identifying myocardial injury following cardiac trauma. An acceptable alternative that is not as sensitive or specific is determination of blood levels of CK-MB isoenzyme fraction.

F. Echocardiography. Blood or effusion in the pericardial space can be detected by echocardiography. Regurgitant valvular lesions, aortic-atrial or ventricular fistulae, and VSD can produce left ventricular dilatation or hypercontractility in the echocardiogram. Valvular regurgitation and shunt flow can be detected and quantitated by a Doppler study. Myocardial contusion and MI result in regional hypokinesis or akinesis.

G. Radionuclide studies. Regions of myocardial injury can often be identified by myocardial scintigraphy with technetium 99m–labeled antimyosin antibodies or technetium 99m–labeled pyrophosphate. Ventricular aneurysms can be identified by radionuclide ventriculography, and intracardiac shunts secondary to fistulae or VSD can be identified and measured by radionuclide angiocardiography.

H. Catheterization and angiography. A variety of hemodynamic findings can be observed in patients with cardiac trauma, depending on the type of injury incurred. Patients may demonstrate the pathophysiologic patterns of tamponade (see Chapter 19), left ventricular failure, right ventricular failure, acute VSD (see Chapter 15), acute valvular regurgitation (see Chapter 16), or MI. VSDs, fistulae, and ventricular or aortic aneurysms can be visualized by angiography. Aortic disruption usually occurs just above the aortic valve or just distal to the left subclavian artery.

I. Protocol for the diagnosis of cardiac trauma

1. Because of the many types of cardiac trauma with differing natural histories, it is hard to envision one diagnostic protocol for all lesions. Fig. 25-1 is a suggested diagnostic protocol for patients suspected of having cardiac traumatic injuries (dashed arrows indicate optional steps). There are a number of branches to this protocol corresponding to the diagnostic strategies used in the various types of cardiac traumatic injury. Patients with life-threatening injuries such as hemopericardium or aortic rupture may require emergency surgical treatment without any diagnostic information other than a brief history and physical examination.

2. Criteria used in the diagnosis. Cardiac traumatic injury is diagnosed in patients with a history of trauma, usually involving the chest, in whom physical examination, ECG, or chest roentgenogram discloses an abnormality consistent with cardiac trauma. Confirmation of the diagnosis de-

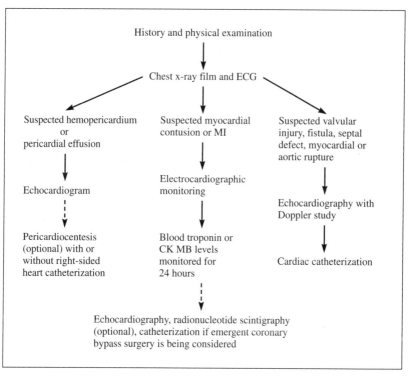

FIG. 25.1. Protocol for the diagnosis of cardiac trauma. Dashed arrow indicates optional procedures.

pends on the demonstration of at least one of the following: (i) elevated serum activity of troponin or CK-MB, (ii) pericardial fluid by echocardiography, (iii) myocardial injury by radionuclide scintigraphy, and (iv) anatomic abnormality such as valvular regurgitation, septal defect, fistula, or aortic or ventricular rupture by echo-Doppler study or catheterization after chest trauma.

3. Differential diagnosis. Because of the setting in which the diagnosis of cardiac trauma is considered, it is unlikely to be confused with other entities. Therefore, diagnostic problems revolve around identifying specific lesions that result from the traumatic event. Pericardial injuries present with prominent rubs or cardiac tamponade. Echocardiography demonstrates fluid in the pericardial space. Myocardial contusion resembles infarction in natural history; presenting complaint; and serologic, physical, ECG, and roentgenographic findings. Residual left ventricular damage is less with contusion than with infarction. Fistulae, VSD, and valvular disruption present with murmurs with or without evidence of left or right ventricular failure. Aorta-to–right heart fistulae produce continuous murmurs and right ventricular failure. VSD and atrioventricular valvular injury with resultant regurgitation cause prominent systolic murmurs, whereas pulmonic and aortic valvular disruption and regurgitation produce diastolic murmurs. Patients with injury to the conduction system usually have some form of heart block. Those with aortic rupture often complain of severe chest and midscapular pain associated with dyspnea,

increased pulse amplitude, and upper extremity hypertension. Identification of cardiac traumatic injuries occurs only if the physician maintains a high index of suspicion when facing patients who have suffered an episode of chest trauma.

III. Therapy

A. Medical treatment. Medical therapy may involve only preoperative volume replacement in a patient with aortic rupture awaiting momentary operative repair. On the other hand, the therapy of cardiac contusion is completely medical, resembling that of non–Q wave myocardial infarction.

1. Arrhythmias. Patients with cardiac traumatic injuries frequently manifest atrial or ventricular arrhythmias. These usually can be controlled with routine antiarrhythmic regimens (see Chapters 3 and 15).

2. Heart failure. Left and right ventricular failure usually can be managed with conventional antifailure regimens, including vasodilators, diuretics, and, on occasion, digitalis.

3. Posttraumatic pericarditis. The treatment of posttraumatic pericarditis resembles that for postinfarction pericarditis. Salicylates, ibuprofen, or other nonsteroidal antiinflammatory agents are used initially, followed by corticosteroids if pericarditis persists (see Chapter 19).

4. Heart block. Transient or permanent conduction disturbances may require temporary or permanent transvenous pacing.

5. Cardiac tamponade. Tamponade is usually the result of hemopericardium in patients with cardiac trauma. Pericardiocentesis should be performed once or several times while the patient is being readied for thoracotomy.

B. Surgery

1. Cardiac traumatic injuries often demand urgent or delayed surgical repair. It is best if repair can be delayed a few weeks to allow for some healing; however, many patients (e.g., those with aortic rupture) require emergency surgical intervention. Patients with valvular disruption may need valve replacement, although repair of the valve is successful in many patients. Fistulae and VSDs usually must be closed unless the flow through them is small. Spontaneous closure of small traumatic VSDs can occur.

2. Laceration or rupture of a coronary vessel, a cardiac chamber, or the aorta requires urgent surgical repair. If a coronary artery has been injured, MI can be ameliorated or prevented if coronary bypass or coronary arterial stenting is performed promptly.

3. Patients with permanent second- or third-degree heart block should receive a permanent pacemaker.

SELECTED READINGS

Adams JE, Davila-Roman VG, Bessey PQ, et al. Improved detection of cardiac contusion with cardiac troponin I. *Am Heart J* 1996;131:308–312.
Troponin I levels help to detect cardiac contusion after blunt chest trauma.
Feghali NT, Prisant LM. Blunt myocardial injury. *Chest* 1995;108:1673–1677.
A concise review of the diagnosis and management of blunt cardiac trauma.
Ferjani M, Droc G, Dreux S, et al. Circulating cardiac troponin T in myocardial contusion. *Chest* 1997;111:427–433.
Troponin was slightly more useful than CK-MB in diagnosing myocardial contusion.
Guest TM, Ramanathan AV, Tuteur PG, et al. Myocardial injury in critically ill patients: a frequently unrecognized complication. *JAMA* 1995;273:1945–1949.
Myocardial injury as diagnosed by elevated cardiac troponin levels is more common than previously thought in critically ill patients in intensive care units.
Hassett A, Moral J, Sabiston DC, et al. Utility of echocardiography in the management of patients with penetrating missile wounds of the heart. *J Am Coll Cardiol* 1986;7:1151–1156.
Two-dimensional echocardiography is useful in finding penetrating missiles that have entered the heart.

Jensen PJ, Thomsen PEB, Bagger JP, et al. Electrical injury causing ventricular arrhythmias. *Br Heart J* 1987;52:279–283.
Patients who sustain electrical injury in which the current passes through the thorax should be monitored for ventricular arrhythmias for 24 hours or more.

Lichtenberg R, Dries D, Ward K, et al. Cardiovascular effects of lightning strikes. *J Am Coll Cardiol* 1993;21:531–536.
Lightning strikes can result in significant myocardial injury and potentially fatal arrhythmias.

Maron BJ, Poliac LC, Kaplan JA, Mueller FO. Blunt impact to the chest leading to sudden death from cardiac arrest during sports activities. *N Engl J Med* 1995; 333:337–342.
Sudden death due to blunt impact to the precordium is the result of malignant ventricular arrhythmias induced by the traumatic blow.

Pretre R, Chilcott M. Blunt trauma to the heart and great vessels. *N Engl J Med* 1997;336:626–632.
Concise review of blunt traumatic injuries to the heart and great vessels and their management.

Smith MD, Cassidy JM, Souther S, et al. Transesophageal echocardiography in the diagnosis of traumatic rupture of the aorta. *N Engl J Med* 1995;332:356–362.
Transesophageal echo is a highly sensitive and specific technique for detecting traumatic injury of the aorta.

Voyce SJ, Becker RB. Diagnosis, management and complications of nonpenetrating cardiac trauma: a perspective for practicing physicians. *J Intensive Care Med* 1993;8:275.
Extensive review of the clinical features of nonpenetrating cardiac trauma.

Weiss RL, Brier JA, O'Connor W, et al. The usefulness of transesophageal echocardiography in diagnosing cardiac contusions. *Chest* 1996;109:73–77.
Cardiac contusions diagnosed with transesophageal echo are associated with a high mortality. Right ventricular contusions were twice as common as left ventricular contusions.

26. PREGNANCY AND HEART DISEASE

I. Introduction. Pregnancy produces a number of alterations in cardiovascular function. The end result of these alterations is increased cardiac work. The patient with heart disease who becomes pregnant, therefore, places two stresses on her heart: the demands of pregnancy and the demands of heart disease. To understand the effect of pregnancy on forms of heart disease, it is necessary to understand the cardiovascular alterations imposed by pregnancy.

II. Cardiac and circulatory changes with normal pregnancy. Pregnancy results in increased cardiac output, heart rate, blood volume, peripheral venous pressure, and right-sided heart pressures (Table 26-1).

A. Cardiac output rises progressively during pregnancy. By 32 weeks of pregnancy, resting cardiac output and blood volume are increased by approximately 50%.

1. Increases in cardiac output are the result of increases in both stroke volume and heart rate.

2. Increases in resting heart rate during pregnancy average approximately 10 beats per minute at term.

B. Blood volume rises approximately 40% to 50% during normal pregnancy. Most of this increase represents an augmentation of plasma volume. Hemoglobin concentration therefore diminishes during pregnancy.

C. Peripheral vascular resistance decreases during pregnancy, but arterial blood pressure changes relatively little because cardiac output increases.

D. Peripheral venous pressure increases during pregnancy, particularly in the legs, because of pressure from the enlarging uterus on the inferior vena cava.

1. Greater peripheral venous pressure commonly results in peripheral edema, hemorrhoids, and varicose veins even in healthy pregnant women.

2. Total body water increases during pregnancy.

E. Right-sided heart pressures are modestly elevated at rest in healthy pregnant women. Left-sided heart pressures are unaffected by pregnancy.

F. Labor with attendant anxiety, exertion, and recurrent Valsalva maneuvers produces marked increases in systemic arterial and venous pressures, right ventricular pressure, heart rate, and cardiac output. All these alterations disappear after delivery. Blood volume and venous pressure return to normal almost immediately after delivery. Other parameters return to normal within hours to days after delivery.

III. Alterations in clinically observable phenomena. During pregnancy, the physiologic alterations just noted produce a number of changes in the physical examination, ECG, chest x-ray film, and echocardiogram of the healthy pregnant woman.

A. Physical examination. Systolic murmurs and continuous venous flow murmurs of no clinical significance are often heard during pregnancy. Diastolic murmurs occur rarely and usually signify the presence of heart disease. The intensity of P2 is increased, and a physiologic third heart sound also may be present. Peripheral edema is a common concomitant of normal pregnancies. Physical findings that may be observed in healthy pregnant women are recorded in Table 26-2.

B. ECG. The ECG remains normal during pregnancy, but some modest changes occur: increased heart rate, shift of the frontal plane axis to the left, and minor T wave changes. Occasional atrial or ventricular premature beats do not imply that organic heart disease is present (Table 26-3).

C. Chest x-ray examination. Radiographic studies should be kept to a minimum in pregnant women to protect the fetus from radiation. Chest x-ray pictures remain normal in healthy pregnant women with clear lung fields and normal heart size. Pulmonary blood vessels become more prominent secondary to increased blood volume (Table 26-3).

TABLE 26-1. HEMODYNAMIC CHANGES DURING PREGNANCY

Increased blood volume
Increased cardiac output
   Increased renal blood flow
   Increased uterine blood flow
   Increased skin blood flow
Decreased peripheral vascular resistance
Increased myocardial contractility
Obstruction of the inferior vena cava
Increased right-sided heart pressures
Increased heart rate

    D. Echocardiogram. Modest changes within the range of normal are noted in the echocardiograms of healthy pregnant women. Thus, heart rate increases, and left and right ventricular end-diastolic dimensions and left ventricular mass increase (Table 26-3).

IV. Effect of pregnancy on patients with heart disease. The circulatory changes that occur in healthy pregnant women (Table 26-1) represent an additional strain on the cardiovascular system of women with preexisting heart disease. Symptoms and signs of heart disease usually increase during pregnancy. In general, patients with heart disease can expect worsening by one clinical class during pregnancy. Thus, patients who are New York Heart Association (NYHA) class I before pregnancy develop class II symptoms during pregnancy. Individuals who are class II before pregnancy move into class III during pregnancy, and so forth. Specific forms of heart disease may require medical or even surgical therapy during pregnancy.

    A. Valvular heart disease. Valvular heart disease is the most common cardiovascular condition in pregnant women, with mitral stenosis predominant. Murmurs of valvular heart disease increase in intensity during pregnancy and are sometimes first noticed at this time. Risk to the fetus and mother increases with increasing clinical class, being in an acceptable range only for patients who are class I or II before pregnancy. Potential complications in pregnant patients with valvular heart disease include pulmonary edema, infectious endocarditis, pulmonary embolism, and supraventricular arrhythmias. A number of women with prosthetic heart valves have had successful pregnancies. Problems in these individuals usually revolve around managing their anticoagulation during pregnancy, delivery, and postpartum (see Section **V.A.3.**).

TABLE 26-2. PHYSICAL FINDINGS DURING NORMAL PREGNANCY

Systolic murmurs: often ejection murmur at the base
Diastolic murmurs: physiologic tricuspid flow murmurs are rarely heard; the presence of a diastolic murmur usually implies that significant heart disease is present
Continuous murmurs
   Venous hum
   Mammary souffle
A physiologic third heart sound may be present and does not necessarily imply that heart disease is present
Fourth heart sound (seldom)
Splitting of first heart sound common
Increased P2
Hyperdynamic pulses
Peripheral edema
Varicose veins

TABLE 26-3. ALTERATIONS OBSERVED IN COMMON CARDIAC TESTS DURING NORMAL PREGNANCY

ECG
  Increased heart rate
  Shift of frontal plane QRS axis to the left
  Minor shift in T wave axis
  Occasional atrial or ventricular premature beats

Chest x-ray film
  Normal heart size and clear lung fields
  Increased prominence of pulmonary vasculature
  Shift of heart to a more horizontal position late in pregnancy

Echocardiogram
  Increased left and right ventricular end-diastolic dimensions compared with previous echo in the nonpregnant state
  Increased left ventricular mass
  Normal left ventricular ejection phase indexes

B. Congenital heart disease. Women with repaired congential heart defects usually have no difficulty with pregnancy; however, women with pulmonary hypertension are at high risk for sudden death during pregnancy. For these women, pregnancy should be avoided or terminated. Patients with Eisenmenger's syndrome can expect a mortality of approximately 25% from pregnancy, regardless of the underlying congenital defect. Very few of such individuals carry a fetus successfully to term. Women with unrepaired asymptomatic or minimally symptomatic congenital heart disease usually do well during pregnancy. Patients with cyanotic congenital heart disease are at increased risk for fetal and/or maternal morbidity and mortality.

Women with coarctation of the aorta and Marfan's syndrome have an increased risk of aortic rupture or dissection during pregnancy.

C. Pulmonary embolism. Pregnancy increases the risk of women with or without heart disease to develop venous thrombosis and pulmonary embolism. Anticoagulation is often difficult to manage in such patients (see Section **V.A.3.**).

D. Perinatal cardiomyopathy. An unusual entity is primary myocardial disease occurring late in pregnancy or in the early postpartum period (postpartum or perinatal cardiomyopathy; see Chapter 18). This entity occurs more often in multiparous malnourished women, especially if the pregnancy has been complicated by toxemia. Arterial and venous embolism and left ventricular failure are common in these women, with resultant high mortality.

E. Hypertension. Elevated arterial blood pressure deserves careful attention during pregnancy because toxemia may develop with resultant high risk for the patient and her fetus. Blood pressure, urinalysis, and even serum blood urea nitrogen or creatinine should be monitored regularly. If acceleration in hypertension occurs (toxemia) with attendant edema, albuminuria, or retinal changes, the patient should be admitted to the hospital for urgent therapy (see Section **V.A.5.**).

V. Management of pregnant women with heart disease
  A. Medical treatment
    1. Heart failure. Signs and symptoms of heart failure in the pregnant patient with heart disease should be managed by decreased activity (or even a brief period of bed rest), decreased salt intake, digitalization, and diuresis (see Chapter 4). Afterload reduction may be administered in the form of oral hydralazine. Angiotensin-converting enzyme inhibitors should not be given because they increase the incidence of stillbirths. Interruption of the pregnancy should be considered and discussed with the obstetrician

if heart failure is refractory to medical therapy or difficult to manage. Patients with stabilized heart failure often fare best if hospitalized during the final 2 to 3 weeks of their pregnancy.

2. Cardiac arrhythmias. Pregnant patients with heart disease are prone to develop supraventricular and ventricular arrhythmias. Arrhythmias are usually best managed in the hospital with conventional therapies (see Chapter 3). Electrical cardioversion and pacemakers can be used as required, with the same indications and precautions as in nonpregnant patients. Amiodarone is contraindicated, but beta-blockers or verapamil may be administered.

3. Anticoagulation. Pregnant patients with deep venous thrombosis, pulmonary or arterial embolism, or prosthetic heart valves should be treated with anticoagulants. Heparin is the drug of choice: Because the molecule is too large to cross the placenta, the fetus is protected from simultaneous anticoagulation. Anticoagulation therapy should be discontinued for 1 to 3 days before delivery. Subcutaneous low-molecular-weight heparin is particularly useful in pregnant patients because of ease of administration and efficacy.

   Long-term (greater than 1 to 2 months) heparin therapy results in osteoporosis. Therefore, patients with prosthetic heart valves or those in whom anticoagulation must continue for more than 2 months should receive oral anticoagulants (warfarin).

   a. Because warfarin crosses the placenta, it should be avoided during the first trimester, when it predisposes to hemorrhage and fetal developmental abnormalities. The drug should be stopped again during the last 3 weeks before term to allow fetal clotting mechanisms to return to normal before delivery. Heparin (usually subcutaneous low-molecular-weight heparin) is substituted for warfarin during periods when the latter is discontinued.

   b. Oral anticoagulants can be restarted after delivery, but patients should not breast-feed because warfarin is excreted in the milk.

4. Antibiotic prophylaxis. Patients with valvular and congenital heart disease (except atrial septal defect) and an infection involving the reproductive organs or vagina should receive 600,000 U of procaine penicillin twice a day, starting with the onset of labor, together with 1 g of intramuscular streptomycin daily, beginning immediately after delivery. Both antibiotics are continued for 3 days. Alternative antibiotic regimens for penicillin-sensitive individuals are listed in Chapter 16. Patients who do not have vaginal or reproductive organ infections do **not** require endocarditis prophylaxis.

5. Antihypertensive therapy. Patients who are hypertensive during pregnancy should be treated in an effort to prevent toxemia. The drug regimens used usually involve some combination of alpha-methyl-dopa, beta-blockers, diuretics, verapamil, and/or hydralazine (see Chapter 12).

   Patients with toxemia should be admitted to the hospital and treated vigorously (antihypertensive or anti–heart failure regimens or both). Renal function should be monitored closely (see Chapter 13).

B. Surgery

   1. Interruption of pregnancy. Therapeutic abortion should be considered for patients with pulmonary hypertension or symptoms of NYHA class III (moderately severe) or IV (severe) heart failure or angina during the first trimester.

   2. Delivery. Cesarean section or forceps-assisted delivery is usually not necessary, even for symptomatic patients. Vaginal delivery is usually preferred, with caesarian section reserved for patients with obstetrical indications for this intervention.

      a. A number of drugs commonly used during labor are relatively contraindicated in patients with heart disease (e.g., atropine, scopolamine, and ergot derivatives).

b. Early ambulation is encouraged after delivery to decrease the risk of deep venous thrombosis and pulmonary embolism.

3. Cardiac surgery. Cardiac surgical intervention during pregnancy carries an increased risk for both mother and fetus. Fortunately, it is rarely necessary.

Mitral valvuloplasty or replacement is the most common cardiac surgical procedure considered during pregnancy. Surgery should be performed only in women with severe disabling signs and symptoms of pulmonary congestion despite intensive medical therapy. Balloon valvuloplasty can usually be performed safely during pregnancy in patients who become markedly symptomatic.

SELECTED READINGS

Born D, Martinez EE, Almeida PAM, et al. Pregnancy in patients with prosthetic heart valves: the effects of anticoagulation on mother, fetus, and neonate. *Am Heart J* 1992;124:413–417.
Pregnancy in a patient with a prosthetic heart valve is a high-risk situation for both mother and fetus.
Burlew BS. Managing the pregnant patient with heart disease. *Clin Cardiol* 1990;13: 757–762.
Careful review of the physiology of normal pregnancy and its effects on the normal and diseased cardiovascular system.
Chambers CE, Clark SL. Cardiac surgery during pregnancy. *Clin Obstet Gynecol* 1994;37:316–323.
Review of various aspects of the care of pregnant patients before, during, and after cardiac surgery.
Elkayam U, Ostrzega E, Shotan A, et al. Cardiovascular problems in pregnant women with the Marfan syndrome. *Ann Intern Med* 1995;123:117–122.
A clinical review of cardiovascular problems and their management in pregnant patients with Marfan's syndrome.
Harvey WP. Alterations of the cardiac physical examination in normal pregnancy. *Clin Obstet Gynecol* 1975;18:51–63.
Changes in cardiac physical examination that occur in women with normal hearts during pregnancy.
Hunter S, Robson SC. Adaptation of the maternal heart in pregnancy. *Br Heart J* 1992;68:540–543.
Physiological and anatomical adaptations to pregnancy.
Lampert MB, Lang RM. Peripartum cardiomyopathy. *Am Heart J* 1995;130:860–870.
A thorough review of peripartum cardiomyopathy
Martinez-Reding J, Cordero A, Kuri J, et al. Treatment of severe mitral stenosis with percutaneous balloon valvotomy in pregnant patients. *Clin Cardiol* 1998;21:659–663.
Percutaneous mitral balloon valvotomy is safe and effective in pregnant patients.
Midei MG, DeMent SH, Feldman AM, et al. Peripartum myocarditis and cardiomyopathy. *Circulation* 1990;81:922–928.
A review of the clinical and pathological features of 18 patients with peripartum cardiomyopathy.
Nolte JE, Rutherford RB, Nawaz S, et al. Arterial dissections associated with pregnancy. *J Vasc Surg* 1995;21:515–520.
A clinical review of diagnosis and management of arterial dissection in pregnant patients.
Page RL. Treatment of arrhythmias during pregnancy. *Am Heart J* 1995;130:871–876.
A review of the management of various arrhythmias during pregnancy.
Perloff JK. Pregnancy and congenital heart disease. *J Am Coll Cardiol* 1991;18: 340–342.
Outcomes for pregnant women with congenital heart disease.
Pitkin RM, Perloff JK, Koos BJ, et al. Pregnancy and congenital heart disease. *Ann Intern Med* 1990;112:445–454.

Review of various clinical aspects of pregnancy complicating congenital heart disease.

Roth A, Elkayam U. Acute myocardial infarction associated with pregnancy. *Ann Intern Med* 1996;125:751–762.

Management of acute MI in pregnant patients.

Sibai BM. Treatment of hypertension in pregnant women. *N Engl J Med* 1996;335: 257–265.

A thorough review of the management of hypertension during pregnancy.

Toglia MR, Weg JH. Venous thromboembolism during pregnancy. *N Engl J Med* 1996; 335:108–113.

Outcomes in pregnant patients with venous thromboembolism.

Vered Z, Poler SM, Gibson P, et al. Noninvasive detection of the morphologic and hemodynamic changes during normal pregnancy. *Clin Cardiol* 1991;14:327–334.

Serial echocardiography was performed in 15 healthy patients during various phases of pregnancy. The changes in left ventricular function are described.

27. NONCARDIAC SURGERY IN PATIENTS WITH HEART DISEASE

I. **Introduction.** Approximately one third of patients over 35 years of age who undergo surgery have some form of cardiovascular disease, including hypertension. Surgery poses a stress for the cardiovascular system that may be dangerous in individuals with severe or unstable heart disease. A number of factors have been identified that can adversely affect patients with heart disease who undergo surgery:

Hemorrhage→hypovolemia→hypotension and ischemia
Impaired ventilation→hypoxia→ischemia
Increased serum proteins and bedrest after surgery, which predispose to venous thrombosis and pulmonary embolism
Healing and infection, which require increased cardiac output
Myocardial depressant effects of essentially all general anesthetics
Ether and cyclopropane, which produce increased sympathetic nerve stimulation (increased circulating norepinephrine)
Spinal anesthesia→vasodilatation→hypovolemia→hypotension and ischemia

Surgical risk for patients with heart disease is the same with general and spinal anesthesia.

Over the years, a number of investigators have developed various indices or scoring systems that correlate with postoperative risk for cardiovascular morbidity and mortality. Many clinicians use these indices in their daily assessment of patient risk. The **Suggested Readings** section of this chapter contains references that will enable interested individuals in locating these indices. Gilbert et al (*Ann Intern Med* 2000;133:356–359) compared four different instruments of preoperative risk assessment to see which was the most predictive of morbidity and mortality. They found no significant difference between the four instruments, which were as follows: (i) the American Society of Anesthesiologists score, (ii) the cardiac risk index of Goldman et al (see **Suggest Readings**), (iii) the modified Goldman Index of Detsky, and (iv) the American College of Physicians Index. There was considerable room for improvement in these indices for predicting perioperative morbid and mortal events. Areas under the receiver operating characteristic (ROC) curves were only 0.625, 0.642, 0.601, and 0.654, respectively. Thus, a substantial portion of the risk was missed by the four indices.

II. **Risk of surgery in patients with coronary artery disease (CAD)**

A. **Myocardial infarction (MI).** Patients with previous MI have increased risk (4% to 8%) of infarction during surgery compared with that of individuals without prior infarction (0.1% to 0.7%). Mortality from postoperative MI is higher in patients with previous infarction (25% to 70%) compared with those without prior infarction (10% to 25%).

B. **Angina pectoris.** Surgical risk is essentially the same for patients with stable angina pectoris as it is for individuals with remote MI (more than 6 months earlier). A number of factors increase surgical risk in patients with CAD (Table 27-1). In addition to the factors mentioned there, the risk of postoperative MI and death is higher in individuals who undergo surgery of the great vessels, lung, or upper abdomen compared with other types of operations. Surgical mortality rises with increasing age in patients with CAD (Table 27-2). Obviously, elective nonessential surgery should be avoided, if possible, in patients with CAD who demonstrate one or more of the factors listed in Table 27-1.

Patients with negative exercise tolerance tests or pharmacological radionuclide stress tests are better surgical risks than individuals with S–T segment depression after exercise or with perfusion defects. Some authorities advocate that patients with a history suggesting CAD undergo ECG exercise testing or

TABLE 27-1. FACTORS INCREASING SURGICAL RISK IN PATIENTS WITH CORONARY ARTERY DISEASE

Factor	Approximate % mortality in patients with specified factor
No factor increasing surgical risk, age >50 years	3
Operation within 3 months of MI	100
Operation 3–6 months after MI	50
Operation >6 months after MI	3–14
Angina pectoris	3–14
Inhalation anesthesia	10
Spinal anesthesia	10
NYHA clinical classification	
I	4
II (not requiring digitalis/diuretics)	9
II (requiring digitalis/diuretics)	12
III (not requiring digitalis/diuretics)	19
III (requiring digitalis/diuretics)	27
IV	67
Presence of third heart sound or elevated neck veins	20
>5 premature ventricular contractions/minute	14
Atrial arrhythmias including atrial premature beats	9

MI, myocardial infarction; NYHA, New York Heart Association.

a pharmacological radionuclide stress test. Individuals with strongly positive tests are usually referred for cardiac catheterization with an eye to angioplasty or coronary artery bypass grafting.

In general, however, most patients with stable CAD can be assessed for risk from clinical information alone, without the need for any specialized test such as an exercise test. All forms of stress testing or diagnostic echo or catheterization are reserved for potentially unstable patients (severe angina or heart failure) or individuals in whom risk assessment is unclear after collection of routine clinical data. The clinical database should contain the following information for the clinician to decide if the patient's preoperative cardiovascular risk is increased:

1. The patient's functional status—the poorer the status, the higher the risk for cardiovascular events and death.
2. The patient's age—the higher the patient's age (especially ages greater than 80 years), the higher the risk for cardiovascular events and death. Increasing age correlates with a higher rate of perioperative complications and mortality as well as longer length of stay in older patients (especially those over age 80) who undergo noncardiac surgery. However, despite increased risk for morbidity and mortality, the mortality rate

TABLE 27-2. EFFECT OF AGE ON SURGICAL MORTALITY IN PATIENTS WITH AND WITHOUT CORONARY ARTERY DISEASE

Age (yr)	With coronary artery disease (%)	Without coronary artery disease (%)
50–59	10	3
60–69	15	7
>70	23	14

remains low: ages 50 to 59 years, 0.3%; 60 to 69 years, 0.8%; 70 to 79 years, 0.9%; and 80 to 89 years, 2.6%.

3. The presence of comorbid conditions such as diabetes mellitus, peripheral vascular disease, renal dysfunction, and chronic pulmonary disease increases the risk for cardiovascular events and death.

4. The type of surgery also helps to determine the cardiovascular risk: The bigger the procedure—e.g., intraabdominal, intrathoracic, or major head and neck procedures—the higher the cardiovascular risk for events or death.

III. Risk of surgery in patients with hypertensive heart disease

A. Mild to moderate uncomplicated hypertension. Surgical risk in this group of patients is the same as in patients without heart disease.

B. Hypertensive heart disease. Surgical risk in patients with hypertension accompanied by symptoms and signs of heart failure is similar to that for patients with CAD. Thus, patients with clinically evident hypertensive heart disease have approximately a 13% mortality risk with all operations and a 26% mortality risk with intraabdominal or intrathoracic procedures. Angina in combination with hypertensive heart disease does not increase the risk. Old MI in combination with hypertensive heart disease increases the risk of surgical mortality to 18% for all operations and to 31% for intraabdominal and intrathoracic procedures.

IV. Risk of surgery in patients with valvular heart disease. Morbidity and mortality after noncardiac surgery is proportional to the patient's preoperative functional classification. Patients with well-compensated mitral valve disease have a surgical mortality of 5% to 6% when all operations are considered. Patients with moderate to severe aortic stenosis have a surgical risk of 10% to 13% for all surgery, a value similar to that noted in patients with CAD.

V. Preoperative management of patients with heart disease undergoing noncardiac surgery

A. Antihypertensive medications. The techniques of modern anesthesia enable the physician to continue antihypertensive medication up to the moment of surgery. If patients are not to take anything by mouth after surgery, intravenous or transcutaneous antihypertensive therapy can be administered until the patient can take oral medications.

B. Antianginal medications. Isolated cases have been reported of accelerated angina or MI following abrupt discontinuation of beta-blockade. Although such incidents are almost certainly unusual, it is best to continue beta-blockers until a few hours before surgery. Thus, most patients receive their last dose of beta-blocker early in the morning before surgery. Long-acting nitrates are similarly discontinued shortly before surgery. Transcutaneous nitrates can be continued during surgery.

C. Anti–heart failure medications. Patients with signs and symptoms of heart failure should have vasodilators, diuretics, and digoxin continued until a few hours before surgery. Patients with more severe degrees of heart failure may have pulmonary arterial and systemic arterial catheters inserted before surgery, although data supporting this practice are minimal at best.

1. Prophylactic digitalization/beta-blockade. Considerable controversy surrounds the issue of prophylactic, preoperative digitalization in elderly patients or in individuals with heart disease but without signs or symptoms of heart failure. Arguments in favor of prophylactic digitalization include the following: (i) digitalis counteracts the negative inotropic actions of anesthetic agents; (ii) digitalis-induced increases in myocardial contractility are beneficial during the postoperative period when metabolic demands are increased; and (iii) digitalis may decrease postoperative atrial arrhythmias or lessen ventricular response, should such an arrhythmia occur. However, beta-blockade is more effective than digitalis preparations in preventing postoperative atrial arrhythmias, including atrial fibrillation. The main argument against prophylactic digitalization is that digitalis administration may result in postoperative digi-

talis toxicity. Indications for prophylactic digitalization are summarized in Table 27-3. Many cardiologists today prefer prophylactic administration of beta-blockers rather than digitalis preparations in this setting. A number of randomized blinded studies have shown that prophylactic administration of beta-blockade decreases the likelihood of postoperative supraventricular arrhythmias.

D. Pacemakers. Some authorities advise preoperative placement of a temporary transvenous pacing catheter in asymptomatic patients with bifascicular block (right bundle branch with left anterior or posterior hemiblock; left bundle branch block) with or without first-degree atrioventricular (AV) block. However, most evidence supports the concept that progression to higher grades of AV block with consequent serious bradycardia is very unusual during or after surgery in such patients. Therefore, prophylactic pacemaker insertion is not recommended in patients with bifascicular block with or without first-degree AV block. The presence of bundle branch block on the ECG is **not** associated with a high incidence of postoperative cardiovascular complications in patients undergoing noncardiac surgery. Perioperative mortality is **not** increased in patients with right bundle branch block. Mortality is increased in patients with left bundle branch block. However, when one corrects for other risk factors such as age and the presence of chronic heart failure, left bundle branch block is **not** an independent risk factor for complications or death.

Perioperative pacing is indicated in patients with second- or third-degree AV block or **symptomatic** sick sinus syndrome.

E. Endocarditis prophylaxis. Antibiotic prophylaxis is indicated in patients with a variety of congenital and valvular cardiovascular conditions (see Chapter 16).

F. Anticoagulation. Low-dose (unfractionated or low-molecular-weight) heparin therapy is advised for patients with heart disease who are to undergo procedures requiring more than 1 or 2 days of bedrest. The dosage is 5000 U subcutaneously of unfractionated heparin or low-molecular-weight heparin two or three times a day, for example, subcutaneous Lovenox, at a dose of 40 mg every day.

G. Antiarrhythmic medications. Patients with severe ventricular ectopy (frequent couplets, runs) should receive antiarrhythmic medication during and after surgery. Often, intravenous lidocaine is the simplest and most effective agent in this setting. Intravenous procainamide, beta-blockade, or both may also be effective.

H. Hemodynamic monitoring. Patients with moderate or severe heart disease may be managed with the aid of hemodynamic monitoring during induction of anesthesia, during surgery, and during the immediate postoperative period (12 to 48 hours). Such monitoring consists of pulmonary arterial and systemic arterial pressure recording. With this careful monitoring, it is hoped that episodes of hypovolemia and hypervolemia, as well as hypotension and hypertension, might be avoided. However, as noted earlier, the evidence supporting this practice is quite slim (see Chapter 9). The anesthesiologist and

TABLE 27-3. INDICATIONS FOR PROPHYLACTIC DIGITALIZATION/ BETA-BLOCKADE[a]

A history of left ventricular failure

Presence of atrial fibrillation or flutter with ventricular response >90 beats per minute

History of atrial fibrillation or flutter

Patients >50 years who are to undergo an intrathoracic procedure

Patients with significant valvular or myocardial disease who do not demonstrate signs of overt left ventricular failure

[a] Beta-blockade is usually preferred over digitalis preparations for prophylactic preoperative administration.

the surgeon may choose to use various combinations of volume replacement, diuretics, pressors, and vasodilators to prevent or treat the above-mentioned complications.

I. Cardiac surgery/angioplasty. Selected patients with severe CAD or aortic stenosis are best served by undergoing corrective cardiac surgery (coronary artery bypass grafting or aorta valve replacement) or coronary angioplasty before being subjected to major elective, noncardiac surgery (e.g., bowel resection). Patients with very symptomatic CAD despite medical therapy or individuals with a positive electrocardiographic exercise or pharmacological radionuclide stress test should be considered for coronary bypass or angioplasty before being subjected to elective, major, noncardiac surgery. Patients with symptomatic aortic stenosis should undergo aortic valve replacement before elective noncardiac surgical procedures.

J. Overall Strategy. The American College of Cardiology/American Heart Association (ACC/AHA) guidelines for perioperative cardiovascular evaluation for noncardiac surgery recommend only clinical screening for stable patients with cardiovascular disease. Major clinical predictors of perioperative risk that should be addressed are (i) the presence of an unstable coronary syndrome; (ii) the presence of decompensated heart failure; (iii) the presence of clinically significant arrhythmias such as ventricular tachycardia, atrial fibrillation, or other supraventricular arrhythmias with a rapid ventricular response, and second- or third-degree heart block; and (iv) the presence of severe valvular heart disease. Patients with one or more of these syndromes should be considered for further diagnostic and/or therapeutic interventions, for example, cardiac catheterization, angioplasty, and antiarrhythmic medication. Patients undergo their elective surgery when they are stable after the appropriate diagnostic/therapeutic intervention. It is worthwhile reading the executive summary of the ACC/AHA guidelines for perioperative evaluation listed in the **Suggested Readings** for this chapter. This publication contains important and detailed information along with clinical algorithms for the evaluation of patients with cardiovascular disease.

SELECTED READINGS

Bode RH Jr, Lewis KP, Zarich SW, et al. Cardiac outcome after peripheral vascular surgery: comparison of general and regional anesthesia. *Anesthesiology* 1996;84:3–13.
Cardiovascular outcomes were the same after these two different forms of anesthesia.

Boersma E, Poldermans D, Bax, et al. Predictors of cardiac events after major vascular surgery: role of clinical characteristics, dobutamine echocardiography, and beta-blocker therapy. *JAMA* 2001;285:1865–1873.
Echo stress testing is only useful in high risk patients for predicting perioperative cardiovascular events.

Brown KA, Rowen M. Extent of jeopardized viable myocardium determined by myocardial perfusion imaging best predicts perioperative cardiac events in patients undergoing noncardiac surgery. *J Am Coll Cardiol* 1993;21:325–330.
The probability of cardiac events in patients undergoing noncardiac surgery is best predicted by myocardium at risk as reflected on thallium 201 perfusion imaging.

Cutler BS, Wheeler HB, Paraskos JA, et al. Assessment of operative risk with electrocardiographic testing in patients with peripheral vascular disease. *Am J Surg* 1979; 137:484–490.
Prognostic implications of electrocardiographic stress testing in the preoperative evaluation of patients with heart disease who are to undergo noncardiac surgery.

Das MK, Pellikka PA, Mahoney DW, et al. Assessment of cardiac risk before nonvascular surgery: dobutamine stress echocardiography in 530 patients. *J Am Coll Cardiol* 2000;35:1647–1653.
Dobutamine stress echo was useful in predicting perioperative cardiovascular events.

Eagle KA, Brundage BH, Chaitman BR, et al. American College of Cardiology/American Heart Association guidelines for perioperative cardiovascular evaluation for noncardiac surgery. *J Am Coll Cardiol* 1996;27:910–948.

The most complete guidelines for evaluation and management of perioperative patients with cardiovascular disease.

Gersh BJ, Rihal CS, Rooke TW, et al. Evaluation and management of patients with both peripheral vascular and coronary artery disease. *J Am Coll Cardiol* 1991;18:203–214.

A thoughtful review of various diagnostic approaches to risk assessment in patients with CAD who are about to undergo noncardiac surgery.

Gerson MC, Hurst JH, Hertzberg VS, et al. Cardiac prognosis in noncardiac geriatric surgery. *Ann Intern Med* 1985;103:832–837.

Inability to exercise was the most prominent predictor of surgical risk in a geriatric population.

Goldman L, Caldera DL, Nussbaum SR, et al. Multifactorial index of cardiac risk in noncardiac surgical procedures. *N Engl J Med* 1977;297:845–850.

Discussion of a prospectively determined multifactorial index that allows preoperative estimation of cardiac risk independent of direct surgical risk.

Hendel RC, Whitfield SS, Villegas BJ, et al. Prediction of late cardiac events by dipyridamole thallium imaging in patients undergoing elective vascular surgery. *Am J Cardiol* 1992;70:1243–1249.

Dipyridamole thallium imaging is valuable in the prognostic evaluation of patients with CAD who undergo noncardiac surgery.

McFalls EO, Doliszny KM, Grund F, et al. Angina and persistent exercise thallium defects: independent risk factors in elective vascular surgery. *J Am Coll Cardiol* 1993;21:1347–1352.

Angina and the presence of fixed thallium defects after exercise are independent predictors of cardiac risk in patients undergoing elective vascular surgery.

Nahlawi M, Holly TA. *Preoperative consultation.* In: Alpert JS, ed. *Cardiology for the primary care physician.* Philadelphia: Current Medicine, 2001:17–24.

Concise review of preoperative management of patients with cardiovascular disease for noncardiac surgery.

O'Hara DA, Duff A, Berlin JA, et al. The effect of anesthetic technique on postoperative outcomes in hip fracture repair. *Anesthesiology* 2000;92:947–957.

Different anesthetic techniques yield the same cardiovascular outcomes after hip fracture surgery.

Pasternack PF, Grossi EA, Baumann FG, et al. Beta blockade to decrease silent myocardial ischemia during peripheral vascular surgery. *Am J Surg* 1989;158:113–116.

Preoperative beta-blockade decreases episodes of silent myocardial ischemia during and after peripheral vascular surgery.

Pastore JO, Yurchak PM, Janis KM, et al. The risk of advanced heart block in surgical patients with right bundle branch block and left axis deviation. *Circulation* 1978; 57:677–680.

Temporary pacemaker insertion is rarely necessary in patients with chronic right bundle branch block and left axis deviation who require noncardiac surgery.

Takase B, Younis LT, Byers SL, et al. Comparative prognostic value of clinical risk indexes, resting two-dimensional echocardiography, and dipyridamole stress thallium 201 myocardial imaging for perioperative cardiac events in major nonvascular surgery patients. *Am Heart J* 1993;126:1099–1106.

Noninvasive testing was better at predicting risk for cardiac events than was clinical risk indexes in patients with CAD who underwent noncardiac surgery.

28. DISEASES OF THE AORTA

I. **Introduction.** Atherosclerotic aortic aneurysms and dissection of the aorta are, at present, the main diagnostic conditions affecting the major artery of the body. Congential abnormalities are occasionally seen; tertiary syphilis involving the aorta is quite rare.

II. **Dissection of the aorta.** Not a true aneurysm, dissection of the aorta is a hematoma that dissects for a variable distance along the aortic media. The dissection may involve almost the entire length of the aorta, or it may consist only of a localized area of intramural aortic hematoma. Dissection occurs when the aortic intima is disrupted and the media is exposed to the intraluminal pressure of the aorta. In predisposed individuals with degenerative changes (cystic medial necrosis) of the aortic media, blood enters the aortic media, creating a plane of dissection for a variable distance. Factors that predispose to the development of cystic medial necrosis areas follows:

Aging
Hypertension
Pregnancy
Atherosclerosis
Aortic valve disease
Coarctation of the aorta
Marfan's syndrome
Other connective tissue abnormalities

The prognosis for untreated dissection of the aorta is poor. Approximately 70% of affected individuals die within the first week after dissection, and 90% die within the first month.

Aortic dissections often originate in intimal tears at two sites: just above the aortic valve and just distal to the left subclavian artery. Aortic intimal disruption in the first case often results in dissection of the ascending aorta, aortic arch, and descending aorta (ascending aortic dissection), whereas intimal disruption distal to the left subclavian artery usually causes dissection of the descending aorta alone (descending aortic dissection). Complications of ascending aortic dissection can include interruption of coronary, arm, and cerebral arteries, as well as aortic insufficiency and hemopericardium with tamponade. Complications of descending aortic dissection can include interruption of arterial supply to the spinal cord, kidneys, and legs.

A. **Diagnosis**

1. **History.** Patients with dissection report the sudden onset of excruciating anterior or posterior (or both) chest pain. The pain is maximal in intensity at its onset, in contradistinction to the discomfort of myocardial infarction (MI), which begins as a mild sensation and gradually builds in intensity. Ascending and descending aortic dissections can both produce anterior and posterior chest pain. Characterizations of the pain of dissection as ripping or tearing are usually retrospective, occurring after the diagnosis has been established. An occasional patient (particularly if Marfan's syndrome is present) develops dissection of the aorta without pain. Most patients come to the physician within a few hours of the onset of pain, but sometimes a person seeks medical attention days to weeks after dissection. Patients with descending aortic dissection tend to be older and have more associated medical diseases (hypertension, diabetes mellitus, preexisting heart disease) than do individuals with ascending aortic dissection.

Patients may present with complaints secondary to obstruction of an artery to the heart, brain, or limbs. Dyspnea secondary to the development of acute aortic insufficiency, or hypotension secondary to hemopericardium with cardiac tamponade or rupture of the dissection into the pleural space may be a prominent feature at presentation.

2. Physical examination. Hypotension secondary to hemopericardium with cardiac tamponade is common in patients with ascending aortic dissection. Evidence of compromised arterial supply to the heart, brain, or limbs also is often observed in patients with ascending aortic dissection. Moreover, a murmur of aortic insufficiency may be noted in these individuals. Patients with descending aortic dissection are not usually hypotensive, nor do they have involvement of coronary, cerebral, or arm arteries. Aortic insufficiency does not develop in patients with descending aortic dissection. Peripheral pulse inequalities may be observed. Physical findings in patients with aortic dissection include the following (not all findings are present in all patients with dissection):

   Hypotension
   Sinus tachycardia
   Elevated jugular venous pressure (unilateral or bilateral)
   Brisk arterial upstroke
   Pulsation of either sternoclavicular joint
   Pericardial rub
   Murmur of aortic insufficiency
   Pulse inequalities (e.g., absent or decreased carotid, brachial, or
      femoral pulse)
   Symptoms secondary to cerebral or spinal cord ischemia (e.g., hemiplegia, paraplegia)

3. ECG. The ECG findings in patients with dissection are usually nonspecific: sinus tachycardia and nonspecific ST–T changes. Often, absence of signs of MI by ECG suggests the diagnosis of dissection in a patient with excruciating chest discomfort. A rare patient with ascending aortic dissection develops obstruction of a coronary artery with resultant MI. In such circumstances, the diagnosis of dissection may be suspected from chest roentgenographic findings.

4. Chest x-ray examination. The chest x-ray film often suggests the diagnosis of dissection. Progressive widening of the aortic shadow on the posteroanterior or anteroposterior chest film is specific for aortic dissection, although one cannot predict whether the dissection is in the ascending or descending aorta. Mediastinal widening on a single chest film also suggests dissection, as does an increased distance (greater than 1 cm) from aortic intimal calcification to the outer edge of the aortic shadow. A thoracic computed tomography (CT) or magnetic resonance imaging (MRI) scan usually demonstrates the dissection clearly.

5. Echocardiography. Reduplication of aortic wall echoes has been reported in patients with dissection. Unfortunately, this finding also may be seen in many individuals without dissection. In some patients, the intimal tear and the dissection itself may be seen in the echocardiogram. This is often the case if transesophageal echocardiography is used.

6. CT scanning and MRI. CT and MRI are both accurate techniques for identifying aortic dissection.

7. Catheterization and angiography. Aortography of the ascending and descending aorta is the gold standard for confirmation of the diagnosis of dissection. Angiography allows the site of origin and extent of the dissection to be defined. In addition, aortography can demonstrate compromised peripheral arteries and aortic insufficiency.

   Aortography is usually required for planning appropriate surgical intervention, although selected patients can undergo surgical intervention after transesophageal echocardiography, CT, or MRI scanning.

8. Protocol for the diagnosis of aortic dissection
   a. **The testing sequence** for making the diagnosis of aortic dissection is as follows:

   History and physical examination
   ↓
   ECG
   ↓
   Chest x-ray film with or without CT/MRI scan or transesophageal two-dimensional echocardiography
   ↓
   Aortography

   b. Criteria for making the diagnosis. The diagnosis of aortic dissection is made in patients who almost invariably present with severe chest or back pain.

   The physical examination may be unremarkable, or it may reveal evidence of cardiac tamponade, aortic insufficiency, or compromised arterial supply to brain, spinal cord, or limbs. The ECG usually shows only nonspecific changes, but the chest x-ray film essentially always reveals mediastinal widening or progressive widening of the aortic shadow. Aortography, CT scanning, MRI imaging, or transesophageal echocardiography demonstrate the dissection.

   c. Differential diagnosis. A number of conditions can mimic aortic dissection.
      (1) Atherosclerotic aneurysm of the aorta. This is a chronic condition. Evidence for its presence usually can be found on earlier chest x-ray films.

      Aortography often is indicated in patients with chronic aortic aneurysms, and this test can generally distinguish dissection from other forms of aortic aneurysm.

      (2) Arterial embolism. Thrombus released from the left side of the heart or proximal aorta embolizes to the peripheral circulation, often producing signs and symptoms secondary to ischemia of brain or limbs. Arterial embolism can be distinguished from aortic dissection by the normal width of mediastinal and aortic shadows on the chest x-ray film and by the absence of dissection on aortography or noninvasive imaging techniques. In addition, aortography in patients with arterial embolism reveals embolic obstruction of peripheral arteries.

      (3) MI. Patients with severe chest pain may have suffered an MI. The correct diagnosis in patients with aortic dissection is suggested by absence of infarction on the ECG, mediastinal or aortic widening on the chest x-ray film, and demonstration of dissection by aortography, CT scanning, MRI imaging, or transesophageal echocardiography.

      (4) Massive pulmonary embolism. The diagnosis of pulmonary embolism is often entertained in patients with central chest pain and hypotension. The correct diagnosis is made when acute right ventricular failure (acute cor pulmonale) is recognized on physical examination and ECG in patients with pulmonary embolism, and when mediastinal or aortic widening is noted in the chest x-ray pictures of patients with dissection. Aortography or noninvasive imaging confirms the diagnosis of dissection. Pulmonary angiography, spiral CT scanning, or ventilation-perfusion scanning confirms the diagnosis of pulmonary embolism.

B. Therapy
   1. Medical treatment
      a. Antihypertensive therapy. Patients with dissection who are elderly, debilitated, or otherwise at high surgical risk (e.g., with severe comor-

bid conditions) should receive medical therapy aimed at lowering the systolic arterial blood pressure to 100 to 110 mm Hg and at blunting the rate of rise of the aortic pressure wave. Intravenous antihypertensive therapy is preferred, regulated with the aid of intraarterial pressure monitoring. Two regimens have been used with success: (i) trimethaphan (a ganglionic blocker) with or without concomitant beta-blockage and (ii) nitroprusside (a vasodilator) after prior beta-blocker administration. Intramuscular reserpine also has been used with success, but this agent is more difficult to regulate than the intravenous regimens. Oral therapy is initiated rapidly (including beta-blockers unless specifically and strongly contraindicated). A variety of oral antihypertensive agents may be used (see Chapter 12). Contraindications to medical therapy include normal to low arterial blood pressure, cardiac tamponade, compromise of a major artery, aortic insufficiency, and left ventricular failure.

    b. General measures. Pain should be relieved with morphine or another opiate analgesic, and a mild tranquilizer should also be administered unless the patient is somnolent or stuporous. Patients with dissection should be managed in an intensive care unit with careful monitoring of intraarterial blood pressure and urine output.

  2. Surgery. Patients with ascending aortic dissection are best treated surgically, particularly if any of the contraindications to medical therapy (Section **II.B.1.a.**) exist. Even elderly patients with ascending aortic dissections should be considered for surgery. The surgical mortality for repair of an ascending aortic dissection is 10% to 20%.

    a. Surgery involves transection of the ascending aorta above the coronary ostia. The intimal tear (almost invariably in this region) is resected, and both ends of the aorta are oversewn, thus obliterating the false channel in the aortic media. A small woven Dacron graft is then used to reconnect the two sections of the aorta.

    b. Patients with descending aortic dissection are often older and more infirm than those with ascending aortic dissection. Therefore, patients with descending aorta dissection may be greater surgical risks (50% to 60% mortality) compared with patients with ascending aortic dissection (10% to 20% mortality).

      For this reason, in the absence of contraindications, medical therapy is usually attempted in patients with descending aortic dissection. Recurrent pain or evidence of extension of the dissection during medical therapy should be considered a strong indication for operative repair of the dissection. Some authorities favor urgent surgical repair of both ascending and descending aortic dissections.

    c. Patients who survive medical or surgical therapy of dissection should be discharged from the hospital on an aggressive antihypertensive regimen that includes beta-blockade.

III. Aneurysms of the aorta. Aortic aneurysms may develop in the thoracic or abdominal aorta (Table 28-1) secondary to a variety of etiologies. However, atherosclerosis is the commonest cause of aortic aneurysm at the present time. Aneurysms are usually of two morphologic types: fusiform (spindle shaped) and sacciform (pouch shaped).

  A. Diagnosis

    1. History. Both thoracic and abdominal aortic aneurysms are often detected by physical examination or roentgenography at a time when the patient is asymptomatic; however, both types of aneurysms may present with a bewildering variety of clinical syndromes (Table 28-2).

    2. Physical examination. Thoracic aneurysms may be difficult to detect on physical examination. An occasional patient with thoracic aortic aneurysm demonstrates tracheal deviation or tug or pulsation of the right sternoclavicular joint. Most abdominal aortic aneurysms are palpable in the periumbilical area, often slightly to the left of the midline. Definite expansile

TABLE 28-1. ETIOLOGY OF ANEURYSMS OF THE AORTA

Thoracic aneurysms
   Atherosclerosis
   Infection (mycotic)
   Trauma
   Syphilis
   Marfan's syndrome
   Aortic stenosis
   Coarctation of the aorta
   Patent ductus arteriosus
   Relapsing polychondritis

Abdominal aneurysms
   Atherosclerosis
   Syphilis infection (mycotic)
   Trauma
   Relapsing polychondritis

movement of the aneurysm usually can be detected. Abdominal bruits may be audible, and associated lower extremity pulse deficits may be noted. Physical findings in patients with aortic aneurysms are listed in Table 28-3. Patients with aortic aneurysm complicating Marfan's syndrome may demonstrate arachnodactyly, ectopia lentis, high arched palate, tall stature, and kyphoscoliosis.

3. ECG. ECG findings in patients with aortic aneurysms are the result of associated heart disease (e.g., nonspecific ST–T changes or infarction patterns in patients with coronary artery disease; left ventricular hypertrophy in individuals with hypertension or aortic regurgitation). The ECG is often normal in patients with aortic aneurysm.

4. Chest x-ray examination, CT, and MRI. Thoracic aneurysms are often first suspected because of an abnormally enlarged aortic shadow on the

TABLE 28-2. SYNDROMES AND SYMPTOMS CAUSED BY AORTIC ANEURYSMS

Thoracic aneurysms
   Anterior or posterior chest pain
   Dysphagia (esophageal compression)
   Hoarseness (vocal chord paralysis secondary to compression of the recurrent laryngeal nerve)
   Superior vena caval syndrome (compression of the superior vena cava)
   Cough, dyspnea, or both (pulmonary arterial or tracheal compression)
   Hemoptysis (erosion of aneurysm into pulmonary parenchyma or rupture of aneurysm into a bronchus)
   Shock (rupture of aneurysm into pleural space)
   Angina (ostial lesions of syphilitic aortitis)

Abdominal aneurysms
   Midabdominal, lumbar, or pelvic pain
   Shock (rupture of aneurysm into peritoneal cavity)
   Intestinal obstruction (duodenal compression)
   Peripheral edema (inferior vena caval compression)
   Gastrointestinal bleeding (rupture of aneurysm into duodenum)
   High-output heart failure (rupture of aneurysm into vena cava)
   Arterial insufficiency of legs (thrombosis of aneurysm or embolization of thrombus to legs)

TABLE 28-3. PHYSICAL FINDINGS IN PATIENTS WITH AORTIC ANEURYSMS

Thoracic aneurysms
  Tracheal tug (pulsation)
  Tracheal deviation
  Vocal cord paralysis
  Superior vena caval syndrome
  Pulsation of right sternoclavicular joint
  Visible and palpable pulsation of anterior chest wall (usually second or third
    intercostal space on the right or higher up on the left)
  Inequality of upper extremity pulses or blood pressure (or both)

Abdominal aneurysms
  Palpable expansile mass in periumbilical area, often to left of midline
  Abdominal systolic bruit
  Decreased lower extremity pulses
  Continuous abdominal bruit and high-output heart failure (rupture of aneurysm
    into inferior vena cava)

chest x-ray film. Patients with syphilitic aortic aneurysms have characteristic linear ("eggshell") calcifications of the ascending aorta. An abnormally enlarged aortic shadow may be seen along the left or right sternal border. Tortuosity, buckling, or kinking of the aorta may cause similar findings in the chest film. Poststenotic dilatation of the ascending aorta in patients with aortic stenosis can also produce a similar roentgenographic picture. CT and MRI scans of the thorax and/or abdomen are highly accurate in demonstrating aortic aneurysms.

Abdominal aortic aneurysms may be clearly outlined on anteroposterior and lateral roentgenograms of the abdomen if calcification is present in the aortic wall. They are also clearly demonstrated by abdominal ultrasound. Patients with retroperitoneal rupture of an abdominal aortic aneurysm may demonstrate obliteration of the margin of the psoas muscle in the anteroposterior abdominal x-ray film. A CT or MRI scan of the abdomen or chest will clearly delineate an aortic aneurysm.

5. Laboratory tests. Roughly 70% to 90% of patients with syphilitic aortic aneurysms have positive screening serologic reactions for syphilis (Wassermann, Hinton, Venereal Disease Research Laboratory). More sensitive and specific tests, the treponemal immunologic tests (Reiter's protein complement fixation test, fluorescent treponemal antibody absorption test), are useful in diagnosing syphilitic aortitis. Patients with atherosclerotic aortic aneurysms often have abnormal serum lipids.

6. Echocardiography. Transthoracic echocardiography may demonstrate a dilated aortic root in patients with thoracic aortic aneurysm. On the other hand, the transthoracic echocardiogram may be normal. Transesophageal echocardiography may demonstrate a thoracic aortic aneurysm when the transthoracic echo study is normal. Abdominal cross-sectional echocardiography usually visualizes abdominal aortic aneurysms with such clarity that accurate measurements of the diameters of the aneurysms can be obtained. The growth of abdominal aortic aneurysms can be followed with serial cross-sectional echocardiograms.

7. Angiography. Aortography frequently provides definitive evidence of the location, extent, and diameter of thoracic or abdominal aortic aneurysms. Aortography occasionally is misleading, however, because the lumen of the aneurysm is filled with laminated thrombus.

8. Protocol for the diagnosis of aortic aneurysm
    a. **The testing sequence** for making the diagnosis of aortic aneurysm is recorded in Fig. 28-1. (Dashed arrows indicate optional steps.)

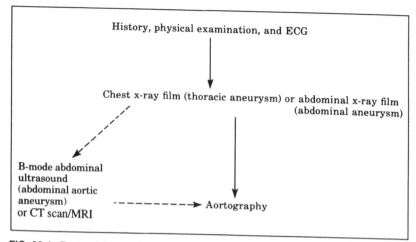

FIG. 28-1. Protocol for the diagnosis of aortic aneurysm. *Dashed arrows* indicate optional procedure.

   b. Criteria for making the diagnosis
     (1) Thoracic aortic aneurysm. Thoracic aortic aneurysm is diagnosed in a symptomatic or asymptomatic individual with an abnormal aortic shadow on posteroanterior and lateral chest roentgenogram, as well as by demonstration of a thoracic aortic aneurysm on CT, MRI, or aortography.
     (2) Abdominal aortic aneurysm. Abdominal aortic aneurysm is diagnosed in a symptomatic or asymptomatic individual with a palpable pulsatile abdominal mass and confirmatory visualization of the aneurysm on abdominal anteroposterior and lateral x-ray, cross-sectional ultrasound study, or abdominal CT or MRI scan. Aortography is performed preoperatively only as an aid to the vascular surgeon extirpating the aneurysm.
   c. Differential diagnosis. Because a variety of agents can produce aortic aneurysms, it is important to search for syphilis, hypertension, and associated valvular or congenital heart disease (Table 28-1).
     (1) Tortuous or kinked aorta. Patients with buckling, tortuosity, or kinking of the aorta secondary to atherosclerosis, aging, or hypertension may have roentgenographic findings similar to those noted in individuals with thoracic aortic aneurysm. If the patient is a surgical candidate, CT, MRI, or aortography should be used to distinguish these two entities.
     (2) Chest neoplasms. Various malignant and benign tumors of the lung and mediastinum may simulate thoracic aortic aneurysm on the chest x-ray film. CT, MRI, and occasionally aortography is usually required to rule out aortic aneurysm; thoracotomy or mediastinoscopy may be necessary to identify the type of neoplasm involved.
     (3) Chronic aortic dissection. Some patients survive the acute episode of aortic dissection and develop chronic dissection with or without an associated true aortic aneurysm. Careful CT, MRI, or aortographic study is required to distinguish chronic dissection with or without true aortic aneurysm from the more common atherosclerotic or hypertensive aortic aneurysm.

    (4) Mycotic aneurysm. Atherosclerotic aortic aneurysms can become secondarily infected. Rarely, primary bacterial invasion of the aorta produces a mycotic aortic aneurysm. Fever, leukocytosis, and positive blood cultures in the absence of cardiac murmur point toward the diagnosis of mycotic aneurysm. CT, MRI, or aortography demonstrates the aortic aneurysm.

    (5) Acute abdomen. Rupture of an abdominal aortic aneurysm can simulate a variety of acute abdominal catastrophes. A pulsatile abdominal mass in a patient in shock complaining of severe abdominal or back pain suggests the diagnosis of ruptured abdominal aortic aneurysm. An x-ray film, ultrasound study, or CT or MRI of the abdomen often confirms the presence of an abdominal aortic aneurysm when calcification in the wall of the aneurysm is observed.

B. Therapy

  1. Medical treatment

    a. Patients with thoracic and abdominal aortic aneurysms should be rendered normotensive by an antihypertensive drug regimen. In Laplace's law (tension = pressure times radius), the tension in the wall of the aneurysm is directly proportional to the blood pressure within the aneurysm.

      Increased tension in the wall of an aneurysm results in more rapid expansion and earlier rupture of the aneurysm. If tolerated, systolic arterial blood pressure should be kept at or below 120 mm Hg. A beta-adrenergic blocking agent should be used as part of the antihypertensive regimen if the patient can tolerate this agent.

    b. Aneurysmal diameter is monitored noninvasively (physical examination, x-ray study, ultrasound, CT, MRI) or invasively (aortography) in patients with aortic aneurysms. Determination of an aneurysmal diameter is usually performed at 6-month intervals. Disagreement exists concerning the minimum size that asymptomatic aneurysms should be allowed to attain before surgical extirpation is undertaken. In general, abdominal aortic aneurysms larger than 5 to 6 cm in diameter should be removed, although aneurysms as small as 4 cm in diameter occasionally rupture. Smaller thoracic aortic aneurysms are often excised, even in the absence of symptoms. Clearly, the patient's general health and vigor are the most important factors in deciding whether surgical therapy of aortic aneurysm is indicated.

    c. Associated conditions should be treated appropriately before aneurysmectomy is attempted. Thus, hyperglycemia should be controlled in patients with diabetes mellitus, and angina pectoris should be stabilized by medical, catheter, or surgical therapy before elective surgery for aortic aneurysm.

      Patients with frank or impending rupture of an aortic aneurysm should undergo excision of the aneurysm without delay.

    d. Patients with aortitis or aortic aneurysm secondary to syphilis should be treated with 2.4 million U of intramuscular benzathine penicillin per week for 3 weeks (total, 7.2 million U); or 600,000 U of intramuscular aqueous procaine penicillin G per day for 15 days (total, 9 million U); or 500 mg of oral tetracycline four times a day for 30 days (total, 60 g); or 500 mg of oral erythromycin four times a day for 30 days (total, 60 g).

  2. Surgery. Symptomatic aortic aneurysms of any size or asymptomatic aneurysms greater than 5 to 6 cm in diameter should be excised and replaced by a woven Dacron graft. Patients who are otherwise in good health have a surgical risk of approximately 5% to 10% for ascending and descending thoracic aortic aneurysms and 15% or higher for thoracoabdominal or aortic arch aneurysms. Surgical risk for resection of an

abdominal aortic aneurysm averages 5%. Patients with heart disease who undergo elective resection of an abdominal aortic aneurysm have a mortality of approximately 13%; those without heart disease who have the same operation have a mortality of 2%.

SELECTED READINGS

Ballal RS, Nanda NC, Gatewood R, et al. Usefulness of transesophageal echocardiography in assessment of aortic dissection. *Circulation* 1991;84:1903–1914.
Transesophageal echocardiography is a very accurate test for identifying aortic dissection.

Chan KL. Impact of transesophageal echocardiography on the treatment of patients with aortic dissection. *Chest* 1992;101:406–410.
Many patients will not need aortography if a clear picture of the aortic dissection is obtained by transesophageal echocardiography.

Clouse WD, Hallett JW, Schaff HV, et al. Improved prognosis of thoracic aortic aneurysms: a population-based study. *JAMA* 1998;280:1926–1929.
Overall survival for thoracic aortic aneurysms has improved significantly over recent years.

Erbel R, Alfonso F, Boileau C, et al. Diagnosis and management of aortic dissection: recommendations of the Task Force on Aortic Dissection, European Society of Cardiology. *Eur Heart J* 2001;22:1642–1681.
Extensive review of pathophysiology, diagnosis, and management of aortic dissection.

Fink HA, Lederle FA, Roth CS, et al. The accuracy of physical examination to detect abdominal aortic aneurysm. *Arch Intern Med* 2000;160:833–836.
Abdominal palpation has only moderate overall sensitivity for detecting abdominal aortic aneurysm of any size but has good sensitivity for detecting aneurysms large enough to warrant surgical intervention.

Glower DD, Fann JI, Speier RH, et al. Comparison of medical and surgical therapy for uncomplicated descending aortic dissection. *Circulation* 1990; 82 (Suppl IV): IV39–IV46.
Medical and early surgical therapy are equivalent in outcome for patients with descending aortic dissection.

Hagan PG, Nienaber CA, Isselbacher EM, et al. The international registry of acute aortic dissection (IRAD). new insights into an old disease. *JAMA* 2000;283:897–903.
Acute aortic dissection presents with a wide range of manifestations. Classic findings are often absent, and in-hospital mortality remains high.

Januzzi JL, Movsowitz HD, Choi J, et al. Significance of recurrent pain in acute type B aortic dissection. *Am J Cardiol* 2001;87:930–933.
Recurrent pain in patients with descending aortic dissection does not necessarily mean extension of the dissection and is not necessarily associated with a poor prognosis.

Melchior T, Hallam D, Johansen BE. Aortic dissection in the thrombolytic era: early recognition and optimal management is a prerequisite for increased survival. *Int J Cardiol* 1993;42:1–6.
A careful review of diagnostic strategies and clues to aortic dissection. Emphasis is placed in distinguishing dissection for MI.

Meszaros I, Morocz J, Szlavi J, et al. Epidemiology and clinicopathology of aortic dissection: a population-based longitudinal study over 27 years. *Chest* 2000;117: 1271–1278.
Aortic dissection continues to be markedly underdiagnosed on initial presentation.

Newman AB, Arnold AM, Burke GL, et al. Cardiovascular disease and mortality in older adults with small abdominal aortic aneurysms detected by ultrasonography: the cardiovascular health study. *Ann Intern Med* 2001;134:182–190.
Total mortality, cardiovascular disease mortality and concomitant cardiovascular disease rates are higher in patients with abdominal aortic aneurysm than in patients without this condition.

Salo JA, Soisalon-Soininen S, Bondestam S, et al. Familial occurrence of abdominal aortic aneurysm. *Ann Intern Me.* 1999;130:637–642.

Aging brothers of patients with known abdominal aortic aneurysm are at the highest risk for developing this condition.

Song JK, Kim HS, Kang DH, et al. Different clinical features of aortic intramural hematoma versus dissection involving the ascending aortic. *J Am Coll Cardiol* 2001;37:1604–1610.

Clinical features allow one to distinguish acute aortic intramural hematoma from acute aortic dissection.

Svensson LG, Crawford ES, Hess KR, et al. Dissection of the aorta and dissecting aortic aneurysms: improving early and long-term surgical results. *Circulation* 1990;82 (Suppl IV): IV24–IV38.

Surgical management of dissection has improved dramatically over the last 20 years.

Von Kodolitsch Y, Schwartz AG, Nienaber CA. Clinical prediction of acute aortic dissection. *Arch Intern Med* 2000;160:2977–2982.

Three easily determined clinical variables were highly predictive of the presence of acute aortic dissection.

29. PERIPHERAL VASCULAR DISEASE

I. Introduction. Many clinicians equate peripheral vascular disease with arteriosclerosis obliterans (AO), which affects the major arteries of the lower extremities.
   Lymphatic and venous diseases, however, also are encompassed by the term **peripheral vascular disease.** This chapter examines the two most common forms of peripheral vascular disease: AO and thrombophlebitis (TBP).

II. AO. The pathophysiology and risk factors for AO resemble those of ischemic heart disease, with the symptom of intermittent claudication comparable to that of angina pectoris. Both symptoms are the result of ischemia in muscle (skeletal versus cardiac) secondary to an imbalance between supply and demand of blood borne oxygen and nutrients. The severity of ischemia and of intermittent claudication is related to the extent of the atherosclerotic arterial narrowing, and to the size and amount of work done by skeletal muscles distal to the arterial obstruction.

   A. Diagnosis
      1. History. Most patients with AO of the lower extremities complain of exertional pain in the toes, feet, calves, thighs, or buttocks. The earliest sign of AO of the legs is exertion-induced (usually walking) intermittent claudication of the calves or feet. Claudication ordinarily is described as a heaviness, numbness, weakness, aching, or cramping in the muscles themselves. Claudication of calf muscles implies obstruction to flow in the femoropopliteal arteries, whereas claudication in the thighs or buttocks suggests that aortoiliac disease is present. More severe degrees of AO usually produce claudication that is more easily precipitated and longer lasting. Claudication disappears when the individual rests or walks more slowly. Ischemic injury to peripheral nerves, which results in ischemic neuropathy and gangrene or pregangrene, produces great discomfort in the toes. Such discomfort occurs at rest and is usually a late symptom in patients with AO.

         The prognosis of patients with AO is largely affected by the presence or absence of associated ischemic heart disease. Some studies report a mortality as high as 6% per year, mostly as a result of myocardial infarction or sudden death. Amputation rates for AO of the lower extremities range from 4% to 12% over 5- to 10-year follow-up periods. The amputation rate is higher in diabetics, who usually have more extensive arterial disease than do nondiabetics.

      2. Physical examination. Absent or markedly decreased peripheral pulses are the sine qua non of AO of the lower extremities. Other physical findings in this disorder are

         Disappearance of peripheral pulses after strenuous exertion
         Systolic or diastolic bruits over lower abdomen or groin
         Blanching of the foot during elevation and redness (rubor) during dependency
         Poor capillary filling after skin compression
         Prolonged venous filling time (greater than 15 seconds) with dependency
         Loss of hair on the dorsum of the foot
         Trophic changes of the skin and nails
         Ischemic ulceration (occurs first at tips of toes)
         Gangrene of toes
         Temperature differences between affected and unaffected foot

      3. ECG. The ECG may be normal, or it may demonstrate findings secondary to associated ischemic heart disease (see Chapter 15).
      4. X-ray examination. The chest roentgenogram may be normal, or findings secondary to associated ischemic heart disease (see Chapter 15) or arteriosclerotic aortic aneurysm (see Chapter 28) may be noted. Abdominal and lower-extremity roentgenograms frequently demonstrate vascular calcification in patients with AO.

5. Echocardiography. Echocardiography may be normal, or findings related to associated ischemic heart disease (see Chapter 15) may be noted. A number of noninvasive procedures have been developed to document the presence of AO of the legs. Measurement of blood pressure at the ankle before and after exercise, determination of peripheral arterial pulse amplitude, quantitation of blood flow in leg muscles before and after exercise by plethysmographic or radionuclide clearance techniques, and Doppler ultrasound examination of the peripheral arterial system are all sensitive and specific techniques for confirming the presence of AO of the lower extremities.

6. Radionuclide tests. Myocardial scintigraphy and radionuclide angiography may demonstrate findings that are the result of associated ischemic heart disease. Clearance of radioactive tracers after injection into skeletal muscle is directly proportional to that muscle's blood flow. A number of radionuclides (xenon 133, iodine 131) have been injected intramuscularly to measure lower-extremity muscle blood flow before, during, and after exercise or induced reactive hyperemia. Patients with AO of the lower extremities almost invariably demonstrate reduced clearance and hence reduced muscle blood flow during such examinations.

7. Cardiac catheterization and angiography. Catheterization may be performed in patients with AO to define the extent and severity of associated ischemic heart disease. On occasion, angiography of the abdominal aorta and peripheral arteries will be performed at the same time because of concern for the condition of the latter vessels. For example, patients with significant left main coronary arterial stenosis or markedly reduced left ventricular function may be candidates for intraaortic balloon counterpulsation. This pumping device is inserted into the aorta through the femoral and iliac arteries; the adequacy of these vessels to accept the balloon catheter may be assessed by angiography at the time of cardiac catheterization. In addition, interventional therapy such as stent placement may be performed in the peripheral arteries at the time of cardiac catheterization.

   A thorough angiographic study of the distal aorta and peripheral arteries is performed in patients who are candidates for arterial reconstructive surgery or peripheral vascular angioplasty.

8. Protocol for the diagnosis of AO

   a. Testing sequence for making the diagnosis. A protocol for making the diagnosis of AO is as follows (dashed arrow indicates optional step):

   History and physical examination
   ↓
   Roentgenogram of lower extremities
   ↓
   Noninvasive test of arterial sufficiency (radionuclide clearance, plethysmography, Doppler)
   ↓
   Angiography of distal aorta and peripheral arteries (optional; usually performed only before reconstructive arterial surgery or angioplasty)

   b. Criteria for making the diagnosis. The diagnosis of AO is made in patients with a history of exercise-induced leg muscle discomfort (claudication) or rest pain in the distal foot who demonstrate abnormal peripheral leg pulses. Confirmation of the diagnosis is obtained by a noninvasive test of arterial sufficiency (radionuclide clearance, plethysmography, Doppler).

   Roentgenograms of the lower extremities are helpful in defining the extent of arterial calcification. Angiography of the peripheral circulation is reserved for patients who are candidates for arterial reconstructive surgery or angioplasty.

    c. Differential diagnosis

        (1) Arterial embolism. Acute and frequently severe arterial insufficiency of the legs results when a thrombus from the left atrium, left ventricle, or proximal aorta lodges in the peripheral circulation. This condition is differentiated from AO by history (acute onset, no history of claudication) and angiography (acute interruption of an otherwise normal or near normal artery). Differentiation is important because patients with arterial embolism should undergo embolectomy with a Fogarty catheter and receive systemic anticoagulants (see Chapter 22).

        (2) Arteritis. Arterial insufficiency may be the result of arteritis (Takayasu's, collagen vascular disease, giant cell). Arteritis patients usually demonstrate one or more of the following findings: fever, malaise, weight loss, rash, areas of cutaneous gangrene, and elevated erythrocyte sedimentation rates. Risk factors for arteriosclerosis are likely to be absent in patients with arteritis. Peripheral pulses may be surprisingly normal or absent.

        (3) Osteoarthritis of the lower spine or leg joints. Pain from osteoarthritic involvement of the lower back or joints of the leg may occur only with exertion. This entity usually can be distinguished from AO by history (pain localized to joints or lower back and not to muscles) and physical examination (normal pulses and arthritic deformities).

        (4) Thromboangiitis obliterans (Buerger's disease). Thromboangiitis obliterans occurs almost exclusively in men who smoke heavily and who are less than 35 years of age. This unusual condition is characterized by an intense inflammatory reaction in veins and small- to medium-sized arteries. Thus, patients often present with migratory superficial TBP and gangrene of the tips of the toes. The upper extremities frequently are involved along with the legs.

B. Therapy

  1. Medical treatment

    a. Protection of the skin. Prophylactic measures to protect the skin of the feet and toes are necessary to retard the development of gangrene. Such measures include the following:

      Avoidance of all forms of foot trauma
      Use of comfortable, carefully fitted footwear
      Avoidance of exposure of feet to excessive heat or cold
      Careful trimming of toenails
      Bunions, calluses, and corns cared for by a podiatrist or physician
      Application of lanolin cream (or similar agent) to dry skin
      No application of patent medicines to feet
      No application of adhesive plaster to feet
      Prompt therapy of any foot infection, including dermatophytosis (athlete's foot)

    b. Tobacco. All forms of tobacco use should be immediately and completely discontinued.

    c. Lowering of serum lipids. The low-cholesterol/low-saturated-fat diet advocated by the American Heart Association is strongly advised for patients with AO. Lipid-lowering medications, for example, statins or fibrates, are often required as well to bring serum cholesterol and triglyceride values down into the normal range or below.

    d. Exercise. Daily exercise (walking or bicycling) to claudication and beyond has been shown to improve exercise tolerance and even to increase blood flow in leg muscles distal to arterial obstruction. Patients should exercise 30 to 60 minutes daily.

e. Vasodilators and other medical therapy. There is minimal evidence that vasodilator drugs are of any benefit in patients with AO. Such medications may even cause harm by improving blood flow in areas with normal arterial supply at the expense of zones with arterial insufficiency. The vasodilator/antiplatelet drug cilostazol (100 mg twice a day), has been shown to be effective in increasing walking distance in patients with intermittent claudication. Pentoxifylline (400 mg three times a day) increases red cell flexibility and decreases blood viscosity. This latter agent also increases walking distance in claudication patients, but the beneficial effect is modest at best. Patients with Raynaud's phenomenon often benefit from therapy with nifedipine, 10 to 40 mg three or four times a day. Modest improvement in exercise tolerance has been observed in patients who receive oral pentoxifylline (400 mg three times a day with meals). This agent apparently improves blood flow through stenotic peripheral arteries by decreasing blood viscosity. In general, the best program for a patient with intermittent claudication consists of smoking cessation, daily exercise, lipid lowering medication, control of hypertension, and aspirin. There is some evidence (the Clopidogrel Versus Aspirin in Patients at Risk of Ischemic Events [CAPRIE] study) that clopidogrel is more effective than aspirin in preventing cardiovascular events in patients with peripheral vascular disease.

Several studies have reported benefit in patients with claudication from oral propionyl-L-carnitine therapy (1 g twice a day).

f. Ischemic ulcers. A serious complication of AO, ischemic ulcers should be treated with bed rest and lower-extremity dependency (elevation of head of bed), as well as measures to debride and cleanse the ulcer (soaks in mild disinfectant solutions two or three times a day and frequent change of sterile dry dressings). Cultures of the ulcer are obtained, and antibiotics are administered if evidence of infection is noted. Rest pain usually is relieved by aspirin or codeine (often in combination). Severe rest discomfort may require opiates for analgesia. Surgical or angioplasty revascularization is usually indicated.

g. Anticoagulation. Anticoagulants are of no proved benefit in patients with AO.

2. Surgery

a. Arterial reconstructive surgery and angioplasty. Patients with extremely limiting claudication, rest pain, or gangrene may be candidates for arterial reconstruction if intervention is not contraindicated by associated disease.

Saphenous vein bypass of severely stenotic or occluded arterial segments has been quite successful. Endarterectomy has been used successfully in patients with reasonably localized aortic or iliac arterial obstruction. Percutaneous transluminal catheter dilatation of a stenotic arterial segment with or without stenting can also be performed in selected patients. It is important to remember that AO is usually a slowly progressive and nonfatal disease with well-tolerated symptoms. Interventional therapy should be reserved for patients who are quite symptomatic or who have a limb that is threatened by severe ischemia. Surgical mortality for aortoiliac reconstruction is approximately 5%; mortality for femoropopliteal arterial surgery is approximately 2%.

b. Sympathectomy. Sympathectomy does not ameliorate intermittent claudication. It is probably of little benefit in patients with rest pain or gangrene and therefore plays little role in the management of patients with AO.

c. Amputation. When gangrene cannot be controlled medically or surgically, or when the risk involved in arterial reconstructive surgery is excessive, amputation may be necessary. Preservation of the knee (or below-the-knee [BK] amputation) is of importance in speeding rehabilitation of the amputee. Prosthesis fitting and use in the immediate postoperative period speeds the rehabilitation process.

III. TBP. Earlier clinicians often distinguished three related conditions that affected peripheral veins: TBP, phlebothrombosis, and phlebitis. Current attitudes combine all three under the single term *thrombophlebitis*. Venous thrombosis occurs through the interaction of three factors: stasis of flow, hypercoagulability of the blood, and injury to venous endothelium, as pointed by Virchow in the nineteenth century. TBP is associated with a number of diseases that produce one or more of these initiating factors (Table 29-1). Venous thrombosis rarely affects the nutritional state of the tissues drained by the thrombosed vein due to the extensive system of collateral venous channels. Arterial blood flow into a limb with TBP is normal unless the entire venous system of a limb becomes thrombosed (phlegmasia cerulea dolens), with resultant arterial insufficiency.

A. Diagnosis

1. History. TBP can affect superficial or deep veins. In the former case, the condition is generally benign; in the latter, the outcome is often pulmonary embolism, a condition that may be fatal (see Chapter 22). Patients with superficial TBP complain of localized pain and tenderness over the region of the thrombosed vein. Those with lower-extremity deep vein TBP may be asymptomatic, or they may describe swelling, pain, or tenderness of the calf. Symptoms (and signs) are usually unilateral.

2. Physical examination. Superficial TBP is associated with erythema, induration, and tenderness over the involved region. Deep venous TBP may be associated with a normal physical examination or with peripheral edema, venous distention, or local tenderness to palpation of the calf or the course of the involved vein. Physical findings in superficial and deep TBP are summarized in Table 29-2.

3. ECG. The ECG is usually normal in patients with TBP unless associated cardiac disease or pulmonary embolism is present (Chapter 22).

4. Chest x-ray examination. The chest roentgenogram is usually normal in patients with TBP unless associated cardiac disease or pulmonary embolism is present (see Chapter 22).

5. Blood tests. The high-sensitivity D-dimer test is quite sensitive in diagnosing intravascular thrombosis. However, specificity is lower because many systemic illnesses, for example, sepsis, can lead to microscopic intravascular coagulation and hence a positive D-dimer test.

6. Echocardiography. Echocardiography is normal unless associated heart disease or pulmonary embolism is present (see Chapter 22).

A number of noninvasive tests have been devised to assess the adequacy of **peripheral venous function** and to aid in the diagnosis of TBP. A high percentage of patients with venous thrombosis of the leg will have an abnormal result if one of these examinations is performed. Three such tests are the Doppler venous flow determination, impedance plethysmography, and phleborheography. Impedance plethysmography is the most commonly used test. Combination of the results of one of these tests with the results of a serum D-dimer test is an accurate way to diagnose deep venous thrombosis.

7. Radionuclide tests. Myocardial scintigraphy and radionuclide angiography are normal in patients with TBP unless they have associated heart disease. A radionuclide technique, the ^{125}I fibrinogen test, is quite accurate in detecting calf and thigh TBP. The calf and thigh are scanned shortly after the intravenous administration of ^{125}I-labeled fibrinogen. Areas of increased tracer uptake delineate regions of venous thrombosis. The technique is not useful in detecting upper femoral and iliac TBP, nor are the results valid when hematomas or healing wounds are present in the leg. There is a very slight chance that patients will develop

TABLE 29-1. ETIOLOGY OF THROMBOPHLEBITIS

Stasis of flow
    Heart failure
    Postoperative
    Postpartum
    Varicose veins
    Prolonged travel in car, bus, train, plane
    Bed rest
    Debilitating disease

Hypercoagulability of blood
    Malignancy
    Postoperative
    Polycythemia
    Thrombocytosis
    Oral contraceptives/pregnancy/hormone replacement therapy
    Sepsis

Injury to venous endothelium
    Trauma
    Thromboangiitis obliterans (Buerger's disease)

Systemic lupus erythematosus
    Septic thrombophlebitis
    Intravenous catheters
    Intravenous administration of medication

---

    serum hepatitis after this test, because pooled plasma is used to obtain the fibrinogen.
8. Cardiac catheterization and angiography. Catheterization and angiography are unremarkable in patients with TBP unless associated cardiac disease or pulmonary embolism is present (see Chapter 22). Angiography of the venous system, termed **venography** or **phlebography,** accurately delineates venous thrombosis. This test is safe and can be performed rapidly. Routine venography may result in inadequate visualization of soleal venous sinuses, anterior tibial veins, and the profunda femoral and iliofemoral venous systems. Venography is the gold standard to which various noninvasive tests for venous thrombosis are compared.

TABLE 29-2. PHYSICAL FINDINGS IN THROMBOPHLEBITIS

Superficial
    Erythema
    Tenderness
    Induration along course of involved vein

Deep
    Low-grade fever
    Malaise
    Tenderness to deep palpation or along course of involved vein (or both)
    Induration of overlying muscle
    Venous distention (superficial)[a]
    Peripheral edema[a]
    Cyanosis[a]
    Findings of associated pulmonary embolism (see Chapter 22)

[a] Uncommon manifestations.

9. Protocol for the diagnosis of TBP
   a. Testing sequence for making the diagnosis. A protocol for making the diagnosis of TBP is as follows (dashed arrow indicates optional step):

   History and physical examination
   ↓
   Noninvasive test of venous function (Doppler, plethysmography, phleborheography) with or without a serum D-dimer test
   ↓
   Venography (optional; performed if diagnosis still in doubt after noninvasive testing)

   b. Criteria for diagnosis. The diagnosis of TBP is made in the following patients:
      (1) Patients are asymptomatic or complain of calf or medial thigh tenderness and have abnormal results (usually unilateral) on one of the noninvasive tests of venous function (Doppler, plethysmography, phleborheography). The serum D-dimer test is positive.
      (2) Patients are asymptomatic or symptomatic and demonstrate venous thrombosis by venography.
      (3) Patients have documented pulmonary embolism (see Chapter 22) and abnormal results on noninvasive or invasive (venography) evaluation of peripheral venous potency.
   c. Differential diagnosis
      (1) Lymphedema. Lymphedema is the result of a number of pathologic processes (infection, trauma, hypersensitivity, malignancy), all of which obstruct or obliterate lymphatic channels. It is differentiated from TBP by its more gradual onset of edema and by the lack of venous distention, cyanosis, or discomfort. Noninvasive tests of venous function are normal in lymphedema.
      (2) Cellulitis and lymphangitis. These entities are the result of bacterial infection and are frequently associated with high fever, chills, and malaise. The involved limb is erythematous, feels warm to the touch, and often demonstrates the red streaks of lymphangitic spread of the infection. Regional lymph nodes are usually enlarged and tender.
         Noninvasive tests of venous function are normal.
      (3) Arterial embolism. Severe arterial insufficiency secondary to peripheral arterial embolism may superficially resemble TBP; however, acute arterial insufficiency is not associated with edema or venous distention. Moreover, weak or absent pulses, a pale and cool extremity, and decreased peripheral sensation are all usually found in patients with acute arterial insufficiency.
B. Therapy
   1. Medical treatment
      a. Prophylaxis. It is far better to prevent venous thrombosis than to treat it once the condition has developed. Preventive measures include early ambulation during medical and surgical illnesses; leg exercises; elastic stockings; low-dose heparin administration (5000 U subcutaneously two or three times a day or, once or twice daily subcutaneous injections of low-molecular-weight heparin); and warfarin, dextran, or aspirin administration.
      b. Anticoagulation. Localized superficial TBP rarely, if ever, requires anticoagulant therapy. Extensive or progressive superficial TBP and deep venous thrombosis, however, should be managed with 7 to 10 days of intravenous heparin therapy (continuous or intermittent).

Heparin regimens are detailed in Chapter 22. Most clinicians favor 3 to 6 months or more of oral warfarin therapy after the initial 7 to 10 days of heparin. Occasional patients with extensive TBP (often complicated by pulmonary embolism) are treated with thrombolytic agents (see Chapter 22). However, thrombolytic therapy can be complicated by excessive bleeding and acute pulmonary embolism.

Home therapy with subcutaneous administration of low-molecular-weight heparin, for example, enoxaparin (1 mg/kg subcutaneously q12h or 1.5 mg/kg subcutaneously for 4 to 7 days, followed by oral warfarin therapy) has been shown to be both efficacious and safe. Patients are frequently grateful if they do not have to be admitted to the hospital.

 c. Analgesics, heat, and elevation. Analgesics such as aspirin (650 mg four times a day) or ibuprofen (300 mg three or four times a day), elevation of the affected limb, and moist heat help alleviate discomfort in patients with TBP. Usually a regimen of analgesics, heat, and elevation is all that is required for individuals with superficial TBP.

 d. Elastic stockings. Elastic supportive stockings are beneficial for patients with persistent edema. Individuals who develop chronic venous insufficiency (edema, stasis dermatitis, ulcers) after TBP should be fitted with full-length elastic stockings (Jobst stockings).

2. Surgery

 a. Venous interruption. Inferior vena caval interruption (clip, ligation, umbrella) should be considered for patients in whom TBP recurs or extends during therapy. Venous interruption also is indicated in patients with deep venous TBP and a strong contraindication to anticoagulation (e.g., active gastrointestinal bleeding). Patients with deep vein TBP and massive pulmonary embolism may be candidates for venous interruption (see Chapter 22).

 b. Thrombectomy. Thrombectomy has been shown to be of benefit only in patients with phlegmasia cerulea dolens.

SELECTED READINGS

Beebe HG, Dawson DL, Cutler BS, et al. A new pharmacological treatment for intermittent claudication: results of randomized, multicenter trial. *Arch Intern Med* 1999;159:2041–2050.
Long-term use of cilostazol improved walking distance in patients with intermittent claudication.

Boccalon H, Elias A, Chale JJ, et al. Clinical outcome and cost of hospital vs home treatment of proximal deep vein thrombosis with a low molecular weight heparin: the Vascular Midi-Pyrenees Study. *Arch Intern Med* 2000;160:1769–1773.
Home treatment of deep venous thrombosis with low-molecular-weight heparin is both safe and efficacious.

Brevetti G, Diehm C, Lambert D, et al. European multicenter study on propionyl-L-carnitine in intermittent claudication. *J Am Coll Cardiol* 1999;34:1618–1624.
Oral propionyl-L-carnitine therapy produced longer walking distances in patients with intermittent claudication.

Burek KA, Sutton-Tyrrell K, Brooks MM, et al. Prognostic importance of lower extremity arterial disease in patients undergoing coronary revascularization in the Bypass Angioplasty Revascularization Investigation (BARI). *J Am Coll Cardiol* 1999;34:716–721.
Patients with peripheral arterial disease who undergo coronary revascularization have a worsened prognosis compared with that of patients without peripheral vascular disease.

Crique MH, Coughlin SS, Fronek A. Noninvasively diagnosed peripheral arterial disease as a predictor of mortality: results from a prospective study. *Circulation* 1985; 72:768–773.

Noninvasive evidence of peripheral vascular disease correlates directly with mortality over a mean follow-up period of 4 years.

Criqui MH, Fronek A, Barrett-Connor E, et al. The prevalence of peripheral arterial disease in a defined population. *Circulation* 1985;71:510–515.

Objective assessment of peripheral vascular function discloses many individuals with asymptomatic peripheral vascular disease.

Criqui MH, Fronek A, Klauber MR, et al. The sensitivity, specificity, and predictive value of traditional clinical evaluation of peripheral arterial disease: results from noninvasive testing in a defined population. *Circulation* 1985;71:516–522.

An abnormal posterior tibial pulse is the best predictor of the presence of peripheral vascular disease.

Criqui MH, Langer RD, Fronek A, et al. Mortality over a period of 10 years in patients with peripheral arterial disease. *N Engl J Med* 1992;326:381–386.

Patients with large-vessel peripheral arterial disease have a high cardiovascular mortality.

Girolami B, Bernardi E, Prins MH, et al. Treatment of intermittent claudication with physical training, smoking cessation, pentoxifylline, or nafronyl. *Arch Intern Med* 1999;159:337–345.

Physical training was the most effective therapy for patients with intermittent claudication.

Grady D, Wenger NK, Herrington D, et al. Postmenopausal hormone therapy increases risk for venous thromboembolic disease: the Heart and Estrogen/Progestin Replacement Study. *Ann Intern Med* 2000;132:689–696.

Postmenopausal hormone therapy increases the risk for venous thromboembolism.

Heit JA, Mohr DN, Silverstein MD, et al. Predictors of recurrence after deep vein thrombosis and pulmonary embolism: a population-based cohort study. *Arch Intern Med* 2000;160:761–768.

Venous thromboembolism recurs frequently especially during the 6 to 12 months after initial diagnosis.

Hertzer NR. The natural history of peripheral vascular disease: implications for its management. *Circulation* 1991;83(Suppl I): I12–I19.

A review of the natural history of peripheral vascular disease in light of different management strategies.

Hiatt WR. Medical treatment of peripheral arterial disease and claudication. *N Engl J Med* 2001;344:1608–1621.

A thorough review of current therapy for peripheral arterial disease.

Hiatt WR, Regensteiner JG, Hargarten ME, et al. Benefit of exercise conditioning for patients with peripheral arterial disease. *Circulation* 1990;81:602–609.

Exercise training significantly improved walking distance in patients with peripheral arterial disease.

Hull RD, Carter CJ, Jay RM, et al. The diagnosis of acute, recurrent, deep vein thrombosis: a diagnostic challenge. *Circulation* 1983;67:901–906.

Noninvasive detection of deep venous thrombosis is accurate and clinically useful.

Isner JM, Rosenfeld K. Redefining the treatment of peripheral artery disease: role of percutaneous revascularization. *Circulation* 1993;88:1534–1537.

An extensive review of the results and role of percutaneous arterial angioplasty in the management of patients with peripheral arterial disease.

Perone N, Bounameaux H, Perrier A. Comparison of four strategies for diagnosing deep vein thrombosis: a cost-effectiveness analysis. *Am J Med* 2001;110:33–40.

The combination of a venous ultrasound study, the clinical presentation, and a high-sensitivity D-dimer test results in accurate diagnosis of deep venous thrombosis.

Pilger E, Decrinis M, Stark G, et al. Thrombolytic treatment and balloon angioplasty in chronic occlusion of the aortic bifurcation. *Ann Intern Med* 1994;120:40–444.

Thrombolytic therapy followed by peripheral vascular angioplasty may avoid the need for surgery in patients with aortoiliac disease.

Radack K, Deck C. Beta adrenergic blocker therapy does not worsen intermittent claudication in subjects with peripheral arterial disease: a metaanalysis of randomized controlled trials. *Arch Intern Med* 1991;151:1769–1776.

Beta-blockers can be safely used in patients with peripheral arterial disease.

Radack K, Wyderski RJ. Conservative management of intermittent claudication. *Ann Intern Med* 1990;113:135–146.

A review of conservative, medical management of patients with intermittent claudication

Schulman S, Lindmarker P. Duration of Anticoagulation Trial Investigators: incidence of cancer after prophylaxis with warfarin against recurrent venous thromboembolism. *N Engl J Med* 2000;342:1953–1958.

The risk for developing cancer is elevated for 2 years after an episode of venous thromboembolism.

Schweizer J, Kirch W, Koch R, et al. Short- and long-term results after thrombolytic treatment of deep venous thrombosis. *J Am Coll Cardiol* 2000;36:1336–1343.

Thrombolytic therapy gives better short and long-term results compared with anticoagulation in patients with deep venous thrombosis; however, serious bleeding and pulmonary embolism are more common after thrombolytic therapy, thereby limiting its usefulness.

30. CENTRAL NERVOUS SYSTEM INVOLVEMENT IN CARDIOVASCULAR DISEASE

I. **Introduction.** The central nervous system (CNS) frequently is affected by cardiac disease or by the same pathologic processes (e.g., atherosclerosis) that affect the heart. A number of different cardiovascular diseases can produce signs and symptoms of CNS dysfunction:

Atherosclerotic cerebrovascular disease
Hypertensive cerebrovascular disease (encephalopathy, hemorrhage)
Cerebral atrioventricular malformation
Berry aneurysm
Cerebral embolism (thrombus, fat, air); see list below
Infectious and marantic endocarditis
Dissection of the aorta
Arteritis (Takayasu's, polyarteritis nodosa, giant cell, lupus erythematosus)
Migraine
Rheumatic fever (Sydenham's chorea)
Tachyarrhythmias and bradyarrhythmias

II. **Diagnosis**
   A. **History.** A complete description of all neurologic syndromes that result from the entities just listed is beyond the scope of this manual. Both focal and diffuse neurologic syndromes are seen.

   Patients with **cerebral embolism** usually present with a sudden, focal neurologic deficit. Headache may occur just before or at the same time that the neurologic deficit develops. The nature of the focal deficit depends on the vessel involved. Cerebral emboli lodge, in decreasing order of frequency, in the distributions of the following cerebral arteries: middle cerebral, posterior cerebral, vertebral, cerebellar, and anterior cerebral. Seizures are common as an initial manifestation of cerebral embolism. Cerebral embolism often occurs during vigorous activity. The prognosis for recovery from an embolic cerebrovascular accident is usually better than that from a cerebral thrombosis or hemorrhage. Entities that can cause cerebral embolism are

   Myocardial infarction (MI)
   Left ventricular aneurysm or pseudoaneurysm
   Rheumatic heart disease
   Infectious or marantic endocarditis
   Cardiomyopathy
   Sick sinus syndrome with atrial arrhythmias
   Thyrotoxicosis with atrial fibrillation
   Paroxysmal or sustained atrial fibrillation
   Cardiac tumors
   Mitral valve prolapse
   Prosthetic heart valves
   Congenital heart disease with right-to-left shunt (paradoxical embolism)

   Syncope is often the result of tachyarrhythmias or bradyarrhythmias (see Chapter 24).
   B. **Physical examination.** As already noted, a variety of neurologic findings (focal and diffuse) may result from the cardiovascular diseases that affect the CNS. The nature of the neurologic findings depends on the location of CNS involvement.
      1. Patients with increased intracranial pressure commonly demonstrate arterial hypertension and bradycardia.
      2. Signs and symptoms of neurologic dysfunction may be stuttering in progression, with the completed lesion taking hours to days to develop, or

the ultimate deficit may evolve over minutes. Episodes of transient neurologic deficit that subsequently clear are called transient ischemic attacks (TIAs). If such episodes repeatedly involve the same area of the nervous system, they are probably the result of fixed atherosclerotic cerebrovascular disease. Involvement of different regions of the brain by TIAs suggests recurrent episodes of cerebral embolism.

C. ECG. ECG findings in patients with CNS involvement vary according to the underlying cardiovascular disease. A pattern of MI may be seen in patients with cerebral embolism. Left ventricular hypertrophy may be observed in patients with hypertensive cerebrovascular disease or infectious endocarditis. Right ventricular hypertrophy may be noted in patients with mitral stenosis. A variety of arrhythmias may be seen secondary to sick sinus syndrome, rheumatic heart disease, cardiomyopathy, or ischemic heart disease.

1. Primary ECG changes (deeply inverted T waves and/or nonspecific ST–T wave changes) have been observed in patients with subarachnoid hemorrhage, intracerebral hemorrhage, or head injuries, especially those with loss of consciousness.

2. Tachyarrhythmias and bradyarrhythmias can produce signs and symptoms of diffuse CNS dysfunction secondary to reduced cardiac output and arterial blood pressure. Hospital or ambulatory (Holter) monitoring identifies such rhythm disturbances (see Chapter 24).

D. X-ray examination. Roentgenographic findings in patients with CNS manifestations of cardiovascular disease reflect the underlying cardiac disease. For example, patients with hypertensive intracerebral hemorrhage often demonstrate left ventricular enlargement and prominence of the aortic shadow on routine chest roentgenography; an individual with cerebral embolism secondary to mitral stenosis might have left atrial and right ventricular enlargement and pulmonary vascular redistribution on the chest film. Individuals with dissection of the aorta reveal marked mediastinal widening.

Computed tomography (CT) scanning and magnetic resonance imaging (MRI) are particularly adept at separating cerebral infarction from hemorrhage. MRI can also be used to define the lumina of the extra- and intracerebral arteries by means of magnetic resonance arteriography.

E. Echocardiography. Just as findings in the ECG and the chest roentgenogram vary according to the underlying cardiovascular condition, abnormalities in the echocardiogram of patients with neurologic involvement reflect cardiac pathological conditions: Abnormal mitral valve motion and structure are seen in patients with mitral stenosis and cerebral embolism; valvular vegetations may be observed in patients with infectious or marantic endocarditis; and the characteristic echoes of left atrial tumor may be seen in patients with myxoma. A patent foramen ovale may be detected in patients with paradoxical arterial embolism.

A number of noninvasive techniques can document abnormally reduced carotid arterial blood flow or pressure secondary to stenosis of the artery. Such tests are helpful in deciding when transient symptoms are secondary to recurrent cerebral embolism and when they are the result of fixed stenosis of the carotid artery. Two commonly used tests are ocular pneumoplethysmography (measuring the arterial pressure in a branch of the internal carotid artery, the ophthalmic artery) and the cerebrovascular ultrasound and Doppler examination (measuring the velocity of flow and the patency of branches of the carotid artery).

F. Radionuclide studies. The diagnosis of cardiac conditions that produce neurologic symptoms can be aided by radionuclide studies. For example, recent MI with secondary cerebral embolism may be documented by technetium myocardial scintigraphy.

Adequacy of carotid arterial blood flow can be tested by a radionuclide cerebral flow study. The results are occasionally helpful in distinguishing neurologic signs and symptoms secondary to cerebrovascular disease from those that are caused by cerebral embolism or other entities.

G. Catheterization and angiography. Catheterization findings vary depending on the underlying cardiac lesion. Carotid angiography is used to define the anatomic location and extent of atherosclerotic lesions. This procedure usually is performed in preparation for carotid arterial surgery or angioplasty. On occasion, carotid angiography is used to differentiate atherosclerotic from embolic cerebrovascular disease.

H. Protocol for the diagnosis of CNS involvement

1. Testing sequence for making the diagnosis. Because a variety of cardiovascular conditions can produce CNS manifestations, no single protocol can define all entities. In general, a careful cardiovascular and neurologic history and physical examination followed by an ECG, chest x-ray film, and echocardiogram will furnish enough information to define most cardiovascular conditions that produce CNS manifestations. Special cardiovascular (radionuclide, angiographic) or neurologic (ocular pneumoplethysmographic, Doppler, radionuclide, CT/MRI, angiographic) examinations may be required to distinguish primary cerebrovascular disease from cardiovascular disease with secondary involvement of the CNS. The major distinction often revolves around the question: Are CNS signs and symptoms the result of primary vascular disease or arterial embolism from the heart?

2. Criteria for distinguishing arterial embolism to the brain from other cardiovascular causes of neurologic signs and symptoms. Patients with cerebral embolism often, but not always, have neurologic symptoms that commence suddenly without prodrome. Seizures are common. Neurologic findings may be localized or diffuse secondary to showers of emboli to different cerebral zones. Recurrent symptoms from different areas of the brain suggest cerebral embolism.

Thrombotic, calcific, or cholesterol emboli may be identified in retinal vessels during ophthalmoscopic examination. Documentation of one of the conditions predisposing to cerebral embolism is strong evidence in favor of that diagnosis.

In a young patient without risk factors for atherosclerosis and with either a normal cerebral echo-Doppler study or a normal ocular pneumoplethysmography, the diagnosis of cerebral embolism is likely. Such emboli may originate in the venous circulation and cross to the arterial vascular system through an atrial septal defect or patent foramen ovale (paradoxical embolism). A CT scan is helpful in ruling out cerebrovascular atrioventricular malformation with secondary hemorrhage. Carotid angiography often is required to confirm the diagnosis of arterial embolism.

3. Differential diagnosis of cardiovascular conditions that cause CNS signs and symptoms

a. Cerebral embolism. The most important differentiation to be made is the separation of primary neurologic and cerebrovascular diseases from cerebral embolism. This separation is discussed in Section **II.A.**

b. Cerebrovascular disease. If cerebral embolism is unlikely, a primary cerebrovascular disease (atherosclerotic, hypertensive, congenital) should be sought. Ocular pneumoplethysmography, cerebral echo-Doppler studies, radionuclide brain scanning, CT scanning, MRI, or carotid angiography may be required. Unusual conditions such as dissection of the aorta or arteritis have a number of specific features (absent pulses, skin lesions, etc.) that distinguish them from the more common forms of cerebrovascular disease. The presence of carotid bruits favors the diagnosis of primary cerebrovascular disease.

c. Arrhythmias. Excessively rapid or slow heart rate can result in hypotension and cerebral ischemia with resultant symptoms. Neurologic signs and symptoms (dizziness, confusion, obtundation) are invariably diffuse rather than focal. Hospital or ambulatory (Holter) ECG monitoring usually discloses the abnormal rhythm (see Chapter 3).

d. Ménière's syndrome. Dizzy spells may be the result of brain stem TIAs (vertebral-basilar circulation), or such spells may be secondary to Ménière's syndrome. Tinnitus, deafness in one ear, and lack of other signs or symptoms of brainstem involvement (diplopia, facial numbness, dysarthria) all suggest that the dizzy spell was the result of Ménière's syndrome or another disease of the peripheral labyrinthine apparatus.

III. Therapy

A. Medical treatment

1. Anticoagulation. Patients who have an episode of cerebral embolism should be anticoagulated first with heparin (7 to 10 days) and then with warfarin for as long as the predisposing cardiovascular condition lasts. Anticoagulation should **not** be used in individuals with infectious and marantic endocarditis or cardiac tumors. Patients with TIAs frequently benefit from daily therapy with platelet anticoagulants (e.g., aspirin, 650 mg twice a day; clopidogrel, 75 mg per day; or a fixed combination of aspirin and dipyridamole known as Aggrenox). Individuals with TIAs also will have fewer attacks if treated with warfarin; however, warfarin therapy carries a greater risk of bleeding complications than does treatment with aspirin.

   Considerable controversy surrounds the timing of anticoagulant therapy in patients with arterial embolism. One school of thought favors waiting for 24 hours after the onset of symptoms before anticoagulating the patient with heparin. Other neurologists prefer waiting 7 to 10 days after the embolic episode before initiating anticoagulant therapy. CT scanning is often helpful in this situation because it can separate cerebral infarction from hemorrhage. Thus, anticoagulation would be initiated in patients whose CT scan was consistent with infarction without hemorrhage.

   Patients with acute ischemic stroke benefit from intravenous tissue plasminogen activator administered within 3 hours of the onset of symptoms. Streptokinase therapy has not been shown to be beneficial in these patients. Before thrombolytic therapy is administered, an emergency CT scan must be obtained to visualize any cerebral hemorrhage that would contraindicate thrombolytic therapy.

2. Specific measures. Because a variety of cardiovascular conditions produce CNS manifestations, different specific therapeutic regimens are required to treat these entities. For example, antibiotics are indicated in infectious endocarditis, antihypertensive medications in hypertensive cerebrovascular disease, and steroids in giant cell arteritis.

3. Vasodilators. There is no evidence that vasodilators are of any benefit in patients with cerebrovascular disease.

4. Risk factor reduction. Patients with atherosclerotic cerebral vascular disease should receive therapy aimed at reducing or interrupting the atherosclerotic disease process. Such measures include smoking cessation, control of hypertension, control of serum lipids (statin or fibrate drugs), weight reduction, and control of diabetes.

B. Surgery

1. Carotid surgery/angioplasty. Carotid arterial endarterectomy is indicated in patients with frequent TIAs or waxing and waning neurologic signs and symptoms secondary to a significant (greater than 70%) carotid arterial stenosis. Patients with asymptomatic carotid stenosis probably **should not** undergo carotid endarterectomy. Carotid arterial angioplasty with or without stent placement is performed by some interventional cardiologists in lieu of carotid endarterectomy.

The use of **intracranial bypass surgery** (anastomosing a branch of the external carotid artery to either the middle cerebral artery or the vertebral artery) for the treatment of lesions not accessible to standard endarterectomy is controversial. Some clinicians advocate its use in selected patients, whereas others feel that there is no evidence of benefit.

2. Specific surgical measures. A number of specific surgical procedures can be of considerable benefit in patients with a variety of cardiovascular conditions that produce neurologic signs and symptoms. A few examples are berry aneurysmectomy or coating, repair of aortic dissection, left ventricular aneurysmectomy, excision of atrial myxoma, and insertion of a demand pacemaker.

SELECTED READINGS

Barnett HJM, Taylor W, Eliasziw M, et al. Benefit of carotid endarterectomy in patients with symptomatic moderate or severe stenosis. *N Engl J Med* 1998;339: 1415–1425.
Symptomatic patients with greater than 70% carotid arterial stenosis benefited from carotid endarterectomy.

Brott T, Bogousslavsky J. Treatment of acute ischemic stroke. *N Engl J Med* 2000; 343:710–721.
Authoritative review of current therapy for acute ischemic stroke.

Couch JR. Antiplatelet therapy in the treatment of cerebrovascular disease. *Clin Cardiol* 1993;16:703–710.
Antiplatelet therapy reduces the risk of stroke in patients with cerebrovascular disease.

Crouse JR 3rd. Assessment and management of carotid disease. *Annu Rev Med* 1992;43:301–316.
Review of epidemiology, diagnosis, and management of patients with carotid artery disease.

Fisher M, Bogousslavsky J. Further evolution toward effective therapy for acute ischemic stroke. *JAMA* 1998;279:1298–1303.
Thrombolytic therapy is effective in the early treatment of patients with acute ischemic stroke.

Goldstein LB, Adams R, Becker K, et al. Primary prevention of ischemic stroke: a statement for healthcare professionals from the stroke council of the American Heart Association. *Circulation* 2001;103:163–182.
The recommended program for the primary prevention of stroke.

Hu FB, Stampfer MJ, Colditz GA, et al. Physical activity and risk of stroke in women. *JAMA* 2000;283:2961–2967.
Regular physical activity is associated with a reduced risk of stroke in women.

Inzitari D, Eliasziw M, Gates P, et al. The causes and risk of stroke in patients with asymptomatic internal carotid artery stenosis. *N Engl J Med* 2000;342:1693–1700.
The risk of stroke among patients with asymptomatic carotid artery stenosis is relatively low.

Kreus KE, Kemila SJ, Takala JK. Electrocardiographic changes in cerebrovascular accidents. *Acta Med Scand* 1969;185:327–334.
Electrocardiographic ST–T changes in patients with cerebrovascular accidents.

Kwiatkowski TG, Libman RB, Frankel M, et al. Effects of tissue plasminogen activator for acute ischemic stroke at one year. *N Engl J Med* 1999;340:1781–1787.
Acute administration of this thrombolytic agent reduced stroke disability at 1 year.

McGovern PG, Burke GL, Sprafka JM, et al. Trends in mortality, morbidity, and risk factor levels for stroke from 1960 through 1990: the Minnesota Heart Survey. *JAMA* 1992;268:753—759.
There has been a 50% reduction in stroke mortality from 1960–1990 that is attributable to both primary and secondary preventive measures.

Roubin GS, New G, Iyer SS, et al. Immediate and late clinical outcomes of carotid artery stenting in patients with symptomatic and asymptomatic carotid artery stenosis: a 5-year prospective analysis. *Circulation* 2001;103:532–537.

Carotid stenting can be performed safely and with excellent results in experienced hands.

Sacco RL, Elkind, MS. Update on antiplatelet therapy for stroke prevention. *Arch Intern Med* 2000;160:1579–1582.

A discussion of antiplatelet therapy in patients at risk for stroke.

White HD, Simes J, Anderson NE, et al. Pravastatin therapy and the risk of stroke. *N Engl J Med* 2000;343:317–326.

Therapy with this statin drug reduces the risk of stroke.

Wolf PA, Grotta JC. Cerebrovascular disease. *Circulation* 2000;102(Suppl IV): IV75–IV80.

State of the art summary of advances in the diagnosis and therapy of cerebrovascular disease.

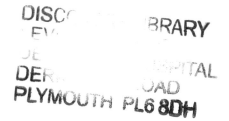

SUBJECT INDEX

Note: Page numbers followed by f refer to illustrations; page numbers followed by t refer to tables.

A

A wave, 4–6, 5f, 6f
ABCD survey, 135–136
Abdomen, acute, vs. aortic aneurysm, 385
Abdominojugular (hepatojugular or abdominal) test, 9–11, 10f, 11f
Abortion, therapeutic, 369
Accelerated idioventricular rhythm, 45
ACE inhibitors. *See* Angiotensin-converting enzyme (ACE) inhibitors
Acebutolol, in hypertension, 177, 182
ACLS (advanced cardiac life support), 135–136
Action potential, 32
Activity
  in angina pectoris, 234
  in aortic regurgitation, 262
  in aortic stenosis, 257
  in mitral regurgitation, 252
  in mitral stenosis, 244
  after myocardial infarction, 219–220, 219t
  after pulmonary embolism, 344
Adenosine
  in myocardial infarction, 213t
  in paroxysmal supraventricular tachycardia, 39
Adrenal arteriography, in hypertension, 174
Advanced cardiac life support (ACLS), 135–136
Adventitious heart sounds, 15
A-H interval, 46–47
Alcohol intake, hypertension and, 184
Alcohol septal ablation, in hypertrophic cardiomyopathy, 299
Aldactone (spironolactone)
  in heart failure, 72, 75t
  in hypertension, 177, 178t
Aldomet (methyldopa), 177, 179t, 197t
Aldosterone sampling, in hypertension, 174
Aldosteronism, primary, 185
Alpha-adrenergic blockers, in hypertension, 177
Alprazolam, in myocardial infarction, 218
Aminophylline, in pulmonary edema, 98
Amiodarone, 45

  in arrhythmias, 57–58
  in myocardial infarction, 213t, 216t
  in ventricular tachycardia, 45
Amitriptyline (Elavil), 160t, 161–162
Amputation, in arteriosclerosis obliterans, 391–392
Amrinone, 81
Amyl nitrite, in auscultation, 20t, 22t
Analgesics
  in myocardial infarction, 218
  in thrombophlebitis, 395
Anemia
  echocardiography in, 26t
  heart failure with, 66t
Aneurysm
  aortic. *See* Aortic aneurysm
  sinus of Valsalva, 287–288
Angina pectoris, 226–235
  in aortic stenosis, 253
  diagnosis of, 227–232, 229t
    protocol for, 231–232
  electrocardiography in, 228–229, 229t
  exercise and, 150
  after myocardial infarction, 225
  noncardiac surgery and, 372–374, 373t
  Prinzmetal's, 228, 231
  prognosis for, 227, 227t, 228t
  stable, 227
  syncope with, 123
  treatment of, 232–235, 233t
  unstable, 227–228, 232
  vs. pericarditis, 316–317
Angiography. *See* Cardiac catheterization with angiography
Angioplasty, in arteriosclerosis obliterans, 391
Angiotensin-converting enzyme (ACE) inhibitors
  in heart failure, 77t–79t, 85
  in hypertension, 181t, 182–183
  in myocardial infarction, 218
Anomalous venous return, partial, 277–278
Antianxiety drugs, 160t, 161
Antiarrhythmic agents
  in angina pectoris, 234
  in aortic regurgitation, 262
  in cardiopulmonary resuscitation, 136
  in congestive cardiomyopathy, 302

405